MW01256278

Integrative Preventive Medicine

Integrative Medicine Library

Published and Forthcoming Volumes

SERIES EDITOR

Andrew Weil, MD

Integrative Preventive Medicine

EDITED BY

Richard H. Carmona, MD, MPH, FACS

17th Surgeon General of the United States
Vice Chairman, Canyon Ranch
Distinguished Professor of Public Health
Mel and Enid Zuckerman College of Public Health
University of Arizona

Mark Liponis, MD

Chief Medical Officer, Health and Healing
Canyon Ranch

To my Friend, colleague and fellow high school drop out!

It is a pleasure to know and work with you. Your extraording health care leadership makes a difference everyday. MAYO is fortunate to have you as a leader.

Rich

OXFORD
UNIVERSITY PRESS

OXFORD

UNIVERSITY PRESS

Oxford University Press is a department of the University of Oxford. It furthers
the University's objective of excellence in research, scholarship, and education
by publishing worldwide. Oxford is a registered trade mark of Oxford University
Press in the UK and certain other countries.

Published in the United States of America by Oxford University Press
198 Madison Avenue, New York, NY 10016, United States of America.

© Oxford University Press 2018

All rights reserved. No part of this publication may be reproduced, stored in
a retrieval system, or transmitted, in any form or by any means, without the
prior permission in writing of Oxford University Press, or as expressly permitted
by law, by license, or under terms agreed with the appropriate reproduction
rights organization. Inquiries concerning reproduction outside the scope of the
above should be sent to the Rights Department, Oxford University Press, at the
address above.

You must not circulate this work in any other form
and you must impose this same condition on any acquirer.

CIP data is on file at the Library of Congress
ISBN 978-0-19-024125-4

This material is not intended to be, and should not be considered, a substitute for medical or other
professional advice. Treatment for the conditions described in this material is highly dependent on
the individual circumstances. And, while this material is designed to offer accurate information with
respect to the subject matter covered and to be current as of the time it was written, research and
knowledge about medical and health issues is constantly evolving and dose schedules for medications
are being revised continually, with new side effects recognized and accounted for regularly. Readers
must therefore always check the product information and clinical procedures with the most up-to-
date published product information and data sheets provided by the manufacturers and the most
recent codes of conduct and safety regulation. The publisher and the authors make no representations
or warranties to readers, express or implied, as to the accuracy or completeness of this material.
Without limiting the foregoing, the publisher and the authors make no representations or warranties
as to the accuracy or efficacy of the drug dosages mentioned in the material. The authors and the
publisher do not accept, and expressly disclaim, any responsibility for any liability, loss or risk that
may be claimed or incurred as a consequence of the use and/or application of any of the contents of
this material.

1 3 5 7 9 8 6 4 2
Printed by Webcom, Inc., Canada

CONTENTS

FOREWORD

ANDREW WEIL, M.D.

A main reason that the U.S. health care system is in crisis is its lopsided focus on disease management rather than on prevention and health promotion. Sadly, conventional medicine does not manage well the most prevalent chronic diseases, most of which result from poor lifestyle choices. They drain much of the money we spend on health care and could be prevented if we would teach and incentivize people to improve habits of eating and exercise, get adequate rest and sleep, neutralize harmful effects of stress, attend to mental and emotional wellness, and practice self- care.

Given that we now spend upwards of 18 percent of our gross domestic product (GDP) on health care – more than any other country – yet have the poorest health outcomes of all developed nations, one would think the U.S. would try to do better at preventing disease and promoting health. We don't for the simple reason that prevention doesn't pay. As dysfunctional as our health care system is, it generates rivers of money – money that flows into few pockets: those of Big Pharma, the manufacturers of medical devices, and insurers. We happily pay for medications and procedures; we do not reimburse physicians for counseling patients about nutrition or exercise or teaching them how to breathe. Until our priorities of reimbursement change, health care providers trained to practice integrative medicine are at a great disadvantage.

In the past, preventive medicine has concerned itself with sanitation, immunization, and disease screening – all worthy enterprises but not what I consider the most important aspects of prevention and health promotion: the influence of lifestyle choices on health and risks of disease and the ways health professionals and society can encourage people to change them for the better. A new field of lifestyle medicine is coming into being. Integrative practitioners are trained in it, and preventive medicine must embrace it.

The effectiveness of preventive medicine has also been limited by the same deficiencies that weaken conventional medicine in general – namely, attending only to the physical body and not to the whole person (including mind and spirit), undervaluing the intrinsic healing potential of human beings, ignoring the useful ideas and practices of other systems of treatment (like traditional Chinese medicine), and not doing enough to improve the health of communities and the environment.

This volume is a milestone in the development of a new paradigm of preventive medicine. My longtime friend and colleague, Dr. Richard Carmona, has assembled a stellar roster of contributors from diverse fields of expertise to give readers a sense of what is possible. The alliance of integrative medicine and preventive medicine is logical and natural. Each can learn from and enrich the other. I am confident that *Integrative Preventive Medicine* will help strengthen that alliance and lead to better health outcomes in our society.

ACKNOWLEDGMENT

We'd especially like to thank Patricia Maxwell for her indispensable help in coordinating the entire process of writing and publishing this text and also Kathryn Duffy whose assistance was tremendously helpful. Without their persistence, patience, stamina and hard work this wonderful book would not have been possible. Thanks to the tireless efforts of both Ms. Maxwell and Duffy we are blessed to be able to share the expertise and insights presented in the textbook of Integrative Preventive Medicine.

CONTRIBUTORS

Kim Aikens, MD, MBA
CEO, Aikens Approach
West Palm Beach, FL

Meredith A. Banasiak, MArch, EDAC
Design researcher
Boulder Associates Architects
Senior instructor
University of Colorado
Program in Environmental Design
Boulder, Colorado

Steven Brewer, MD
Medical Director
Canyon Ranch in Tucson
Canyon Ranch
Tucson, AZ

Josephine P. Briggs, MD
Director, National Center for
    Complementary and Integrative
    Health
National Institutes of Health
Bethesda, MD

Benjamin R. Brown, MD
Associate Clinical Professor, University
    of California San Francisco
Medical Director
Ornish Lifestyle Medicine
Sausalito, CA;
Director of Integrative Medicine
UCSF Santa Rosa Family Medicine
    Residency Program
Cofounder
IM4Us: Integrative Medicine for the
    Underserved (IM4Us.org)

Jennifer Cabe, MA
Executive Director and Board Member
Canyon Ranch Institute
Tucson, AZ

Edward Calabrese, PhD
Environmental Health Sciences
Department of Public Health
School of Public Health and Health
    Sciences
University of Massachusetts
Amherst, MA

Nancy G. Casanova, MD, MPH
Department of Medicine
University of Arizona, Tucson
Tucson, AZ

Eddie T. Chiang, MA
Department of Medicine
University of Arizona, Tucson
Tucson, AZ

Param Dedhia, MD
Director of Sleep Medicine
Canyon Ranch
Tucson, AZ

Joe G. N. Garcia, MD
Department of Medicine
University of Arizona, Tucson
Tucson, AZ

Cynthia Geyer, MD
Medical Director—Canyon Ranch in
    Lenox
Lenox, MA

Heather Greenlee, ND, PhD
Department of Epidemiology
Mailman School of Public Health
Herbert Irving Comprehensive Cancer
    Center
Columbia University
New York, NY

Wayne B. Jonas, MD
Samueli Institute
Alexandria, VA

**David L. Katz, MD, MPH, FACPM, FACP,
FACLM**
Founder, True Health Initiative
President, American College of
    Lifestyle Medicine
Director, Yale University Prevention
    Research Center
Griffin Hospital
Derby, CT

Casey M. Lindberg, PhD, MArch
Postdoctoral Research Associate
University of Arizona Institute on
    Place and Wellbeing
College of Architecture, Planning, and
    Landscape Architecture
Arizona Center for Integrative
    Medicine
Tucson, AZ

Mark Liponis, MD
Chief Medical Officer
Canyon Ranch
Lenox, MA and Tucson, AZ

Bettina Martin, MD
Integrative Medical Doctor
Canyon Ranch in Lenox
Lenox, MA

Farshad Fani Marvasti, MD, MPH
Director
Prevention, Public Health and Health
    Promotion
Department of Academic Affairs
Assistant Professor
Department of Family, Community
    and Preventive Medicine
University of Arizona College of
    Medicine Phoenix
Medical Director
Healthy Lifestyles Research Center,
    College of Health Solutions
School of Health Promotion and
    Nutrition
Arizona State University
Adjunct Clinical Instructor
Department of Medicine
Stanford School of Medicine

Michael M. Merzenich, PhD
Professor
UCSF School of Medicine
San Francisco, CA

Zelda Moran
Department of Epidemiology
Mailman School of Public Health
Columbia University
New York, NY

Joseph Pizzorno, ND
Editor-in-Chief, *Integrative Medicine:
A Clinician's Journal*

Andrew Pleasant, PhD
Senior Director for Health Literacy
and Research
Canyon Ranch Institute
Tucson, AZ

Jeffrey D. Roizen, MD, PhD, FAAP
Instructor in Pediatrics
Perelman School of Medicine at the
University of Pennsylvania
Attending in Endocrinology
Children's Hospital of Philadelphia
Philadelphia, PA

Michael F. Roizen, MD, FACP
Chief Wellness Officer and Chair
Wellness Institute of Cleveland Clinic
Professor at the Cleveland Clinic
Learner College of Medicine
Case Western Reserve University
Cleveland, OH

Kathleen Sanders, FNP-BC, MPH
Department of Medicine
Division of Hematology/Oncology
Columbia University
New York, NY

David Satcher, MD, PhD
Founding Director and Senior Advisor
to the Satcher Health Leadership
Institute
16th US Surgeon General
Satcher Health Leadership Institute
Morehouse School of Medicine
Atlanta, GA

Eric B. Schoomaker, MD, PhD
Lieutenant General, US Army (Ret)
Professor and Vice Chair for
Leadership, Centers and Programs
Department of Military and
Emergency Medicine
Uniformed Services University of the
Health Sciences
Bethesda, MD

Gary E. Schwartz, PhD
Professor of Psychology, Medicine,
Neurology, Psychiatry and Surgery
Director, Laboratory for Advances in
Consciousness and Health
Department of Psychology
University of Arizona, Tucson
Tucson, AZ

Shauna Shapiro, PhD
Professor of Psychology
Santa Clara University
Santa Clara, CA

Ryan M. Shindler, BSArch
MArch student
University of Arizona College of
Architecture, Planning, and
Landscape Architecture
University of Arizona Institute on
Place and Wellbeing
Tucson, AZ

Esther M. Sternberg, MD
Research Director, Arizona Center for
    Integrative Medicine
Director, University of Arizona
    Institute on Place and Wellbeing
Professor of Medicine
University of Arizona College of
    Medicine
Tucson, AZ

Heather Tick, MA MD
Clinical Associate Professor
Gunn-Loke Endowed Professor for
    Integrative Pain Medicine
Departments of Family Medicine and
Anesthesiology and Pain Medicine
University of Washington
Seattle, WA

Ting Wang, PhD
Department of Medicine
University of Arizona, Tucson
Tucson, AZ

Walter C. Willett, MD, DrPH
Fredrick John Stare Professor of
    Epidemiology and Nutrition
Chair, Department of Nutrition
Harvard T. H. Chan School of Public
    Health
Boston, MA

1

Learning from the History of Integrative Preventive Medicine to Address Our Current Healthcare Challenges

WAYNE B. JONAS, MD, AND EDWARD CALABRESE, PHD

Introduction

Medical practices that were not part of conventional, Western medicine, have been part of all health systems, from the time that Western medicine was itself "complementary and alternative" to Ayurveda in 19th-century India. The division increased after the formalization of professional guilds in the 17th century and the Flexner Report in 1916 that established the domination of a more reductionist prevention and disease management system.[1,2] These practices have been described with a variety of terms including "irregular medicine," "unconventional," "nonmainstream," "unorthodox," "quackery," "folk," "alternative," "complementary," and "adjunctive." In the last 20 years, the terms "complementary and alternative medicine" (CAM) and, more recently, "integrative medicine" (IM) have emerged. While, CAM and IM are the latest terms for practices that are not generally accepted by the dominant medical culture, what has now been included under the term "integrative medicine" has expanded to include many practices already accepted in conventional preventive medicine, such a nutrition, smoking cessation, and physical activity. In addition, IM seeks not only to deliver CAM and conventional practices but also to coordinate their use in such a way as to maximize the benefit they each bring to the prevention and treatment of illness. Thus, integrative preventive medicine (IPM) is the coordinated delivery of evidence-based, conventional and CAM medical practices for the primary, secondary, and tertiary prevention of disease and illness. What can we learn from this evolution for the future of healthcare? What might IPM look like in design and delivery?

Lessons Learned from the History of Integrative Medicine

A detailed summary of the evolution of CAM and IM in the United States was published in a special issue of *Forschende Komplementarmedizin* in 2013.[3] In that article the first author described many of the lessons learned in the mainstreaming of CAM into practice. A key issue for IPM is to pay close attention to the social forces such as power, resources, and scope of practice. Prevention secures less than 5% of the funding in the healthcare industry, despite the large contributions to population health it makes. While also securing only small amounts of public and private funding, CAM enjoys widespread public support, with between 40% to 70% of the public regularly using CAM and often paying out of pocket for its products and services. Much of this public use is for "wellness" and to stay healthy, thus aligning concepts in preventive medicine and CAM in the public's mind.[4] Thus, developing clear communication strategies for the public on what IPM is will be crucial for its success.

Another common feature between CAM and preventive medicine is the nature of "evidence-based medicine" in addressing public health issues. Like many preventive practices, CAM practices often use long-term, complex, and "whole systems" approaches involving self-care and behavior change, where randomized controlled trials (RCTs) are often difficult or the results of RCTs ambiguous. Thus, small studies or epidemiological and observational studies are the only information available. This type of research is often rejected for clinical decision-making or for reimbursement purposes. Without solid science, many CAM therapies are considered "experimental" and thereby not reimbursable by insurers. The emergence of "personalized" or "precision" medicine and an increasing appreciation for whole practice "comparative effectiveness research" (CER) is changing this thinking and allowing the development of new methodologies that may be more useful for IPM.

A concerted effort to do more high-quality research on IPM is also needed. Studies on truly integrated, integrative medical models are rare, so this research gap will plague IPM.[5] Expanding the definition of IPM to include more firmly established preventive practices such as diet and lifestyle practices could bolster the evidence for the field. In addition, solid areas of science showing common ground between prevention and complementary practices should also be explored. The Wellness Initiative for the Nation[6] and the National Prevention Strategy are efforts in the United States to link integrative, lifestyle, and more conventional public health efforts. Later in this chapter, we describe another one of those areas (hormesis and the dose-adaptive response) that forms a scientific foundation for many of the healing practices IPM seeks to advance.

The current healthcare system is dramatically successful for acute, infectious, and mechanically correctable disease. It falls short in prevention, integrative practices, and the management of many chronic diseases; and it is too expensive. Integrative preventive medicine might be able to address these challenges, but it needs a deeper examination of how these practices impact healing. More emphasis on enhanced self-care skills and health promotion are needed. A paradigm for tapping a population's resilience and healing potential must become central to IPM. Healing should be as important as cure. Passage of the Patient Protection and Affordable Care Act of 2010 (ACA) in the United States has brought an opportunity to truly reform our approach to preventive medicine. While ACA is currently focused on expanding coverage for conventional services for those without health insurance, the most far-reaching aspect of the ACA is undoubtedly its potential to lead a shift from sickness to wellness as the organizing principle of our thinking in healthcare delivery. This reunderstanding of the path to health can bring cost savings while simultaneously improving people's lives. The remainder of this chapter explores how these lessons might form the foundation for solving our current healthcare challenges.

The National Prevention Council: A New Era

In 2008, the Samueli Institute released the Wellness Initiative for the Nation (WIN) to advance the process of healing ("salutogenesis") as a formative concept for healthcare in the United States. A core feature of WIN was to establish a platform for health in all national policies.[6] As a result of this and other legislative work, the National Prevention, Health Promotion and Public Health Council (Council) was established. The Council is the most comprehensive effort to date that links prevention, health promotion, public health, and IM. Its members represent 17 cabinet-level agencies and offices, and are advised by a grassroots Advisory Group (AG) on Prevention, Health Promotion, Integrative Medicine and Public Health.[7] The Council is the US federal embodiment of IPM and the principle of health in all policies.

The full names of the Council and AG, while cumbersome, are instructive for IPM, as each body is charged to address the full territory of their name. If the Council is used to its fullest capacity, it can make a great difference in the health of the nation. The charge for the Council includes the following provisions:[8]

   (a) provide coordination and leadership at the Federal level, and among all executive departments and agencies, with respect to prevention, wellness, and health promotion practices, the public health system, and integrative health care in the United States;

   (b) develop . . . a national prevention, health promotion, public health, and integrative health care strategy . . . ;

   (c) provide recommendations to the President and the Congress concerning the most pressing health issues confronting the United States and changes in Federal policy to achieve national wellness, health promotion, and public health goals . . .

   (d) consider and propose evidence-based models, policies, and innovative approaches for the promotion of transformative models of prevention, integrative health, and public health on individual and community levels across the United States.

The central charge for the AG is to "develop policy and program recommendations and advise the Council on lifestyle-based chronic disease prevention and management, integrative health care practices, and health promotion." The primary work of the Council to date has been the creation of a National Prevention Strategy (NPS) and the National Prevention Council Action Plan (AP). It is in the AP that each agency represented on the Council makes specific commitments for activities to be undertaken that implement the vision, goal, priorities, and recommendations in the NPS.

Transforming Our Thinking and Approach to Health

Fulfilling the mission of the Wellness Initiative for the Nation and the National Prevention Council would be transformative for healthcare. Transformation is needed in our approach to health because in the last 100 years a radical change has already occurred in what ails us, largely because of advances in knowledge about preventive medicine. The current and future ailments around the world are chronic, lifestyle and socially caused diseases and diseases of aging. The greatest contemporary dangers to health are our daily habits, the public and private environments we create and how we live in them. Most of us are not dying from outbreaks of infectious diseases, except in some underdeveloped countries and soon, even in those countries, chronic, lifestyle-related diseases will predominate.[9] We are now plagued by chronic diseases that we are largely creating collectively and individually and that come at great economic and human cost. For this reason, it is important that IPM refocus its attention from an acute, disease-oriented system to creation of a health and wellness–oriented system that spans the full spectrum of life. We need to transform our thinking that healthcare, community wellness, and access to medicinal treatment are one and the same. We need to understand that, while medical care is required at times, health is supported or compromised by an array of social determinants, personal choices, and local and national policies.

Three important concepts can help the IPM field understand and achieve the potential of this reorientation.

SALUTOGENESIS AND HEALTH PROMOTION

The first concept is salutogenesis,[10–12] the process of health creation, which stands in contrast to pathogenesis, the mechanisms by which disease occurs. We know a lot about pathogenesis, with medical science having identified more than 8,000 specific disease-causing factors. It is time we focus comparable scientific and public health attention on the routes to health and wellness, and how to use them as individuals, foundations, organizations, communities, and as a nation and a world. Chronic disease management is not about answering a yes/no question to whether someone has a disease. Disease and health exist as a continuum. One does not go from being in good health to being morbidly obese and diabetic overnight. One moves into increasingly problematic states of ill health day by day, and the world has been doing this at an alarming and costly rate. Yet even chronic disease can often be reversed and treated with these same social and behavioral factors—thus integrating prevention and treatment into a unified model. Figure 1.1 illustrates this reorientation and the integration of salutogenesis and pathogenesis.[13]

Research reveals that four specific health-promoting actions can prevent, slow, and even reverse many chronic diseases. No matter one's current stage of life or degree of health/illness, our health potential lies in the access to the following: (1) optimum nutrition and proper substance use; (2) physical exercise and rest; (3) resilience and stress management; and (4) social connectivity and integration. These four factors reflect many of the needs addressed by Abraham Maslow in his 1950s "hierarchy of human needs," which moves from the physiological, to safety, love, belonging, and esteem, culminating in self-actualization.[14] This corresponds also to the full definition of health created by WHO in 1948.[15] However, in Maslow's model the top needs can only be addressed when the prior needs have been met. We now know that humans

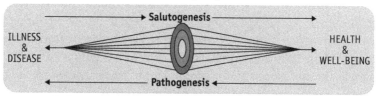

Salutogenesis
The Process of Healing

Salutogenesis: The process through which
health and well-being are produced.

Pathogenesis: The mechanism by which a disease is caused.

FIGURE 1.1 Salutogenesis: The Process of Healing

and communities often attain flourishing through any and all levels with the aspirational component of a personally meaningful life as the core driver, even when some of the other needs are not being met. This calls for a reorganization of the human health model into a systems approach rather than a hierarchy. We illustrate this later in the chapter.

So the first key concept in IPM is the importance of reframing health from a "Salutogenic" perspective and applying that perspective in science, medical care and in public health.

WHOLE SYSTEMS APPROACHES

The second concept for IPM is using whole person and whole systems in contrast to reductionist thinking. Integrative preventive medicine should embrace the realization that all behavior, mental and physical, is inherently health-related, and that national health is best created when government and public health agencies function holistically and collaboratively, sharing and respecting all perspectives and resources. The National Prevention Strategy calls specifically for the integration of clinical and public health in our efforts at prevention and health promotion, recognizing the inherent interrelationship of individual health and community health and the importance of enhancing synergies between these disciplines. For decades, millions of consumers have integrated various natural therapies into their own healthcare. Consumers want access to the best products and practices of alternative, complementary, conventional, and traditional healthcare systems and modalities, and they want the professionals involved to work collaboratively on behalf of the patients' well-being—which is the true meaning of patient-centered care.

Whole systems healthcare also requires that wellness and health promotion practices be facilitated in the full context of the individual and group. Significant differences in health promotion and wellness exist from person to person depending on social, cultural, racial, and historical circumstances. The place they are born and the environment in which they live are often the major drivers in their ability to attain health and engage in productive and prosperous behavior. Educational level, living location, and economic opportunities are three of the largest drivers of health, well-being, and longevity. These contexts enable or inhibit the ability to engage in responsible behavior, even when there is an intention and effort to do so. Thus, both individual and community wellness require these factors be addressed when creating health.[16]

There are systems of medicine that exemplify whole person and whole system thinking. These include Eastern and Western systems, some of ancient origin and others recently developed. These approaches strongly emphasize the importance of good diet, exercise, sleep, harmonious relationships, and methods of managing stress. An Eastern example is Chinese medicine,[17] with its accompanying concepts of balance and prevention. Oriental medicine focuses on identifying the root causes of what may seem from a reductionist perspective to be distinct, even unrelated symptoms. It promotes health by promoting balance—balance within the person, and also between the person and family, community and environment, including being in balance with nature and the seasons. Figure 1.2 illustrates these comparisons between our earth and our bodies.

In Western medicine, a relatively recent approach called functional medicine[18] looks at the influence of lifestyle and environment on genetic vulnerability in the initiation and progression of chronic disease. While conventional diagnoses are certainly recognized, functional medicine aims to identify the underlying causes of disease states, through focusing on a patient's core nutritional imbalances, fundamental physiological processes, environmental inputs, and genetic predispositions.

The systems just mentioned—one Eastern and one Western derived—are examples of whole systems thinking in healthcare and each embodies aspects of what we need in 21st-century healthcare and IPM. Honoring patient requests for collaboration by different kinds of healthcare providers so that the patients may benefit from the strengths of each and can elect health approaches that fit their condition, preference, and disposition is in keeping with Sackett et al's definition of evidence-based medicine as a tripartite approach incorporating "the integration of best research evidence with clinical expertise and patient values."[19]

A key to integration at all levels is collaborative team care. Collaboration at a national level will ensure that tax dollars are being used effectively and

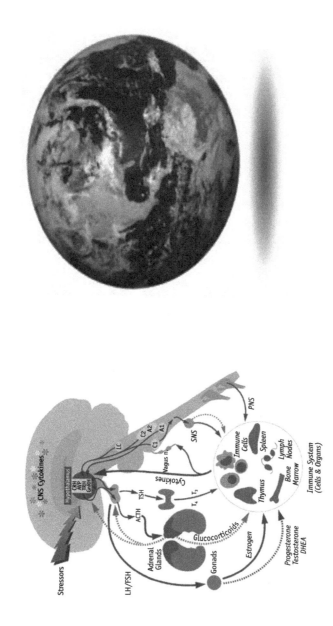

FIGURE 1.2 Whole Persons, Whole Systems: The Ecology of Health Creation

efficiently, with government agencies working to address the same problem through coordinated programs. Collaboration at the provider level can protect patients from receiving inadequate, inappropriate, or contradictory treatments when healthcare professionals remain ignorant of one another's role in the patient's total care. Collaboration at the organizational level would allow for continuous integration of processes while tracking outcomes and making adjustments for optimal care. Collaboration in research integration would mean drawing from multiple methodologies to tap both the brilliance of reductionist science and the wisdom of a whole system and personalized approach, including incorporation of the patients' perspectives. The work of the Patient-Centered Outcomes Research Institute (PCORI) is bringing greater rigor to whole systems research that includes patient input at all phases of research.[20]

The second concept, then, is that IPM be supported by whole systems thinking—an essentially ecological view that sees things in their contexts and relationships, not in isolation.

HARNESSING ADAPTIVE RESPONSES

The concept of a signal or stress-adaption response is another lesson for consideration as a core scientific concept for IPM. The principle derives from the area of hormesis—a dose-response relationship characterized by low-dose stimulation and a high-dose inhibition. This dose response is typically reported in the published literature by either an inverted U or J-shaped dose response, depending on the type of biological effects that are plotted. Multiple large databases using rigorous a priori entry and evaluative criteria have revealed that hormesis is widely observed in the biological and biomedical literature and is independent of biological model, endpoint measured, inducing agent, level of biological organization, cell type, and mechanism.[21-26] Thus, hormesis has very high generality, and is a basic biological concept for a healing-oriented science at the subcellular, cellular, organ, and whole person levels.

The hormetic nature of dose and signal-responses have important clinical and public health implications, since they define the biological constraints within which pharmaceutical agents, herbal treatments, lifestyle changes, mind-body practices, and other medical and public health interventions will work. Detailed evaluations of vast preclinical studies of numerous drug categories and natural products reveal that maximal responses are consistent with the quantitative features of the hormetic dose response. This means that the degree to which drugs and natural products (e.g., anxiolytic, antiseizure, memory, pain, immune-enhancing agents, wound-healing treatments) can improve healing and performance is limited by these constraints of plasticity.

This is also the case regardless of the potency of the agent. Thus, the hormesis concept not only is important to preventive and therapeutic medicine but also is a determining feature of its clinical efficacy. In fact, the optimal dose selected for a clinical trial is typically the optimal hormetic dose reported in the preclinical study.

This feature of dose response is also central to developmental processes, affecting numerous functions including how systems create biological curvatures, as seen with capillary formation, the rounding of the eye and the head of the femur, and numerous other cases.[27] Integrative preventive medicine can use this science to design interventions that precondition (for primary prevention) or postcondition (for secondary prevention). Over the past several decades, the concept of conditioning (both pre and post) for adaptive responses has been revealed to be perhaps the most powerful response to protect biological systems both before and after significant or life-threatening challenges and stresses. That is, a prior conditioning with an agent or stressor within an optimal temporal widow can up-regulate adaptive processes that protect against threats in conditions such as heart attacks, strokes, shock, brain traumatic injury, and other serious conditions. Detailed dose-response assessments of these pre- and post-conditioning studies have revealed that these processes conform to the same quantitative features of the dose response defined by hormesis and are likewise independent of model, endpoint, agent, and mechanism.[28,29] The preconditioning concept is particularly significant because it permits biological systems to create the equivalent of a biological "shield" that can protect itself for specific periods of time from a vast array of life-threatening challenges and then to repeat the process again and again. This concept has the potential to profoundly affect public health practices, including laying a solid scientific basis for the proper use of natural products and numerous lifestyle choices in prevention and throughout treatment as well as during follow-up activities. Thus, it may be a key to elucidating the mechanisms of prevention in integrative and conventional medicine.

One limitation of preconditioning is that it may occur early in development and is active well into adult life, which points to the need for careful integration of these practices with the salutogenic approach. For example, in older, and especially elderly men and women, the capacity for conditioning adaptive responses can profoundly degrade.[30,31] These types of performance degradations also may occur in younger adults when associated with comorbidities such as diabetes, atherosclerosis, and obesity. The degradation of the capacity to induce conditioning adaptive responses may have profound implications on health quality and longevity. Thus, support of health optimization methods such as with smoking cessation, nutrition, sleep, and physical activity become key to the effectiveness of condition as a preventive and therapeutic approach.

Used properly, preconditioning along with salutogenic support could be used to reduce risks of numerous serious conditions such as glaucoma, hearing loss, and bone fractures. Thus, the capacity to optimize physiological processes and build biological shields via the use of dose adaptation represents an important integrative prevention and treatment strategy. Of particular importance is that many preconditioning activities are part of lifestyle choices regardless of income and societal healthcare benefits. As such, these concepts can and should be integrated into health plans and therapeutic strategies.

The third concept, then, is that harnessing adaptive responses for IPM is a powerful vehicle to enhance health and well-being throughout the entire life cycle.

Becoming a Healthy World

Becoming a healthy nation requires a focused effort at all levels, from federal policy to individual daily choices. In the 21st century, when we recognize the central role of human behavior and environments in determining the quality of our health, we need a definition of health that motivates us to take care of ourselves and one another, a vision that recognizes human variation and offers something that is attainable for every individual and community. While the World Health Organization (WHO) definition of health, used since 1948, was a helpful move forward in its time, it does not serve us fully today and has been critiqued by many over the years.[32] That definition, which speaks of "a state of complete physical wellbeing," something unattainable for most, must be replaced with one that speaks to the process of healing and health creation—a process available to us all.

TREATMENT AS WELL AS PREVENTION

Current science indicates that treatments previously thought of largely as prevention or disease management can actually reverse disease. For example, Dean Ornish and others have explored the potential of an intensive program of lifestyle management to improve one's health and reduce or avoid symptoms of heart disease, diabetes, and prostate cancer—the first two being among the most expensive conditions plaguing Americans.[33,34] Subjects in the experimental arms of these trials were asked to adhere to a regimen including a whole foods, low fat, plant-based diet; no smoking; moderate exercise; stress management (often either yoga and /or meditation); and support group attendance. In short, a strong integrative program addressing mind and body.

Results of these and other studies indicate that disease can actually be reversed and costs can be reduced using these approaches.[35] Thus, lifestyle and complementary medicine can be used for treatment of disease, not just for prevention, and so these approaches are a central tenet of IM, yet they are the same practices for IPM.

This growing body of work holds important lessons. First, health promotion efforts sometimes function as prevention and sometimes as disease-reversing treatment. Second, the trajectory of adoption of lifestyle and IPM work illustrates the challenge of translating research findings into primary care and both clinical and community-based public health efforts. Third, these areas demonstrate the importance of investigating complex interventions as whole systems. We recommend support for comparable research on other complex systems like acupuncture and oriental medicine, as well as traditional Chinese and Ayurvedic medicine, naturopathic medicine, and functional medicine—testing the whole system's approach rather than single elements at a time, which would likely lose important synergies.

THE IMPORTANCE OF SOCIAL CONTEXT AND THE ENVIRONMENT

We suggest that health is a physical, mental, emotional, social, and spiritual state of well-being that allows an individual to cope with stresses, contribute to the community, and enjoy a happy life. Since we are all born with different capacities, and different circumstances, the needs to attain optimal health vary from one individual to another. The social, cultural, historical, economic, and physical context must all be considered when seeking to enhance health. With such a holistic definition of health we can move more purposely to attain it, and to reclaim it, through prevention, health promotion, and other public health and clinical efforts.[36]

The Integrative Healthcare Center of the Future

How would these principles be delivered to the public in clinical care? What is the role of the community health center and public health services given this new vision of IPM? What would the clinic deliver? What would an IPM center look like?

Figure 1.3 illustrates the core components of an IPM center of the future.

The primary purpose of this IPM center would be to teach the public about and help deliver to them primary components of salutogenesis. We suggest they are the following:

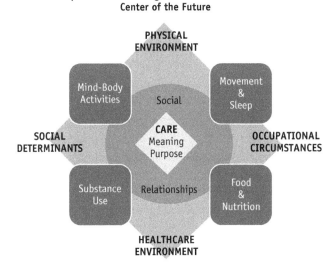

Components of an Integrative Preventive Medicine
Center of the Future

FIGURE 1.3 Components of Human Flourishing for the IPM Center of the Future

Stress Management and Resilience. Research has demonstrated the benefits of achieving a mind-body state that is known to counter the stress
response and to improve receptivity and motivational factors for lifestyle change. Recent research has shown that mind-body practices
can be learned and that they can counter the physical, psychological,
and even genetic effects of stress. They can prevent or alleviate post-
traumatic stress disorder (PTSD), improve fitness and weight management, and enhance cognition and overall physical function—all
of which serve to enhance health and strengthen personal resilience.

Physical Exercise and Sleep. Physical exercise and sleep can reduce
stress, improve brain function, slow aging and heart disease, and help
establish and maintain optimum weight. Fitness, along with proper
rest and sleep, maintains functioning and productivity of the whole
person throughout the lifespan and in any stage of health or illness.

Optimum Nutrition and Substance Use. Ideal weight and optimal physiological function occur best in the context of proper nutrition and
reduced exposure to toxic substances—nicotine, alcohol, drugs—that
impair function. Food and substance management require systematic
motivational structures, environmental controls, food selection training, and family, peer, and community involvement.

Social Cohesion and Service. The social environment is a key to health
and to healing, as is service to self and others. Both health and

happiness are socially contagious. Social bonding and cohesion is not only health enhancing in its own right but also is essential for sustainable behavioral change in any community, whether it is in a combat brigade, a business worksite, a federal agency, or a local school or community. Health promotion can be effectively achieved in any social context, where common values are shared among peers, friends, family, coworkers, and residents. As continued economic pressures add to social stress and disproportionately affect underserved communities, programs of resilience and behavior change offered by the community can help to alleviate stress-inducing factors that lead to illness and premature death.

The Inner and Outer Environments. These behavioral components of human flourishing are embedded in a healthy physical environment and cultivation of a purposeful life. A healthy environment attends to the physical structures and settings that facilitate healing and minimize the adverse impact on the earth. Attention to architecture, art, and exposure to nature, sound, smell, and light are key elements. Building and operating with "green" principles completes the ecological and sustainable nature of an optimal healing environment.

Integrative Medicine. This foundation of core health-producing factors would be supported by a community of care and treatment practitioners whose work facilitates whole-person healing. These practices—sometimes referred to as *holistic* or *integrative medicine*—catalyze and accelerate healing when recovery is stopped or delayed. They also serve as complements to conventional treatment regimens. When effective, these practices can do far more than simply address a disease process or control a single condition, because the whole-person view that guides them can engage multiple levels of healing—mind, body, and spirit.

Conventional Medicine. Elimination of specific diseases with drugs and surgery are a key feature of the new integrative medical home. These interventions are delivered with teams fully coordinated with the lifestyle and CAM practices described above. Vaccines, screening tests, and risk factor modification drawn from evidence-based practices are available in a manner that supports and reinforces the vision of health promotion and IPM embodied in this center.

What might an IPM center of the future actually look like? Figure 1.4a is a rendering of such a "clinic." Notice that the central part of the clinic is a hands-on educational center where the public comes not only to learn about IPM but also to take home knowledge and skills for implementing health-promotion

(a)

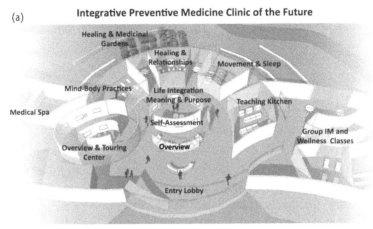

FIGURE 1.4A Integrative Preventive Medicine Clinic of the Future: The Educational Center

behaviors in their life. Figure 1.4a shows the first floor and entryway for such a clinic that holds the primary interventions for all chronic illness, as described previously. Figure 1.4b shows specific treatment modalities—whether conventional (e.g., drugs and surgery) or complementary (e.g., acupuncture or chiropractic) or involving natural products (e.g., homeopathy or herbs). Notice that

(b)

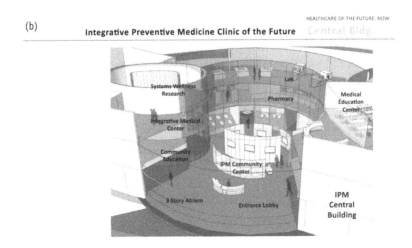

FIGURE 1.4B Integrative Preventive Medicine Clinic of the Future: An Integrated Delivery System

these are second-tier (and second-floor) activities provided only after the core basics of health promotion and self-care are understood and delivered.

Conclusions

All societies flourish by supporting individuals within communities in their pursuit of health and happiness, enabling them to prosper and give back to society. Many nations are declining in key measures of health and wellness. The gap is widening between those who are able to prosper and those that are denied the opportunity. The world continues to spend more of its wealth on healthcare and gets far too little in return. National and global well-being is declining, as evidenced by increasing disparities; decreasing quality of life and life expectancy, educational attainment, and employment readiness; strained military service members, veterans, and their families; rising medical bills and social service costs; and sagging business productivity. The result is a world that is shortchanging its children and undermining the productivity, pre-paredness, peace, and prosperity of its citizens.

Yet, we have a vast storehouse of knowledge and resources that can produce health, wellness, and prosperity. By widely practicing the core components of IPM, people can be more productive, prosperity can spread equitably, and, simultaneously, the costs of poor health, shorter lives, and national debt can be reduced. Recently, there has been a proliferation of efforts focused on cre-ating community health and well-being, and those efforts have come from a number of sectors. Funders, businesses, community leaders, and governments are starting to take bold steps to change the culture of health and move from healthcare to health creation. They are on the right track and now need all sec-tors of the economy across all nations to actively engage. These efforts could benefit by enhanced collective dialogue around the emerging field of IPM.

Acknowledgments

The authors thank Viviane Enslein for assistance in preparation of this chapter.

References

1. Bivins R. *Alternative Medicine? A History.* New York: Oxford University Press; 2008.
2. Flexner A. *Medical Education in the United States and Canada: A Report to the Carnegie Foundation for the Advancement of Teaching.* New York, NY: Cornell University Library; 1910.

3. Jonas WB, Eisenberg D, Hufford D, Crawford C. The evolution of complementary and alternative medicine (CAM) in the USA over the last 20 years. *Forschende Komplementarmedizin (2006).* 2013;20(1):65–72.

4. National Center for Health Statistics. *National Health and Nutrition Examination Survey (NHANES).* 2007. http://wwwn.cdc.gov/nchs/nhanes/search/nhanes07_08.aspx. Accessed January 12, 2016.

5. Khorsan R, Coulter I, Crawford C, Hsiao A. Systematic review of integrative health care research: randomized control trials, clinical controlled trials, and meta-analysis. *Evidence*-Based Complementary and Alternative Medicine: *eCAM.* 2011.

6. Samueli Institute. Wellness Initiative for the Nation (WIN). 2008. https://www.samueliinstitute.org/research-areas/health-policy-communities/wellness-initiative-for-the-nation. Accessed January 11, 2016.

7. HR 3590, Patient Protection and Affordable Care Act, Title IV Subtitle A, Section 4001, P420.

8. HR 3590, Patient Protection and Affordable Care Act, Title IV Subtitle A, Section 4001, P421.

9. World Health Organization. *Global Action Plan for the Prevention and Control of Noncommunicable Diseases, 2013–2020.* Washington, DC: WHO Press.

10. Antonovsky A. The salutogenic perspective: toward a new view of health and illness. *Advances.* 1987;4:47–55.

11. Antonovsky A. *Health, Stress, and Coping.* San Francisco, CA: Jossey-Bass, 1979.

12. Antonovsky A. *Unraveling the Mystery of Health: How People Manage Stress and Stay Well.* Jossey-Bass; 1987.

13. Jonas WB, Chez RA, Smith K, Sakallaris B. Salutogenesis: the defining concept for a new healthcare system. *Global Advances in Health and Medicine: improving healthcare outcomes worldwide.* 2014;3(3):82–91.

14. Maslow A. A theory of human motivation. *Psychol Rev* 1943;50(4):370.

15. *Preamble to the Constitution of the World Health Organization as adopted by the International Health Conference, New York, 19–22 June, 1946; signed on 22 July 1946 by the representatives of 61 States (Official Records of the World Health Organization, no. 2, p. 100) and entered into force on 7 April 1948.*

16. Centers for Disease Control and Prevention. *Social Determinants of Health.* http://www.cdc.gov/socialdeterminants/.

17. Kaptchuk T. *The Web That Has No Weaver: Understanding Chinese Medicine.* New York, NY: Contemporary Books; 2000.

18. Jones D, Hofmann L, Quinn S. *21st Century Medicine: A New Model for Medical Education and Practice.* Gig Harbor, WA: Institute for Functional Medicine; 2009.

19. Sackett D, Straus S, Richardson W, Rosenberg W, Haynes R. *Evidence-Based Medicine: How to Practice and Teach EBM.* Edinburgh, Scotland: Churchill Livingstone; 2000.

20. PCORI. *Methodology Standards.* 2012. http://www.pcori.org/assets/PCORI-Methodology-Standards.pdf.

21. Calabrese EJ. Hormetic mechanisms. *Crit Rev Toxicol* 2013;43(7):580–606.

22. Calabrese EJ, Baldwin LA. The frequency of U-shaped dose responses in the toxicological literature. *Toxicol Sci* 2001;62(2):330–338.

23. Calabrese EJ, Baldwin LA. The hormetic dose-response model is more common than the threshold model in toxicology. *Toxicol Sci* 2003;71(2):246–250.

24. Calabrese EJ, Staudenmayer JW, Stanek EJ, 3rd, Hoffmann GR. Hormesis outperforms threshold model in National Cancer Institute antitumor drug screening database. *Toxicol Sci* 2006;94(2):368–378.

25. Calabrese EJ, Stanek EJ 3rd, Nascarella MA, Hoffmann GR. Hormesis predicts low-dose responses better than threshold models. *Int J Toxicol* 2008;27(5):369–378.

26. Calabrese EJ, Hoffmann GR, Stanek EJ, Nascarella MA. Hormesis in high-throughput screening of antibacterial compounds in E coli. *Hum Exp Toxicol* 2010;29(8):667–677.

27. Fosslien E. The hormetic morphogen theory of curvature and the morphogenesis and pathology of tubular and other curved structures. *Dose-Response* 2009;7(4):307–331.

28. Calabarese E. Preconditioning is hormesis: Part I: Documentation, dose-response features and mechanistic foundations. *Pharmacol Res* 2016;110:242–264.

29. Calabarese E. Preconditioning is hormesis: Part II: How the conditioning dose mediates protection. Dose optimization within temporal and mechanistic frameworks. *Pharmacol Res* 2016;110:265–275.

30. Calabrese EJ, Dhawan G, Kapoor R, Iavicoli I, Calabrese V. What is hormesis and its relevance to healthy aging and longevity? *Biogerontology* 2015;16(6):693–707.

31. Calabrese EJ, Dhawan G, Kapoor R, Iavicoli I, Calabrese V. Hormesis: a fundamental concept with widespread biological and biomedical applications. *Gerontology*. 2016;62:530–535.

32. Huber M, Knottnerus JA, Green L, et al. How should we define health? *BMJ (Clinical Research Ed.).* 2011;343:d4163.

33. Silberman A, Banthia R, Estay IS, et al. The effectiveness and efficacy of an intensive cardiac rehabilitation program in 24 sites. *Am J Health Promot* 2010;24(4):260–266.

34. Ornish D, Lin J, Chan JM, et al. Effect of comprehensive lifestyle changes on telomerase activity and telomere length in men with biopsy-proven low-risk prostate cancer: 5-year follow-up of a descriptive pilot study. *Lancet Oncol* 2013;14(11):1112–1120.

35. Samueli Institute. *Better Health, Lower Cost.* 2016. http://www.samueliinstitute. org/file%20library/health%20policy/better-health-lower-cost-bending-the-cost-curve.pdf.

36. Samueli Institute. *WELL Community Project.* http://www.samueliinstitute.org/ research-areas/health-policy-communities/community-work. Accessed January 11, 2016.

2

Integrative Medicine and the Social Determinants of Health

DAVID SATCHER, MD, PHD

In 2009, the Institute of Medicine (IOM) held its Summit on Integrative Medicine and the Health of the Public. To set the stage for this very important summit, David Katz, MD, MPH, and Ather Ali, ND, MPH, were commissioned by the IOM to develop a paper titled "Integrative Medicine and the Health of the Public."[1] The abstract of this very clear and provocative paper is as follows:

It is interesting that in the same year as the Summit, the World Health Organization (WHO) Commission on Social Determinants of Health (CSDH)—on which I served along with 23 other global health scientists, from 2005 to 2009—presented its final report on the social determinants of health (SDH), *Closing the Gap in a Generation: Health Equity Through Action*[2] to the WHO. In turn, the report was accepted and released by the WHO in 2009.

Thus, it is appropriate to ask the question, "How do social determinants of health interact with and impact integrative, preventive medicine?" My immediate reaction is that the SDH place preventive medicine in a broader context and require a focus on policy, which is critical for impacting SDH.

The term "social determinants of health" was defined by the CSDH thus: "The conditions in which people are born, grow, learn, work, and age."[2] In society, they are most influenced by the distribution of wealth and power. Thus, as a rule, changes in SDH require changes in policy.

Some of the best examples of the impact of SDH are found in the new approach that the Centers for Disease Control and Prevention (CDC) is taking in the prevention and control of HIV/AIDS, viral hepatitis, sexually transmitted infections, and tuberculosis. Perhaps one of the most interesting and challenging examples of moving from a traditional approach to prevention to one that incorporates the SDH, is the CDC transition plan enunciated in 2010. In a series of articles in the July/August 2010 issue of *Public Health Reports*, Drs. Hazel Dean and Kevin Fenton outlined the important transition needed for HIV, sexually transmitted disease (STD), and tuberculosis (TB):[3]

> Individual level determinants including high risk behaviors such as unsafe sex and drug injecting practices are major drivers of disease transmissions and acquisition risk. However, it is also clear that the pattern and distribution of these infectious diseases in the population are further influenced by the dynamic interplay among the prevalence of the infectious agents, the effectiveness of the prevention and control interventions, and an array of social and structural environmental factors.

Many of these conditions arise because of the circumstances in which people grow, live, work, socialize, and form relationships, and because of the system often put in place to deal with illness, all of which, in turn, are shaped by political, social, and economic factors. This means that behaviors do not occur in a vacuum with respect to sexually transmitted infections (STIs). Individual sexual risk behaviors occur within the context of a sexual partnership or partnerships, which are, in turn, part of a wider social network. For other infections, or infectious diseases, including TB, while physical environment can influence patterns and opportunities for interpersonal contact, social mixing, and the probability of onward transmission of infectious agents, all of these determinants of transmission risk also occur within the context of a wider social and structural network. The authors later discussed the social impact of stigma on the spread of a disease such as TB. This is interesting because of our work on mental health and how we noted and communicated the impact of stigma on health-seeking behaviors in individuals and families dealing with mental disorder.

Fenton and Dean point out how the growing recognition of the social and structural barriers to prevention and control efforts for HIV, viral hepatitis, STI, and TB have allowed prevention experts to employ more comprehensive approaches to these interventions. I find especially interesting programs of social mobilization to oppose harmful traditions of practice, which often interfere with good health practices.

But structural factors include those physical, social, cultural, organizational, community, or economic and legal policy aspects of the environment that impede or inform all efforts to avail disease transmission. Social factors are the economic and social conditions that influence the health of people and communities as a whole. They include conditions of early childhood development, education, employment, income and job security, as well as food security, health services, access to services, housing, social inclusion, and stigma. The stigma surrounding TB has become a major factor in the diagnosis and treatment of this disease.

In an article in the 2010 issue of *Public Health Reports*, "Prisons as Social Determinants of Hepatitis C Virus and Tuberculosis Infections" by Niyi Awofeso,[4] a discussion takes place about the effects of prisons as social institutions that contribute to the health status and health outcomes of the incarcerated population. Sexual practices, often common in prison, dramatically increase the spread of HIV. In turn, the communities from which these prisoners come and to which they return, are impacted with an increased risk for the spread of HIV. Already the growing shortages of males in these communities lead to the potential for one male infecting several female sexual partners.

In the same issue of *Public Health Reports*, Anna Satcher Johnson and her colleagues examine and compare the patterns of infections and spread of HIV in native-born American blacks versus foreign-born American blacks.[5] First, they found major differences in the modes of spread in foreign-born blacks versus native-born blacks (predominantly male to male sexual spread). Second, they found that the rate of diagnosis of HIV in foreign-born black women was nearly equal to that of men and considerably higher than in native-born black women. Third, they found that foreign-born blacks were more likely than native-born blacks to be diagnosed with AIDS within 1 year of the HIV diagnoses. These findings reflect historical social differences in these two populations, who end up together in this country—thus showing the impact of history and experience.

Reed and colleagues examined the context of economic insecurity and debts among female sex workers in India.[6] Economic status and debts were associated with experiences of violence and sexual risk factors for HIV in this population. As one would expect, this describes an association between education and STI diagnoses among young black and white women. They found an inverse relationship between education and STIs, with the association, however, modulated between racial groups. The authors suggest that other factors besides education play an intricate role in determining STI risk for young black women. Surely the plight of black men must be a factor in the risk, for even educated black women, as implied in looking at the high incarceration rates in communities and the return from incarceration by these men to communities where men are in short supply.

As former directors of the CDC, Bill Foege and I were asked to submit commentary (Satcher) and viewpoints (Foege) on this topic relative to actions that could be taken to address social determinants. In my commentary, I suggested four areas for interventions to successfully address SDH. I commented on (1) the importance of "health in all policies"[7] and an approach recognizing that nearly all social determinants are outside the direct control of the health sector; (2) the need for public health to build stronger partnerships with nontraditional partners; (3) the need to conduct equity-effectiveness analyses along with cost-effectiveness analyses in all public health work; and (4) the need to expand resources to address all the SDH.

Bill Foege introduced his concept of "the last mile," identifying the specific outcomes to be achieved by addressing SDH.[8] He also proposed to develop a matrix for health and to incorporate prevention as part of medical practice allowing for reimbursements for preventive medicine.

During the development of the Affordable Care Act (ACA),[9] a Prevention Council was assembled, from all agencies of the federal government, with a special focus on responding to the SDH and health in all policies. The Prevention Council, chaired by the then-surgeon-general Dr. Regina Benjamin, developed specific recommendations—a Prevention Agenda,[10] as well as a budget, to be incorporated into the CDC budget going forward. The budget would start at 500 million dollars in 2011, and rise to two billion dollars per year by 2015, continuing at that level through 2020. This proposed budget has never been fully allocated as proposed, so the Prevention Council Proposal, for targeting the SDH, has not yet been realized.

In a 2009 article, "Don't Forget About the Social Determinants of Health" in the *Journal of Health Affairs*,[11] Gail Wilensky and I challenged the incoming Obama administration to respond to the CSDH's report by promoting and implementing policies that will expedite healthy conditions for babies growing in the womb. We pointed out that maternal nutrition virtually sculpted the developing brain of the child in utero. We were pleased that the underfunded Prevention Agenda of the ACA built on this recommendation. However, the impact of social conditions on health does not end but instead escalates at birth and continues throughout life.

Targeting the SDH could be very helpful in the area of obesity and overweight. This problem and related conditions are responsible for a very large component of Medicare costs in this country.[12] People who do not engage in adequate physical activity and practice good nutrition, will suffer from many chronic diseases, requiring care by the time they are eligible for Medicare.

In December 2001, *The Surgeons General's Call to Action to Prevent and Decrease Overweight and Obesity*[13] was released. We were especially concerned about how this condition was impacting children. It led us to refer to overweight and obesity as an "epidemic"—a term that had previously been reserved for infectious diseases. We found that, between 1980 and 2000, the problem of overweight and obesity in children had almost tripled in this country. Given that 80% of children who are obese at the age of 12, would be obese as adults, the *Call to Action* was long overdue. Thus, we attempted to clearly define those areas where action was both needed and feasible.

We first identified settings that could and should be targeted: (1) families and communities; (2) schools, where the average child spends eight or more hours a day, and where the health care system provides a powerful setting for intervention; (3) media and communications; and (4) worksites. In each of these settings, we applied the acronym "CARE" to define opportunities for intervention. The "C" stood for Communication, where we felt there were tremendous opportunities for improvement; "A" stood for Action that could be taken in the various settings; "R" for Research; and "E" for Evaluation.

Using this approach we were able to make specific recommendations for what could be done in these settings. Many of these recommendations have been implemented with some evidence of impact, especially for children under the age of 5. We have seen a stabilization of overweight and obesity, and in some states like Mississippi and Georgia, evidence of significant reductions.

However, *The Call to Action* was released before the *World Health Organization's Report on Social Determinants of Health*. In 2001, the CSDH had not been formed to look at the impact of SDH, but many of the major barriers to progress were in the area of the SDH, which require in most cases changes in policy. For example, we recommended that Americans consume at least five servings of fruits and vegetables a day, but at the time, the Department of Agriculture's "Free Breakfast and Lunch Program"[14] did not comply with this recommendation. It was not until the "Child Nutrition Reauthorization Healthy, Hunger-Free Act of 2010" [15] that this began to be corrected.

In many communities, there was no easy access to fresh fruits and vegetables because there were no grocery stores nearby. Louisville, Kentucky, would pass zoning laws requiring that all communities have access to grocery stores, and thus fresh fruits and vegetables, clearly illustrating that change in the SDH almost requires a change in policy.

The Wellness Policy, as established by the Child Nutrition and WIC Reauthorization Act of 2004,[16] requires that schools return to physical education K-12, and while many school boards have followed through, others have not. Some have pointed to their inability to employ physical education teachers, stating that funds were needed to teach science and math instead.

In 2005, when I was chair of the board for "Action for Healthy Kids,"[17] we released a report that incorporated research showing that physically active children who ate a good breakfast performed better in school, including on standardized exams in science and math. So, hopefully in time, more schools will appreciate the value of regular physical activity and good nutrition to school performance, and the fact that children who are physically active and engaged in good nutrition exercise better discipline in class. As shown in the

National Football League– and National Dairy Council–funded program Fuel Up to Play 60,[18] some innovative approaches to achieving the goal have been implemented by schools, and even by some individual teachers in the schools.

While people realize the importance of regular physical activity, fear and threat of violence are and have been major barriers to walking and jogging programs in some communities. Notably, some communities have been innovative in creating safe environmental opportunities for physical activity. Again, the Prevention Agenda of the ACA included funding that provided for virtually every child to have access to safe places to be physically active. Unfortunately, as previously stated, those funds have not been sufficiently allocated through the CDC budget as was planned.

One of the early participants in the Satcher Health Leadership Institute Health Policy Fellowship Program moved into a nearby community, where she was told it was not safe to continue to go outside in the early mornings to walk or jog. She responded by developing a community walking group, and ultimately acquiring police support in making their walking path safer. Increasingly, churches are doing similar things.

The worksite may well present one of the greatest areas of success. Businesses/corporations that provide health insurance coverage for employees, have begun to provide incentives for employees to be healthy and to engage in healthy activities. They have supported smoking cessation and/or weight loss programs, and have rewarded those who have participated. The employees' component of the premium has decreased where workers have quit smoking or lost weight. Of course, many businesses, such as Johnson and Johnson, which won a top national award in corporate health improvement in 2012,[19] have also saved millions of dollars in their health plans by implementing these programs encouraging smoking cessation, weight loss, and physical activity.

Spelman College, whose campus I can see from my office window, a few years ago gave up competitive sports to focus on the need for all students to engage in regular physical activity versus the 5% or so who engaged in competitive sports. They have developed a campus wellness program that includes a state-of-the-art wellness center.[20] Spelman has dramatically changed its social environment in favor of regular physical activity, for all students, providing both the opportunity and the incentive for such.

In the healthcare arena, many physicians have attempted to write prescriptions for food and physical activity where indicated, with varying degrees of success. As I discuss these issues with physicians, especially young physicians, the question that is asked over and over again is, "How do I, as a practicing physician, deal with and take into consideration the social determinants of health?" Through integrative, preventive medicine, physicians have worked to influence their patients' behavior in the areas of physical activity, nutrition, and avoidance of toxins as well as their sexual behavior and sleep and relaxation routines. But now we are saying that physicians must go even further and work to influence their patients' social conditions, as the conditions in which they live, work, and play. As I interact with young physicians around these questions, I suggest three areas of potential intervention to enhance social conditions impacting the health of patients and their families: (1) education of patients and their communities; (2) partnership with community institutions, especially those in the workforce, education, and government; and (3) interactions with policy and policy makers to ensure the support for these interactions.

Just as physicians can educate their patients about lifestyles that are best for their health, they are now called on to educate them about how the social environment can impact their health. We know there are social environments that are not conducive for people who suffer from addictions. And patients in recovery should avoid such social interactions. Likewise, there are social environments that enhance healthy behaviors. Clearly, there are children with asthma who thrive better in some environments than others. Sadly, some children still live in apartment buildings where they are exposed to tobacco smoke from neighbors.

Some community environments are not safe for either children or adults. Exposure to violence seems to increase the risk that children who grow up in these areas are themselves more prone to violence.[21] This is in addition to the fact that such environments are not safe for families. From a positive perspective, children and families need safe places to get outdoors and be physically active, and patients need to be educated about this. By the same token, families need to live in areas where there is safe, clean water to drink. Exposure to lead is dangerous for any age group but especially so for the developing brain.

The *Surgeon General's Prescription*, which I released in 1999 at the World Health Conference on Health Promotion and Disease Prevention, is a card that I always carry with me to pass out when I speak. In addition to encouraging people to avoid toxins, such as tobacco, and practice responsible sexual behavior, including abstinence as appropriate, it calls for moderate physical activity at least 5 days a week for at least 30 minutes per day. It also calls for good nutrition, especially 3–5 servings of fruits and vegetables per day. However, again, this will only happen if families have access to fresh fruits and vegetables. Some communities require innovation to compensate for the absence of grocery stores.

One of the most interesting and challenging leadership development programs at the Satcher Health Leadership Institute at the Morehouse School of Medicine (SHLI/MSM) is the Smart and Secure Children (SSC)/Quality Parenting Program. We believe that parents contribute the most important social environments for their children, and this begins with pregnancy. Because of this, we consider parents the most important leaders in the community. Each year, The SSC Program engages about 100 parents from low-income, predominately black communities, for a 12-week program dealing with child development from 0 to 5 years. We seek to measure developmental landmarks while influencing nutrition and early parent-to-child communication. The program was designed to measure changes in the children, not the parents; however, the parents expressed concern about any possible impact on them. Since depression has been increasing in black women in urban communities,[22] we decided to measure the impact, if any, of program participation on depression in the female participants. We were pleased to find that the risk for depression went down among the women who participated in the program. Positive outcomes in the children, relative to developmental landmarks, have also been noted.

We have recommended that physicians should educate parents about improving the social conditions in which their children are developing, especially early communication with the children, including reading, singing, and other forms of communication. The National Institutes of Health (NIH) is now supporting the replication of the SSC Program in 12 states; we are already working in seven of them.

But education of patients about opportunities and dangers inherent in interaction with the social environment or social conditions of the environment is not the only contribution physicians can make relative to integrative prevention. Physicians can also partner with community institutions such as schools, churches, and workplaces to positively impact SDH. Pediatric residents, of which I was one, at Strong Memorial Hospital in Rochester, New York, in the early 1970s, were not allowed to make the diagnosis of attention deficit hyperactive disorder (ADHD), without having visited the home and school of the child to discuss the child's behavior with its parents and teachers in different settings. This helped to create a more positive environment for the child and also improved the teacher's level of comfort with the child. But it was also noted that some children who seemed hyperactive at home were not so at school.

Doctors, especially primary care physicians, are now partnering with teachers and parents for the early diagnosis of autism and autism spectrum disease. The Clinical Research Center of the Morehouse School of Medicine Transdisciplinary Collaborative Center (TCC), is working with a church in the Atlanta community, to help congregation members manage their diabetes. This effort is based on the theory and belief that a supportive environment expedites lifestyle/behavior changes of diabetic patients in a predominately black, low-income community and congregation. These kinds of social interactions seem to support both behavioral change and adherence to treatment plans in the patient population. So, clearly, there are opportunities for partnering with community institutions to improve the SDH.

Five years ago, at SHLI/MSM, we initiated a program in Community Health Leadership with a focus on health promotion and disease prevention. We invited community pastors, community businesses, county commissioners, city council members, and heads of nonprofit organizations to recommend people from their organizations who could spend 12 weeks (1 day/week) with us preparing to provide health promotion and disease prevention leadership in their communities. We felt we could also learn (shared learning) how to better interact with the community in our efforts to improve its health. So it was shared learning that took us from integrative prevention to integrative prevention in the context of SDH. When members of the CDC Reach Program (a national program to reduce racial and ethnic health disparities) heard about our program, they asked if they could participate. Since our program was local, it did not require travel or lodging costs, so we had no funds for the REACH program to participate. But in response, the CDC offered to fund lodging and travel, allowing members of their REACH Program, from 40 different communities, to participate. We have now graduated over 300 people from the Community Health Leadership Program, including more than 30 pastors who referred themselves, as opposed to, or in addition to, other members of their congregations. Many of the pastors have now developed positive programs in their churches and surrounding communities, including HIV/AIDS education and screening, violence prevention, and community safety for physical activity and community interaction.

Several county commissioners and at least 10 mayors have completed the Community Health Leadership Program, as well as several other people who are community leaders. We are now working with the mayors to develop a special program to support their involvement in this component of the program. The original director of this program was recently hired by the City of New Haven, Connecticut, in an effort to develop and expand the program throughout that city; we are anxious to see how this progresses.

There are many opportunities for physicians to partner with communities, to improve the social environment and the SDH, with tremendous impact on overall health and well-being. Physicians can also partner effectively with government to improve the social environment for the health of individuals and the community. Government, as represented by public health, is dependent on physicians and other healthcare providers for all three of the main functions of public health: assessment, assurance, and policy development.

For many years, from 1873 to 1954, the Public Health Service (PHS) was led by a physician. The surgeon general, who oversaw all aspects of the PHS, was trained in medicine until that time. During the period from 1873 to 1954, when the surgeon general had the major administrative responsibility of the PHS, there was very little direct communication between the surgeon general and the American people. However, in 1954, the function of the surgeon general changed when the position of head of the PHS was separated from the Office of the Surgeon General and the position of Secretary of Health, Education and Welfare was created and later became the Secretary of Health and Human Services.

This integration of health, education, and welfare, and later health and human services was in many ways a major step forward. It is perhaps no coincidence that 10 years later, the nation received its first direct and official report from the surgeon general, titled *Smoking and Health*.[23] Since its release in 1964, this report and subsequent follow-ups are estimated to have saved almost 10 million lives—a period in which the percentage of Americans who smoke on a regular basis, has fallen from 43% to 16% today.

In 1987, recognizing smoking as a SDH, California became the first state to prohibit smoking in public places and now over half of the states in the country have such legislation.[24] This is an excellent example of physicians partnering with government at the highest level, but there are opportunities for such partnerships at every level. Physicians certainly have the responsibility to help their patients quit smoking, but we get the biggest bang when physicians interact with government to impact the SDH.

At the local level, physicians have impacted educational policy, either by participating on school boards or serving as very credible advocates for local policies that are in the best interest of the health of children and the community. If we are ever to reach the goal of assuring that every child has a safe place to be physically active and have access to good nutrition, physicians in communities will have to get involved and to provide leadership where applicable. The most critical requirement for effective partnerships is the sharing of the community vision and goals. Physicians can also take the kind of social histories that will allow them to help patients deal better with their social environment.

Health equity will not be achieved until we work together to respond to the need, of all citizens, for access to quality healthcare and also quality living environments. The expertise of physicians committed to preventive medicine will be critical to reaching the goal of health equity. Furthermore, we must remember that access to healthcare is itself a SDH. When physicians and other health professionals choose to practice in underserved communities, they positively impact the SDH in that community. Though indirectly, when physicians live and/or work in a community, it raises income and even education levels—two major SDH. Conversely, it is difficult to get physicians to live or work in communities that are underserved, because environments of poverty and violence have such negative impacts on SDH, including income and education.

But wherever physicians live and/or practice, if they are practicing IPM, they must be concerned about the SDH that may be limiting factors for patients attempting to change their lifestyles. As we have noted, SDH may be rate-limiting factors in the motivation and/or ability of patients to lead healthy/ healthful lifestyles. Income and education together impact the kinds of social environment that one can enjoy. Income and education can buy leisure time, into which can be built health-promoting activities including access to safe places to walk, run, bike, swim, play tennis, or other healthy behaviors. On the other hand, low-income and/or poverty greatly limit access to safe environments, as well as to fresh fruits and vegetables. At the same time, low income and poverty can enhance the risk of violence in communities.

Finally, and perhaps most importantly, we know that SDH can only be changed by changes in policy. Thus, physicians must partner with policy makers to help assure that the policies put in place are in the best interest of the health of the community. We often refer to the McKinlay Model,[25] which is built on a model for improving the nutrition of children. It shows the points of intervention as: *downstream, midstream,* and *upstream.* In this model, *downstream* is where we deal with individuals, their health, and their behavior. *Midstream* is community, and it is where we come together in communities to improve the health of the community and the health-promoting environment of the community. And finally *upstream* is where we make policy, and physicians increasingly must be involved in informing policy and developing relationships with policy makers that would enhance communications around health promotion policies in the community. So upstream, ultimately, must be our target, and examples of that include the *Surgeon General's Report on Overweight and Obesity* in 2001, which led to Congress passing the Child Nutrition and WIC Reauthorization Act, establishing the Wellness Policy in 2004. Then of course later, Congress passed the Child Nutrition Reauthorization Healthy, Hunger-Free Kids Act in 2010.

It must be pointed out that sometimes it is much easier to make policies than it is to implement them. The implementation of policy is the ultimate goal. We know, for example, that many schools that adopted the Wellness Policy, did not follow up and implement physical education K-12 accompanied by good nutrition. So, whether it is the making of policy or its implementation, when it comes to the social determinants of health, there is a role for physicians and other health professionals.

References

1. Katz DL, Ali A. *Preventive Medicine, Integrative Medicine and the Health of the Public.* Commissioned for IOM, February, 2009.
2. Commission on Social Determinants of Health (CSDH). *Closing the Gap in a Generation: Health Equity Through Action on the Social Determinants of Health.* Final Report of the Commission on Social Determinants of Health. Geneva, Switzerland: World Health Organization; 2008.

3. Dean HD, Fenton KA. Addressing social determinants of health in the prevention and control of HIV/AIDS, viral hepatitis, sexually transmitted infections, and tuberculosis. *Public Health Rep* 2010;125(Suppl 4):1–5.
4. Awofeso N. Prisons as social determinants of hepatitis C virus and tuberculosis infections. *Public Health Rep* 2010;125(Suppl 4):25–33.
5. Johnson-Satcher A, Hu X, Dean HD. Epidemiologic differences between native-born and foreign-born black people diagnosed with HIV infection in 33 U.S. states, 2001–2007. *Public Health Rep* 2010;125(Suppl 4):61–69.
6. Reed E, Gupta J, Biradavolu M, et al. The context of economic insecurity and its relation to violence and risk factors for HIV among female sex workers in Andhra Pradesh, India. *Public Health Rep* 2010;125(Suppl 4):81–89. Epub 2010/07/16.; PubMed Central PMCID: PMC2882978.
7. Rudolph L, Caplan J, Ben-Moshe K, et al. *Health in All Policies: A Guide for State and Local Governments*. Washington, DC, and Oakland, CA: American Public Health Association and Public Health Institute; 2013.
8. Nguyen J. *The Task Force for Global Health: 2013 Annual Report*. April 21, 2014.
9. *Learn About the Affordable Care Act*. http://www.hhs.gov/healthcare/.
10. Shearer G. *APHA Issue Brief: Prevention Provisions in the Affordable Care Act*. Washington, DC: American Public Health Association; 2010. https://www.apha.org/~/media/files/pdf/topics/aca/prevention_aca_final.ashx.
11. Wilensky G, Satcher D. Don't forget about the social determinants of health. *Health Affair* 2009;28(2):194–198.
12. Lakdawalla DN, Dana P, Goldman DP, et al. The health and cost consequences of obesity among the future elderly. *Health Affairs*. Published online September 26, 2005.
13. US Department of Health and Human Services. *The Surgeon General's Call to Action to Prevent and Decrease Overweight and Obesity*. Rockville, MD: US Department of Health and Human Services, Public Health Service, Office of the Surgeon General. Washington, DC: US GPO; 2001.
14. US Department of Agriculture and Nutrition Service. *National School Lunch Program (NSLP)*. http://www.fns.usda.gov/nslp/whats-new.
15. US Department of Agriculture and Nutrition Service. School Meals. *Healthy Hunger-Free Kids Act of 2010*. http://www.fns.usda.gov/school-meals/healthy-hunger-free-kids-act.
16. US Department of Agriculture and Nutrition Service. *Team Nutrition: Local School Wellness Policy*. Available from http://www.fns.usda.gov/tn/local-school-wellness-policy.
17. *Action for Healthy Kids Annual Report 2005–2006*. http://www.actionforhealthykids.org/storage/documents/AFHK_Annual_Report_2005-2006_FINAL.pdf.
18. *Fuel Up to Play 60*. https://www.fueluptoplay60.com/about/about-the-program.
19. National Business Group on Health. *Johnson & Johnson's Fikry Isaac, MD, Honored with 2013 Global Leadership in Corporate Health Award*. https://www.businessgrouphealth.org/pressroom/pressRelease.cfm?ID=215.

20. Spelman College Vision, Mission, and Goals. *Our Vision: Embracing Wellness for the Health of I*t. http://www.spelman.edu/about-us/wellness-center/vision-and-mission.

21. Office of the Surgeon General (US); National Center for Injury Prevention and Control (US); National Institute of Mental Health (US); Center for Mental Health Services (US). *Youth Violence: A Report of the Surgeon General.* Rockville, MD: Office of the Surgeon General, 2001.

22. US Department of Health and Human Services. Office of Minority Affairs. *Mental Health and African Americans.* http://minorityhealth.hhs.gov/omh/browse.aspx?lvl=4&lvlid=24.

23. US Department of Health, Education and Welfare. Public Health Service Office of the Assistant Secretary for Health. Office of Smoking and Health. *Smoking and Health: Report of the Advisory Committee to the Surgeon General of the Public Health Service.* Publication No. (PHS) 79–50066. 1964.

24. American Nonsmokers' Rights Foundation. *US Tobacco Control Laws Database: Research Applications.* http://www.no-smoke.org/goingsmokefree.php?id=519.

25. McKinlay JB. The new public health approach to improving physical activity and autonomy in older populations. In: Heikkinen E, ed. *Preparation for Aging.* New York: Plenum Press, 1995:87–103.

3

Health Literacy and Cultural Competence in Integrative Preventive Health and Medicine

ANDREW PLEASANT, PHD, AND JENNIFER CABE, MA

Introduction

As the United States and the world continue to experience unsustainable growth in the rates of chronic disease and rising healthcare costs, most urgently needed are upstream solutions—far before the point of people needing and seeking medical treatment. The reality is that in the United States, we do not have a healthcare system, we have a sick care system.

In the United States, what is clearly required to address this untenable situation is a shift in the underlying premises of the health and medical philosophies and resulting infrastructure. This chapter proposes that an evidence-based solution lies in a convergence between an integrative approach to health and medicine and health literacy. That convergence inherently embraces cultural competency and leads health systems, healthcare professionals, and the people they serve—often referred to as "patients"—to work together as a newly integrated whole that is greater than the sum of the parts. By renewing and recombining various parts of the current sick care system into an integrative team, this approach can prevent and reverse chronic disease and lower the cost of care.

Recent efforts in the field of health literacy reflect this trend, which we later exemplify through the work of Canyon Ranch Institute, toward integrating health literacy into all policies and practices—and, as we explain, inherently moving toward an integrative approach to health as a result. Examples of this trend include the National Academy of Sciences,

Engineering, and Medicine's Roundtable on Health Literacy in the United States embracing and supporting the "two-sided" nature of health literacy for the past several years. Originally cast by some as a deficit in the public that health professionals had to endure and address, health literacy is now widely seen as an issue of supply *and* demand so that healthcare systems have a responsibility to lower health literacy barriers as well. (See www.nationalacademies.org/hmd/Activities/PublicHealth/HealthLiteracy.aspx.)

Other examples of this trend include the Calgary Charter on Health Literacy's definition of health literacy that explicitly embraces the two-sided nature of health literacy.[1] Later work, such as the conceptual basis for the European Health Literacy Survey effort (see healthliteracyeurope.net) reflect this ongoing trend around the world. The approach of the Ophelia Project—optimizing health literacy and access to health information and services—conceived and promoted by Richard H. Osborne largely in Southeast Asia and Australia, also approaches health literacy as a multidimensional concept. The Ophelia Project uses an integrated approach as the basis for both measurement and community-based interventions (see www.Ophelia.net.au). Finally, across the United States since the advent of the Patient Protection and Affordable Care Act of 2010, a large and growing number of health literacy organizations, such as Health Literacy Missouri or Wisconsin Health Literacy, are actively working to lower health literacy barriers to finding, understanding, evaluating, communicating about, and selecting (using) health insurance policies. That has produced a dramatic gain in the number of individuals in the United States with health insurance—often a necessary first step toward bringing people into actively seeking to address their health issues. All of this work—ongoing around the world—is developing and proving ways to redesign, reform, and refinance healthcare by merging health literacy with a robust conception of health while addressing a range of social, political, and environmental determinants of health, including culture, in order to lower barriers to healthcare, prevent chronic disease, improve health, and lower costs.

In the ongoing efforts of Canyon Ranch Institute, a 501c(3) nonprofit public charity based in Tucson, Arizona, we have worked to develop, refine, and prove the viability, effectiveness, and efficiency of this approach. In this chapter, we provide an overview of how to operationalize that approach and detail some of the many outcomes of the effort, which has produced healthier people, happier and more productive health care professionals, improved health system performance, and better relationships between health systems and the communities they serve.

Health Literacy

We start with a brief explanation of health literacy. Initially, a concept that focused on the public's lack of success at understanding and navigating complex health knowledge and health systems, the idea of health literacy has since expanded to include the challenges created by health systems and healthcare professionals. In the approach taken at Canyon Ranch Institute, we employ health literacy as an evidenced-based path to behavior change for the public, health professionals, and health systems.[1-3]

Health literacy is how people can—or how they can be helped and supported to—find, understand, evaluate, communicate, and then use information to make an informed decision about their health and health behaviors.[1,4] This is a move beyond the history of health communication, health promotion, and health education that all too often stopped at the goal of helping people understand information. That limited approach does nothing to help people to bridge the gap between what they know and what they actually do in practice. The approach we detail in this chapter has documented success at supporting people to make and maintain healthy behavior changes.

Relationship of Health Literacy and Cultural Competence

Before health literacy emerged as an area of interest, practice, and expertise, cultural competency had addressed the abilities of individuals to successfully navigate the varying and often difficult terrain when different cultural perspectives encounter each other. While some practitioners are continuing to maintain a distinction between health literacy and cultural competence, we suggest that is the less productive path.

If there is a golden rule to both health literacy and cultural competency, it is to directly engage with people as early and often as possible. The two approaches are deeply linked in an underpinning priority to the importance of individuals, their capacities, their perspectives, their beliefs, their knowledge, their practices, and their worldviews.

The early focus within health literacy on limitations to people's skills and the idea of "plain language" as the solution may have been unsettling to practitioners of cultural competence as they felt individuals were being undervalued. Alternatively, the many (but far from all) of the early proponents of health literacy who came from medical and health professions may have felt the critical perspective of cultural competency as unacceptable and unnecessary within their healthcare practices.

Culture is most profoundly expressed through language and other modes of human communication. Health literacy is most focused on the uses of language and other modes of communication as well. The two fields should not only be in sync, they should be indistinguishable. The best practices of health literacy should always align with the best practices of cultural competency and vice versa. Nothing else will succeed in helping people to improve their health and helping health systems and healthcare professionals to help people accomplish that widely shared and highly valued goal of freedom from unnecessary disability and early death that are brought on by the myriad of preventable factors.

From that perspective, we address health literacy and cultural competency as a singular entity. We most often use the phrase "health literacy," but readers should know that we do not distinguish between a health literate and a cultural competent approach. They are one and the same.

Integrative Preventive Health and Medicine

The third area of our focus is integrative approaches to health and medicine and how those can enhance prevention. First, to clarify, we assert that the distinction between health and medicine is still warranted. In the United States, our current healthcare system is largely focused on medicine—care for people after they fall ill. Health is a larger area of activity including health and medical professionals as well as people in their everyday lives. We would hope that distinction would one day be less severe as health and medical professionals adopt the best practices of health literacy (including, as discussed, cultural competency) and shift their focus to prevention versus solely treatment—especially in the context of chronic disease. That day is yet to arrive.

The approach to integrative health and medicine we employ at Canyon Ranch Institute is a focus on mind, body, spirit, and emotion. Often we encounter efforts that only list mind, body, and spirit in this equation. We suggest the importance of emotions in relation to behavior change is so critically important that it is a significant error to omit emotions from the definition and practice of integrative health and medicine.

Further, an approach to integrative health and medicine that firmly and robustly embraces the four components of mind, body, spirit, and emotion also produces a perfect partnership with health literacy and cultural competency. This is not a coincidence but is by design. Sadly, in the time that Americans spend with a healthcare professional they are most regularly treated as either a body carrying a problem or, if they are experiencing mental or behavioral health issues, they are treated as a mind carrying a problem. In both approaches they are distinctly not treated as a whole, complex person.

This is an outcome the design and incentives of the financial model underpinning our current sick systems as well as the current approach to training healthcare professionals to staff those systems. For example, if the stakeholders across a health system desire to shift their focus to prevention, they will find little reimbursement from payers (private and government insurance companies). That means the savings their efforts may create will not benefit their financial well-being, but instead will benefit the financial well-being of the insurance companies who experience the savings from the successful prevention of disease. That is, to be sure, not always the case, as examples of alternative possibilities are increasing in number; but the status quo majority remains entrenched in an approach that does not encourage either an integrative approach to health and medicine or a focus on prevention, or an equitable distribution of savings accrued by preventing chronic disease. The world does not have to operate in this mode.

How Health Literacy, Cultural Competency, and Integrative Health and Medicine Lead to Prevention

The merger of health literacy and cultural competency when combined with a mind, body, spirit, and emotion approach to integrative health and medicine inherently demands of health systems and professionals that they address the people seeking their support and assistance from a whole-person approach. If health and medical professionals and institutions engage with people early and often; if they pay attention to not only a current health issue but to an entire life—what comes forward is a universal precautions approach to health literacy and respect for culture. This is the moment when healthcare professionals start to inherently and easily approach health and medicine from an integrative perspective and shift their focus from treating a disease to collaborating with a person to achieve better health and greater overall fulfillment in life.

This shift was summed up very nicely by Winston Wong, MD, our colleague on the National Academy of Sciences (NAS) Roundtable on Health Literacy and Medical Director, Community Benefit and Director, Disparities Improvement and Quality Initiatives at Kaiser Permanente, when he suggested during a recent NAS meeting that what medical care providers should ask patients, especially when they see them for such a little time each year, is "What does a good day mean to you?"

The discussion that led to that observation and suggested question had focused on expanding the relationship between medical care providers and the people they serve to move beyond what hurts—to how to help people live a better life. The possible result is an empowered person who is also more satisfied with the relationship they have with their health and medical professional—that professional becomes not just a "provider," but is a true health partner with the person seeking to lie a healthier, happier life.[5]

The Canyon Ranch Institute Approach to Partnership

At Canyon Ranch Institute, our approach to partnership is a model that embraces the integrative health approach, health literacy, and cultural competency as one. In this approach, the whole is greater than the sum of the parts, and no part of the equation can be delinked from the others. The Canyon Ranch Institute PRIMES model is based on our experience that the most effective way to address the currently broken sick care system is to engage in multisectorial partnerships that include all of the people and institutions that have a stake in the outcomes of health and healthcare in the United States and globally.

PRIMES stands for Partner, Require Radical Equity, Insist on Infrastructure, Make it Known, Evaluate, and Sustain.

At Canyon Ranch Institute, we have three levels of engagement—Partner, Join, and Connect. What other organizations might call lead, we call Partner, and it is in our partnerships that we develop, hone, and evolve our programs and methodologies that advance health literacy to ensure that all people can become educated, inspired, and empowered to prevent disease and embrace a life of wellness. We discuss the Partner level of engagement more in this chapter. The "Join" and "Connect" levels are those in which we join with other like-minded people and organizations in coalitions, roundtables, convenings, associations, and the like, and also in which we simply introduce people to others who may be able and willing to answer questions and provide other supportive resources.

The "P" in PRIMES is Partner. At the Partner level, we follow a clearly delineated process to discuss and document shared understandings about our mutual missions and goals, so that we can have a pathway to as efficiently as possible make integrative health and health literacy the tools that we apply in our partnerships and programs to help people and systems advance health and well-being in novel and measurable ways. We have experienced that this up-front commitment to ethical and partnership development by all parties contributes to a long-term view of the relationships. These partnerships connect all of our work, across multiple programs, geographic regions, healthcare systems, cultures, languages, and more.

Next, the "R" in PRIMES stands for Radical Equity. The idea of radical equity across sectors and systems is a concept that we have not been able to find thus far in other organizations or systems. Our unique insistence at Canyon Ranch Institute on the idea that all sectors of society can help improve the social determinants of health and the overall health and well-being of individuals, families, and communities has led us to bring together low-income people who need access to healthy living opportunities; large corporate entities, healthcare professionals and the systems they work within; public, private, and charter schools; colleges and universities; government entities; a wide range of faith-based organizations across the broad spectrum of spirituality and religion that inform much of American life and culture; sports and athletic teams and organizations; restaurants, grocery stores, food banks, and other food-service organizations; nonprofit entities; media companies; and a wide range of other sectors of society that are important to people and their health. We bring all of these sectors together to communicate about their best practices with one another, specifically in the context of a program that we have all decided to explore and implement together focused on the integrative health model and advancing health literacy. This concept of radical equity applies to all of the partners in any Canyon Ranch Institute endeavor, and is inherent to our ability to ensure the integrative approach. That approach relies on the resources and strengths that certain people, organizations, and industries can bring to bear to help improve individual and community health.

Infrastructure is the "I" in PRIMES, and refers to the need for organizations engaged in advancing best practices in health, including and especially in integrative health and health literacy, to have stable infrastructure. That infrastructure, while often not the core business of such an organization, is essential to partnership development and sustainability. The legal, financial, governance, and logistical aspects of an organization make the mission-driven programmatic work possible.

Make it Known refers to the need for strategic communications planning, execution, and measurement to ensure accurate and consistent messaging about both integrative health and health literacy concepts and programs. This "M" is PRIMES is necessary for two main reasons. The first is that the integrative approach and health literacy are not already widely accepted aspects of society. The second reason is the extensive and unrelenting competition for attention by a wide range of topics unrelated to health, and certainly unrelated to integrative health and health literacy. By conveying accurate and reliable information across a range of dissemination platforms, including online and in person, partnerships and the organizations that nurture them are not only sharing the best practices of health literacy but also modeling those practices.

Evaluate—is the "E" in PRIMES and focuses on the utility and necessity of rigorously tracking progress and outcomes of a partnership. We approach evaluation as a subset of scientific research—thus evaluation should produce usable, valid, and reliable evidence. Among the many possible and desired outcomes of conducting rigorous evaluation of a partnership are to inform participants of the changes they have made or not made; provide valid and reliable evidence of success or failure; justify the program to funders and management; document need for additional resources—support future funding efforts/sustainability; indicate areas requiring program modification and improvement—continuous quality improvement; inform policy; and facilitate the sharing of best practices.

Sustainability is the "S" in PRIMES and refers to the desired result of the PRIMES model. Sustainability does not refer to sustaining a particular project, program, or annual event. Rather, it focuses on sustaining the integrity of the mission of the organization engaged in each of the previous aspects of the PRIMES model. Achieving sustainability is both the highest purpose and a crucial necessity for organizations such as Canyon Ranch Institute that are involved in making a positive difference in the lives of people globally, through partnerships that educate, inspire, and empower people to prevent disease and embrace a life of wellness.

The Canyon Ranch Institute Life Enhancement Program*

We now turn to the Canyon Ranch Institute Life Enhancement Program (CRI LEP), an example of how a true healthcare system might function by focusing on health literacy and an integrative approach to health and medicine with the goal of preventing and reversing chronic disease. The CRI LEP is developed and implemented in partnership with a community-based healthcare organization. Staff members—representing specialists with backgrounds in nutrition, physical activity, behavior change, sense of purpose, integrative health, stress management, and social support—join together to form an integrative Core Team to provide the CRI LEP to their patient population. They work together as a team so that CRI LEP participants experience the entire range of the integrative health model in a coordinated and effective fashion. Those staff members participate in a two-part training program that focuses on the best practices of health literacy and integrative health and medicine in practical ways that help people help themselves to better health.

*Canyon Ranch Institute is now part of Health Literacy Media in St. Louis, MO.

The program itself comprises at least 40 hours of group sessions and a minimum of 4 hours of one-on-one consultations with healthcare professionals. The group sessions include presentations and discussions on all aspects of the integrative model—mind, body, spirit, and emotion—as well as sessions focused on nutrition, cooking, physical activity, behavioral health, spirituality, pharmacology, oral health, and a grocery-store tour. The one-on-one consultations allow participants to explore deeper connections with their own health in conversations with accredited healthcare professionals who were trained by Canyon Ranch Institute experts in the best practices of integrative health and health literacy. These one-on-one consultations include, at a minimum, at least four 1-hour conversations and hands-on activities focused on integrative health, nutrition, physical activity, and behavioral health.

Each CRI LEP is rigorously evaluated toward constant quality improvement of the program and to document program outcomes, including behavior changes and physical and physiological health changes. This evaluation is—at most sites—conducted at baseline, post-program, 3-month post program, and 1-year post program. Some sites are adding a 2-year post program evaluation as well. The evaluation includes blood work (cholesterol panel, blood glucose, and C-reactive protein), exercise (sit-ups, push-ups, flexibility, and a treadmill test), physical measurements (waist, hips, height, and weight), and an extensive knowledge, attitudes, behaviors, and beliefs individual interview.[6,7] (See http://www.canyonranchinstitute.org/partnerships-a-programs/cri-life-enhancement-program/cri-lep-overview.)

Health Literacy Best Practices

Uniquely, the CRI LEP is tailored to each partner site. To accomplish this tailoring, Canyon Ranch Institute staff members conduct extensive formative research in each community prior to the training of the partner's Core Team and the launch of the CRI LEP. This formative research consists of individual in-depth interview conducted with community leaders and representatives from businesses and organizations that reflect the integrative model—mind, body, spirit, and emotion. Additionally, individuals who reflect the population who would participate in the CRI LEP are directly engaged in a series of focus group discussions. The findings of the formative research are used as a basis to tailor program materials, the training of the core team that will provide the program, and the content and framing of presentations within the program.

A particular aspect of this tailoring of the program to the cultural, environmental, social, and political realities of each community involves the use of narratives as an approach to demonstrating the viability of change in that environment. Narratives are perhaps the most powerful means for individuals to construct coherent accounts of their lives.[8,9] Most often, the sense-making activity associated with health literacy takes the shape of a narrative.[9,10] Narrative structure consists of an opening situation, a moment of transformation, and a closing situation wherein all change presented is depicted as a new and coherent reality. The moment of transformation is what makes narrative a strong element of a behavior change model.

The CRI LEP materials include a participant guide, which is given to each participant. In this book, there are—by design—a series of narratives about the lives of different individuals that run throughout the length of the volume, beginning in the second chapter and culminating in the final chapter. These narratives are drawn from the formative research. We gather stories of success and failure in each community, then use those details to craft narratives that involve individuals that reflect the population that we are targeting in each community. The narratives involve challenges to health that are common within the community and then—through the narrative structure—demonstrate how those challenges can be successfully addressed in the lives of individuals that reflect the lives of participants in the program. Thus, participants in the CRI LEP are directly exposed to a linguistic structure of positive change based on the lives of real individuals in each community. As a result, participants often reflect that they are reading about people just like them who are struggling with—and overcoming—the same challenges to living a healthier and happier life.

Training Health Professionals in Best Practices of Health Literacy

We also use the formative research as a basis for training of the healthcare professionals in each community who will actually deliver the CRI LEP to the participants in that community. In this training, we merge the realities of each community with the best practices of health literacy and the full model of integrative health and medicine that underpin the CRI LEP.

In particular, the health literacy best practices we focus on in the training include:

- The approach to health literacy as a theory of behavior change rather than health literacy as simply focused on plain language and numeracy skills.[1,4,7]
- The need to improve health literacy versus simply removing complexity, as integrative health and medicine are, indeed, complex and we

need to assure that participants effectively embrace that complexity in their lives.

- The need to adopt universal precautions versus highlighting the dominant yet incomplete and potentially damaging "deficit model" of health literacy. That is, we focus on the skills people already have and are using, and work to expand and improve those skills, rather than focus solely on what skills people do not have. This approach supports even people who have low or nonexistent health literacy to identify manageable goals and behavior changes they can make and sustain.

- Transforming the skills and abilities of healthcare professionals from talking at or to people to talking with people. This transformation, which is truly a change in philosophy and behaviors and not merely additive to other thought processes and activities, reflects the underlying principle that while educating people has a value, the overarching goal is not only to help people increase their knowledge but also to decrease the gap between what they know and what they do.[11]

- An effective approach to use of the teach-back technique. In particular, we focus on shifting the need to use the teach-back not to reflect the participant's potential lack of understanding but to see the lack of usage of health information to make informed decisions about health to actually be caused by the healthcare professional. By making this switch, we tap into the healthcare professional's desire to improve their own skills and we elicit the participation of the people who are experiencing the CRI LEP to help the healthcare professionals reach that goal.

- A simulated participant exercise in which the healthcare professionals interact with an individual trained to fulfill the role of a CRI LEP participant. The guide for the simulated participant is rewritten in each community to incorporate particular aspects of the determinants of health, surrounding natural and built environment, and local culture that is encountered during the formative research. In particular, during this exercise Core Team members are encouraged and trained to listen first, then speak; address the whole person's life, not just a diagnosis of a health condition; use the teach-back technique in order to "chunk and check" information that is shared during the session, engage directly with the simulated participant to collaborate on the identification of viable small-step goals focusing on healthier behavior change.

Individual-Level Outcomes

The CRI LEP's application of that robust approach to integrative health—mind, body, spirit, and emotions—combined with the best practices of health literacy has produced dramatic health outcomes for participants across a broad range of cultural settings and contexts to date. Put simply, people are healthier, happier, and leading fuller lives as a result of their participating in the program. Specifically, outcome data combined from seven disparate sites to date—in Arizona, Missouri, Ohio, New York, Georgia, and Massachusetts—show statistically significant healthy changes across numerous indicators reflecting the underlying approach to integrative health and medicine. For example, a brief look at outcomes for the over 900 participants to date at sites across the United States includes:

- A self-reported gain, on average, of seven healthy days each month. If that sustains for a year, participants will gain 84 healthy days—nearly three months more of health per year.
- For those with high blood pressure at baseline, a drop in blood pressure on average of 14.7/10.3.
- An average increase of 66 minutes of exercise each week.
- A drop in depression, using the PHQ-9 depression scale of 9.1 points for participants who were at risk for depression at baseline (PHQ-9 score of 15 or higher). That is roughly a 45% drop in depression.
- A 111% increase in health literacy scores using our new measurement tool based on the Calgary Charter on Health Literacy.
- A 78% increase in health knowledge regarding nutrition, stress management, physical activity, integrative health, and personal health.
- This all occurs with a savings, in comparison to other interventions to achieve the same health gains using a Quality-Adjusted Life Year approach, of $188,395.77 on average.

Community-Level Outcomes

The impacts of the CRI LEP go far beyond changes in individual health status for participants and extend into the communities where the program is offered and into the careers of the healthcare professionals who offer the program. One of the earliest community-level impacts of the program came at the first site with a premier federally qualified community health center, Urban Health Plan, Inc., located in the South Bronx, New York. During the program start-up and training phase, it became clear there was a problem. The South Bronx, at the time, was essentially a food desert. You could talk to people about eating a balanced diet including vegetables—but there was not a fresh vegetable to be found for sale at any market or restaurant in the entire community. To address this huge problem, the CEO of Urban Health Plan essentially guaranteed sales with a small market located next to the clinic. As a result, that store started selling a small tableful of fresh vegetables. Fast-forward to today, now that small store only sells fresh fruits and vegetables, there is a new grocery store on the next block. That grocery store offers a robust produce section, with a wide range of fresh fruit and vegetables for sale at affordable prices, and there are now two farmer's markets in the community, both offer cooking demonstrations that provide credits to shoppers for observing the demonstrations. Those credits can be used to purchase goods at the farmer's markets. In addition, the farmer's market doubles the value of all state- and federally sponsored food benefits.

At that same site, Urban Health Plan, the introduction of health literacy via the CRI LEP has led the organization to establish its own health literacy center—a unique feature for a federally qualified health center. This awareness and integration of health literacy principles and practices extends into a workforce development program for the community, and into having health educators as a part of pediatrics, OB/GYN, adult medicine, and school-based health programs.

The members of the Core Teams for the CRI LEP programs across the country have also grown internally and spread that growth across the healthcare system of which they are a part. For example, the integrative health Core Team member and leader of medical education for the hospital system he is part of recently called his experience as a CRI LEP core team member "the most meaningful experience" in his medical career. Time after time, we find that exposing professionals in medical systems to the CRI LEP—and giving them the ability to truly interact with participants outside of the medical model focused solely on disease diagnosis and treatment—reminds them of why they went into health and medicine in the first place and reignites their internal drive to excel. As a result, we continually hear from our partners how the presence of the CRI LEP has changed the way they interact with all of the people who come seeking care, not just the participants in the CRI LEP.

For example, one Core Team member recently told us,

"I think the excitement of it all in our connection and our conversations that we have with each other, it's kind of bubbled up more my excitement and the passion for what I do with my work. And so I have more conversations. I try to fill it into more groups that I'm running, into more one-on-one conversations with patients that I'm working with. And even with my co-workers. Which then can sometimes shift and change the way we operate as a team and gets back into what the patients get."

A participant in the CRI LEP also recognized how this program has shifted not only their own health status but also their perception of the healthcare organization that is offering the CRI LEP in their community, saying in a recent focus group, "And it's like a new side to them. It's like you walk in the front door and they're like, 'Oh, my gosh! I'm so glad you're here!' And it makes you want to come back." This occurred in a community where the formative research conducted prior to the arrival of the CRI LEP revealed a significant amount of antipathy of the local hospital system, which was most frequently referred to as the place where people in the community went to die.

Those effects have continued to diffuse across not only the healthcare delivery organizations that offer the CRI LEP but also the lives and communities of participants. The focus of the CRI LEP is on reaching the people at the lower levels of health in a community. Improving their health is the surest way to improve the overall health of a community.

What has happened as a result is not only an improvement in community health but also an empowerment of individuals within the community to not only take control of their own lives but also begin work to empower others in their community to improve their own health and well-being. That move, on each participant's own part, has often resulted in some significant transformations in their own lives—and as a result reaching everyone else in their lives. For example, numerous participants in the CRI LEP are now employed by the healthcare delivery organization where they experienced the program. This level of engagement ranges from being a patient greeter to a member of the board of directors.

A stellar example, which we will tell in greater detail elsewhere in the future, is the story of Reginald Franklin of Savannah, Georgia. "Reggie" was a member of the first group of participants in the CRI LEP in Savannah, which was a partnership with Curtis V. Cooper Primary Health Care, Inc.—a federally qualified health center. When Reggie started the program he was obese, depressed, and, during the baseline assessment for the CRI LEP, learned he had type 2 diabetes. By the end of the program, Reggie had lost over 20 pounds. Two years later, he has tripled that weight loss. He has started regular practice of yoga, runs nearly every day, and continues to work with the exercise specialists and nutritionists he met during the CRI LEP. Further, he is now a member of the Core Team offering the CRI LEP in Savannah working to support participants, and is now the vice chair of the board of directors of Curtis V. Cooper Primary Health Care, Inc. His new personal motto is "No U-Turns," and Reggie is working every day to continue his own personal health journey and inspire the entire Savannah community through a video documentary of his transformation to health as well as documenting his story in newspaper articles and speaking engagements.

Finally, the CRI LEP has influenced both Canyon Ranch Institute and our partners to develop a suite of healthy lifestyle programs based on the best practices of integrative health and health literacy in order to prevent and reverse chronic disease. These include, but are not limited to, the CRI Theater for Health program, which uses interactive theater in a community to change health behaviors. The initial pilot of this program was held in a shantytown of Lima, Peru, through a partnership with Clorox. The outcomes of the effort include a reduction of *e Coli* and *listeria* in the cooking areas within the shantytown.[12] Additionally, CRI has developed a CRI Healthy Table program (focused on healthy cooking), the CRI Healthy Community program (for parents and their children), the CRI Healthy Garden program (healthy gardening and stress management focus), and variations of the CRI LEP—the CRI LEP for Families, which focuses on young children and their caregivers, and the CRI LEP for Teens, which focuses on teens and their caregivers.

Conclusion

The success of the CRI LEP is grounded in many elements. Two primary elements are our approach to partnership and the best practices of health literacy being infused throughout the program. The partnerships we develop based on the PRIMES model become self-sustaining, award-winning, and create transformation among the partners. Health literacy is infused throughout the tailoring of the program and training of the Core Teams that provide the program in their community. The words, approaches, and tools used become an injection of health literacy, health, and well-being. The dosage and manner of application are tailored to each participant and community. That content and style, much like an immunization, seeks out and modifies or replaces the ideas and habits causing poor health. The CRI LEP content is embedded within participants' hearts and minds. In turn, the participants go out and share what they have learned and changed in their lives with friends, family, and their entire community. Through that process of diffusion, the CRI LEP metastasizes, in a healthy manner, to far more people than directly participate in the program experience the positive health effects in their lives as well. This is how we can turn the world's health around for the better.

As noted earlier, the CRI LEP is one of a growing number of examples of efforts to merge the best practices of health literacy into a universal precaution approach. This approach, as noted, inherently addresses a person's entire life rather than just their symptoms and the diagnosis of the day. This approach explicitly addresses culture, knowledge, communication ability, self-efficacy, empowerment, and the entire range of social, political, and environmental determinants of an individual's, a community's, and the world's health and well-being. We close by suggesting that the approach we have described is perhaps the most financially sustainable, cost-efficient, equitable, and effective manner to truly achieve health in all policies and health for all.

Suggested Reading Materials

- Health Literacy Around the World: Part 1 Health Literacy Efforts Outside of the United States
  Andrew Pleasant
  http://www.ncbi.nlm.nih.gov/books/NBK202445/
- Health Literacy Around the World: Part 2 Health Literacy Efforts Within the United States and a Global Overview
  Andrew Pleasant
  https://www.nationalacademies.org/hmd/~/media/Files/Activity%20 Files/PublicHealth/HealthLiteracy/Commissioned-Papers/ Health%20Literacy%20Around%20the%20World%20Part%202.pdf
- A Prescription Is Not Enough: Improving Public Health with Health Literacy
  Andrew Pleasant, Jennifer Cabe, Laurie Martin
  https://www.nationalacademies.org/hmd/~/media/Files/Activity%20 Files/PublicHealth/HealthLiteracy/Commissioned-Papers/A-Prescription-Is-Not-Enough-Improving-Public-Health-with-Health-Literacy.pdf
- Health Literacy Research and Practice: A Needed Paradigm Shift
  Andrew Pleasant, Jennifer Cabe, Kavita Patel, Jennifer Cosenza, Richard Carmona
  http://www.ncbi.nlm.nih.gov/pubmed/26372030
- A Health Literacy Fable for Tomorrow: Help the World Be Healthy with Health Literacy
  Andrew Pleasant
  https://nam.edu/perspectives-2014-a-health-literacy-fable-for-tomorrow-help-the-world-be-healthy-with-health-literacy/
- A Tale of Two Health Literacies: Public Health and Clinical Approaches to Health Literacy
  Andrew Pleasant, Shyama Kuruvilla
  http://heapro.oxfordjournals.org/content/23/2/152.full

- Advancing Health Literacy: A Framework for Understanding and Action
  Christina Zarcadoolas, Andrew Pleasant, David Greer
  http://www.wiley.com/WileyCDA/WileyTitle/productCd-0787984337.html

References

1. Coleman C, Kurtz-Rossi S, McKinney J, Pleasant A, Rootman I, Shohet L. Calgary Charter on Health Literacy. 2009. http://www.centreforliteracy.qc.ca/Healthlitinst/Calgary_Charter.htm. Accessed July 13, 2010.
2. Zarcadoolas C, Pleasant A, Greer D. Advancing Health Literacy: A Framework for Understanding and Action. San Francisco, CA: Jossey Bass; 2006.
3. Zarcadoolas C, Pleasant A, Greer D. Understanding health literacy: An expanded model. *Health Promot Int* 2005;20:195–203.
4. Pleasant A, Cabe J, Patel K, Cosenza J, Carmona R. Health literacy research and practice: A needed paradigm shift. *Health Commun* 2015;30(12):1176–1180.
5. Roundtable on Health Literacy; Board on Population Health and Public Health Practice; Institute of Medicine; The National Academies of Sciences E, and Medicine. Health literacy: Past, present, and future: Workshop summary. Washington, DC: Roundtable on Health Literacy; Board on Population Health and Public Health Practice; Institute of Medicine; The National Academies of Sciences, Engineering, and Medicine; 2015.
6. Pleasant A, Kuruvilla S, Zarcadoolas C, Shanahan J, Lewenstein B. A Framework for Assessing Public Engagement with Health Research. Geneva, Switzerland: World Health Organization; 2003.
7. Pleasant A. Health literacy: an opportunity to improve individual, community, and global health. *New Dir for Adult and Cont Educ.* 2011;2011(130):43–53.
8. Labov W. Some further steps in narrative analysis. *J Narrat Life Hist* 1997;7:395–415.
9. Shanahan J, Pelstring L, McComas K. Using narratives to think about environmental attitude and behavior: an exploratory study. *Soc Natur Resour* 1999;12:405–419.
10. Fisher WR. Narration as a human communication paradigm: the case of public moral argument. *Commun Monogr* 1984;51(1):1–22.
11. Pang T, Sadana R, Hanney S, Bhutta Z, Hyder A, Simon J. Knowledge for better health—a conceptual framework and foundation for health research systems. *B World Health Organ* 2003;81:815–820.
12. Pleasant A, de Quadros A, Pereira-Leon M, Cabe J. A qualitative first look at the Arts for Behavior Change Program: Theater for Health. *Arts Health* 2015;7(1):54–64.

4

Genomics, Epigenetics, and Precision Medicine in Integrative Preventive Medicine

NANCY G. CASANOVA, TING WANG, EDDIE T. CHIANG,
AND JOE G. N. GARCIA

Synopsis: We briefly review the use of genomewide screening for early detection, treatment, and prevention and the utility of genome-based biomarkers as a tool for precision medicine and its application to population and integrative preventive medicine.

Introduction

The holistic approach of integrative preventive medicine (IPM) convenes the integration of proactive prevention with the purpose of prolonging health, preventing chronic diseases, improving life quality, decreasing healthcare expenses, limiting the risk of adverse interactions, and reducing gaps in care. At the core of IPM primary prevention are integrative modalities effective in health promotion, including lifestyle counseling, dietary guidance, stress mitigation techniques, interventions to improve sleep quality, and use of nutriceuticals and herbal supplements. The exact mechanisms by which these modalities influence health are poorly understood; however, there is increasing evidence that these strategies may involve common genomic and epigenetic effects. Integrative preventive medicine is well positioned in modern healthcare to incorporate the vast, rapidly advancing, and increasingly available genomic-related data to benefit individual-level clinical care and to improve population interventions and preventive medicine. The integration of genetic, epigenetic, and precision medicine strategies into IPM approaches has the very real potential to maximize health benefits, minimize harm, and possibly avoid unnecessary healthcare costs.

Leveraging the most advanced scientific evidence is an essential process to understanding complex systems, such as development, homeostasis, and responses to the environment.[1] Likewise, understanding the impact of genetics and epigenetics on human health advances our insights into human pathobiology, particularly complex diseases. David Hilbert, the brilliant 20th-century German mathematician, said, "rapid advances come from the development of sharper tools for exploration." Indeed, a critical consequence of the human genome project was the rapid and continued development of multiple high-throughput technologies including rapid whole-genome sequencing, genomewide association studies (GWAS), ChIP-Seq, RNA-Seq, epigenetics, transcriptomics, and mass spectroscopy-based proteomics. These tools have generated a different vision of genome functionality that has retreated from the notion of a single gene causing a single disease. State-of-the-art healthcare delivery is rapidly incorporating these high-throughput tools to enable accurate risk prediction and therapeutic targeting. Precision medicine and clinical translational medicine are elements of this integrative concept, a concept that enables individualized approaches to health and complex disease.

Precision Medicine

Precision medicine is revolutionizing the manner by which one improves health and alleviates suffering from disease, by considering individual genetic differences as well as differences in lifestyles and environment.[2] This visionary approach is built on the premise that treatment decisions should be based on individual genetic variability, taking advantage of already available large-scale genomic, metabolomics, and proteomic databases. The National Institutes of Health (NIH) Precision Medicine Initiative (PMI)[3] aims to integrate a national longitudinal research cohort with social, racial/ethnic diverse backgrounds representing the nation demographics. This cohort will provide genetic data, biological samples, and other health information to researchers and translational clinicians.

GENOMIC BIOMARKERS OF HEALTH AND DISEASE

Biological markers or biomarkers are indicators of normal biological and pathological processes. Measurements such as blood pressure, body mass index, and cholesterol levels have been successfully correlated with metabolic diseases. Disease biomarkers are used to diagnose various phases of disease, monitor severity of disease and responses to therapy, and serve as potential predictors of prognosis and responses to therapy.[4] Multiple methodologies have been applied for biomarker detection in biological fluids and tissues (serum, cerebral spinal fluid, bronchoalveolar lavage fluid, etc.) using enzyme-linked immunosorbent assays (ELISA), proteomic analysis, and mass spectrometry.

Molecular biomarkers have been applied in detection, screening, diagnosis, treatment, and monitoring of cancer. These biomarkers can be macromolecules such as proteins or other biomolecules such as messenger RNAs (mRNAs), microRNAs (miRNAs), or other metabolites. Peripheral blood provides easy access for obtaining levels of these biomarkers and for assessment of organs that are ordinarily difficult to access. Multiple biomarkers have been identified from preclinical research, but few have been proven useful in clinical practice. Despite limitations, the use of biomarkers to enhance accurate diagnosis and prediction of disease activity remains a focal point in routine clinical care and preventive medicine. Criteria used to evaluate the value of disease biomarkers include disease-associated specificity, sensitivity, traceability, stability, repeatability, and reliability.[4,5] These markers must be detectable in the blood, since the blood is in contact with all organs; however, biomarker validation is complex, often requiring validation in human tissues, with overexpression of targeted candidates correlated with dysfunction of specific organs or tissues.[6] Likewise, in order to assess the transition from health to disease, biomarker assessment should occur in a longitudinal manner, with each individual serving as his/her own control for the changing levels of biomarkers in the blood.

Gene expression-based microarrays and RNA sequencing strategies provide opportunities to discover novel disease mechanisms.[7] Microarray technology allows the simultaneous measurement of mRNA transcripts for assessment of gene expression across the entire genome providing insight into the overall level of gene activity and protein expression.[8] A gene signature is a group of genes derived from a specific tissue or biological fluid, whose combined expression pattern is characteristic of a biological, cellular, or molecular phenotype. The signature is composed of a set of genes whose expression is dysregulated (either increased or decreased expression) compared to normal tissues. Gene expression signatures are potentially powerful tools that can reveal a range of biologically and clinically important characteristics of biological samples[9] and are used to differentiate diseases phenotypes, including disease severity.[10] For example, sepsis is an important cause of hospitalization and death. Recently the reactive oxygen species (ROS)-associated molecular signatures were assessed as biomarkers to predict survival in sepsis. *In silico* analyses of gene expression profiles allowed the identification of a 21-gene ROS-associated molecular signature that predicts survival in sepsis patients.[11]

Likewise, we analyzed genomewide gene expression in peripheral blood mononuclear cells (PBMCs) in sarcoidosis patients and identified a gene signature that distinguishes complicated versus uncomplicated sarcoidosis.[12,13] This signature revealed a predictive accuracy when classifying sarcoidosis patients from healthy controls in two independent external cohorts.[12,13] Figure 4.1 provides an example of using gene signature for diagnosis.[14] Similarly, PBMC gene expression profiles were compared in patients with either sarcoidosis or sickle cell disease with a goal of identifying those with concomitant pulmonary hypertension, a serious complication of both disorders. Two gene signatures were identified;[15,16] however, comparison of both signatures failed to identify overlap between the gene signatures, suggesting that the mechanisms for development of pulmonary hypertension in sarcoidosis may be distinct from sickle cell disease.

PHARMACOGENOMICS

The integration of genome-generated big data has spawned new fields within precision medicine, transforming the traditional clinical therapeutic approach. Pharmacogenomics is defined as the science of determining benefit–risk balance based on race- and ethnic-specific genomic variants of the patient's germ line and/or diseased tissue.[17] The hallmark of pharmacogenomics is to target a specific drug to a precise patient subphenotype.

Single nucleotide polymorphisms (SNPs) are gene variations occurring approximately every 500–1000 base pairs of the genome that serve as biological markers and potentially predict drug responses, susceptibility to certain toxins, or predisposition to disease. As an example, the class of drugs known as the statins comprises HMG-CoA reductase inhibitors commonly used to treat hypercholesterolemia. Statins are well tolerated, but elicit myalgias and creatinine kinase elevation in a percentage of users and, in rare cases, induce rhabdomyolysis. Studies to date indicate that statins induce blood and tissue coenzyme Q-10 (CoQ10) depletion, which may be prevented by supplemental CoQ10.[18] Two SNPs in the *COQ2* gene, a gene involved in the coenzyme Q (ubiquinone) biosynthetic pathway, have been linked to statin-induced myopathy.[19,20] Other SNPs in genes involved in statin pharmacokinetics (*SLCO1B1* and *OATP1B1*) are genetic risk factors for myopathy.[20]

Another example of the impact of pharmacogenomics is cystic fibrosis (CF), an autosomal recessive condition affecting the lungs and the digestive systems. Although the mutated chloride channel is well known, CF now can be subclassified according to the defective channel characteristics. Ivacaftor is a drug only effective in a subset of CF patients in whom the channel reaches the

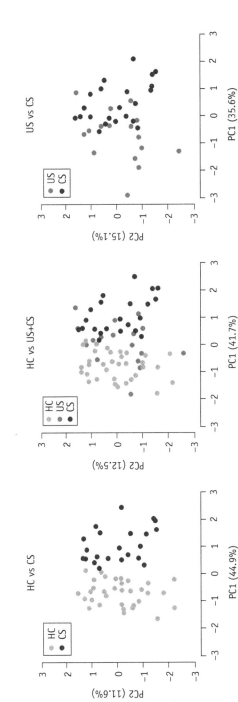

FIGURE 4.1 Example of using a 20-gene signature for the diagnosis of sarcoidosis.[14] Identifying gene signatures in sarcoidosis. Principal component analysis on expression values of the 20-gene signature. X-axis: principal component 1 with eigenvalue; Y-axis: principal component 2 with eigenvalue. Left panel: patients with complicated sarcoidosis and healthy controls; middle panel: patients with complicated sarcoidosis, uncomplicated sarcoidosis, and healthy controls; and right panel: patients with complicated sarcoidosis and uncomplicated sarcoidosis. HC: healthy controls; US: patients with uncomplicated sarcoidosis; and CS: patients with complicated sarcoidosis

surface.[21] Drug development research is currently taking advantage of genomic signatures to stratify patients for phase III trials. Genomic signatures may also be useful in identifying subjects likely to benefit from adjuvant dietary strategies such as probiotics and prebiotics, which have shown initial promise in improving CF-related chronic inflammation.[22]

Precision oncology is an area where pharmacogenomics has achieved significant progress due to the now-routine incorporation of molecular testing into clinical care. For example, oncogene-targeted therapies based on tumor-borne mutations have led to clinically validated therapies targeting genes in pathways related to proliferation or apoptosis inhibition.[23,24]

Epigenetics in Disease Development

Epigenetics is an important mechanism for gene expression during uterine development, childhood, and aging. At the cellular level, epigenetic mechanisms are involved in regulation of cell cycles and DNA repair secondary to carcinogen exposures. Therefore, epigenetics is also viewed as the interface modulator between the genome and the environmental stressors and endogenous factors that may promote tumor development and disease progression.[25] Epigenetics controls transcriptional output and, therefore, traits. Correlating epigenomic and transcriptomic information can be highly informative[1] in order to corroborate the etiology of many diseases and the influence of elements such as environment, diet, chemicals, drugs and pharmaceutical products.

EPIGENETIC MECHANISMS

Independent modifications to the linear DNA sequence, include DNA methylation, histone acetylation, methylation, phosphorylation, ubiquitination, citrullination, sumoylation, and ADP ribosylation.[26] Histone modification influences DNA methylation, thus, gene expression is controlled by activation and repression mechanisms. An example is the effects of decreased dietary folate intake on DNA methylation and biosynthesis. This results in reduced levels of S-adenosylmethionine (SAM) leading to DNA hypomethylation and inappropriate protoconcogene activation, activation of latent transposons, and chromosome rearrangement and instability, commonly seen in colorectal cancer.[27] The effects of folate and methionine in DNA methylation are depicted on Figure 4.2.

Epigenetic features can control transcriptional output, and DNA methylation and demethylation are the best-characterized epigenetic modifications. Methylation/demethylation of DNA involves the addition or deletion of a

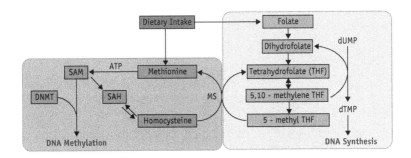

FIGURE 4.2 Folate and methionine metabolism effects on DNA methylation. DNMT, DNA methyltransferases; SAH, S-adenosyl homocystein; MS, methionine synthase; SAM, S-adenosyl methionine

methyl group at the 5' position on the pyrimidine ring of cytosines, creating 5-methylcytosine (5-mC).[28]

Functionally, the methylation primarily prevents the binding of specific transcription factors to DNA at the gene promoter region, thereby suppressing gene expression,[29] although hypermethylation may also induce enhanced expression.[30] Additionally, DNA methylation interferes with alternative splicing, thereby generating splicing variants.[31] The DNA methyltransferases (DNMT) are responsible for maintenance of DNA methylation[32] with four known types of DNMTs: DNMT1, DNMT2, DNMT3a, and DNMT3b, all of which utilize S-adenosylmethionine as the methyl donor.[32] (Figure 4.3).

DISEASES ASSOCIATED WITH ALTERATIONS IN DNA METHYLATION

The DNA methyltransferase–mediated altered methylation of the genome is associated with increasing age and increased cancer risk.[33,34] Hypermethylation of tumor suppressor gene promoter sites may lead to increased carcinogenesis, while oncogene hypomethylation stimulates tumor growth. Therapeutic modification of DNA methylation may contribute to better outcomes in integrative medicine or IPM. For example, one rodent study confirmed that offspring from mothers supplemented with methyl donors were brown in color and lean compared to nonsupplemented mothers who produced yellow, obese offspring, with increased incidence of diabetes and cancer.[33]

Owing to the relative simplicity of the assay, methylation levels in the long interspersed nucleotide element-1 (LINE-1) have commonly been used as a surrogate measurement of cellular global DNA methylation. LINE-1 hypomethylation is shown to be associated with more chromosomal instability in

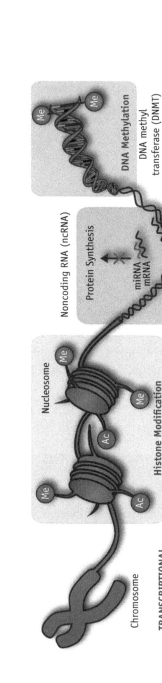

FIGURE 4.3 Overview of the various epigenetic mechanisms. Epigenetics include the interplay between DNA methylation, histone modification, and RNA-mediated post-transcriptional regulation that alters the generation and stability of transcripts

colorectal cancer.[35] The LINE-1 hypomethylation is also associated with poor outcome in several cancer types.[36-38] Average LINE-1 methylation levels in colorectal tumors decline as tumors progress.[39] With regard to IPM, LINE-1 methylation may be a risk factor[40] for colorectal cancer, with LINE-1 hypomethylation indicating an aggressive subtype, prevented by adequate folate intake and avoidance of alcohol.[41]

Another key component of epigenetic regulation of gene expression is histone modification. The DNA is tightly packed into the nucleus as chromatin consisting of 147 base pairs of DNA wrapped around a histone octamer. When DNA transcription occurs, the histones are required to open to allow access to the DNA. Modifications on histone proteins control transcription through phosphorylation, acetylation, sumoylation, methylation, ubiquitylation, prolyl-isomeryzation, and ADP-ribosylation, and these enzymes rely on a number of cofactors and metabolites.[42] The most well studied of these modifications is histone acetylation, with increased histone acetylation enhancing active transcription while decreased acetylation tightens histone structures with reduced active transcription.[42] Histone acetylation and deacetylation are catalyzed by two groups of enzymes called histone acetyltransferases (HATs) and histone deacetylases (HDACs). Acetyl coenzyme A serves as donor of the acetyl group, which is transferred to lysines of histone tails by HATs.[43] There are five groups of HATs and four classes of HDACs, due to structural and activity differences.[44] Due to the complexity of histone modifications and number of different enzymes that can occur on histones regulating DNA transcription, substantial research is still required to determine clinical relevance. Nevertheless, the histone acetylation regulation via HDAC implicates metabolic control in human disease.[45-47]

Cigarette smoking is a major environmental hazard associated with lung cancer development. Studies using epigenome-wide association studies (EWASs) have identified 1,450 smoking-associated CpG sites.[48,49] Genomewide association studies confirmed associations with smoking for a previously identified CpG site within the KLF6 gene and identified 12 novel sites located in 7 genes: *STK32A, TERT, MSH5, ACTA2, GATA3, VTI1A,* and *CHRNA5* (FDR < 0.05).[49] These examples demonstrate the progress in understanding of epigenetics and its relevance to IPM.

Complementary Alternative Medicine Epigenetic Effects

The use of complementary and alternative medicine (CAM) approaches to clinical care is a common practice and includes herbs, dietary treatment, meditation, relaxation, homeopathy, hypnotherapy, aromatherapy, and multivitamins.[50] While the combined use of alternative and conventional medicine has been deemed to be beneficial in improving psychological distress and adjustment, the sole use of CAM as an alterative to standard of care in cancer patients carries the potential for treatment delays, increased recurrence, and death.[51] As highlighted later, the key gap is the absence of sufficient numbers of clinical trials conducted to assess the efficacy of CAM approaches and any untoward risk in such approaches.

CANCER CHEMOPREVENTIVE AGENTS

Cancer chemopreventive agents include resveratrol, a phytoalexin found in grapes, berries, and peanuts, which exhibits chemopreventive activity in three different stages: tumor initiation, promotion, and progression.[52] Resveratrol acts as a selective estrogen receptor modulator (SERM) and regulates proteins involved in DNA synthesis and cell cycle, such as p53 and Rb/E2F, and cyclins. Cyclin-dependent kinases affect the activity of transcriptional factors involved in proliferation and stress responses, such as NF-kB, AP1, and Egr1.[53,54]

Epidemiological studies have shown that a soy-rich diet decreases the incidence of some human cancers, including breast and prostate cancers. Genistein, the active component found in soy, exerts its cancer preventive effects by targeting various pathways relevant in the development of cancer, and may affect cancer progression.[55,56] Curcumin, a compound found in the Asian spice known as turmeric, exhibits anticancer properties via acetylation of lysine residues that regulates NF-κB, including transcriptional activation, DNA binding affinity, I-κBα degradation, and NF-kB nuclear translocation.[57,58] Curcumin-treated cells demonstrate inhibition of epigenetic regulators such as the histone deacetylases: HDAC1, HDAC3, and p300/, which decreases NF-κB and Notch1 activity with significant inhibition of cell proliferation. The effect of curcumin on HDACs and HATs was partially due to increased proteasomal degradation.[57]

Organosulfur compounds present in allium vegetables, such as garlic, chives, and leeks, are used to improve immunity and cardiovascular health, responses to radiation, cancer protection, and as hypoglycemic agents in traditional medicine.[55] Risk of stomach and colon cancers is significantly reduced if allium vegetables are consumed regularly,[59] attributed to organosulfur compounds such as diallyl sulfide [DAS], diallyl disulfide [DADS], and diallyl trisulfide [DATS] that induce cell cycle arrest and apoptosis and inhibit cancer growth, angiogenesis, and metastasis.[60] The epigenetic modulation of some phytochemicals is summarized in Table 4.1.

Table 4.1 Dietary Agents as Epigenetics Modulators

Agent	Source	Epigenetic Effect	Disease Correlation	References
Resveratrol	Grapes, peanuts, apples, some berries	Histone modification—decrease acetylation of histone H3K9 by inducing SIRT1 expression, DNMT down-regulation, miRNA modulation	Tumor suppression, antimetastasis	52,55,61,62
Curcumin	Turmeric	DNMT1 inhibition, Histone modulation—HDAC1, HDAC3, and NF-kB decreased activity; miRNA expression modulation	Cancer protection	55,57,63
Catechins	Green, black tea	DNMT1 inhibition, folate cycle disruption and increased SAM level, modify expression of miRNAs	Cancer protection	55,64
Sulfora-phane	Broccoli, sprouts, kale, cabbage	DNMT1 down regulation, Histone modulation—increased acetylation H3 and H4 and HDAC decreased activity	Tumor suppression, cardiovascular protection	55,65,66
Organo-sulfurs	Garlic	Histone acetylation induction—H3 and H4 increased binding on promoter of p21	Cancer, cardiovascular protection	55,60,67
Genistein	Soy	DNMT inhibition, cell growth inhibition	Cancer protection	55,56

Similarly, high consumption of fish oil or ω-3 PUFAs, including docosa-hexaenoic acid (DHA), reduces the risk of colon, pancreatic, and endometrial cancers by inducing human cancer cell apoptosis without limited toxicity. In addition, DHA enhanced the efficacy of anticancer drugs by increasing drug uptake and suppressing survival pathways in cancer cells.[68]

IMMUNOMODULATORS

Inflammation is a common feature across many chronic diseases including diabetes, heart disease, digestive disorders, and cancer. Dietary patterns modify inflammation, and the traditional Mediterranean diet (fruit, green vegetables, legumes, nuts, whole grains, moderate consumption of olive oil and alcohol, low consumption of red meat and butter) has been demonstrated to reduce inflammation.[69,70] In addition, the Mediterranean diet exerts cardiovascular protection over a 10-year period of observation.

Myriocin is a natural product derived from a type of entomopathogenic fungus *Isaria sinclairii* (vegetative wasp), with strong immunosuppressant effects through inhibition of serine palmitoyl transferase, the initial enzyme in the biosynthesis of sphingolipids. This natural product led to the discovery of Fingolimod FTY720,[71] a chemically modified myriocin. Fingolimod is now recognized as an immunosuppressant[72] via specific receptor ligation.[73,74] Fingolimod undergoes rapid phosphorylation in vivo by sphingosine kinase 2 to produce phosphor-FTY720 or fingolimod-phosphate,[75] a structural analog of natural sphingosine-1-phosphate (S1P), which binds and activates S1P receptors with high affinity to exert biological effects.[76] This leads to internalization of S1P receptor 1 (S1PR1) in lymphocytes, inhibiting the migration of lymphocytes toward S1P, an immunosuppressive mechanism highly effective in multiple sclerosis[76,77] and proposed for use in other inflammatory lung diseases[74] and chronic inflammatory demyelinating polyneuropathy.[78] Interestingly, genetic variation within S1P receptors exert strong effects on receptor function, therapeutic efficacy of FTY720, and disease outcome.[79,80] Genetic screening of SNPs in S1P receptor genes will significantly enhance precision medicine approaches to prescribing FTY720 as an immunosuppressant therapy.

Probiotics regulate immune responses by inhibiting pathogen growth in colonic mucosa via bacteriocin production, toxin inactivation, and interference with pathogen adherence. Lactobacillus strains, such as *Lactobacillus* GG and *Saccharomyces. boulardii*, demonstrate significant strain- and dose-dependent clinical benefit in the treatment of acute watery diarrhea.[81-83]

Chinese traditional herb medicine, used for thousands of years in China and Asian countries, have selectively been proven effective, with a recent Nobel Prize in Physiology or Medicine (2014), shared by Chinese scientist Youyou Tu for her development of an effective antimalarial treatment derived from the wormwood plant, *Artemisia annua*. Although clinical outcomes are inconsistent, modern genetic techniques show epigenetic effects of traditional Chinese herbs via influences on gene expression. Hsieh et al. found 36% of 3,294 medicinal herbs analyzed influenced histone-modifying enzymes, chromatin condensation, or miRNA- or methyl CpG-binding proteins.[84] Effects of Chinese herb medicine on epigenetic gene expression regulation and potential health effects are summarized in Table 4.2.

Adjuvant Preventive Modalities in Integrative Preventive Medicine

As noted throughout this book, IPM modalities may influence health via common genomic and epigenetic impact and effects. Acupuncture at the SJ5 acupoint exerts neuroprotective effects via increased expression of Bcl-2, an antiapoptotic gene and Birc1b mRNA.[98] Acupuncture in ischemic stroke patients specifically alters brain function in regions associated with sensation, vision, and motion, whereas this generally activates brain areas associated with insomnia and other functions in normal individuals.[99] Acupuncture increased the glucose metabolism in local cerebral regions in patients with cerebral infarction measured by positron emission computer tomography (PET/CT).[100]

Personalized Medicine Applied to Population Health

The concept of population health is a true integration of numerous biologic molecular data points, cellular and phenotypic measurements, and individual genome sequences.[5] The balance between individual and population interventions for improving health[101] considers assessing micro- and macro-level factors as determinants of health and disease through complex population-based, longitudinal epidemiologic studies that consider endogenous factors, such as gene expression; individual factors, such as dietary intake and exercise habits; and socioeconomic factors.[102] However, a new phenomenon is observed with regard to our ability to generate and analyze "omics" data that may delay

Table 4.2 Chinese Herb Medicines as Epigenetic Modulators (2010–2016)

Agent	Epigenetic Effect	Clinical/Biological Outcome	References
Andrographis paniculata	Increased expression of 22 miRNAs and decrease of 10 miRNAs	Inhibition on hepatoma tumor growth	85
Hedyotis diffusa plus Scutellaria barbata	miR-155 reduction	Induction of bladder cancer cell apoptosis	86
Herb-partitioned moxibustion	miR-147 and miR-205 down-regulation	Protection against Crohn's disease	87
Radix Astragali	miR-375 up-regulation	Neuroprotective effects in cerebral ischemia/ reperfusion	88
Chinensis Franch, Astragalus membranaceus, and Lonicera japonica	Down-regulation of miR29-b	Sustained antidiabetic effects	89
Salvia miltiorrhiza	Upregulation of miR-133 expression	Protection against hypoxic cardiac myocytes	90
Salvia miltiorrhiza	Reduced acetylation of histone H3	Therapy and prevention of breast cancer	91
Tripterygium wilfordii Hook f	Reduced demethylation of histone H3 lysine 9	Antifertility and anticancer effects	92–94
Acanthopanax senticosus	HDAC inhibition	Inducing apoptosis of leukemia cells	95
Trichosanthes kirilowi	DNA demethylation via DNMT1 inhibition	Human cervical cancer suppression	96
Radix Angelicae Sinensis	DNA demethylation via DNA methyltransferase inhibition	Anticancer effect	97

the transition to personalized medicine application to population health. Currently, availability of "omics" facilities are heterogeneous, with personalized medicine likely to widen the growing disparity/equity in health systems between high- and low-income populations.[103] There is a dramatic challenge for academic medicine to merge integrative approaches into the educative model for future generations of physicians and health professionals, thereby optimizing health and well-being through evidence-based, sustainable, integrative approaches.

Precision Medicine Integrated in Preventive Models

We have entered an era in disease-prevention approaches, disease treatment, and prevention, that now takes into account the issues of individual variability in genes, environment, and lifestyle for each person. However, as prevention is an area that has received less emphasis in precision medicine,[21] the integrative model offers an opportunity to mine the interface between genomics and risk assessment, family health history, and clinical decision support. The availability of abundant genomic data sets collected in cell and animal models provides the opportunity for integration into a clinically meaningful and practical use that could be translated into population risk management.

DATA INTEGRATION

The critical challenge of integrating and sharing personal health information in a secure way is a global concern. Countries such as Denmark, United Kingdom, Belgium, Norway, and Estonia have developed large-scale research data set of genomic data linked to electronic medical records. Examples include the EasyGenomics cloud in Beijing Genomics Institute (BGI), and "Embassy" clouds as part of the ELIXIR project in collaboration with multiple European countries.[26] In the United States, academic centers, government organizations such as the National Human Genome Research Institute, and private industry have obtained massive data sets derived from a variety of genomic platforms. Data identifying genetic variants from individuals willing to share their electronic medical records with the aim of fostering clinical and genomic discovery is growing exponentially.

Biologists have studied specific proteins and molecular pathways individually, describing local interactions and perturbations in detail, with understanding the individual components as an important first step. However, to truly understand complex biological systems requires an integrated approach.[5] The ability to share genomic data and clinical data and both integrate and translate these data into healthcare models and population health policies will pose a challenge for clinicians, scientists, and biostatisticians and public health policy makers. This integrated preventive model conceives a level of integration that requires incorporating "omics" data in the preventive intervention platform according to the level of risk of certain groups (Figure 4.4).

Increased cost-effectiveness is one potential advantage of precision medicine in the preventive field, where genome sequencing identifies *actionable gene variants*, defective genes with potential negative health effects.[5] A recent study in familial hypercholesterolemia revealed that DNA testing for known family mutations and LDL-cholesterol levels is more cost-effective than current primary prevention.[104] Likewise, US Preventive Services Task Force (USPSTF) current guidelines recommend genetic risk assessment and BRCA mutation testing for breast and ovarian cancer susceptibility in women with increased risk who have family members with breast, ovarian, tubal, or peritoneal cancer.[105] Although BRCA 1-2 mutation gene testing remains cost-prohibitive in many circumstances, the charge is likely to decrease once the testing market is available in more labs.[106]

Complex illnesses involve the interplay of environmental, genetic, and epigenetic factors. Genomic-derived biomarkers are useful tools in the preventive model to predict disease susceptibility and implement directed therapy to avoid future disease-related complications. Similarly, allele frequency estimation, studied in population genetics, is relevant to define public health policies for common and rare but lethal diseases in certain groups at risk, such as African Americans and Hispanics. Ashkenazi Jews are a good example, in which preconception carrier prescreening is recommended[107] for certain rare conditions (Tay-Sachs, alpha and beta thalassemia, etc.).

Conclusions

A key goal of integrative medicine is to provide the availability of diverse and appropriate options for patients, ultimately blurring the boundaries between conventional care and CAM. Genomic and epigenetic approaches exist within those blurred boundaries. Although the strength of current scientific evidence is incomplete, IPM in the modern healthcare era is well positioned to lead the integration of the vast and rapidly proliferating genomic-related information to improve population interventions in preventive medicine. Future research strategies are needed to more fully integrate the application of genomic and epigenetic data into synergies of integrative medicine and primary, secondary,

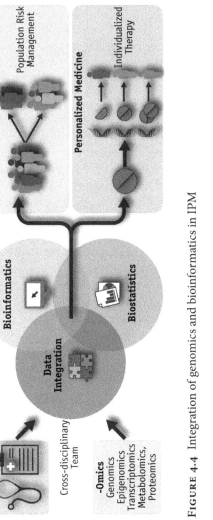

FIGURE 4-4 Integration of genomics and bioinformatics in IPM

and tertiary prevention levels. In doing so, IPM will have even greater capacity to maximize health benefits, minimize harm, and prevent unnecessary health-care costs. As scientific findings begin to advance from a purely translational, genome-research phase to full clinical application, the regulatory and reimbursement policies barriers will need to be circumvented as well as legislative protections for privacy for systemwide adoption[108] for the full application of genomic and personalized medicine in preventive medicine.

References

1. Hawkins RD, Hon GC, Ren B. Next-generation genomics: an integrative approach. *Nat Rev Genet* 2010;11:476–486. doi:10.1038/nrg2795.
2. The White House, Office of the Press Secretary. *Fact Sheet: President Obama's Precision Medicine Initiative.* https://www.whitehouse.gov/the-press-office/2015/01/30/fact-sheet-president-obama-s-precision-medicine-initiative. Accessed January 30, 2015.
3. Fradkin JE, Hanlon MC, Rodgers GP. NIH precision medicine initiative: implications for diabetes research. *Diabetes Care* 2016;39:1080–1084. doi:10.2337/dc16-0541.
4. Wang X, Ward PA. Opportunities and challenges of disease biomarkers: a new section in the Journal of Translational Medicine. *J Transl Med* 2012;10:240. doi:10.1186/1479-5876-10-240.
5. Hood L. Systems biology and p4 medicine: past, present, and future. *Rambam Maimonides Med J* 2013;4:e0012. doi:10.5041/rmmj.10112.
6. Cooke CR, Erickson SE, Watkins TR, Matthay, MA, Hudson LD, Rubenfeld GD, Age-, sex-, and race-based differences among patients enrolled versus not enrolled in acute lung injury clinical trials. *Crit Care Med* 2010;38:1450–1457. doi:10.1097/CCM.0b013e3181de451b.
7. Casanova N, Zhou, T, Knox KS, Garcia JG. Identifying novel biomarkers in sarcoidosis using genome-based approaches. *Clin Chest Med* 2015;36:621–630. doi:10.1016/j.ccm.2015.08.005.
8. Sealfon SC, Chu TT. RNA and DNA microarrays. *Methods Mol Biol* 2011;671:3–34. doi:10.1007/978-1-59745-551-0_1.
9. Chang JT, et al. SIGNATURE: a workbench for gene expression signature analysis. *BMC Bioinformatics* 2011;12:443. doi:10.1186/1471-2105-12-443.
10. Wen Q, Kim CS, Hamilton PW, Zhang SD. A gene-signature progression approach to identifying candidate small-molecule cancer therapeutics with connectivity mapping. *BMC Bioinformatics* 2016;17:211. doi:10.1186/s12859-016-1066-x.
11. Bime C, et al. Reactive oxygen species-associated molecular signature predicts survival in patients with sepsis. *Pulm Circ* 2016;6:196–201. doi:10.1086/685547.
12. Akahoshi M, et al. Association between IFNA genotype and the risk of sarcoidosis. *Hum Genet* 2004;114:503–509.
13. Zhou T, et al. GSE37912: Peripheral blood gene expression as a novel genomic biomarker in complicated sarcoidosis. *Gene Expression Omnibus* 2012. https://www.ncbi.nlm.nih.gov/geo/query/acc.cgi?acc=GSE37912

14. Zhou T, et al. Peripheral blood gene expression as a novel genomic biomarker in complicated sarcoidosis. *PLoS One* 2012;7:e44818. doi:10.1371/journal.pone.0044818.

15. Desai AA, et al. A novel molecular signature for elevated tricuspid regurgitation velocity in sickle cell disease. *Am J Respir Crit Care Med* 2012;186:359–368. doi:10.1164/rccm.201201-0057OC.

16. Singla S, et al. Expression profiling elucidates a molecular signature for pulmonary hypertension in sarcoidosis. *Pulm Circ NA* 2016;6:465–471. doi:0.1086/688316.

17. Simon R, Wang SJ. Use of genomic signatures in therapeutics development in oncology and other diseases. *Pharmacogenomics* 2006;6:166–173. doi:10.1038/sj.tpj.6500349.

18. Littarru GP, Langsjoen P. Coenzyme Q10 and statins: biochemical and clinical implications. *Mitochondrion* 2007;7 Suppl:S168–S174. doi:10.1016/j.mito.2007.03.002.

19. Oh J, Ban MR, Miskie BA, Pollex RL, Hegele RA. Genetic determinants of statin intolerance. *Lipids Health Dis* 2007;6:7. doi:10.1186/1476-511X-6-7.

20. Vladutiu GD. Genetic predisposition to statin myopathy. *Curr Opin Rheumatol* 2008;20:648–655. doi:10.1097/BOR.0b013e328314b7b4.

21. Ashley EA. The precision medicine initiative: a new national effort. *JAMA* 2015;313:2119–2120. doi:10.1001/jama.2015.3595.

22. Li L, Somerset S. The clinical significance of the gut microbiota in cystic fibrosis and the potential for dietary therapies. *Clin Nutr* 2014;33:571–580. doi:10.1016/j.clnu.2014.04.004.

23. Hanahan D, Weinberg RA. Hallmarks of cancer: the next generation. *Cell* 2011;144:646–674. doi:10.1016/j.cell.2011.02.013.

24. Zugazagoitia J, et al. Current challenges in cancer treatment. *Clin Ther* 2016;38:1551–1566. doi:10.1016/j.clinthera.2016.03.026.

25. Herceg Z. Epigenetic mechanisms as an interface between the environment and genome. *Adv Exp Med Biol* 2016;903:3–15. doi:10.1007/978-1-4899-7678-9_1.

26. Marx V. Biology: the big challenges of big data. *Nature* 2013;498:255–260. doi:10.1038/498255a.

27. Lamprecht SA, Lipkin M. Chemoprevention of colon cancer by calcium, vitamin D and folate: molecular mechanisms. *Nat Rev Cancer* 2003;3:601–614. doi:10.1038/nrc1144.

28. Razin A, Riggs AD. DNA methylation and gene function. *Science* 1980;210:604–610.

29. Miller CA, Sweatt JD. Covalent modification of DNA regulates memory formation. *Neuron* 2007;53:857–869. doi:10.1016/j.neuron.2007.02.022.

30. Silva FP, et al. Enhanced methyltransferase activity of SMYD3 by the cleavage of its N-terminal region in human cancer cells. *Oncogene* 2008;27:2686–2692. doi:10.1038/sj.onc.1210929.

31. Lyko F, et al. The honey bee epigenomes: differential methylation of brain DNA in queens and workers. *PLoS Biol* 2010;8:e1000506. doi:10.1371/journal.pbio.1000506.

32. Mastroeni D, et al. Epigenetic changes in Alzheimer's disease: decrements in DNA methylation. *Neurobiol Aging* 2010;31:2025–2037. doi:10.1016/j.neurobiolaging.2008.12.005.

33. Davis CD, Uthus EO. DNA methylation, cancer susceptibility, and nutrient interactions. *Exp Biol Med (Maywood)* 2004;229:988–995.

34. Johansson A, Enroth S, Gyllensten U. Continuous aging of the human DNA methylome throughout the human lifespan. *PLoS One* 2013;8:e67378. doi:10.1371/journal.pone.0067378.

35. Ogino S, et al. LINE-1 hypomethylation is inversely associated with microsatellite instability and CpG island methylator phenotype in colorectal cancer. *Int J Cancer* 2008;122:2767–2773. doi:10.1002/ijc.23470.

36. Bae JM, et al. ALU and LINE-1 hypomethylations in multistep gastric carcinogenesis and their prognostic implications. *Int J Cancer* 2012;131:1323–1331. doi:10.1002/ijc.27369.

37. Hoshimoto S, et al. AIM1 and LINE-1 epigenetic aberrations in tumor and serum relate to melanoma progression and disease outcome. *J Invest Dermatol* 2012;132:1689–1697. doi:10.1038/jid.2012.36.

38. Pattamadilok J, et al. LINE-1 hypomethylation level as a potential prognostic factor for epithelial ovarian cancer. *Int J Gynecol Cancer* 2008;18:711–717. doi:10.1111/j.1525-1438.2007.01117.x.

39 Sunami E, de Maat, M, Vu A, Turner RR, Hoon DS. LINE-1 hypomethylation during primary colon cancer progression. *PLoS One* 2011;6:e18884. doi:10.1371/journal.pone.0018884.

40. Ogino S, et al. Molecular pathological epidemiology of epigenetics: emerging integrative science to analyze environment, host, and disease. *Mod Pathol* 2013;26:465–484. doi:10.1038/modpathol.2012.214.

41. Schernhammer ES, et al. Dietary folate, alcohol and B vitamins in relation to LINE-1 hypomethylation in colon cancer. *Gut* 2010;59:794–799. doi:10.1136/gut.2009.183707.

42. Delage B, Dashwood RH. Dietary manipulation of histone structure and function. *Annu Rev Nutr* 2008;28:347–366. doi:10.1146/annurev.nutr.28.061807.155354.

43. Marmorstein R, Roth SY. Histone acetyltransferases: function, structure, and catalysis. *Curr Opin Genet Dev* 2001;11:155–161.

44. Lardenoije R, et al. The epigenetics of aging and neurodegeneration. *Prog Neurobiol* 2015;131:21–64. doi:10.1016/j.pneurobio.2015.05.002.

45. Su X, Wellen KE, Rabinowitz JD. Metabolic control of methylation and acetylation. *Curr Opin Chem Biol* 2016;30:52–60. doi:10.1016/j.cbpa.2015.10.030.

46. Shimazu T, et al. Suppression of oxidative stress by beta-hydroxybutyrate, an endogenous histone deacetylase inhibitor. *Science* 2013;339:211–214. doi:10.1126/science.1227166.

47. Kim DY, et al. Ketone bodies are protective against oxidative stress in neocortical neurons. *J Neurochem* 2007;101:1316–1326. doi:10.1111/j.1471-4159.2007.04483.x.

48. Bauer M, et al. Tobacco smoking differently influences cell types of the innate and adaptive immune system-indications from CpG site methylation. *Clin Epigenetics* 2015;7:83. doi:10.1186/s13148-016-0249-7.

49. Gao X, Jia M, Zhang Y, Breitling LP, Brenner H. DNA methylation changes of whole blood cells in response to active smoking exposure in adults: a systematic review of DNA methylation studies. *Clin Epigenetics* 2015;7:113. doi:10.1186/s13148-015-0148-3.

50. Adams M., Jewell AP. The use of complementary and alternative medicine by cancer patients. *Int Semin Surg Oncol* 2007;4:10. doi:10.1186/1477-7800-4-10.

51. Chang EY, Glissmeyer M, Tonnes S, Hudson T, Johnson N. Outcomes of breast cancer in patients who use alternative therapies as primary treatment. *Am J Surg* 1997;192:471–473. doi:10.1016/j.amjsurg.2006.05.013x.

52. Jang M, et al. Cancer chemopreventive activity of resveratrol, a natural product derived from grapes. *Science* 1997;275:218–220.

53. Shakibaei M, Harikumar KB, Aggarwal BB. Resveratrol addiction: to die or not to die. *Mol Nutr Food Res* 2009;53:115–128. doi:10.1002/mnfr.200800148.

54. Signorelli P, Ghidoni R. Resveratrol as an anticancer nutrient: molecular basis, open questions and promises. *J Nutr Biochem* 2005;16:449–466. doi:10.1016/j.jnutbio.2005.01.017.

55. Thakur VS, Deb, G, Babcook MA, Gupta S. Plant phytochemicals as epigenetic modulators: role in cancer chemoprevention. *AAPS J* 2014;16:151–163. doi:10.1208/s12248-013-9548-5.

56. Banerjee S, Li Y, Wang Z, Sarkar FH. Multi-targeted therapy of cancer by genistein. *Cancer Lett* 2008;269:226–242. doi:10.1016/j.canlet.2008.03.052.

57. Chen Y, et al. Curcumin, both histone deacetylase and p300/CBP-specific inhibitor, represses the activity of nuclear factor kappa B and Notch 1 in Raji cells. *Basic Clin Pharmacol Toxicol* 2007;101:427–433. doi:10.1111/j.1742-7843.2007.00142.x.

58. Greene WC, Chen LF. Regulation of NF-kappaB action by reversible acetylation. *Novartis Found Symp* 2004;259:208–217; discussion 218–225.

59. Druesne N, et al. Diallyl disulfide (DADS) increases histone acetylation and p21(waf1/cip1) expression in human colon tumor cell lines. *Carcinogenesis* 2004;25:1227–1236. doi:10.1093/carcin/bgh123.

60. Ariga T, Seki T. Antithrombotic and anticancer effects of garlic-derived sulfur compounds: a review. *Biofactors* 2006;26:93–103.

61. Tili E, et al. Resveratrol modulates the levels of microRNAs targeting genes encoding tumor-suppressors and effectors of TGFbeta signaling pathway in SW480 cells. *Biochem Pharmacol* 2010;80:2057–2065. doi:10.1016/j.bcp.2010.07.003.

62. Papoutsis AJ, Lamore SD, Wondrak GT, Selmin OI, Romagnolo DF. Resveratrol prevents epigenetic silencing of BRCA-1 by the aromatic hydrocarbon receptor in human breast cancer cells. *J Nutr* 2010;140:1607–1614. doi:10.3945/jn.110.123422.

63. Marcu MG, et al. Curcumin is an inhibitor of p300 histone acetylatransferase. *Med Chem* 2006;2:169–174.

64. Fix LN, Shah M, Efferth T, Farwell MA, Zhang B. MicroRNA expression profile of MCF-7 human breast cancer cells and the effect of green tea polyphenon-60. *Cancer Genom Proteom* 2010;7:261–277.

65. Traka M, et al. Transcriptome analysis of human colon Caco-2 cells exposed to sulforaphane. *J Nutr* 2005;135:1865–1872.

66. Clarke JD, Dashwood RH, Ho E. Multi-targeted prevention of cancer by sulforaphane. *Cancer Lett* 2008;269:291–304. doi:10.1016/j.canlet.2008.04.018.

67. Seki T, et al. Anticancer effects of diallyl trisulfide derived from garlic. *Asia Pac J Clin Nutr* 2008;17 Suppl 1:249–252.

68. Song EA, Kim H. Docosahexaenoic acid induces oxidative DNA damage and apoptosis, and enhances the chemosensitivity of cancer cells. *Int J Mol Sci* 2016;17:1–10. doi:10.3390/ijms17081257.

69. Panagiotakos DB, et al. Exploring the path of Mediterranean diet on 10-year incidence of cardiovascular disease: the ATTICA study (2002-2012). *Nutr Metab Cardiovasc Dis* 2015;25:327–335. doi:10.1016/j.numecd.2014.09.006.

70. Sofi F, Cesari F, Abbate R, Gensini GF, Casini A. Adherence to Mediterranean diet and health status: meta-analysis. *BMJ* 2008;337:a1344. doi:10.1136/bmj.a1344.

71. Zecri FJ. From natural product to the first oral treatment for multiple sclerosis: the discovery of FTY720 (Gilenya)? *Curr Opin Chem Biol* 2016;32:60–66. doi:10.1016/j.cbpa.2016.04.014.

72. Fujitac T, et al. Simple compounds, 2-alkyl-2-amino-1,3-propanediols have potent immunosuppressive activity. *Bioorg Med Chem* 1995;Lett 5:6.

73. Natarajan V, et al. Sphingosine-1-phosphate, FTY720, and sphingosine-1-phosphate receptors in the pathobiology of acute lung injury. *Am J Respir Cell Mol Biol* 2013;49:6–17. doi:10.1165/rcmb.2012-0411TR.

74. Wang L, et al. FTY720 (s)-phosphonate preserves sphingosine 1-phosphate receptor 1 expression and exhibits superior barrier protection to FTY720 in acute lung injury. *Crit Care Med* 2014;42:e189–e199. doi:10.1097/CCM.0000000000000097.

75. Billich A, et al. Phosphorylation of the immunomodulatory drug FTY720 by sphingosine kinases. *J Biol Chem* 2003;278:47408–47415. doi:10.1074/jbc.M307687200.

76. Chun J., Hartung HP. Mechanism of action of oral fingolimod (FTY720) in multiple sclerosis. *Clin Neuropharmacol* 2010;33:91–101. doi:10.1097/WNF.0b013e3181cbf825.

77. Chiba K. [A new therapeutic approach for autoimmune diseases by the sphingosine 1-phosphate receptor modulator, fingolimod (FTY720)]. *Nihon Rinsho Meneki Gakkai Kaishi* 2009;32:92–101.

78. Erdener SE, Nurlu G, Gocmen R, Erdem-Ozdamar S, Kurne A. Remission with fingolimod in a case of demyelinating polyneuropathy. *Muscle Nerve* 2014;50:615–617. doi:10.1002/mus.24311.

79. Obinata H, et al. Individual variation of human S1P(1) coding sequence leads to heterogeneity in receptor function and drug interactions. *J Lipid Res* 2014;55:2665–2675. doi:10.1194/jlr.P054163.

80. Sun X, et al. Functional promoter variants in sphingosine 1-phosphate receptor 3 associate with susceptibility to sepsis-associated acute respiratory distress syndrome. *Am J Physiol Lung Cell Mol Physiol* 2013;305L467–L477. doi:10.1152/ajplung.00010.2013.

81. Guandalini S. Probiotics for prevention and treatment of diarrhea. *J Clin Gastroenterol* 2011;45 Suppl:S149–S153. doi:10.1097/MCG.0b013e3182257e98.

82. Floch MH, et al. Recommendations for probiotic use-2011 update. *J Clin Gastroenterol* 2011;45 Suppl, S168–S171. doi:10.1097/MCG.0b013e318230928b.

83. McFarland LV. From yaks to yogurt: the history, development, and current use of probiotics. *Clin Infect Dis* 2015;60 Suppl 2:S85–S90. doi:10.1093/cid/civ054.

84. Hsieh HY, Chiu PH, Wang SC. Epigenetics in traditional Chinese pharmacy: a bio-informatic study at pharmacopoeia scale. *Evid Based Complement Alternat Med* 2011;2011:816714. doi:10.1093/ecam/neq050.

85. Lu B, Sheng Y, Zhang J, Zheng Z, Ji L. The altered microRNA profile in andrographolide-induced inhibition of hepatoma tumor growth. *Gene* 2016;588:124–133. doi:10.1016/j.gene.2016.05.012.

86. Pan LT, Sheung Y, Guo WP, Rong ZB, Cai ZM. Hedyotis diffusa plus Scutellaria barbata induce bladder cancer cell apoptosis by inhibiting Akt signaling pathway through downregulating miR-155 Expression. *Evid Based Complement Alternat Med* 2016;2016:9174903. doi:10.1155/2016/9174903.

87. Wei K, et al. Herb-Partitioned Moxibustion and the miRNAs Related to Crohn's Disease: A Study Based on Rat Models. *Evid Based Complement Alternat Med* 2015;2015:265238. doi:10.1155/2015/265238.

88. Wang Y, et al. Downregulated RASD1 and upregulated miR-375 are involved in protective effects of calycosin on cerebral ischemia/reperfusion rats. *J Neurol Sci* 2014;339:144–148. doi:10.1016/j.jns.2014.02.002.

89. Zhao HL, et al. Sustained antidiabetic effects of a berberine-containing Chinese herbal medicine through regulation of hepatic gene expression. *Diabetes* 2012;61:933–943. doi:10.2337/db11-1164.

90. Zhang L, et al. Tanshinone IIA improves miR-133 expression through MAPK ERK1/2 pathway in hypoxic cardiac myocytes. *Cell Physiol Biochem* 2012;30:843-852. doi:10.1159/000341462.

91. Gong Y, Li Y, Abdolmaleky HM, Li L, Zhou JR. Tanshinones inhibit the growth of breast cancer cells through epigenetic modification of Aurora A expression and function. *PLoS One* 2012;7:e33656. doi:10.1371/journal.pone.0033656.

92. Xiong J, et al. Male germ cell apoptosis and epigenetic histone modification induced by Tripterygium wilfordii Hook F. *PLoS One* 2011;6:e20751. doi:10.1371/journal.pone.0020751.

93. Wen L, et al. Triptolide induces cell apoptosis by targeting H3K4me3 and down-stream effector proteins in KM3 multiple myeloma cells. *Curr Pharm Biotechnol* 2015;17:147–160.

94. Zhao F, et al. Role of triptolide in cell proliferation, cell cycle arrest, apoptosis and histone methylation in multiple myeloma U266 cells. *Eur J Pharmacol* 2010;646:1–11. doi:10.1016/j.ejphar.2010.05.034.

95. Wang QY, et al. A preliminary study on epigenetic regulation of Acanthopanax senticosus in leukemia cell lines. *Exp Hematol* 2016;44:466–473. doi:10.1016/j.exphem.2016.03.002.

96. Huang Y, et al. Trichosanthin inhibits DNA methyltransferase and restores methylation-silenced gene expression in human cervical cancer cells. *Mol Med Rep* 2012;6:872–878. doi:10.3892/mmr.2012.994.

97. Su ZY, et al. Epigenetic reactivation of Nrf2 in murine prostate cancer TRAMP C1 cells by natural phytochemicals Z-ligustilide and Radix angelica sinensis via promoter CpG demethylation. *Chem Res Toxicol* 2013;26:477–485. doi:10.1021/tx300524p.

98. Lin D, Lin LL, Sutherland K, Cao CH. Manual acupuncture at the SJ5 (Waiguan) acupoint shows neuroprotective effects by regulating expression of the anti-apoptotic gene Bcl-2. *Neural Regen Res* 2016;11:305–311. doi:10.4103/1673-5374.177740.

99. Chen J, et al. Acupuncture at Waiguan (TE5) influences activation/deactivation of functional brain areas in ischemic stroke patients and healthy people: a functional MRI study. *Neural Regen Res* 2013;8:226–232. doi:10.3969/j.issn.1673-5374.2013.03.004.

100. Liu ET, et al. [Effect of needling at waiguan (SJ5) on brain glucose metabolism in patients with cerebral infarction]. *Zhongguo Zhong Xi Yi Jie He Za Zhi* 2013;33:1345–1351.

101. Khoury MJ, Gwinn ML, Glasgow RE, Kramer BS. A population approach to precision medicine. *Am J Prev Med* 2012;42:639–645. doi:10.1016/j.amepre.2012.02.012.

102. Khoury MJ, Gwinn M, Bowen MS, Dotson WD. Beyond base pairs to bedside: a population perspective on how genomics can improve health. *Am J Public Health* 2012;102:34–37. doi:10.2105/AJPH.2011.300299.

103. Alyass A, Turcotte M, Meyre D. From big data analysis to personalized medicine for all: challenges and opportunities. *BMC Med Genomics* 2015;8:33. doi:10.1186/s12920-015-0108-y.

104. Nherera L, Marks D, Minhas R, Thorogood M., Humphries SE. Probabilistic cost-effectiveness analysis of cascade screening for familial hypercholesterolaemia using alternative diagnostic and identification strategies. *Heart* 2011;97:1175–1181. doi:10.1136/hrt.2010.213975.

105. Moyer VA; US Preventive Services Task Force. Risk assessment, genetic counseling, and genetic testing for BRCA-related cancer in women: U.S. Preventive Services Task Force recommendation statement. *Ann Intern Med* 2014;160:271–281. doi:10.7326/M13-2747.

106. McCarthy AM, Armstrong K. The role of testing for BRCA1 and BRCA2 mutations in cancer prevention. *JAMA Intern Med* 2014;174:1023–1024. doi:10.1001/jamainternmed.2014.1322.

107. Jewish Genetic Diseases Consortium. http://www.jewishgeneticdiseases.org/jewish-genetic-diseases/ (NA).

108. Ginsburg GS, Willard HF. Genomic and personalized medicine: foundations and applications. *Transl Res* 2009;154:277–287. doi:10.1016/j.trsl.2009.09.005.

5

The Concept of Mindfulness in Integrative Preventive Medicine

KIM AIKENS AND SHAUNA SHAPIRO

The widespread clinical applications of mindfulness are based on a few general principles whose simplicity and power have sparked a literature examining the integration of mindfulness into psychology and medicine. Our intention is to explore the applications of mindfulness, specifically within an integrative preventive medicine context. Our goal is to demonstrate that the multidimensional nature of mindfulness has far-reaching applications for prevention in healthcare.

And yet, if mindfulness is to be integrated into Western medicine, we must find ways of translating its nonconceptual, nondual and paradoxical nature into a language that physicians, patients, scientists, scholars—all of us—can understand and agree on. Although the concept of mindfulness is most often associated with Buddhism, its phenomenological nature is embedded in most religious and spiritual traditions, as well as Western philosophical and psychological schools of thought.[1] And yet more importantly, mindfulness is a universal human capacity that transcends culture and religion.

"Mindfulness" is the English translation of the Pali word *Sati* combined with *Sampajañña*, which as a whole can be translated as "awareness, circumspection, discernment, and retention." Bhikku Bodhi, Theravadan scholar and monk, integrates these multiple definitions of mindfulness as meaning to remember to pay attention to what is occurring in one's immediate experience with care and discernment.[2]

We define mindfulness as the awareness that arises through intentionally attending in an open, caring, and discerning way.[3]

Mindfulness comprises three core elements: intention, attention, and attitude.[4] Intention, attention, and attitude are not separate processes or

Box 5.1 Attitude

Nonjudging: impartial witnessing, observing the present moment without evaluation and categorization.[2]

Nonstriving: non-goal-oriented, remaining unattached to outcome or achievement.

Nonattachment: letting go of grasping and clinging to outcome, and allowing the process to simply unfold.

Acceptance: seeing and acknowledging things as they are in the present moment.

Patience: allowing things to unfold in their time.

Trust: developing a basic trust in your experience.

Openness (Beginner's Mind): seeing things freshly, as if for the first time

Curiosity: A spirit of interest, investigation, and exploration.

Letting go: nonattachment, not holding on to thoughts, feelings, experience.

Gentleness: a soft, considerate, and tender quality; however not passive, undisciplined, or indulgent.

Nonreactivity: ability to respond with consciousness and clarity instead of automatically reacting in a habitual, conditioned way.

Lovingkindness: a quality embodying friendliness, benevolence, and love.

stages—they are interwoven aspects of a single cyclic *process* and occur simultaneously, the three elements informing and feeding back into each other (see Box 5.1). Mindful practice *is* this moment-to-moment process.

Intention

Intention is simply knowing why we are practicing mindfulness meditation, what is our aspiration and motivation for practice. When Western psychology attempted to extract the essence of mindful practice from its original religious/cultural roots, to some extent we lost the aspect of the *intention* of the practice, which for Buddhism was freedom from suffering for oneself and all beings. While this was a logical attempt at ethical neutrality on the part of the original Western interpreters; the concept of intention continues to be overlooked in some contemporary definitions.[5] However intention (i.e., *why* one is practicing) is highlighted in Buddhist teachings as a central component of mindfulness and thus considered crucial to understanding the process as a whole.

In order to understand mindful practice accurately and deeply, it is essential to explicitly reincorporate the aspect of intention.[6] As Kabat-Zinn writes, "Your intentions set the stage for what is possible. They remind you from moment to moment of why you are practicing in the first place."[7(P32)] He continues, "I used to think that meditation practice was so powerful . . . that as long as you did it at all, you would see growth and change. But time has taught me that some kind of personal vision is also necessary."[7 (P46)] This personal vision, or intention, is often dynamic and evolving. For example, a therapist may begin a mindful practice to decrease her own stress. As her mindful practice continues, she may develop an additional intention of relating to patients in a more empathic, present way.

The role of intention in meditation practice is exemplified by Shapiro's study,[8] which explored the intentions of meditation practitioners and found that as meditators continued to practice, their intentions shifted along a continuum from self-regulation, to self-exploration, and finally to self-liberation[1]/selfless-service.[8] Further, the study found that outcomes correlated with intentions. Those whose goal was self-regulation and stress management attained self-regulation, those whose goal was self-exploration attained self-exploration, and those whose goal was self-liberation moved toward self-liberation and compassionate service. Similar results were found by Mackenzie, Carlson et al when they interviewed cancer patients who had been practicing meditation for several years.[9] At first, the practice was used to control specific symptoms such as tension and stress, but later on, the focus became more about spirituality and personal growth. These findings correspond with our definition of intentions as dynamic and evolving, which allows them to change and develop with deepening practice, awareness, and insight. As meditation teacher and psychotherapist Jack Kornfield puts it, "Intention is a direction not a destination."

Not only is it important to be clear about one's intentions, it is necessary to reflect on whether they are wholesome or unwholesome, for the benefit or harm of self and others. Value issues are often seen as problematic in Western scientific traditions since modernist theory viewed science as objectively neutral. However, postmodernism and science and technology studies challenge that assumption—there are always values driving behavior. So it's not a question of whether values are operating—in the individual, in the client-therapist interaction, in society—but how and to what extent we can bring these values to consciousness.

Mindful practice helps us (1) bring unconscious/nonconscious values to awareness; (2) decide whether they are really the values we want to pursue—whether they are wholesome, or merely biologically reflexive or culturally conditioned; (3) develop wholesome and skillful values and to decrease unwholesome ones. Intentions should also be differentiated from the concept of "striving" or "grasping" for certain outcomes from meditation practice. Intentions are not seen as goals or outcomes one actively strives toward during each meditation practice. Intentions are not a destination, they are a direction. Our intention sets the compass of our heart in the direction we want to head.

Attention

A second fundamental component of mindfulness is *attention*, observing the operations of one's moment-to-moment, internal and external experience. This is what Husserl refers to as a "return to things themselves," that is, suspending (and/or noting) all the ways of interpreting experience and attending to experience itself, as it presents in the here and now. In this way, one learns to attend not only to the surrounding world but also to the *contents* of one's consciousness, moment by moment.

Attention has been suggested in the field of psychology as critical to the healing process. Mindfulness involves a deep and penetrating attention, not simply grazing the surface. As Bhikku Bodhi notes, "whereas a mind without mindfulness 'floats' on the surface of its object the way a gourd floats on water, mindfulness sinks into its object the way a stone placed on the surface of water sinks to the bottom" (from the *Dhammasangani Malatika*).[2]

Mindful practice involves a dynamic process of learning how to cultivate attention that is discerning and nonreactive, sustained and concentrated, so that we can see clearly what is arising in the present moment (including our emotional reactions, if that's what comes up.) As Germer notes, "An unstable mind is like an unstable camera; we get a fuzzy picture."[10]

Attitude

How we attend is also essential. According to Kabat-Zinn, mindfulness is understood "not just as a bare attention but as an *affectionate* attention."[11] The *qualities* one brings to attention have been referred to as the attitudinal foundations of mindfulness.[6,7,12,13] Siegel (2007) used the acronym COAL to refer to a similar list of qualities: curiosity, openness, acceptance, and love.[13]

Often, the quality of mindful awareness is not explicitly addressed. However, the qualities, or attitude, one brings to the act of paying attention are crucial. For example, attention can have a cold, critical quality, or it can include an open-hearted compassionate quality. It is helpful to note that the Japanese characters for mindfulness are composed of two interactive figures: one is mind, and the other, heart. Therefore, perhaps a more accurate translation of "mindfulness" from the Asian languages is heart-mindfulness, which underlines the importance of including "heart" qualities in the attentional practice of mindfulness.

We posit that, with practice and right effort, persons can learn to attend to their own internal and external experiences, without evaluation or interpretation, and practice acceptance, kindness, and openness even when what is occurring in the field of experience is contrary to deeply held wishes or expectations. This attitudinal dimension of mindfulness must be explicitly introduced as part of the practice.

Attending without bringing the attitudinal qualities into the practice may result in practice that is condemning or judgmental of inner (or outer) experience. Such an approach may well have consequences contrary to the intentions of the practice; for example, cultivating patterns of judgment and striving instead of equanimity and acceptance. The field of neuroplasticity demonstrates that our repeated experiences shape our brain. If we continually practice meditation with a cold, judgmental, and impatient attention, these are the pathways that will get stronger. Our intention instead is to practice with an attitude of open, caring attention.

The attitudinal qualities do not add anything to the experience itself, but rather infuse the container of attention with acceptance, openness, caring, and curiosity. For example, if while practicing mindfulness impatience arises, the impatience is noted with acceptance and kindness. However, these qualities are not meant to be substituted for the impatience or to make the impatience disappear, they are simply the container. These attitudes are an essential part of the mindful practice as Kabat-Zinn states, "The attitude with which you undertake the practice of paying attention . . . is crucial"[(p31)] and "Keeping particular attitudes in mind is actually part of the training itself."[7(p32)] The attitudes are not an attempt to make things be a certain way, they are an attempt to relate to whatever *is* in a certain way.

With intentional training, one becomes increasingly able to take interest in each experience as it arises and also to allow what is being experienced to pass away (i.e., not held onto). By intentionally bringing the attitudes of patience, compassion, and nonstriving to the attentional practice, one relinquishes the habitual tendency of continually striving for pleasant experiences, or of pushing aversive experiences away. Instead, bare awareness of whatever exists in that moment occurs, but within a context of gentleness, kindness, and acceptance.

Mindfulness Meditation, Mindfulness, and Preventive Medicine

Simply put, meditation is about learning to do one thing at a time. It is a practice of concentrated focus on an object such as the breath, sound, a visualization, or physical sensation. Contrary to "zoning out," mindfulness meditation is a way to "zone in" on one's experience. During mindfulness meditation using breath focus, for example, thoughts and emotions may arise, which can be observed with curiosity, in a nonjudgmental way, as part of one's experience in the moment. In this way, mindfulness meditation uses the focus object as a means to harness and train the mind, ultimately leading to greater awareness of mental processes. It involves learning to watch thoughts, feelings, and sensations as they arise and pass, without becoming caught up in them.

The practice of mindfulness meditation helps to cultivate general mindfulness in everyday life. However, mindfulness is much more than a specific meditation technique. Mindfulness refers to one's moment-to-moment awareness, and is more a way of being than a specific practice. It is about being fully present and aware of what you are thinking, feeling, or doing whether you are walking the family dog, talking to a friend or loved one, or doing the dishes. This is mindfulness in action.

Fundamentally, we view mindfulness as a natural human capacity that can be cultivated and strengthened. Seen through this lens, mindfulness can become an important component in integrative preventive medicine since mindfulness has the potential to help prevent illness and increase optimal health.

HEALTH AND PREVENTIVE MEDICINE

Health is difficult to define but important in the light of both mindfulness and preventive medicine. The World Health Organization defines health as the "state of complete physical, mental, and social well-being and not merely the absence of disease or infirmity."[14] Preventive medicine works to improve the lives of individuals by enabling them to enhance their health. The literature suggests that mindfulness can be a crucial adjunct to preventive medicine strategies aimed at improving health and well-being from both a health promotion and disease management standpoint.

Traditionally, preventive medicine has been viewed as enhancing health through strategies targeted at three different levels.[15] Primary prevention seeks to prevent the advent of disease by either eliminating the causes of disease or by increasing disease resistance. Secondary prevention targets early detection and treatment of presymptomatic disease in order to avoid symptom onset. Lastly, tertiary prevention strives to curtail the physical, mental, and social consequences of established symptomatic disease.[16] Goldston describes these levels as "prevention, treatment, and rehabilitation," although the terms "primary," "secondary," and "tertiary" continue to prevail today.[17]

MINDFULNESS-BASED INTERVENTIONS

Research shows that mindfulness skills can be taught and can be beneficial to health.[18,19] Mindfulness-based stress reduction (MBSR) was the first mindfulness-based intervention (MBI) to be introduced in a Western medical setting. Originally developed in 1979 by Jon Kabat-Zinn, MBSR teaches core mindfulness concepts through training in formal mindfulness meditation practices and gentle mindful yoga.[7] In addition, MBSR provides education on the effects of stress on health and well-being. Various adaptations of MBSR have been developed for other conditions, including mindfulness-based cognitive therapy (MBCT) for recurrent depression.[20] In general, MBSR, which primarily focuses on the manifestations of stress, has typically been used for chronic medical conditions such as cancer, chronic pain, heart disease, and fibromyalgia. On the other hand, MBCT focuses on cognition and has been used in the treatment of mental health and eating disorders as well as in burnout. Acceptance and commitment therapy (ACT) is another common mindfulness-based intervention, which teaches mindfulness concepts but lacks instruction in formal meditation practices.[21]

Primary Prevention and Mindfulness

The goal of primary prevention is the reduction of disease incidence through risk factor identification and modification or through the enhancement of disease resistance. Directed at the predisease level, primary prevention includes activities of health promotion, which enhance generalized, nonspecific wellness as well as specific protection, targeted to prevent a specific disease type.[16] Health promotion activities are principally lifestyle focused and geared toward decreasing known risk factors prior to the establishment of the disease process. Examples include healthy nutrition, increased physical activity, smoking cessation, and stress mitigation. In general, the goal of health promotion is to increase well-being while modifying risk factors in order to prevent disease inception. Specific protection, on the other hand, is targeted to a specific disease with the goal of preventing said disease from occurring. Examples include immunization against flu and fluoridation of water to prevent dental caries.

Health Promotion

Health promotion, through healthy lifestyle, nutrition, and environment, is a crucial step toward mitigation of disease.[22] Human behavior regarding health habits is a critical element in health promotion. Modifiable lifestyle behaviors such as cigarette smoking, poor diet, lack of exercise, poor sleep hygiene, and chronic stress strongly contribute to many of the primary causes of death today, both worldwide and in the United States.[23] For example, unhealthy dietary habits and physical inactivity are important modifiable risk factors in the development of cardiovascular disease, the current leading cause of death globally,[24] as well as major contributors to the early development of obesity, metabolic syndrome, type II diabetes, and stroke.[25-27] Promoting sustainable change in these behaviors is a significant public health challenge. In light of this, six health behaviors are currently recommended for overall health promotion:[28]

- Regular physical activity
- Tobacco abstinence
- Stress management
- Limitation of dietary fat, particularly saturated and trans fat
- Consumption of at least five servings of fruits and vegetables daily
- Weight loss (if needed)

Novel approaches to health promotion have significant potential to improve both public and individual health. Mindfulness is one such novel approach that has the potential to yield significant results in the realm of health promotion. The mainstreaming of MBIs reflects the quality and quantity of scientific studies done over recent decades. Of interest to primary prevention are the results of this work as it pertains to health promotion and lifestyle.

MINDFULNESS AND DIET

Good dietary choices are critical to both the maintenance of health and the prevention of disease. The study of mindfulness with regard to dietary intake, although preliminary, shows promise. Dispositional mindfulness, or the basic human capability to be aware and to bring nonjudgmental acceptance to present moment experience, is a basic human trait, which can be innately present at varying levels.[18] A study of morbidly obese adults and diabetics found that those with higher levels of dispositional mindfulness exhibited more restrained and less emotional eating.[29,30] With regard to the effect of MBIs on diet, early research has shown mixed results with some studies remaining inconclusive[31] or showing no effect on the dietary intake of energy, fat, sugar, fruit, or vegetables.[32] Diet has been principally evaluated in studies, which involve MBSR programs. For example, a recent analysis by Salmoirago-Blotcher et al. of 174 participants who completed an MBSR program showed improvement in overall dietary behaviors with reduction in the number of desserts eaten, fast-food meal intake, consumption of sweetened beverages, and use of fats.[33] In addition, a recent randomized controlled trial (RCT) of a Web-based mindfulness program found significant increases in fruit and vegetable intake as well as a decrease in fast food consumption following the mindfulness intervention.[34] Furthermore, a program in MBSR, delivered in conjunction with a vegetable-based dietary intervention, led to decreased saturated fat intake and an increased intake of vegetable protein in men with prostate cancer.[35-37]

MINDFULNESS AND OBESITY

Over the past several decades, the rate of obesity, with its association to chronic disease[38,39] and decreased life expectancy,[40] has increased significantly with 33.9% of US adults considered overweight and 41.5% obese.[41] Consequently, the effect of mindfulness as a primary prevention weight loss strategy is intriguing. Recent research in a large population ($N = 63,628$) has shown that men and women with higher levels of dispositional mindfulness are more physically active and less obese. In this study, overall mindfulness in women was associated with lower odds of being overweight, and to an even greater extent, obese. In men, higher mindfulness was associated with lower odds of obesity only.[42] Further research has shown that dispositional mindfulness may be inversely associated with both obesity and central adiposity,[43] reported serving sizes of energy dense foods,[44] binge eating,[45] and unhealthy eating habits.[46]

Although mindfulness is an inherent trait, research shows that it is modifiable and can be trained.[18,19] Mindfulness-based therapies help to cultivate a nonreactive and nonjudgmental form of awareness in the face of aversive experience, such as stressors, unpleasant thoughts, emotions, and sensations. The development of less reactivity and enhanced self-efficacy, which can result from mindfulness training, may lead to a decreased dependency on the unhealthy behaviors previously used to cope with stress and negative emotion.[47] For example, emotional and stress eating, in addition to food craving and binge eating, are well known obesity-related eating behaviors, which may be impacted by mindfulness training.[48,49] Furthermore, ongoing mindfulness practice may lead to decreased stress and emotional sensitivity, which may help prevent relapse to unhealthy behaviors, thereby helping to support long-term weight maintenance.[47]

Research has evaluated the impact of MBIs on obesity, with weight loss shown in some but not all studies. A review by Katterman et al. that examined only studies in which mindfulness was the primary treatment modality (e.g., MBSR and MBCT), found that effects on weight at postintervention were small and mainly nonsignificant.[49] However, those studies in which weight was the principle outcome, and mindful eating an important interventional component, did report significant weight loss among mindfulness participants.[50-52] A later review, which focused on MBIs for obesity-related eating behaviors, also found efficacy, with 9 out of 10 studies demonstrating either weight loss or weight stabilization with a small effect size (Cohen's $d = .19$).[53] However, this review included studies with and without control groups. The most recent review by Olsen et al. of randomized controlled trials and observational studies, in which weight loss was a primary outcome, found significant decreases in 13 out of 19 mindfulness interventions. However, researchers concluded that methodological weaknesses limited evidence strength.[54] Furthermore, studies using control groups have shown that MBIs positively impact eating behaviors such stress-related eating,[31] diet composition,[33,37] emotional eating,[48] food craving,[55,56] and binge eating.[48] In general, evidence points to a floor effect such that those participants with higher weight, or those who are attempting to lose weight, may have greater benefit from mindfulness interventions.[57]

MINDFULNESS AND PHYSICAL ACTIVITY

Physical activity can have a major impact on healthy lifestyle and is associated with positive health benefits, improved quality of life,[58] happiness,[59] and increased life satisfaction.[60] Epidemiological evidence supports a direct relationship between volume of physical activity and health as well as an inverse relationship to cardiovascular and overall mortality.[61] With regard to mindfulness and physical activity, research is mixed. For example, a study of 441 college women did not show a relationship between dispositional mindfulness and exercise frequency although mindfulness did strongly predict physical health.[46] This is in contrast to studies in which mindfulness was positively associated with physical activity levels, satisfaction and enjoyment of physical activity,[62] exercise maintenance over time,[63] and perception of overall health.[45,62,64]

To date, the effect of MBIs on physical activity has not been extensively researched. Current results have been mixed with some studies showing no increase in activity levels either during or after a mindfulness intervention.[34,65] This is in contrast to research in men with prostate cancer, in which a composite mindfulness training, delivered together with an exercise and dietary intervention, significantly increased physical activity levels at 3 months post training.[36,37,66] In addition, Salmoirago-Blotcher et al. found partial changes in sedentary behavior following MBSR training with increases in participant strength and flexibility scores.[33] Interventions using ACT have also been studied, with three out of four RCTs finding significant positive effects on physical activity outcomes.[67-70]

MINDFULNESS AND SMOKING

Tobacco smoking is a common cause of preventable premature death and is responsible for one out of five deaths in the United States each year.[71] Furthermore, it is estimated that smoking results in a decreased average life expectancy of at least 10 years for smokers as compared to nonsmokers.[72] Although some forms of behavioral smoking cessation therapy have shown efficacy, only approximately 5% to 20% of smokers will remain cigarette free at 6 months following a cessation attempt.[73] Initial research suggests that mindfulness may be linked to improved smoking cessation outcomes. For example, Vidrine et al. found that higher levels of dispositional mindfulness were inversely associated with nicotine dependence and withdrawal severity. In addition, mindfulness was positively associated with self-efficacy in smoking avoidance as well as greater expectation in the ability to control emotion without the assistance of smoking.[74] Furthermore, Hepner et al. found that African American smokers with greater mindfulness had a greater likelihood of abstinence up to 26 weeks post quit.[75] Additional studies have shown the importance of dispositional mindfulness in the reduction of smoking frequency in adolescents.[76]

Mindfulness training has also shown promise as therapy for smoking cessation. A recent literature review by Weiss de Souza et al. examined 13 controlled studies on mindfulness and smoking through April 14, 2014. The majority of studies examined in this review showed positive effects of mindfulness on quit rates when compared with controls despite heterogeneity in methodology.[77] For example, Brewer et al. compared mindfulness training to the American Lung Association's standard Freedom From Smoking (FFS) program and found that mindfulness training resulted in a greater decrease in the number of cigarettes smoked, which was maintained at 17-week follow-up. In addition, mindfulness participants had significantly higher abstinence at 4 months as compared with the FFS group, with rates of 31% versus 6%, respectively.[78] An additional study by Davis et al. in low-income adults also found significantly higher abstinence rates in participants who received mindfulness training plus nicotine replacement (38.7%) versus those who were given quit line counseling plus nicotine replacement (20.6%) at 24 weeks.[79] Phone app[80] or Web-based[81] MBIs have also been found to be effective with smoking abstinence rates for a Web-based intervention group significantly greater than controls at 3-month follow-up.

MINDFULNESS AND STRESS MANAGEMENT

Chronic, long-term stress in daily life can have serious health consequences and is associated with detrimental health behaviors such as alcoholism, smoking, and obesity.[82,83] In addition, exposure to prolonged periods of acute and chronic stress is a risk factor in many disease states including upper respiratory infections,[84] cardiovascular disease,[85-87] stroke,[88] autoimmune disorders,[89,90] and total mortality.[91,92] Stress also leads to an increased risk of mental health problems including depression[93-95] and chronic anxiety.[96] Higher levels of dispositional mindfulness have been found to be associated with better mental health including lower levels of perceived stress, depression, and anxiety.[97-99] In addition, greater mindfulness is strongly associated with greater well-being[100] as well as perceived physical and psychological health.[99] Research suggests that the buffering effect of mindfulness against the negative effect of stress on mental health is cross-generational, and has been found in an adolescent population[101] as well as in young adults and the elderly.[102]

With regard to the impact of mindfulness training, MBSR programs, in particular, have shown strong potential for increasing well-being and decreasing stress-related complaints. A recent review of studies from 2009–2014 found positive changes in stress-related psychological or physiological measures in 15 out of 17 studies, while two studies had mixed results. However, only two studies out of the 15 with positive changes used randomized control designs. Despite study limitations, this review concluded that MBSR is a promising intervention for stress reduction in a healthy population.[103] This echoed the 2009 review findings by Cheisa et al, who found similar positive results regarding the efficacy of MBSR on stress.[104]

MINDFULNESS AND CARDIOVASCULAR DISEASE RISK

Individuals with good cardiovascular health have healthy levels of seven known cardiovascular risk factors, including blood pressure, total cholesterol, fasting glucose, body mass index, smoking, diet, and physical activity.[105] Preliminary research shows that dispositional mindfulness, principally through its association with BMI, smoking, fasting glucose, and physical activity, is positively associated with good cardiovascular health. For example, a study of 382 individuals found that those with high versus low dispositional mindfulness had an 86% higher likelihood of having good cardiovascular health. In this study, sense of control and depressive symptomatology were potential mediating mechanisms.[106] It has been suggested that more mindful individuals have greater awareness and pay more attention to their behavior, which results in improved capability to initiate or prevent the behavior.[18,107] The net result may be an increased capability of maintaining healthy lifestyle behaviors. In addition, both mindfulness interventions and dispositional mindfulness are related to positive affect including lower levels of anxiety and depression.[97,108] Depression is an independent risk for pathophysiologic progression of cardiovascular disease (CVD) and is associated with an increased incidence of cardiovascular morbidity and mortality.[109] Furthermore, depressed patients may be less likely to adhere to heart healthy behaviors, such as smoking cessation and dietary changes, leading to further increases in CVD risk.[110] Consequently, the positive impact of mindfulness on depression may be a significant factor in decreasing CVD risk.

Research on the effect of MBIs on CVD risk is currently in a nascent phase with mixed results and general tendency to poor methodology and small sample size.[47] Overall, however, intervention studies regarding the association of mindfulness with CVD health appear promising, particularly in regard to smoking, blood pressure, obesity, diabetes, diet, and physical activity. Loucks at al. propose that mindfulness exerts its effect on CVD health through three different pathways: (1) attention control, which allows increased ability to hold attention to physical sensation related to CVD risk—for example, smoking, overeating; (2) emotional regulation with reduced stress response and ability to manage cravings; and (3) heightened awareness of physical sensation, thoughts, and emotions.[57]

Secondary Prevention and Mindfulness

Secondary prevention includes activities such as screening, case finding, and appropriate treatment in order to keep disease from becoming symptomatic.[22] Mindfulness interventions have the potential to enhance secondary prevention, particularly in diseases with strong lifestyle or mental health components.

MINDFULNESS AND BLOOD PRESSURE

A mindfulness program as potential treatment for a patient with presymptomatic hypertension is an example of mindfulness training as a secondary prevention strategy. The research is promising, although not definitive, for mindfulness training as an adjunct in hypertension therapy. A recent review and meta-analysis of four randomized controlled trials of mindfulness-based interventions for hypertension found significant, although moderate, effects for Systolic Blood Pressure (Standardized Mean Difference – 0.78, p = .03) and Diastolic Blood Pressure (Standardized Mean Difference - 067, p = .03).[111] However, the studies included in this analysis showed high heterogeneity and included participants with unmedicated prehypertension,[112] unmedicated grade 1 hypertension,[113] a combination of unmedicated grade 1 and 2 hypertension,[114] and participants at high risk for diabetic complications.[115] Further analysis excluding the RCT by de la Fuente et al. in which effect sizes were significantly higher, resulted in no significance for either SPB or DBP, although intervention was still favored.[111] The difference in effect sizes between these studies may pertain to floor effects, in which those participants with the highest blood pressure (unmedicated stage 1 or 2 hypertension) showed the greatest response to intervention, possibly indicating that mindfulness training may be most beneficial to those with the highest baseline blood pressure.[111] Consequently, although promising, mindfulness training as a secondary treatment strategy for asymptomatic hypertension requires further rigorous methodological research.[116]

MINDFULNESS, DIABETES, AND GLUCOSE REGULATION

Several studies have evaluated the effect of mindfulness training in the treatment of diabetes. To date, studies that used standard mindfulness training programs, such as MBSR[115] and MBCT,[117,118] have not influenced glucose regulation. However, interventions that provided mindfulness training, in addition to education regarding diet, physical activity, glucose monitoring, and medication usage, significantly improved glucose regulation, with resultant reductions in HbA-1C and fasting glucose.[119,120]

Tertiary Prevention and Mindfulness

The goal of tertiary prevention is to curtail the physical, psychological, and social damage that is the consequence of chronic symptomatic disease. Tertiary prevention consists of two components; disability limitation with specific treatment to limit damage from or progression of disease and rehabilitation.[22] Typically, there is no cure for the illnesses in which tertiary prevention is applicable and symptoms of stress, depression, and anxiety are common. Consequently, mindfulness has gained in popularity as an adjunct therapy in chronic care and is particularly applicable to the rehabilitation component of tertiary prevention.

MINDFULNESS AND CHRONIC PAIN

A meta-analysis by Veehof et al. in 2010, which included 22 studies (nine randomized controlled trials (RCT), five controlled clinical trials (CCT), five non-controlled) of mindfulness in chronic pain, showed small but significant effects for pain intensity, depression, anxiety, physical well-being, and quality of life in mindfulness participants. When analysis was restricted to the nine RCTs, small but significant effects were found for pain intensity and depression. This review concluded that mindfulness therapies, including MBSR and ACT, had small to moderate effects that were comparable to cognitive-behavioral therapy (CBT) on physical and mental health in chronic pain patients.[121] A review of fibromyalgia patients also found significant improvements in quality of life and depression as a result of MBSR.[122] However, a meta-analysis for low back pain did not show significant improvements in pain or disability when compared to a program in health education.[123]

MINDFULNESS AND CARDIOVASCULAR DISEASE

The effectiveness of MBSR and MBCT in individuals with cardiovascular disease was analyzed in a review by Abbott et al., which included 9 RCTs and 578 participants. Overall, evidence was found for significant decreases in stress, anxiety, and depression with medium effect sizes.[111]

MINDFULNESS AND CANCER

An overview of systematic reviews with meta-analysis of 12 mindfulness RCTs in cancer patients found significant changes in psychological health but not in physical health. Significant improvements were consistently found for depression, anxiety, quality of life, and stress, with a dose response between enhanced mood and meditation time. In addition, participants who attended more mindfulness training sessions showed greater reduction in stress levels.[124]

MINDFULNESS AND DEPRESSION

A review and meta-analysis by Cheisa et al. of MBCT in mental health disorders, suggested that MBCT plus treatment as usual (TAU) has an additive effect when compared to TAU alone in major depressive disorder (MDD). Analysis showed that MBCT plus TAU resulted in a significant reduction in relapse rates occurring over 1 year in patients with three or more major depressive episodes. Findings also suggested that MBCT, when combined with the gradual discontinuation of antidepressants, was similar to antidepressant continuation for prevention of depression relapse over 1 year. Kuyken et al., who randomized 424 recurrently depressed patients to either MBCT with antidepressant discontinuation or antidepressant maintenance over 2 years, echoed these findings. Rates of relapse/recurrence over the study period indicated no difference between conditions, suggesting that MBCT provided relapse protection on par with maintenance antidepressant pharmacotherapy.[125] In addition, a meta-analysis by Piet et al. found that, in the subgroup of participants with three or more depressive episodes, the relapse rate for MBCT treated patients was 36% as compared to 63% for controls, with an associated risk reduction ratio of 43% in favor of MBCT. This study concluded that that MBCT is an effective intervention for relapse prevention in individuals with major MDD in remission.[126]

MINDFULNESS, CHRONIC DISEASE, AND PSYCHOLOGICAL DISTRESS

As previously stated, the goal of tertiary prevention is to curtail not only the physical consequences of chronic disease but also the psychological and social damage. Unsurprisingly, higher levels of psychological distress are more common in patients with chronic disease. This is illustrated by a study done in Australia, which examined clients in a community health services program. This study found that 20% of patients with chronic disease reported very high levels of psychological distress[127] as compared to only 2.4% of the general population.[128] In general, chronic disease places a significant psychological adjustment burden on the patient. Some individuals adjust well to this ongoing challenge, while others encounter serious decline from an emotional and interpersonal standpoint. Adjustment is a multifaceted and often difficult process. Stanton et al. has conceptualized this adjustment as consisting of five different constructs: (1) absence of psychological disorder, (2) low negative affect, (3) maintenance of functional status, (4) learning and mastery of disease-specific tasks, and (5) perceived quality of life.[129] In addition, the presence or absence of associated depression is significant, as depression has been shown to adversely effect functional status[130] while increasing the risk of noncompliance with medical regimens in chronic disease patients.[131] Furthermore, maintenance of positive mood, and an ongoing sense of meaning and purpose in life, have been shown to be positive indicators of adjustment.[129] The mindfulness literature suggests that mindfulness-based interventions can significantly enhance overall adjustment to chronic disease through their positive effects on stress coping, depression, anxiety, mood, and quality of life. These interventions may work through multiple mechanisms of action. For example, they may work through enhancement of self-regulation and an increased sense of control in which thoughts, sensations, and emotions are observed as passing events that are not always acted on. In addition, they may work through the development of increased emotional regulation and "positive reappraisal" in which difficult circumstances or events are reconstructed as positive or meaningful. Furthermore, they may work through enhancement of self-awareness combined with an enhanced ability to "decenter" and observe experiences as they arise and pass away with a sense of nonjudgmental awareness and acceptance.[132]

As the literature demonstrates, mindfulness-based interventions, including both MBSR and MBCT, are well suited as tertiary prevention strategies with the potential for significant benefit. A 2010 review by Merkes looked at 13 studies of MBSR in patients with chronic disease of varying types and showed overall positive change with enhanced coping, improved well-being, and increased quality of life among MBSR participants. Anxiety was measured in eight studies, with all eight showing significant reductions following MBSR. Of the eight studies, which looked at depression, six showed significant improvements in MBSR participants, while two reported no changes. In the six articles that looked at quality of life and well-being, all showed improvements and four were statistically significant.[133] A more recent 2015 systemic review and meta-analysis by Gotink et al. of 115 unique mindfulness-based RCTs and 8,683 individuals concluded that MBSR and MBCT had significant positive effects in chronic pain, cardiovascular disease, cancer treatment, somatic disorders, depression, and anxiety. Improvements were due to increased quality of life, improved physical outcomes, and decreased anxiety, stress, and depression found in the intervention groups.[124] Overall, the evidence indicates that mindfulness training can minimize disability and impairment from chronic disease, particularly on a psychological and quality of life level.

Mindfulness as Prevention for Psychological Health

Mindfulness as a practice may have broad benefits on mental health, sense of well-being, mood, self-acceptance, and ability to cope with stressful situations.

MINDFULNESS AND PSYCHOLOGICAL HEALTH

Although methodological limitations exist within each body of literature, there is good evidence suggesting that mindfulness is positively associated with healthy lifestyle as well as improvements in depressive symptoms, stress, anxiety, quality of life, and selective physical outcomes. However, as previously noted, health is not only defined by the absence of disease but is hallmarked by physical, mental, and social well-being.[14] Certainly, "well-being" is a key-word embedded within this definition. Although it is obvious that physical well-being has a large impact on morbidity and mortality, the literature also shows that psychological well-being is critical to positive health outcomes.[134] For example, a quantitative review and meta-analysis by Chida et al. found that positive affect, including energy, happiness, vigor, emotional well-being, positive mood, and joy, as well as positive trait-like outlooks such as hopefulness, optimism, sense of humor, and life satisfaction were associated with decreased overall mortality (19% reduction in hazard ratio) and cardiovascular mortality (29% reduction) in healthy populations.[135] Furthermore, a study by Xu et al. found that subjective well-being and positive feelings, including positive affect and satisfaction with life, significantly predicted longevity in a population of 6586 individuals followed over 28 years.[136] Consequently, in order to be fully aligned with the view of prevention as enhancing health, it is critical to consider the ramifications of mindfulness on positive psychological constructs that potentially improve not only physical but also psychological well-being.

To date, numerous studies have pointed to an association between self-reported mindfulness and psychological health. For example, higher levels of trait mindfulness have been associated with increased levels of well-being,[137-142] positive affect,[143,144] life satisfaction,[145] agreeableness,[146,147] conscientiousness,[146] spirituality,[148,149] self-compassion,[150-152] self-esteem,[97,153] resilience,[34] vigor,[34] optimism,[97] forgiveness,[154] hope,[137] and empathy[137,155] in both clinical and nonclinical populations. Furthermore, current evidence suggests that these changes could be robust and tend to be maintained over time.[152] Trait mindfulness has also been negatively correlated with depression,[97,156] rumination,[157,158] experiential avoidance,[141,144] social anxiety,[153] cognitive reactivity,[159,160] neuroticism,[155] and overall psychological distress.[149,161]

MINDFULNESS, WELL-BEING, AND POSITIVE AFFECT

Well-being can be simply defined as a state of optimal functioning and experience.[162] Traditionally, philosophers such as Aristotle have differentiated well-being into hedonic and eudaimic frameworks.[163] Hedonic well-being focuses on pleasure and happiness[164] and is reflected in a commonly used scale of subjective well-being (SWB), which measures the emotional quality of daily life, including the balance of positive to negative emotions such as joy, sadness, affection, or anger, in addition to life satisfaction.[162,165] The eudaimic approach, on the other hand, focuses on meaning, personal growth, and self-realization.[162] Consistent with the eudaimic construct, Ryff et al. formulated a model of psychological well-being (PWB), which encompasses personal growth, purpose in life, self-acceptance, environmental mastery, and autonomy.[166,167] Research suggests that mindfulness positively impacts both SWB and PWB.[168] For example, Kong et al. examined mindfulness and well-being in 290 healthy university students in China. Behavioral studies showed that higher levels of student dispositional mindfulness were related to greater SWB, in the form of higher positive affect and lower negative affect, as well as higher PWB. In addition, neuroimaging studies provided initial evidence for links between individual differences in mindfulness and spontaneous brain activity in the left orbitofrontal cortex, left parahippocampal gyrus, and right insula, suggesting a possible neurobiological mechanism for the mindfulness/well-being connection.[168] Likewise, research by Singleton et al. examined PWB in participants who had completed an 8-week course in MBSR. Neuroimaging studies showed that the more PWB improved, the greater the increase in observed gray matter concentration in areas of the brainstem responsible for the synthesis and release of the neurotransmitters norepinephrine and serotonin. Since these neurotransmitters are involved in the modulation of arousal and mood as well as basic functions such as sleep and appetite, this preliminary study suggests that enhanced PWB has a neural correlate.[169] Furthermore, Hollis-Walker et al. found that mindfulness was significantly correlated with PWB, as well as self-compassion, agreeableness, and openness, and accounted for 57% of the predictive variance in PWB in a sample of nonmeditating subjects.[147]

With regard to SWB, the balance of positive affect (PA) to negative affect (NA) is critical. Not only is the presence of PA a strong predictor of meaning in life,[170] but research also suggests it is protective against the development of mental health disorders.[171,172] Mindfulness has been found to be positively associated with PA. For example, in a 2012 meta-analysis on the effects of different forms of meditation, Erbeth et al. found that MBSR led to significant increases in PA in nonclinical populations.[173] In addition, a study by Cousin et al. of healthy adults found a significant increase in PA following an 8-week MBCT course. This increase in PA was mediated by decreases in the use of disengagement coping strategies, such as wishful thinking, problem avoidance, self-criticism, and social withdrawal, when facing daily stressors.[144] Furthermore, a recent RCT by Batink et al. examining the effect of affect, as well as cognitive variables (worry, rumination), in patients with depression found that increases in PA mediated 61% of the effect of MBCT on depressive symptoms.[143]

MINDFULNESS, COMPASSION, AND SELF-COMPASSION

Compassion can be defined as the feeling that arises when seeing the suffering of others, which engenders a subsequent desire to help.[174] Self-compassion turns compassion inward, allowing an attitude of caring and kindness for oneself in the face of one's suffering.[175] As defined by Neff, self-compassion encompasses three primary components: self-kindness, a sense of common humanity, and a balanced awareness of one's emotional experience (mindfulness).[176] Research findings have revealed an association between self-compassion and positive well-being, happiness, optimism, positive affect, and life-satisfaction[177] as well as with lower levels of psychopathology.[178] Furthermore, self-compassion, and the ability to care for self, is closely linked to compassion or the ability to care for others.[179] With regard to mindfulness, there is growing evidence showing an association between mindfulness and self-compassion. Research has shown that MBIs frequently lead to increased self-compassion in both adults[147,151,152] and adolescents.[180,181] A recent meta-analysis by Gu et al. concluded that there is preliminary, though still inconsistent, evidence for the mediating effect of self-compassion on the psychological outcomes of MBIs.[159] In addition, Cheisa suggests that, although improvements in both mindfulness and self-compassion may mediate clinical outcomes, self-compassion could be a stronger predictor of outcomes than changes in mindfulness.[152] Furthermore, a 2012 study by Keng et al. on a nonclinical, nonmeditating sample found that increases in mindfulness independently mediated effects of MBSR on emotional regulation, while increases in self-compassion independently mediated intervention effects on worry. Researchers concluded that mindfulness and self-compassion may have different impacts on clinical and psychological outcomes, allowing these constructs to work together to produce observed improvements.[182]

There is also evidence that mindfulness practices can facilitate the development of compassion in adults.[183,184] A recent study by Condon et al. examined compassionate responses in a group of 69 undergraduate students who were randomized to either a Web-based mindfulness meditation program or an active control group using a Web-based cognitive training program. Results showed that participants in the mindfulness program showed significantly higher compassion and were 37% more likely to exhibit altruistic behavior by giving up their seat to someone perceived to be in pain than did active controls (14%).[183]

MINDFULNESS AND ADAPTIVE COPING

The ability to cope effectively with adversity is important when dealing with health issues. In general, individuals tend to use either engagement (approach) or disengagement (avoidant) strategies when coping with stressors.[185] Avoidance strategies are characterized by responses that provide distance from the stressor and avoidance of the problem. Individuals who exhibit avoidant behavior may react with heightened levels of negative feelings, such as intense anxiety, or maladaptive behaviors, such as substance abuse or aggression, which are aimed at avoiding or minimizing the difficult feelings related to a distressing event.[186] Evidence indicates that avoidant strategies tend to be associated with decreased overall well-being as well as increased psychopathology.[186] In addition, avoidant strategies have been negatively correlated with improvements in treatment outcomes.[187] Engagement, on the other hand, includes strategies such as acceptance, problem-solving, and social support, which allows movement toward the stressor and the emotional and cognitive reactions related to it.[144]

Mindfulness may facilitate the use of adaptive coping strategies, thereby protecting well-being, particularly in the face of difficult and distressing circumstances. Key to mindfulness practice is the adoption of a stance of curiosity as well as an accepting, nonjudgmental attitude to all experience, whether or not it is pleasant or aversive.[188] In addition, mindfulness encourages attention to the present moment, allowing for greater awareness of positive experiences and emotions, which may be present in the midst of adversity. Furthermore, potentially distressing mental content may be moderated through the cognitive process of stepping back from thoughts, emotions, and sensations. Such perspective shifting, also known as decentering[189] or reperceiving,[4] allows the viewing of thoughts and emotions as passing mental events rather than accurate images of reality. This mental shifting, with the concomitant ability to recognize and let go of automatic thoughts and repetitive negative thinking, may result in change mechanisms such as self-regulation, values clarification, cognitive flexibility, and exposure.[4] Such mechanisms, when present, may allow for the development of effective coping as well as more efficient recovery from distressing events.

Current research suggests multiple ways in which mindfulness may lead to adaptive coping. For example, evidence suggests an inverse relationship between mindfulness and experiential avoidance, although some discrepant results have been observed. Moreover, some studies point to the possible superiority of mindfulness to other treatments in reducing avoidant coping strategies.[152] In addition, an RCT by Cousin et al. found that decreased avoidance mediated improvements in positive affect following MBCT.[144] The literature also suggests other mechanisms of action that may help facilitate adaptive coping. For instance, investigators have found an association of both state and trait mindfulness to an increased use of positive reappraisal.[190-193] The use of positive reappraisal, in which stressful events are actively reinterpreted as benign, beneficial, or meaningful,[194] has been associated with positive mental health outcomes.[195] For example, a heart attack may be initially perceived as life ending but later be construed as a wake up call, leading to improved lifestyle and a renewed appreciation for life. In addition, mediation analysis performed by Gu et al. concluded that decreased repetitive negative thinking, including worry and rumination, was a unique mediator of the effects of MBIs on clinical outcomes. Researchers have also found that decreased emotional and cognitive reactivity, or the degree to which a mildly dysphoric state retriggers repetitive negative thinking and emotional patterns, is another significant mediator of mindfulness training on outcomes.[159] Such decreases in negative thought patterns and rumination, combined with decreased cognitive and emotional reactivity, may enhance the ability to engage with, and adapt to, difficult stressors. Ultimately, these combined mechanisms may allow enhanced navigation of adversity, thereby improving self-efficacy, emotional self-regulation, resiliency, well-being, and quality of life. In fact, greater mindfulness has been associated with resilience,[196,197] with increased resiliency levels found following mindfulness-based interventions.[34,198,199] It is possible that the ability to bounce back from stressful situations may be, at least in part, due to the use of mindfulness coping, which may be characterized by a decentered stance, broadened awareness, heightened insight, cognitive flexibility, and positive reappraisal.

Conclusion and Future Directions

The potential applications of mindfulness to preventive integrative medicine are far reaching, and the fruits of such work are already visible. Decades of research demonstrate that mindfulness-based therapies have significant beneficial effects for a wide array of preventive and health-enhancing applications. In addition, innovative clinical applications are underway with the development of new MBIs for specific populations. Further, mindfulness practice shows promise for cultivating positive psychological qualities previously given little attention by Western researchers. Mindfulness can help enlarge our paradigm of health and healing, deepen the intentions we aspire toward, and expand our vision of what is possible. The field of mindfulness is still young, and the possibilities for its integration into Western healthcare are vast.

Notes

1. Self-liberation refers to the experience of transcending (i.e., becoming free of or dis-identifying from) the sense of being a separate self.
2. These categories are offered heuristically, reflecting the general idea that there are mindfulness qualities that characterize the attention during the mindfulness practice.

References

1. Walsh RN. *Essential Spirituality: The 7 Central Practices to Awaken Heart and Mind.* New York: Wiley; 1999.
2. Wallace AB, Bodhi, B. The nature of mindfulness and its role in Buddhist meditation: a correspondence between B. Alan Wallace and the venerable Bhikkhu Bodhi. In: Wallace BA, ed. Santa Barbara, CA: Santa Barbara Institute for Consciousness Studies; 2006.
3. Shapiro SL, Carlson LE. *The Art and Science of Mindfulness: Integrating Mindfulness into Psychology and the Helping Professions.* 2nd ed. Washington, DC: American Psychological Association; 2017.
4. Shapiro SL, Carlson LE, Astin JA, Freedman B. Mechanisms of mindfulness. *J Clin Psychol* 2006;62(3):373–386.
5. Bishop SL. Mindfulness: a proposed operational definition. *Clin Psychol* 2004;11:230–241.
6. Shapiro SL, Schwartz GE. Chapter 8—The role of intention in self-regulation: toward intentional systemic mindfulness. In: Pintrich PR, Zeidner M, eds. *Handbook of Self-Regulation.* San Diego: Academic Press; 2000:253–273.
7. Kabat-Zinn J, University of Massachusetts Medical Center/Worcester. Stress Reduction Clinic. *Full Catastrophe Living: Using the Wisdom of Your Body and Mind to Face Stress, Pain, and Illness.* New York, NY: Delacorte Press; 1990.
8. Shapiro DH Jr. Adverse effects of meditation: a preliminary investigation of long-term meditators. *Int J Psychosomatics* 1992;39(1-4):62–67.
9. Mackenzie MJ, Carlson LE, Munoz M, Speca M. A qualitative study of self-perceived effects of mindfulness-based stress reduction (MBSR) in a psychosocial oncology setting. *Stress Health* 2007;23(1):59–69.
10. Germer CK, Siegel RD, Fulton PR. *Mindfulness and Psychotherapy.* 1st ed. New York: Guilford Press; 2005.
11. Cullen M. Mindfulness: The heart of buddhist meditation? A conversation with Jan Chozen Bays, Joseph Goldstein, Jon Kabat-Zinn, and Alan Wallace. *Inq Mind* 2006;2:4–7.
12. Shapiro SL, Schwartz, GE. The role of intention in self-regulation: toward intentional systemic mindfulness. In: Boekaerts M, Pintrich, PR, Zeidner M, eds. *Handbook of Self-Regulation.* New York, NY: Academic Press; 2000:253–273.

13. Siegel D. *The Mindful Brain: Reflection and Attunement in the Cultivation of Well-Being*. New York, NY: Norton; 2007.

14. World Health Organization. *Constitution of the World Health Organization—Basic Documents*. 45th ed. Supplement ed. October 2006.

15. Leavell HR, Clark EG. *Preventive Medicine for the Doctor in His Community: An Epidemiologic Approach*. New York: McGraw-Hill, Blakiston Division, McGraw-Hill; 1965.

16. Katz DL. *Epidemiology, Biostatistics, and Preventive Medicine Review*. Philadelphia: Saunders; 1997.

17. Goldston SE. *Concepts of Primary Prevention: A Framework for Program Development*. Sacramento, CA: Department of Mental Health. Office of Prevention; 1987.

18. Brown KW, Ryan R, Creswell JD. Mindfulness: theoretical foundations and evidence for its salutary effects. *Psychol Inq* 2007;18(4):211–237.

19. Park T, Reilly-Spong M, Gross CR. Mindfulness: a systematic review of instruments to measure an emergent patient-reported outcome (PRO). *Qual Life Res* 2013;22(10):2639–2659.

20. Segal ZV. *Mindfulness-Based Cognitive Therapy for Depression: A New Approach to Preventing Relapse*. New York: Guilford Press; 2002.

21. Hayes SC, Levin ME, Plumb-Vilardaga J, Villatte JL, Pistorello J. Acceptance and commitment therapy and contextual behavioral science: examining the progress of a distinctive model of behavioral and cognitive therapy. *Behav Ther* 2013;44(2):180–198.

22. Jekel JF, Jekel JF. *Epidemiology, Biostatistics, and Preventive Medicine*. 3rd ed. Philadelphia: Saunders/Elsevier; 2007.

23. World Health Organization. *Global Health Risks: Mortality and Burden of Disease Attributable to Selected Major Risks*. World Health Organization; 2009.

24. Go AS, Mozaffarian D, Roger VL, et al. Executive summary: heart disease and stroke statistics—2013 update: a report from the American Heart Association. *Circulation* 2013;127(1):143–152.

25. Glasgow RE, Kaplan RM, Ockene JK, Fisher EB, Emmons KM. Patient-reported measures of psychosocial issues and health behavior should be added to electronic health records. *Health Affair (Project Hope)* 2012;31(3):497–504.

26. Feigin VL, Norrving B. A new paradigm for primary prevention strategy in people with elevated risk of stroke. *Int J Stroke* 2014;9(5):624–626.

27. Anderson LH, Martinson BC, Crain AL, et al. Health care charges associated with physical inactivity, overweight, and obesity. *Prev Chronic Dis* 2005;2(4):A09.

28. Ory MG, Jordan PJ, Bazzarre T. The Behavior Change Consortium: setting the stage for a new century of health behavior-change research. *Health Educ Res* 2002;17(5):500–511.

29. Ouwens MA, Schiffer AA, Visser LI, Raeijmaekers NJ, Nyklicek I. Mindfulness and eating behaviour styles in morbidly obese males and females. *Appetite* 2015;87:62–67.

30. Tak SR, Hendrieckx C, Nefs G, Nyklicek I, Speight J, Pouwer F. The association between types of eating behaviour and dispositional mindfulness in adults with diabetes: results from Diabetes MILES; The Netherlands. *Appetite* 2015;87:288–295.

31. Daubenmier J, Kristeller J, Hecht FM, et al. Mindfulness intervention for stress eating to reduce cortisol and abdominal fat among overweight and obese women: an exploratory randomized controlled study. *J Obest* 2011;2011:13.

32. Kearney DJ, Milton ML, Malte CA, McDermott KA, Martinez M, Simpson TL. Participation in mindfulness-based stress reduction is not associated with reductions in emotional eating or uncontrolled eating. *Nutr Res (New York, N.Y.)*. 2012;32(6):413–420.

33. Salmoirago-Blotcher E, Hunsinger M, Morgan L, Fischer D, Carmody J. Mindfulness-based stress reduction and change in health-related behaviors. *J Evid-Based Complement Altern Med* 2013 2013;18(4):243–247.

34. Aikens KA, Astin J, Pelletier KR, et al. Mindfulness goes to work: impact of an online workplace intervention. *J Occup Environ Med* 2014;56(7):721–731.

35. Hébert JR, Hurley TG, Harmon BE, Heiney S, Hebert CJ, Steck SE. A diet, physical activity, and stress reduction intervention in men with rising prostate-specific antigen (PSA) after treatment for prostate cancer. *Cancer Epidemiol* 2012;36(2):e128–e136.

36. Carmody JF, Olendzki BC, Merriam PA, Liu Q, Qiao Y, Ma Y. A novel measure of dietary change in a prostate cancer dietary program incorporating mindfulness training. *J Acad Nutr Diet* 2012;112(11):1822–1827.

37. Carmody J, Olendzki B, Reed G, Andersen V, Rosenzweig P. A dietary intervention for recurrent prostate cancer after definitive primary treatment: results of a randomized pilot trial. *Urology* 2008;72(6):1324–1328.

38. Guh D, Zhang W, Bansback N, Amarsi Z, Birmingham CL, Anis A. The incidence of co-morbidities related to obesity and overweight: a systematic review and meta-analysis. *BMC Public Health* 2009;9(1):88.

39. Williams EP, Mesidor M, Winters K, Dubbert PM, Wyatt SB. Overweight and obesity: prevalence, consequences, and causes of a growing public health problem. *Curr Obesity Reports* 2015;4(3):363–370.

40. Peeters A, Barendregt JJ, Willekens F, et al. Obesity in adulthood and its consequences for life expectancy: a life-table analysis. *Ann Intern Med* 2003;138(1):24–32.

41. Fryar C, Carroll MD, Ogen CL. Prevalence of overweight, obesity, and extreme obesity among adults: United States, 1960–1962 through 2011–2012. *NCHS Health and Stats* 2014.

42. Camilleri GM, Méjean C, Bellisle F, Hercberg S, Péneau S. Association between mindfulness and weight status in a general population from the NutriNet-Santé study. *PLoS One* 2015;10(6):e0127447–e0127447.

43. Loucks EB, Britton WB, Howe CJ, et al. Associations of dispositional mindfulness with obesity and central adiposity: the New England Family study. *Int J Behav Med* 2015; Oct 19;23:224–233.

44. Beshara M, Hutchinson A, Wilson C. Does mindfulness matter? Everyday mindfulness, mindful eating and self-reported serving size of energy dense foods among a sample of South Australian adults. *Appetite* 2013;67:25–29.

45. Roberts KC, Danoff-Burg S. Mindfulness and health behaviors: is paying attention good for you? *J Am Coll Health* 2010;59(3):165–173.

46. Murphy MJ, Mermelstein LC, Edwards KM, Gidycz CA. The benefits of dispositional mindfulness in physical health: a longitudinal study of female college students. *J Am Coll Health* 2012;60(5):341–348.

47. Fulwiler C, Brewer J, Sinnott S, Loucks E. Mindfulness-based interventions for weight loss and CVD risk management. *Curr Cardiovasc Risk Rep* 2015;9(10):1–8.

48. O'Reilly GA, Cook L, Spruijt-Metz D, Black DS. Mindfulness-based interventions for obesity-related eating behaviours: a literature review. *Obes Rev* 2014;15(6):453–461.

49. Katterman SN, Kleinman BM, Hood MM, Nackers LM, Corsica JA. Mindfulness meditation as an intervention for binge eating, emotional eating, and weight loss: a systematic review. *Eat Behav* 2014;15(2):197–204.

50. Dalen J, Smith BW, Shelley BM, Sloan AL, Leahigh L, Begay D. Pilot study: Mindful Eating and Living (MEAL): weight, eating behavior, and psychological outcomes associated with a mindfulness-based intervention for people with obesity. *Complement Ther Med* 2010;18(6):260–264.

51. Miller CK, Kristeller JL, Headings A, Nagaraja H, Miser WF. Comparative effectiveness of a mindful eating intervention to a diabetes self-management intervention among adults with type 2 diabetes: a pilot study. *J Acad Nutr Diet* 2012;112(11):1835–1842.

52. Timmerman GM, Brown A. The effect of a mindful restaurant eating intervention on weight management in women. *J Nutr Educ Behav* 2012;44(1):22–28.

53. O'Reilly GA, Cook L, Spruijt-Metz D, Black DS. Mindfulness-based interventions for obesity-related eating behaviours: a literature review. *Obes Rev* 2014;15(6):453–461.

54. Olson KL, Emery CF. Mindfulness and weight loss: a systematic review. *Psychosom Med* 2015;77(1):59–67.

55. Alberts HJ, Mulkens S, Smeets M, Thewissen R. Coping with food cravings: investigating the potential of a mindfulness-based intervention. *Appetite* 2010;55(1):160–163.

56. Alberts HJ, Thewissen R, Raes L. Dealing with problematic eating behaviour: the effects of a mindfulness-based intervention on eating behaviour, food cravings, dichotomous thinking and body image concern. *Appetite* 2012;58(3):847–851.

57. Loucks EB, Schuman-Olivier Z, Britton WB, et al. Mindfulness and cardiovascular disease risk: state of the evidence, plausible mechanisms, and theoretical framework. *Curr Cardiol Rep* 2015;17(12):112–112.

58. Penedo FJ, Dahn JR. Exercise and well-being: a review of mental and physical health benefits associated with physical activity. *Curr Opin Psychiatr* 2005;18(2):189–193.

59. Wang F, Orpana HM, Morrison H, de Groh M, Dai S, Luo W. Long-term association between leisure-time physical activity and changes in happiness: analysis of the Prospective National Population Health Survey. *Am J Epidemiol* 2012;176(12):1095–1100.

60. Maher JP, Doerksen SE, Elavsky S, et al. A daily analysis of physical activity and satisfaction with life in emerging adults. *Health Psychol* 2013;32(6):647–656.

61. Kokkinos P. Physical activity, health benefits, and mortality risk. *ISRN Cardiology* 2012;2012:718–789.
62. Tsafou K-E, De Ridder DT, van Ee R, Lacroix JP. Mindfulness and satisfaction in physical activity: a cross-sectional study in the Dutch population. *J Health Psychol* 2015.
63. Ulmer CS, Stetson BA, Salmon PG. Mindfulness and acceptance are associated with exercise maintenance in YMCA exercisers. *Behav Res Ther* 2010;48(8):805–809.
64. Zvolensky MJ, Solomon SE, McLeish AC, et al. Incremental validity of mindfulness-based attention in relation to the concurrent prediction of anxiety and depressive symptomatology and perceptions of health. *Cogn Behav Therapy* 2006;35(3):148–158.
65. van Berkel J, Boot CRL, Proper KI, Bongers PM, van der Beek AJ. Effectiveness of a worksite mindfulness-based multi-component intervention on lifestyle behaviors. *Int J Behav Nutr Phy* 2014;11:9–9.
66. Hebert JR, Hurley TG, Harmon BE, Heiney S, Hebert CJ, Steck SE. A diet, physical activity, and stress reduction intervention in men with rising prostate-specific antigen after treatment for prostate cancer. *Cancer Epidemiol* 2012;36(2):e128–e136.
67. Tapper K, Shaw C, Ilsley J, Hill AJ, Bond FW, Moore L. Exploratory randomised controlled trial of a mindfulness-based weight loss intervention for women. *Appetite* 2009;52(2):396–404.
68. Moffitt R, Mohr P. The efficacy of a self-managed acceptance and commitment therapy intervention DVD for physical activity initiation. *Brit J Health Psych* 2015;20(1):115–129.
69. Kangasniemi AM, Lappalainen R, Kankaanpaa A, Tolvanen A, Tammelin T. Towards a physically more active lifestyle based on one's own values: the results of a randomized controlled trial among physically inactive adults. *BMC Public Health* 2015;15:260.
70. Ivanova E, Jensen D, Cassoff J, Gu F, Knauper B. Acceptance and commitment therapy improves exercise tolerance in sedentary women. *Med Sci Sport Exer* 2015;47(6):1251–1258.
71. National Center for Chronic Disease Prevention and Health Promotion, Office on Smoking and Health. Reports of the Surgeon General. *The Health Consequences of Smoking-50 Years of Progress: A Report of the Surgeon General*. Atlanta, GA: Centers for Disease Control and Prevention; 2014.
72. Jha P, Ramasundarahettige C, Landsman V, et al. 21st-century hazards of smoking and benefits of cessation in the United States. *New Engl J Med* 2013;368(4):341–350.
73. Mottillo S, Filion KB, Belisle P, et al. Behavioural interventions for smoking cessation: a meta-analysis of randomized controlled trials. *Eur Heart J* 2009;30(6):718–730.
74. Vidrine JI, Businelle MS, Cinciripini P, et al. Associations of mindfulness with nicotine dependence, withdrawal, and agency. *Subst Abus* 2009;30(4):318–327.
75. Heppner WL, Spears CA, Correa-Fernández V, et al. Dispositional mindfulness predicts enhanced smoking cessation and smoking lapse recovery. *Ann Behav Med* 2016;75:1–11.

76. Black DS, Milam J, Sussman S, Johnson CA. Testing the indirect effect of trait mindfulness on adolescent cigarette smoking through negative affect and perceived stress mediators. *J Subst Use* 2012;17(5-6):417–429.

77. de Souza IC, de Barros VV, Gomide HP, et al. Mindfulness-based interventions for the treatment of smoking: a systematic literature review. *J Altern Complement Med* 2015;21(3):129–140.

78. Brewer JA, Mallik S, Babuscio TA, et al. Mindfulness training for smoking cessation: results from a randomized controlled trial. *Drug Alcohol Depen* 2011;119(1-2):72–80.

79. Davis JM, Goldberg SB, Anderson MC, Manley AR, Smith SS, Baker TB. Randomized trial on mindfulness training for smokers targeted to a disadvantaged population. *Subst Use Misuse* 2014;49(5):571–585.

80. Bricker JB, Mull KE, Kientz JA, et al. Randomized, controlled pilot trial of a smartphone app for smoking cessation using acceptance and commitment therapy. *Drug Alcohol Depen* 2014;143:87–94.

81. Davis J, Manley A, Goldberg S, Stankevitz K, Smith S. Mindfulness training for smokers via web-based video instruction with phone support: a prospective observational study. *BMC Complement Altern Med* 2015;15(1):1–9.

82. Siegrist J. Stress at work. In: *International Encyclopedia of the Social* and *Behavioral Sciences*. New York: Elsevier; 2001:15175–15179.

83. Umberson DL. Stress and health behaviour over the life course. *Adv Life Course Res* 2008;13:19–44.

84. Miller GE, Cohen S. Infectious disease and psychoneuroimmunology. In: Vedhara K, Irwin M, eds. *Human Psychoneuroimmunology*. New York, NY: Oxford University Press; 2005:219–242.

85. Dimsdale JE. Psychological stress and cardiovascular disease. *J Am Coll Cardiol* 2008;51(13):1237–1246.

86. Sharkey SW, Lesser JR, Zenovich AG, et al. Acute and reversible cardiomyopathy provoked by stress in women from the United States. *Circulation* 2005;111(4):472–479.

87. Byrne DG, Espnes GA. Occupational stress and cardiovascular disease. *Stress Health* 2008;24(3):231–238.

88. O'Donnell MJ, Xavier D, Liu L, et al. Risk factors for ischaemic and intracerebral haemorrhagic stroke in 22 countries (the INTERSTROKE study): a case-control study. *Lancet* 2010;376(9735):112–123.

89. Harbuz MS, Richards LJ, Chover-Gonzalez AJ, Marti-Sistac O, Jessop DS. Stress in autoimmune disease models. *Ann NY Acad Sci* 2006;1069:51–61.

90. Kemeny ME, Schedlowski M. Understanding the interaction between psychosocial stress and immune-related diseases: a stepwise progression. *Brain Behav Immun* 2007;21(8):1009–1018.

91. Nielsen NR, Kristensen TS, Schnohr P, Gronbaek M. Perceived stress and cause-specific mortality among men and women: results from a prospective cohort study. *Am J Epidemiol* 2008;168(5):481–496.

92. Ohlin B, Nilsson PM, Nilsson JA, Berglund G. Chronic psychosocial stress predicts long-term cardiovascular morbidity and mortality in middle-aged men. *Eur Heart J* 2004;25(10):867–873.

93. Hammen C. Stress generation in depression: reflections on origins, research, and future directions. *J Clin Psychol* 2006;62(9):1065–1082.

94. Mazure CM. Life stressors as risk factors in depression. *Clin Psychol* 1998;5(3):291–313.

95. Kessler RC. The effects of stressful life events on depression. *Annu Rev Psychol* 1997;48:191–214.

96. Roozendaal B, McEwen BS, Chattarji S. Stress, memory and the amygdala. *Nat Rev Neurosci* 2009;10(6):423–433.

97. Brown KW, Ryan RM. The benefits of being present: mindfulness and its role in psychological well-being. *J Pers Soc Psychol* 2003;84(4):822–848.

98. Carlson LE, Speca M, Faris P, Patel KD. One year pre-post intervention follow-up of psychological, immune, endocrine and blood pressure outcomes of mindfulness-based stress reduction (MBSR) in breast and prostate cancer outpatients. *Brain Behav Immun* 2007;21(8):1038–1049.

99. Branstrom R, Duncan LG, Moskowitz JT. The association between dispositional mindfulness, psychological well-being, and perceived health in a Swedish population-based sample. *Brit J Health Psych* 2011;16:300–316.

100. Harrington R, Loffredo DA, Perz CA. Dispositional mindfulness as a positive predictor of psychological well-being and the role of the private self-consciousness insight factor. *Pers Indiv Differ* 2014;71:15–18.

101. Ciesla JA, Reilly LC, Dickson KS, Emanuel AS, Updegraff JA. Dispositional mindfulness moderates the effects of stress among adolescents: rumination as a mediator. *J Clin Child Adolesc* 2012;41(6):760–770.

102. Prakash RS, Hussain MA, Schirda B. The role of emotion regulation and cognitive control in the association between mindfulness disposition and stress. *Psychol Aging* 2015;30(1):160–171.

103. Sharma M, Rush SE. Mindfulness-based stress reduction as a stress management intervention for healthy individuals: a systematic review. *J Evid Based Complementary Altern Med* 2014;19(4):271–286.

104. Chiesa A, Serretti A. Mindfulness-based stress reduction for stress management in healthy people: a review and meta-analysis. *J Altern Complem Med* 2009;15(5):593–600.

105. Lloyd-Jones DM, Hong Y, Labarthe D, et al. Defining and setting national goals for cardiovascular health promotion and disease reduction: the American Heart Association's strategic impact goal through 2020 and beyond. *Circulation* 2010;121(4):586–613.

106. Loucks EB, Britton WB, Howe CJ, Eaton CB, Buka SL. Positive associations of dispositional mindfulness with cardiovascular health: the New England Family Study. *Int J Behav Med* 2015;22(4):540–550.

107. Chatzisarantis NL, Hagger MS. Mindfulness and the intention-behavior relationship within the theory of planned behavior. *Pers Soc Psychol B* 2007;33(5):663–676.

108. Goyal M, Singh S, Sibinga EMS, et al. Meditation programs for psychological stress and well-being: a systematic review and meta-analysis. *JAMA Intern Med* 2014;174(3):357–368.

109. Musselman DL, Evans DL, Nemeroff CB. The relationship of depression to cardiovascular disease: epidemiology, biology, and treatment. *Arch Gen Psychiat* 1998;55(7):580–592.

110. Evans DL, Charney DS, Lewis L, et al. Mood disorders in the medically ill: scientific review and recommendations. *Biol Psychiat* 2005;58(3):175–189.

111. Abbott RA, Whear R, Rodgers LR, et al. Effectiveness of mindfulness-based stress reduction and mindfulness based cognitive therapy in vascular disease: a systematic review and meta-analysis of randomised controlled trials. *J Psychosom Res* 2014;76(5):341–351.

112. Hughes JW, Fresco DM, Myerscough R, van Dulmen MHM, Carlson LE, Josephson R. Randomized controlled trial of mindfulness-based stress reduction for prehypertension. *Psychosom Med* 2013;75(8):721–728.

113. Blom K, Baker B, How M, et al. Hypertension analysis of stress reduction using mindfulness meditation and yoga: results from the HARMONY randomized controlled trial. *Am J Hypertens* 2014;27(1):122–129.

114. de la Fuente M, Franco, C., Salvador, M. Reduction of blood pressure in a group of hypertensive teachers through a program of mindfulness meditation. *Behav Psychol* 2010;18:533–552.

115. Hartmann M, Kopf S, Kircher C, et al. Sustained effects of a mindfulness-based stress-reduction intervention in type 2 diabetic patients: design and first results of a randomized controlled trial (the Heidelberger Diabetes and Stress-Study). *Diabetes Care* 2012;35(5):945–947.

116. Goldstein CM, Josephson R, Xie S, Hughes JW. Current perspectives on the use of meditation to reduce blood pressure. *Int J Hypertension* 2012: 2012;578397–578397.

117. van Son J, Nyklicek I, Pop VJ, Blonk MC, Erdtsieck RJ, Pouwer F. Mindfulness-based cognitive therapy for people with diabetes and emotional problems: long-term follow-up findings from the DiaMind randomized controlled trial. *J Psychosom Res* 2014;77(1):81–84.

118. Tovote KA, Schroevers MJ, Snippe E, et al. Long-term effects of individual mindfulness-based cognitive therapy and cognitive behavior therapy for depressive symptoms in patients with diabetes: a randomized trial. *Psychother Psychosom* 2015;84(3):186–187.

119. Youngwanichsetha S, Phumdoung S, Ingkathawornwong T. The effects of mindfulness eating and yoga exercise on blood sugar levels of pregnant women with gestational diabetes mellitus. *Appl Nurs Res* 2014;27(4):227–230.

120. Gregg JA, Callaghan GM, Hayes SC, Glenn-Lawson JL. Improving diabetes self-management through acceptance, mindfulness, and values: a randomized controlled trial. *J Consult Clin Psych* 2007;75(2):336–343.

121. Veehof MM, Oskam MJ, Schreurs KM, Bohlmeijer ET. Acceptance-based interventions for the treatment of chronic pain: a systematic review and meta-analysis. *Pain* 2011;152(3):533–542.

122. Kozasa EH, Tanaka LH, Monson C, Little S, Leao FC, Peres MP. The effects of meditation-based interventions on the treatment of fibromyalgia. *Curr Pain Headache R* 2012;16(5):383–387.

123. Cramer H, Haller H, Lauche R, Dobos G. Mindfulness-based stress reduction for low back pain: a systematic review. *BMC Complement Altern Med* 2012;12:162.

124. Gotink RA, Chu P, Busschbach JJV, Benson H, Fricchione GL, Hunink MGM. Standardised mindfulness-based interventions in healthcare: an overview of systematic reviews and meta-analyses of RCTs. *PLoS One* 2015;10(4):e0124344–e0124344.

125. Kuyken W, Hayes R, Barrett B, et al. Effectiveness and cost-effectiveness of mindfulness-based cognitive therapy compared with maintenance antide-pressant treatment in the prevention of depressive relapse or recurrence (PREVENT): a randomised controlled trial. *Lancet (London, England)* 2015;386(9988):63–73.

126. Piet J, Hougaard E. The effect of mindfulness-based cognitive therapy for preven-tion of relapse in recurrent major depressive disorder: a systematic review and meta-analysis. *Clin Psychol Rev* 2011;31(6):1032–1040.

127. Taylor M, Horey D, Swerissen H. *Early Intervention and Chronic Disease* in *Community Health Services Initiative. Statewide evaluation. Final report. Executive Summary.* Melbourne Australia: La Trobe University; 2008.

128. Department of Human Services. *Victorian Population Health Survey 2007. Selected Findings.* Melbourne, Australia; 2008.

129. Stanton AL, Revenson TA, Tennen H. Health psychology: psychological adjust-ment to chronic disease. *Annu Rev Psychol* 2007;58:565–592.

130. DeVellis BM, Revenson TA, Blalock SJ. Rheumatic disease and wom-en's health. In: Gallant S, Keita GP, Royak-Schaler R, eds. *Health Care for Women: Psychological, Social and Behavioral Issues.* Washington, DC: American Psychological Association; 1997:333–347.

131. DiMatteo MR, Lepper HS, Croghan TW. Depression is a risk factor for non-compliance with medical treatment: meta-analysis of the effects of anxiety and depression on patient adherence. *Arch Intern Med* 2000;160(14):2101–2107.

132. Holzel BK, Lazar SW, Gard T, Schuman-Olivier Z, Vago DR, Ott U. How does mindfulness meditation work? Proposing mechanisms of action from a concep-tual and neural perspective. *Perspect Psychol Sci* 2011;6(6):537–559.

133. Merkes M. Mindfulness-based stress reduction for people with chronic diseases. *Aust J Prim Health* 2010;16(3):200–210.

134. Howell RT, Kern ML, Lyubomirsky S. Health benefits: meta-analytically deter-mining the impact of well-being on objective health outcomes. *Health Psychol Rev* 2007/03/01 2007;1(1):83–136.

135. Howell RT, Kern ML, Lyubomirsky S. *Health Benefits: Meta-Analytically Determining the Impact of Well-Being on Objective Health Outcomes.* 2007.

136. Xu J, Roberts RE. The power of positive emotions: it's a matter of life or death—subjective well-being and longevity over 28 years in a general population. *Health Psychol* 2010;29(1):9–19.

137. Shapiro SL, Brown KW, Thoresen C, Plante TG. The moderation of mindfulness-based stress reduction effects by trait mindfulness: results from a randomized controlled trial. *J Clin Psychol* 2011;67(3):267–277.
138. Shapiro SL, Oman D, Thoresen CE, Plante TG, Flinders T. Cultivating mindfulness: effects on well-being. *J Clinl Psychol* 2008;64(7):840–862.
139. Bränström R, Duncan LG, Moskowitz JT. The association between dispositional mindfulness, psychological well-being, and perceived health in a Swedish population-based sample. *Brit J Health Psych* 2011;16(Pt 2):300–316.
140. Singleton O, Hölzel BK, Vangel M, Brach N, Carmody J, Lazar SW. Change in brainstem gray matter concentration following a mindfulness-based intervention is correlated with improvement in psychological well-being. *Front Hum Neurosci* 2014;8:33–33.
141. Branstrom R, Kvillemo P, Brandberg Y, Moskowitz JT. Self-report mindfulness as a mediator of psychological well-being in a stress reduction intervention for cancer patients—a randomized study. *Ann Behav Med* 2010;39(2):151–161.
142. Carmody J, Baer RA. Relationships between mindfulness practice and levels of mindfulness, medical and psychological symptoms and well-being in a mindfulness-based stress reduction program. *J Behav Med* 2008;31(1):23–33.
143. Batink T, Peeters F, Geschwind N, van Os J, Wichers M. How does MBCT for depression work? Studying cognitive and affective mediation pathways. *PLoS One* 2013;8(8):e72778.
144. Cousin G, Crane C. Changes in disengagement coping mediate changes in affect following mindfulness-based cognitive therapy in a non-clinical sample. *Brit J Psychol (London, England: 1953)*. 2015.
145. Kong F, Wang X, Zhao J. Dispositional mindfulness and life satisfaction: the role of core self-evaluations. *Pers Indiv Differ* 2014;56:165–169.
146. Thompson BL, Waltz J. Everyday mindfulness and mindfulness meditation: overlapping constructs or not? *Pers Indiv Differ* 2007;43(7):1875–1885.
147. Hollis-Walker L, Colosimo K. Mindfulness, self-compassion, and happiness in non-meditators: a theoretical and empirical examination. *Pers Indiv Differ* 2011;50(2):222–227.
148. Astin JA. Stress reduction through mindfulness meditation: effects on psychological symptomatology, sense of control, and spiritual experiences. *Psychother Psychosom* 1997;66(2):97–106.
149. Carmody J, Reed G, Kristeller J, Merriam P. Mindfulness, spirituality, and health-related symptoms. *J Psychosom Res* 2008;64(4):393–403.
150. Raab K. Mindfulness, self-compassion, and empathy among health care professionals: a review of the literature. *J Health Care Chaplaincy* 2014;20(3):95–108.
151. Baer R, Lykins ELB, Peters JR. Mindfulness and self compassion as predictors of psychological well-being in long-term meditators and matched non-meditators. *J Posit Psychol* 2012;7(3):230–238.
152. Chiesa A, Anselmi R, Serretti A. Psychological mechanisms of mindfulness-based interventions: what do we know? *Holist Nurs Pract* 2014;28(2):124–148.

153. Rasmussen MK, Pidgeon AM. The direct and indirect benefits of dispositional mindfulness on self-esteem and social anxiety. *Anxiety Stress Copin* 2011;24(2):227–233.

154. Oman D, Shapiro SL, Thoresen CE, Plante TG, Flinders T. Meditation lowers stress and supports forgiveness among college students: a randomized controlled trial. *J Am Coll Health* 2008;56(5):569–578.

155. Dekeyser M, Raes F, Leijssen M, Leysen S, Dewulf D. Mindfulness skills and interpersonal behaviour. *Pers Indiv Differ* 2008;44(5):1235–1245.

156. Cash M, Whittingham K. What facets of mindfulness contribute to psychological well-being and depressive, anxious, and stress-related symptomatology? *Mindfulness* 2010;1(3):177–182.

157. Raes F, Williams JMG. The relationship between mindfulness and uncontrollability of ruminative thinking. *Mindfulness* 2010;1(4):199–203.

158. Deyo M, Wilson KA, Ong J, Koopman C. Mindfulness and rumination: does mindfulness training lead to reductions in the ruminative thinking associated with depression? *Explore* 2009;5(5):265–271.

159. Gu J, Strauss C, Bond R, Cavanagh K. How do mindfulness-based cognitive therapy and mindfulness-based stress reduction improve mental health and wellbeing? A systematic review and meta-analysis of mediation studies. *Clin Psychol Rev* 2015;37:1–12.

160. Raes F, Dewulf D, Van Heeringen C, Williams JM. Mindfulness and reduced cognitive reactivity to sad mood: evidence from a correlational study and a non-randomized waiting list controlled study. *Behav Res Ther* 2009;47(7):623–627.

161. Baer RA, Smith GT, Hopkins J, Krietemeyer J, Toney L. Using self-report assessment methods to explore facets of mindfulness. *Assessment* 2006;13(1):27–45.

162. Ryan RM, Deci EL. On happiness and human potentials: a review of research on hedonic and eudaimonic well-being. *Annu Rev Psychol* 2001;52:141–166.

163. Ross WD. *The Nicomachean Ethics of Aristotle.* New York, NY: Oxford University Press; 1954.

164. Falikowski AF. *Experiencing Philosophy.* Upper Saddle River, NJ: Prentice Hall; 2003.

165. Kahneman D, Deaton A. High income improves evaluation of life but not emotional well-being. *P Natl A Sci* 2010;107(38):16489–16493.

166. Ryff CD. Psychological well-being in adult life. *Curr Dir Psychol Sci* 1995;4(4):99–104.

167. Ryff CD. Happiness is everything, or is it? Explorations on the meaning of psychological well-being. *J Pers Soc Psychol* 1989;57(6):1069.

168. Kong F, Wang X, Song Y, Liu J. Brain regions involved in dispositional mindfulness during resting state and their relation with well-being. *Soc Neurosci* 2015:1–13.

169. Singleton O, Holzel BK, Vangel M, Brach N, Carmody J, Lazar SW. Change in brainstem gray matter concentration following a mindfulness-based intervention is correlated with improvement in psychological well-being. *Front Hum Neurosci* 2014;8:33.

170. King LA, Hicks JA, Krull JL, Del Gaiso AK. Positive affect and the experience of meaning in life. *J Pers Soc Psychol* 2006;90(1):179–196.

171. Davis M, Suveg C. Focusing on the positive: a review of the role of child positive affect in developmental psychopathology. *Clin Child Fam Psych* 2014;17(2):97–124.

172. Etter DW, Gauthier JR, McDade-Montez E, Cloitre M, Carlson EB. Positive affect, childhood adversity, and psychopathology in psychiatric inpatients. *Eur J Psychotraumato* 2013;4.

173. Eberth J, Sedlmeier P. The effects of mindfulness meditation: a meta-analysis. *Mindfulness* 2012;3(3):174–189.

174. Goetz JL, Keltner D, Simon-Thomas E. Compassion: an evolutionary analysis and empirical review. *Psychol Bull* 2010;136(3):351–374.

175. Neff KD MP. Self compassion and psychological resilience among adolescents and young adults. *Self Identity* 2010;9(3):225–240.

176. Neff K. The development and validation of a scale to measure self compassion. *Self Identity* 2003;2:223–250.

177. Bluth K, Blanton PW. Mindfulness and self-compassion: exploring pathways to adolescent emotional well-being. *J Child Fam Stud* 2014;23(7):1298–1309.

178. MacBeth A, Gumley A. Exploring compassion: a meta-analysis of the association between self-compassion and psychopathology. *Clin Psychol Rev* 2012;32(6):545–552.

179. Gilbert PE. *Compassion: Conceptualizations, Research, and Use in Psychotherapy.* New York, NY: Routledge; 2005.

180. Bluth K, Blanton PW. Mindfulness and self-compassion: exploring pathways to adolescent emotional well-being. *J Child Fam Stud* 2014;23(7):1298–1309.

181. Bluth K, Roberson PNE, Gaylord SA. A pilot study of a mindfulness intervention for adolescents and the potential role of self-compassion in reducing stress. *Explore (New York, N.Y.)* 2015;11(4):292–295.

182. Keng S-L, Smoski MJ, Robins CJ, Ekblad AG, Brantley JG. Mechanisms of change in mindfulness-based stress reduction: self-compassion and mindfulness as mediators of intervention outcomes. *J Cogn Psychother* 2012;26(3):270–280.

183. Condon P, Desbordes G, Miller WB, DeSteno D. Meditation increases compassionate responses to suffering. *Psychol Sci* 2013;24(10):2125–2127.

184. Roeser RW, Eccles JS. Mindfulness and compassion in human development: introduction to the special section. *Dev Psychol* 2015;51(1):1–6.

185. Connor-Smith JK, Flachsbart C. Relations between personality and coping: a meta-analysis. *J Pers Soc Psychol* 2007;93(6):1080–1107.

186. Hayes SC, Wilson KG, Gifford EV, Follette VM, Strosahl K. Experimental avoidance and behavioral disorders: a functional dimensional approach to diagnosis and treatment. *J Consult Clin Psych* 1996;64(6):1152–1168.

187. Berking M, Neacsiu A, Comtois KA, Linehan MM. The impact of experiential avoidance on the reduction of depression in treatment for borderline personality disorder. *Behav Res Ther* 2009;47(8):663–670.

188. Kabat-Zinn J. *Wherever You Go, There You Are: Mindfulness Meditation in Everyday Life.* New York: Hyperion Hachette Books; 1994.

189. Teasdale JD, Moore RG, Hayhurst H, Pope M, Williams S, Segal ZV. Metacognitive awareness and prevention of relapse in depression: empirical evidence. *J Consult Clin Psych* 2002;70(2):275–287.

190. Hanley A, Garland EL, Black DS. Use of mindful reappraisal coping among meditation practitioners. *J Clin Psychol* 2014;70(3):294–301.

191. Hanley AW, Garland EL. Dispositional mindfulness co-varies with self-reported positive reappraisal. *Pers Indiv Differ* 2014;66:146–152.

192. Garland E, Gaylord S, Park J. The role of mindfulness in positive reappraisal. *Explore (New York, N.Y.)* 2009;5(1):37–44.

193. Troy AS, Shallcross AJ, Davis TS, Mauss IB. History of mindfulness-based cognitive therapy is associated with increased cognitive reappraisal ability. *Mindfulness (NY)* 2013;4(3):213–222.

194. Lazarus RS, Folkman S. *Stress, Appraisal, and Coping.* New York, NY: Springer; 1984.

195. Helgeson VS, Reynolds KA, Tomich PL. A meta-analytic review of benefit finding and growth. *J Consult Clin Psych* 2006;74(5):797–816.

196. Kemper KJ, Mo X, Khayat R. Are mindfulness and self-compassion associated with sleep and resilience in health professionals? *J Altern Complem Med* 2015;21(8):496–503.

197. Montero-Marin J, Tops M, Manzanera R, Piva Demarzo MM, Álvarez de Mon M, García-Campayo J. Mindfulness, resilience, and burnout subtypes in primary care physicians: the possible mediating role of positive and negative affect. *Front Psychol* 2015;6:1895.

198. Klatt M, Steinberg B, Duchemin A-M. Mindfulness in Motion (MIM): An onsite mindfulness based intervention (MBI) for chronically high stress work environments to increase resiliency and work engagement. *Jove-J Vis Exp* 2015(101):e52359–e52359.

199. Pidgeon AM, Ford L, Klaassen F. Evaluating the effectiveness of enhancing resilience in human service professionals using a retreat-based Mindfulness with Metta Training Program: a randomised control trial. *Psychol Health Med* 2014;19(3):355–364.

6

The Role of Family and Community in Integrative Preventive Medicine

FARSHAD FANI MARVASTI, MD, MPH

Key Concepts

- Integrative preventive medicine (IPM) is the best approach to control and prevent the chronic diseases of our time that account for the vast majority of healthcare expenses and lives lost.
- Integrative preventive medicine provides a shift from acute to chronic disease treatment and prevention with the goal of morbidity compression to extend the period of disease-free high-quality life.
- The role of family and community in IPM is to leverage primary care as the chief means for disseminating and implementing a new integrative model of prevention.
- Integrative preventive medicine shifts the focus of family and community medicine from reactive "sick" acute care to proactive preventive "health" care.
- Integrative preventive medicine for family and community goes beyond simply treating each individual by including an assessment of the larger community and context in the prevention of disease to target key risk factors.
- Integrative preventive medicine changes the patient encounter in family and community medicine to recreate "routine" physical exams as opportunities for primary prevention and patient health education.
- Integrative preventive medicine empowers physicians to go beyond simply following up on prediabetic patients to proactively engaging

> them on an evidence-based lifestyle regimen to prevent the onset of diabetes.
> - Integrative preventive medicine redefines the USPSTF standard for primary prevention guidelines to include proactive engagement and evidence-based integrative prevention of disease beyond routine screening recommendations.
> - Integrative preventive medicine fosters the development of innovation in primary care where the patient is the focus and a relationship over time exists to initiate and follow up on lifestyle interventions to prevent disease and maintain optimal health.

Introduction

Seventy-five cents of every dollar spent on healthcare in the United States is spent on chronic diseases. In fact, cardiovascular disease, cancer, and diabetes are now responsible for 7 out of every 10 deaths among Americans each year and account for up to 75% of the nation's health expenditures.[1] These well-known chronic diseases have modifiable risk factors and are therefore preventable. Integrative preventive medicine (IPM) is the best approach to control and prevent the chronic diseases of our time that account for the vast majority of healthcare expenses and lives lost.

Integrative Preventive Medicine Recognizes the Changes in Epidemiology Toward Chronic Disease

Despite the epidemic of chronic disease, our healthcare system, or more accurately our "sick" care system, is based on an acute care approach that is over 100 years old. The current model is the result of fundamental changes in medical education, research, and practice that took place in the wake of the Flexner Report in 1910.[2] At the time of the report in 1910, acute infectious diseases such as polio and tuberculosis were the major sources of morbidity and mortality.[3] An acute care approach powerfully addressed these conditions through the development of a hospital-based system that successfully treated a non-ambulatory acutely sick patient population. Philanthropic contributions and scientific breakthroughs fueled rapid expansion of this model into the industrial medical complex that now permeates our healthcare system.[4] Despite our success in eradicating and controlling many acute infectious diseases, we now struggle with the changes in disease epidemiology that mandate a new focus on chronic disease management and prevention.

Integrative preventive medicine is based on these changes in disease epidemiology and therefore shifts the focus of our system appropriately from acute to chronic conditions. A shift in focus requires a fundamental understanding of the differences between acute and chronic care as shown in Table 6.1.

While acute conditions usually have a rapid onset and are self-limited in their disease course, chronic diseases have a gradual onset and are progressive over time. One does not "catch" a heart attack like a cold virus; rather a myocardial infarction is the acute exacerbation of the chronic process of atherosclerosis. Evidence of this comes from many sources including atherosclerotic streaks found in Vietnam War veterans in their early to mid-20s.[5] As the pathogeneses of acute and chronic diseases differ, so do their treatments. While acute disease usually involves supportive measures, as in the case of the common cold, or targeted therapies, for clear bacterial infections such as streptococcus pharyngitis, chronic conditions such as type II diabetes (the majority of diabetes cases, accounting for 90%–95% of all diabetes) require more complex multifactorial treatment plans. Integrative preventive medicine recognizes the distinction between chronic and acute conditions and focuses on the chronic diseases of our time. In sync with the pathogenesis of chronic disease, IPM focuses on risk factor modification over time. Integrative preventive medicine therefore emphasizes prevention instead of episodic treatment

Table 6.1 Differences in Acute Versus Chronic Care

Disease Category	Acute	Chronic
Onset	**Rapid onset, runs its course, self-limited**, usually affects one body system	**Gradual slow onset, affects multiple systems**, is not responsive to "curing" treatments, not self-limited but progressive over time
Examples	Influenza, cold virus, strep throat, sprains, fractures, abscess	Diabetes, cardiovascular disease, asthma, obesity, cancer
Treatment	Supportive measures, targeted specific therapies with goal of cure (incision and drainage for abscess, removal of infected appendix or gallbladder)	Symptom management, to prevent but not to cure; multiple complex treatment plans aimed at control and prevention of progression (multiple medications for diabetes and dietary changes and exercise for weight loss)

and risk factor modification instead of simply disease treatment once it is in its later stages.

The Role of Family and Community Medicine in Integrative Preventive Medicine

A new emphasis on preventing the chronic diseases of our time requires a new focus on primary care or family and community medicine (these will be used interchangeably throughout this chapter). Primary care has been underused, underfunded, and underappreciated by both the public and medical professionals. These cultural and professional biases against primary care have contributed in large part to the current shortage of primary care physicians, which has reached crisis levels.[6] Despite these realities, family and community medicine or primary care and public health are critical to the care and prevention of chronic diseases. One main reason for this is the fact primary care occurs over time and is relationship based. It also includes "well" visits from childhood and "wellness" physicals for adults. These non-sick or healthy visits serve as great opportunities for prevention and risk factor modification. Integrative preventive medicine shifts the focus from acute to the chronic care and therefore empowers family and community medicine as the foundation for a new model of care that is based on prevention and health promotion over time. The value of this approach cannot be understated as a means to stem the tide of our current epidemic of chronic disease.

In addition to the implications for the practice of primary care outlined below, IPM also requires a new emphasis on family and community in medical education. Integrative preventive medicine is evidence based and recognizes that 80% of medical education is focused on biology and biological factors in the development of disease. Yet, 60% of premature deaths are actually due to "nonbiologic" factors.[7] These "nonbiologic" factors form the basis for the risk factors of chronic disease and include behavioral choices, lifestyle, and social determinants. Therefore, IPM recognizes the broader social context and community as critical components to the success of any prevention or therapeutic intervention. For example, a diabetic patient may be advised to change her diet but may not be able to afford the healthy food choices that are necessary to control and prevent progression of diabetes through lifestyle changes. Ignoring these economic and social realities will result in ineffective healthcare interventions. Integrative preventive medicine enlists the support and engagement of the larger community to prevent disease by empowering peers and patients to take an active role in their health. For example, community health educators can serve as catalysts for groups of patients with diabetes or even prediabetes and metabolic syndrome to make lifestyle changes. Integrative preventive medicine further empowers family and community medicine by recognizing the need to shift our medical education to reflect the changes in disease epidemiology from acute diseases that require hospital-based care to chronic conditions that are best addressed in ambulatory settings. The need for this shift is well supported by the fact that 80% of clinical education still occurs in inpatient settings, while 80%–90% of medicine is now practiced in outpatient settings.[7] Therefore, IPM recognizes the community and social context as a focal point of care and shifts medical practice to where it is needed most.

Integrative Preventive Medicine Creates a New Model of Family and Community Medicine

To stem the tide of our current epidemic of chronic disease, IPM creates a new model of primary care that is based on prevention and health promotion across the lifespan. Central to this new model is the definition of prevention and its purported goals. The concept of prevention (from the Latin root, *praeventus*, to anticipate) has been articulated since ancient times.[8,9] Disease prevention therefore includes any and all efforts to anticipate the genesis of disease and forestall its progression to clinical manifestations. This definition of disease prevention does not presume to cure disease. Rather than focusing on acute treatment and cure, IPM seeks to compress morbidity and increase the period of disease-free life for as long as possible. The new model of family and community medicine is therefore based on this concept of morbidity compression that was first articulated by James Fries.[10]

In contrast to the goal of morbidity compression that is afforded by IPM, our current primary care system parallels other specialty fields in medicine that are reactive in their approach to treat acute morbidity as efficiently as possible. While optimal acute care is central even to acute exacerbations of chronic diseases such as myocardial infarctions, the chronic care IPM approach seeks to forestall and delay the development of this acute episode that is both potentially fatal and costly. The impact of IPM for family and community is best understood through an understanding of functional capacity and how it changes over time. Functional capacity is defined here as the ability to perform daily activities at a high level with an exceptional quality of life. Most estimates of functional capacity show a significant and steady decline in a number of physiological systems as early as age 45.[11] This decline is accelerated resulting in increased healthcare usage as gleaned by various outcomes such as the percentage of people with prescription medications taken within the last 30 days which jumps from 38% to 67% when comparing individuals aged 18 to 44 with those who are between 45 and 64.[12] This steady decline and persistent morbidity results in decades of hospitalizations and recurrent admissions to rehabilitation centers and ultimately assisted living care facilities that all together account for exorbitant costs and poor quality of life.[12] As bleak as this picture appears, aging experts at the MacArthur Foundation have asserted that only 30% of the characteristics of aging are genetically based and that environmental factors play a more critical role in the process.[13,14] This finding supports the goals of IPM to compress morbidity and lengthen the period of disease-free healthy life by modifying preventable risk factors for the chronic diseases of our time. Therefore, the goal becomes successful aging through the application of IPM in family and community medicine.

Figure 6.1 shows how the application of IPM to healthcare and the development of a prevention model can change the curve of decline in functional capacity with age. Optimizing prevention through the application of evidence-based primary prevention strategies in family and community medicine settings can shift this curve to the right and thereby increase the period of disease-free, high-quality life. Not only does the IPM approach result in increased functional capacity and quality of life but also it prevents hundreds of millions of dollars that are currently being spent on care for the long period of morbidity that affects most of our population. By shifting the graph to the right through the delay of disease progression and morbidity onset, billions

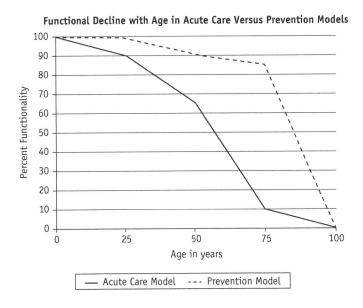

FIGURE 6.1 Functional Decline with Age in Acute Care Versus Precention Models. Developed by Randall S. Stafford and Farshad Fani Marvasti

of dollars now spent on geriatric care can be saved. Thus, the IPM prevention model increases individual quality of life and reduces costs to our healthcare system.

Integrative Preventive Medicine Leverages Primary Care to Disseminate Prevention Strategies

Integrative preventive medicine deployed early in the lifespan through evidence-based application of primary prevention to clinical practice seeks to compress morbidity and extend the period of disease-free, high-functioning life. It uses an integrative and admittedly holistic approach to medical care that is absent in our current family and community settings. Therefore IPM is more proactive than reactive in how it approaches health and disease: going upstream to change the course of these conditions by focusing on prevention.

In established models, prevention has been categorized as primary, secondary, and tertiary.[15] As shown in Table 6.2, prevention efforts need not be limited to patentable medications or a fixed clinical site with episodic visits and diagnostic testing. Prevention involves the entire range of services from modifying behavior for healthy lifestyle changes to community health education interventions to address the "built environment" including underlying social, political, or economic conditions that predispose population members to disease. As noted, our current system emphasizes the optimization of acute care and thereby focuses almost exclusively on secondary and tertiary prevention. The new model of IPM in primary care expands the dissemination of prevention strategies to shift the focus toward primary prevention as an upstream approach to the chronic diseases of our time.

Integrative Preventive Medicine Changes the Patient Encounter in Primary Care to Recreate "Routine" Physicals

As primary care is relationship based and occurs over time, it is the best-suited field for the deployment of an integrative prevention model to address chronic disease. Although our current model focuses on acute treatment and tertiary prevention, IPM shifts the focus to primary and secondary prevention. This shift results in the recreation of "routine" physicals as opportunities for

Table 6.2 A Range of Prevention Efforts

Level	Definition	Examples
Primary Prevention	Activities intended to forestall the development of a disease prior to its clinical diagnosis	Eating a healthy diet and regular exercise to maintain optimal weight, cholesterol, blood pressure, and glucose control in patients with family history of diabetes mellitus type II; population-based health-screening activities such as health promotion activities to address SES, cultural and built environment where disease develops prior to clinical diagnosis.
Secondary Prevention	Activities intended to forestall further developments of existing disease while in its early stages before it results in significant morbidity	Implementing diabetes prevention program with lifestyle changes or low-dose metformin in newly diagnosed diabetic prior to onset of end organ disease. Controlling hypertension through aerobic exercise, the DASH diet, and antihypertensive medications.
Tertiary Prevention	Activities intended to forestall end-stage sequelae of symptomatic clinical disease including significant morbidity leading to functional impairment or death	Treating a diabetic patient with neuropathy and chronic kidney disease with optimal medical management to prevent renal failure and dialysis. Anticoagulants in patients with coronary disease

primary prevention and health education. Instead of merely asking a comprehensive review of systems to find evidence of a latent condition or performing physical exam maneuvers to find an abnormal murmur, IPM transforms these visits to true "wellness" focused encounters. Rather than focusing exclusively on finding latent disease, these visits ought to focus on assessing the patient for risk factors and behaviors that could lead to the development of chronic disease. For example, metabolic syndrome, or syndrome x, has been implicated as a common pathway toward the development of both diabetes and cardiovascular disease.[16] Currently we have little to offer these patients and usually wait until an actual diagnosis is made to address these risk factors. Integrative preventive medicine empowers primary care physicians and their extended team of ancillary healthcare providers to prevent the inevitable progression of metabolic syndrome to disease. For example, motivational interviewing has been identified as a potentially powerful tool for effecting behavioral change.[17] Behavioral change is critical to addressing metabolic syndrome to prevent disease. Its importance is recognized based on the fact that social determinants of disease and not predetermined unchangeable genetics affect our ability to age successfully.[13] These nonbiological factors such as lifestyle choices can be modified. In the IPM model, the social history becomes more extended as a means to find these social determinants and adjust them early on in the process. Therefore, primary prevention and individuals with precursors of disease such as metabolic syndrome become key targets for early intervention to prevent disease diagnosis and progression.

To address metabolic syndrome and early stage chronic disease, IPM expands the use of motivational interviewing and health education. It incorporates well-studied tools such as action planning as part of routine visits to recreate these encounters and initiate a dialogue between the patient and the provider to effect behavioral change. Action planning has been studied in various contexts and has been shown to be particularly effective in healthy behavioral change.[18] Most patients reported making a behavior change based on an action plan, suggesting that action plans may be a useful strategy to encourage behavior change for patients seen in primary care.[19] The Chronic Disease Self-Management Program (CDSMP) developed by Kate Lorig at Stanford uses this model for behavioral change to address chronic disease. The model involves using a systematic approach of setting health goals with patients using a standard template, SLAM,[20] as shown in Table 6.3. Even in 15-minute patient encounters that are characteristic of our acute care model, the SLAM template can initiate an IPM lifestyle change through brief action planning. Subsequent email or phone contact can be made with the patient to assess their progress either by the physician or health coach in a team-based model of care. Success here depends on gaining momentum with small steps toward successful lifestyle changes. Integrative preventive medicine recognizes the critical role that this science of behavior change plays in perpetuating our chronic disease

Table 6.3 SLAM Template Used in the CDSMP Approach
to Setting Health Goals

SLAM	
Specific	Walking
Limited	For 45 minutes
Achievable	Must be 7 out of 10 on confidence scale
Measurable	Walk on Mon/Wed/Fri by next week

epidemic and favors research and education in this area as part of the new prevention model of care.

In addition to action planning and motivational interviewing, providing accurate, evidence-based health education is central to the role of family and community in IPM. The word "doctor" comes from the Latin root *docēre*, which means to teach.[21] In our acute care model, doctors primarily focus on medications and procedural interventions rather than education. The IPM model of care identifies education as a critical tool that is largely untapped by physicians and healthcare providers in our current system. The new prevention model makes education paramount as the primary means for preventing chronic disease through primary care visits and community health education programs. With the preventive model that is proactive rather than reactive, health education materials tailored to each individual patient in the form of an after visit summary and plan of care is emphasized as a key part of the clinical encounter. Using this format of summarizing key insights and patient health goals as a take-home message for patients is a relatively simple way to support individual efforts to make healthy lifestyle changes.

Another tool that has been studied with some success is the use of exercise prescriptions.[22] These prescriptions for physical activity have been found to be effective but are limited when simply given out of context. With IPM, the focus is on prevention and physical activity becomes a central pillar to treatment in addition to medication or other conventional therapies. When given in the context of the after visit summary as part of the patient's health plan and goals set during the visit, exercise prescriptions can be powerful tools for patients to recognize the value of such healthy lifestyle practices. Integrative preventive medicine also expands and tailors exercise prescriptions to include physical therapy routines that are amenable to self-care. For example, the prevalence of low-back pain cause by low-back strain is known to be a common primary care diagnosis. Other sprains and strains also present to the primary care provider. In addition to standard medical therapy such as NSAIDs, exercise regimens have a key role in treating acute injuries to the low back or other joints. These persistent injuries such as low-back strain can be prevented through the use of daily low-back exercises. The expanded routine physical exam that focuses on a needs assessment for patients as part of the IPM model would identify a sedentary lifestyle as a key target for intervention. As most people are now employed in office jobs that require long hours of sitting, low-back injuries are more common. Therefore, exercise prescriptions that include specific low-back exercises to anyone with this sedentary lifestyle can be a powerful tool when widely used in "routine" physical settings to prevent back injury.

Hippocrates is considered to be the founder of Western medicine. He is quoted as advocating for the use of food as medicine and medicine as food.

Recognizing the linkages between diet and chronic disease that are currently building similar to the evidence that clearly linked smoking with lung cancer, food prescriptions can also be used as part of the new IPM model for integrative prevention of chronic disease. For example, there has been well-established evidence for the Mediterranean diet in the prevention of cardiovascular disease.[23] A food prescription for this type of diet with specific examples and food choices such as the use of extra virgin olive oil in healthy portions as part of our diet can be prescribed along side statins or blood pressure medications used to treat risk factors for cardiovascular disease. Integrative preventive medicine providers could also include simple recipes as part of their food prescriptions for easy-to-make foods such as homemade salad dressing to accompany fresh leafy greens. For example, a salad dressing of extra virgin olive oil, sea salt, cayenne pepper and fresh lime or apple cider vinegar can be made in minutes. The benefit of teaching patients how to make delicious foods that are healthy for them cannot be overstated, as this contributes to healthy habits that pay long-term dividends in preventing disease and maintaining health.

Integrative Preventive Medicine Empowers Primary Care Providers

Integrative preventive medicine empowers physicians to go beyond simply monitoring patients with metabolic syndrome or prediabetes to proactively engaging them with the evidence-based lifestyle changes outlined earlier to prevent the onset of diabetes. Evidence-based nutritional advice and exercise counseling can be systematically incorporated into patient encounters over time. Integrative preventive medicine is more strategic and evidence based rather than simply limited to conventional approaches that are confined to the acute care model that continues to be misapplied to the chronic disease burden. Interventions that are more in sync with the IPM approach toward diseases such as obesity include stealth interventions that focus on overall well-being and physical activity instead of simply weight loss as the explicit endpoint.[24] A primary care provider who practices IPM may identify hypertension and obesity as part of a typical patient visit, but will focus on the overall holistic picture of health as the goal of therapy instead of narrowing it down to numerical changes in these measurements. For example, developing a pattern of healthy daily physical activity and following dietary guidelines to ensure at least 5–7 servings of vegetables and fruits every day would be the goal of care. A healthy side effect of behavioral change to achieve this goal would be lowered blood pressure and weight loss to optimal levels. Therefore, IPM shifts the focus from disease-oriented outcomes toward patient-oriented out-comes as a means to achieve chronic disease control and prevention. This shift empowers primary care providers to succeed in behavioral change therapies for their patients.

Integrative Preventive Medicine Redefines Standards to Focus on Primary Prevention

Integrative preventive medicine redefines the US Preventive Services Taskforce (USPSTF) standard for primary prevention guidelines to include proactive engagement and evidence-based integrative prevention of disease beyond routine screening recommendations. Instead of focusing simply on screening for a disease as a means of secondary prevention, IPM seeks to use the best evidence to prevent the disease and extend the period of disease-free high-functioning life for as long as possible. As shown in Table 6.4, a number of conditions with conservative screening recommendations by the USPSTF[25] can be expanded based on known evidence to include proactive primary prevention. According to the CDC, "of cancers that affect both men and women, colorectal cancer is the second leading cause of cancer-related deaths in the United States and the third most common cancer in men and in women."[26] In the case of colorectal cancer screening, the guidelines suggest that nothing is done until age 50 to find occult cancer or precancerous lesions such as polyps via colonoscopy. As early as the 1970s, epidemiological research discovered a direct correlation with red meat consumption and the incidence of colon cancer.[27] Additional evidence has accumulated over the last 40 years to support several basic interventions that are efficacious, safe, cost-effective, and amenable to self-care. Strong evidence exists for decreasing colorectal cancer by increased physical activity of all types and foods containing dietary fiber such as plant foods. Equally strong evidence exists to show an increased risk for colorectal cancer with consumption of red meat, processed meat, alcoholic drinks especially in men, and abdominal fat.[28] Therefore, expanding our approach to address this deadly disease through an IPM framework empowers individuals of all ages to engage in these lifestyle changes to prevent colorectal cancer. Such lifestyle changes based on existing evidence as shown in Table 6.4 have little to no harm associated with them. For these and other conditions IPM moves beyond relying on surveillance to find early stage disease and instead focuses on primary prevention that every patient can engage in at any time.

In support of the shift from limited screening for secondary prevention to proactive primary prevention, the USPSTF has initiated new recommendations

Table 6.4 USPSTF Grades of Evidence: Grade A: Strongly Recommended Grade B Recommended, Grade C No Recommendation (service can improve health outcomes but balance of harm and evidence too close to justify recommendation) Grade D Not Recommended Grade I Insufficient Evidence[18]

Condition	USPSTF Guideline	IPM Expansion
Colorectal Cancer	Adults, beginning at age 50 years and continuing until age 75 years (Grade A)	All ages to increase physical activity, fiber with plant-based foods, decrease red meat and alcohol intake, and smoking cessation
Healthful Diet and Physical Activity to Prevent Cardiovascular Disease (CVD)	Adults BMI>25 with additional CVD risk factors (Grade B) General population (Grade C) Intensive behavioral counseling on lifestyle changes	All ages could benefit greatly from simple behavioral counseling and motivational interviewing with action plans and healthy lifestyle goals
Diabetes Mellitus	Adults, sustained blood pressure (either treated or untreated) greater than 135/80 mm Hg (Grade B)	Screen adolescents and adults with risk factors even if asymptomatic, all ages prevent insulin resistance with diet and physical activity action plans for lifestyle change
Low-Back Pain	Insufficient to recommend for or against the routine use of interventions to prevent low-back pain in adults in primary care settings (Grade 1)	All ages, specific low-back exercises and ergonomic changes for desk-based jobs to strengthen low-back muscles and prevent injury

for the prevention of cardiovascular disease through evidence-based physical activity and dietary changes such as the Mediterranean diet.[23] As shown in Table 6.4, this is given a grade B recommendation for those who are overweight or obese and have specific cardiovascular risk factors. The recommendation is grade C for the same basic lifestyle health education for the general public, and there is a note in both cases on potential harms including "the lost opportunity to provide other services that have a greater health effect." This statement suggests there is a time limit on what can be done with any given patient. Although our current practice of primary care is an episodic approach based on the acute care model of care, much can be done to expand health education and improve health literacy beyond these visits. Although little evidence exists to recommend this by the USPSTF, an IPM perspective questions the relevance of this approach to a basic health education issue. Given the easy accessibility and lack of side effects for these lifestyle changes to prevent cardiovascular disease, there is little to no conceivable harm in sharing this information with patients. In fact, health education of this type will help to thwart the misinformation and false claims of the food industry that continuously bombard the general public through many media outlets. Taking a broader perspective, IPM leverages media and community health education programs to disseminate prevention knowledge such as the Mediterranean diet to the general population. Innovative models of care can be developed to expand this beyond current practices. Therefore, IPM enables physicians and the healthcare team to intervene at multiple levels of patient engagement to promote health throughout the lifespan. Through IPM, primary care physicians attempt to not only detect early stage disease through screening but also discover risk factors in the form of behavioral practices that contribute to the development of chronic disease and thereby focus on primordial prevention beyond traditional primary care visits and restrictive guidelines.

Integrative Preventive Medicine Fosters the Development of Innovation in Primary Care

In redefining the approach to prevention beyond restrictive guidelines, IPM fosters the development of innovative models of primary care where the patient is the focus and the relationship over time is leveraged to optimize chronic disease prevention. Integrative preventive medicine goes beyond diagnosing and treating patients to include lifestyle interventions to prevent disease and promote health. The longitudinal nature of primary care enables it to facilitate behavioral change incrementally over time based on a therapeutic relationship between the provider and the patient. This relationship has come under significant duress in our current system, where providers are pressed for time and unable to delve deeper into the social and nonbiological elements that largely determine the chronic diseases of their patients.[7] Changes in healthcare delivery such as the advent of managed care and the persistence of fee for service reimbursement based on the acute care model has resulted in a volume-based practice structure where primary care physicians move through patients like "hamsters on a treadmill."[29] This model is largely a result of the misapplication of the acute care approach to the current burden of chronic disease. Being overworked and dissatisfied, primary care physicians are powerless to provide adequate access for acute care visits and limited in their ability to provide state-of-the-art chronic care.[30] A shift toward a preventive care model through implementation of IPM in family and community medicine aligns with the emerging shift from volume-based to value-based reimbursement.

By using family and community medicine to prevent disease and maintain health, IPM shifts the focus of care from "sick" to "healthy" visits. Given current models of reimbursement that are based on the acute care system of disease management, most patients do not go to their doctor unless they are sick and experiencing disease symptoms or illness. An integrative prevention-based model requires a shift in reimbursement patterns from fee for service in treating acute conditions to value-based reimbursement that pays primary care provider health systems to keep their patients healthy over time. The move toward value-based reimbursement is likely to accelerate in the coming years to stem the exorbitant costs of care. The shift has already resulted in the emergence of disruptive models of primary care innovation that are currently being studied and discussed in public forums.[31] An initiative funded by the Robert Wood Johnson Foundation known as the LEAP program has identified a team-based approach as a key innovation to improving primary care in the management and prevention of chronic disease.[32] Integrative preventive medicine fosters this type of innovation by recognizing the need for a preventive model of care that is best suited to the chronic diseases of our time. For example, the Diabetes Prevention Program (DPP) has been extensively studied as a community-based approach to preventing diabetes that is efficacious, safe, and cost-effective.[33] Expanding this type of approach beyond traditional sick care visits to include the greater community and healthcare team is a key part of IPM in primary care. Similar to DPP, group visits and workshops can be powerful tools for IPM. Involving health education and the development of peer group dynamics, this format is well suited to chronic disease care and prevention. Such new models of care based on the IPM prevention model will align with value-based changes in healthcare to reinforce the therapeutic relationship as a means to stem the tide of chronic disease through effective dissemination of primary prevention strategies.

Conclusions

Our current system is over 100 years old. It is based on outdated epidemiology and therefore focused on acute care. Our current epidemic of chronic disease demands a new model that shifts the focus from acute treatment to chronic disease prevention. Integrative preventive medicine reinvents family and community medicine to create a new model of care. This model is based on prevention with the goals of morbidity compression and expansion of functional capacity throughout the lifespan. It does not presuppose cure but rather anticipates and forestalls the development of chronic disease through novel evidence-based preventive therapies. The focus of primary care is therefore expanded beyond disease diagnosis and treatment to include primary prevention through lifestyle changes over time. The implications of IPM for family and community medicine are reaching in scope requiring a reevaluation of existing visit structures, screening practices, and reimbursement models. Research in primary prevention strategies needs to be expanded and subsidized to develop evidence-based interventions at all ages that are amenable to self-care, cost-effective, and safe. The science of behavioral change will become critical to identify mechanisms to catalyze the move toward healthy lifestyles on a population level. To support these changes in primary care practice, policy must also be developed to address the social and economic determinants of disease. Such changes will legislate on environmental toxins, the built environment, and the food industry to be accountable for their respective impact on chronic disease and health. The refined IPM model of primary care should be taught as part of medical education to ensure a baseline of competency for providing preventive approaches to patients at risk for chronic disease diagnosis and progression. This will require the expansion of motivational interviewing and health education in the undergraduate medical school curriculum. With these and other changes, the role of family and community medicine will be redefined to serve as the chief means for implementing a new prevention model to stem the tide of lives lost from the chronic diseases of our time.

References

1. *Healthy People 2020*. Washington, DC: US Department of Health and Human Services, 2010. http://www.healthypeople.gov/2020/default.aspx. Accessed August 15, 2015.

2. Fleming D. William H. *Welch and the Rise of Modern Medicine*. Boston: Little, Brown; 1954.

3. Jones DS, Podolsky SH, Greene JA. The burden of disease and the changing task of medicine. *N Engl J Med* 2012;366:2333–2338.

4. Marvasti FF, Stafford RS. From sick care to health care—reengineering prevention into the U.S. system. *N Engl J Med* 2012;367:889–891.

5. McNamara JJ, Molot MA, Stremple JF, Cutting RT. Coronary artery disease in combat casualties in Vietnam. *JAMA* 1971;216(7):1185–1187.

6. Bodenheimer T, Pham HH. Primary care: current problems and proposed solutions. *Health Affair* 2010;29(5):799–805.

7. Schroeder SA. We can do better—improving the health of the American people. *N Engl J Med* 2007;357:1221–1228.

8. Merriam-Webster Dictionary. *Prevent.* http://www.merriam-webster.com/diction-ary/prevent. Accessed March 13, 2011.

9. Vayalil PK, Kuttan G, Kuttan R. Rasayanas: evidence for the concept of prevention of diseases. *Am J Chin Med* 30:155–171.

10. Fries JF. Aging, natural death, and the compression of morbidity. *N Engl J Med* 1980;303:130–135.

11. Archana Singh-Manoux, et al. Timing of onset of cognitive decline: results from Whitehall II prospective cohort study. *BMJ* 2012;344:d7622.

12. Centers for Disease Control and Prevention. *Health United States, 2014: At a Glance.* 2014. http://www.cdc.gov/nchs/data/hus/hus14.pdf. Accessed August 15, 2015.

13. Rowe JW, Kahn RL. Successful aging. *Gerontologist* 1997;37(4):433–440.

14. Brody JE. *Good Habits Outweigh Genes as Key to a Healthy Old Age.* New York Times, February 23, 1996C, 9:1.

15. Katz D, Ather A. *Preventive Medicine, Integrative Medicine and the Health of the Public.* Commissioned for the IOM Summit on Integrative Medicine and the Health of the Public. 2009.

16. Beilby J. Definition of metabolic syndrome: report of the National Heart, Lung, and Blood Institute/American Heart Association Conference on Scientific Issues Related to Definition. *Clin Biochem Rev* 2004;25(3):195–198.

17. Christie D, Channon S. The potential for motivational interviewing to improve outcomes in the management of diabetes and obesity in paediatric and adult populations: a clinical review. *Diabetes Obes Metab* 2014;16(5):381–387.

18. Handley MA, MacGregor K, Schillinger D, Sharifi C, Wong S, Bodenheimer T. Using action plans to help primary care patients adopt healthy behaviors: a descriptive study. *J Am Board Family Med* 2006;19:224–231.

19. MacGregor K, Handley M, Wong S, Sharifi C, Gjeltema K, Schillinger D, Bodenheimer T. Behavior-change action plans in primary care: a feasibility study of clinicians. *J Am Board Family Med* 2006;19:215–223.

20. Lorig K, Holman H, Sobel D, Laurent D, Gonzalez V, Minor M. *Living a Healthy Life with Chronic Conditions.* 4th ed. Bull Publishing Company, 2012. https://www.bull-pub.com/catalog/Living-a-Healthy-Life-with-Chronic-Conditions-4th-Edition

21. OED Online. *Doctor*, n. Oxford University Press. September 19, 2015.

22. Petrella RJ, Koval JJ, Cunningham DA, Paterson DH. Can primary care doctors prescribe exercise to improve fitness? *Am J Prev Med* 2003;24(4):316–322.

23. Estruch R, Ros E, Salas-Salvadó J, et al. Primary Prevention of Cardiovascular Disease with a Mediterranean Diet. *N Engl J Med* 2013; 368:1279–1290, April 4, 2013.

24. Robinson, TN, Sirard JR. Preventing childhood obesity. *Am J Prev Med* 2005;28(Suppl 2):194–201.

25. US Preventive Services Task Force. *Recommendations for Primary Care Practice.* 2015. http://www.uspreventiveservicestaskforce.org/Page/Name/recommendations.

26. Cancer Statistics Working Group. *United States Cancer Statistics: 1999–2012 Incidence and Mortality Web-Based Report.* Atlanta, GA: Department of Health and Human Services, Centers for Disease Control and Prevention, and National Cancer Institute; 2015.

27. Carroll KK. Experimental evidence of dietary factors and hormone-dependent cancers. *Cancer Res* 1975;35:3374–3383.
28. *Colorectal Cancer 2011 Report: Food, Nutrition, Physical Activity and the Prevention of Colorectal Cancer.* American Institute for Cancer Research and World Cancer Research Fund; 2011.
29. Morrison I, Smith R. Hamster health care: time to stop running faster and redesign health care. *BMJ* 2000;321:1541–1542.
30. Bodenheimer, T. Innovations in primary care in the United States. *Brit Med J* 2003;326:796–799.
31. Robert Graham Center. 2014. *Primary Care Forums: Disruptive Innovations in Primary Care.* http://www.graham-center.org/rgc/press-events/events/forums/disruptive-innovations.html.
32. Laden MD, Bodenheimer T, Fishman NW, et al. The emerging primary care workforce: preliminary observations from the primary care team: learning from effective ambulatory practices project. *Acad Med* 2013;88(12):1830–1834.
33. Lawlor MS, Blackwell CS, Isorn SP, et al. Cost of group translation of the diabetes prevention program. *Am J Prev Med* 2013;44(4):S381–S389.

7

Place and Well-Being

The Next Frontier of Integrative Preventive Medicine

CASEY M. LINDBERG, PHD, MARCH, MEREDITH A. BANASIAK,
MARCH, EDAC, RYAN M. SHINDLER, BSARCH, AND
ESTHER M. STERNBERG, MD

Introduction and Framework

Overwhelmingly, evidence shows that health is directly correlated with the environment. Indeed, the World Health Organization has long defined health as more than the absence of disease,[1] yet more recently, other organizations have emphasized the impact of the physical environment on health. In fact, the US Department of Health and Human Services Secretary's Advisory Committee has adopted a *place-based* approach recognizing the physical environment, both natural and built, as a key influence on health.[2,3] It is thus imperative for integrative medicine practitioners to incorporate information about optimal environments in their toolkits for disease prevention.

Despite this emphasis on the importance of place and the environment on health, a 2014 market report, based on a national survey, suggests that less than half of medical professionals are aware of the impact of the built environment on health, and only 15% reported receiving information on design and health connections.[4] This is in contrast to a large majority of design professionals' awareness of this connection.[4] Responding to the challenge to increase awareness of health-environment connections among health professionals and the general public, the design and construction communities aim to connect with medical partners to increase the research and evidence communicated to health professionals, and to make more explicit the alignment between the environment and top rated health risk factors such as obesity and chronic stress.

Among the first attempts to characterize interactions between people and environment was Kurt Lewin's force field analysis, which describes behavior as the function of the individual and the environment.[5] However, Lewin's "environment" was a social environment and abstract in the physical sense. Soon after, the neuropsychologist Donald Hebb noted behavioral improvements in laboratory rats that were taken home as pets to more enriched environments.[6] Over the following decades, several studies reported various characteristics of neurological plasticity resulting from environmental stimulation.[7] More recently, the discovery of adult neurogenesis has revealed that the physical environment continually shapes brain structure and function. Indeed, animal studies indicate that enriched environments are correlated with improved cognitive performance.[7] The latter finding may in part be related to increased activity, and therefore greater physical exercise, of animals placed in enriched environments. These discoveries advanced place-based research on cognition and performance by providing animal models to triangulate relationships between brain, body, and environment.

Evidence-based design (EBD), one means of improving health impacts through the built environment, emerged over the last two decades, drawing on the tradition of evidence-based medicine. In this chapter, we use an EBD approach to describe key linkages, distilled from current research, between health and the physical environment that are most relevant to providing an environment-based health context for clinical practitioners. This material is organized according to the six key areas correlating health and design defined by the American Institute of Architects (AIA): environmental quality, natural systems, sensory environments, physical activity, safety, and social connectedness.[8] Recognizing that the physical environment is interconnected with other determinants of health,[3] this chapter is meant to augment the material provided by other integrative preventive practices defined in this volume.

Importantly, the following sections are not intended to serve as an exhaustive review of the related literature but rather as a snapshot of some of the seminal work as well as some key recent developments. The former would be beyond the scope of this chapter; it is important to note that each section has an associated literature that is quickly growing both in depth and breadth, each with its own implications for recommendations impacting health and well-being.

Environmental Quality

Since the initial epidemiological connection between health and the environment in John Snow's mapping of the water supply and the cholera outbreak in England in 1854,[9,10] the study and regulation of health risks and hazards of the environment have notably expanded to air quality. In fact, when associating connections between health and the environment, medical professionals reported the greatest familiarity with the category of environmental quality concerns relating to acute illness factors such as mold and air pollution.[4] Increased urbanization has led to concentrated and increased risk factors for health risks associated with air pollution from motor vehicles, electricity generation, and industrial pollution, and may account for the deaths of approximately 1.2 million people worldwide each year due to cardiovascular and respiratory diseases.[11] In recent decades, inner cities have been particularly affected with rising asthma rates, especially among children, the cause of which is unknown but could be related to higher amounts of cockroach dust exposure in those areas.[12]

Toxins in the air (in addition to those in water, soil, and food) have a disproportionately high effect on children as, pound for pound, they breathe more air than adults, are less able to deal with toxins, have more disruptable physiological systems due to growth and development, and have more years of life remaining to develop chronic diseases.[13]

Indoor air quality can affect health and well-being just as outdoor air quality can. Humans are an increasingly indoor species, with the developed world spending over 90% of their time indoors.[14] Though the regulatory mechanisms for indoor environmental quality (IEQ) have historically focused on avoiding dangerous levels of certain air quality characteristics, environmental quality has the potential not only to prevent illness and disease but also to *optimize* wellness and psychological well-being. Moreover, recent developments in IEQ literature have signaled a change in direction from the study of specific chemical pollutants and particulate matter to the interaction between the individuals inhabiting a space and design factors.[15]

One commonly measured and monitored chemical in the indoor environment is carbon dioxide (CO_2), a good indicator of the performance of ventilation and the occupancy of a controlled space. Building standards define certain levels of CO_2 that are known to be harmful to human health, and other levels that are associated with reports of stuffiness and drowsiness. Because ventilation accounts for a large proportion of energy use in buildings, natural ventilation (i.e., operable windows) is often offered as a design solution to save on costs. However, such strategies must be carefully applied with climate in mind, as CO_2 levels have been found to readily exceed acceptable levels in seasons when building occupants are unlikely to open windows.[16] Green building designs (e.g., low-polluting building materials, sufficient ventilation rates) have been found to be associated with better occupant health outcomes compared to nongreen building designs, but empirical research is lacking.[17] One recent experiment manipulated CO_2 and volatile organic compound levels, and found that participants exhibited significantly higher performance on an array of cognitive tests under conditions that mirrored green building practices of ventilation compared to nongreen building practices.[18] When ventilation rates went beyond the recommended levels for green building operations, decreased concentrations of CO_2 were still associated with increased cognitive task performance.[18] Similar trends of cognitive performance have also been shown in children during a classroom-setting manipulation of ventilation rates.[19] Ventilation rates are typically based on meeting standards while saving on energy costs, but other indirect human costs are relevant, like employee sick leave, absenteeism, and presenteeism. In one study of 40 buildings within a single company, higher rates of sick leave and IEQ complaints were associated with lower levels of outdoor air supply.[20]

Current advances in personal ventilation technology allow for the increased understanding of how clean air exchange and flow affects human health, well-being, and performance. Personal ventilation directs the flow of clean air to the individual's breathing zone rather than to the volume of the entire room, and has been associated with increased perceived air quality and both subjective and objective measures of performance, all while being an energy-saving model of building operation.[21]

Natural Systems

The physical, mental, and social benefits associated with a connection with nature are widely documented, and attest to the importance of engaging with nature in everyday lives. The effects of nature have been linked with benefits such as improved attention, cognitive functioning and test scores, reduced stress, improved mood and coping skills, and enhanced immune functioning.[22] Children's contact with nature has also been linked with physical and psychological health as well as social, sensory, and creativity benefits.[23] Studies suggest that nature benefits result from both direct contact with nature, such as taking a walk through a park, and passive engagement with nature, such as observing nature through a window. In Roger Ulrich's seminal study in 1984, postoperative patients in rooms with views of nature (versus those viewing a brick wall) stayed fewer days in the hospital and took significantly less pain medication.[24] Similarly Sullivan and Kuo[25] showed less violence and improved social interactions in people randomly assigned to apartments with a view of a grove of trees as compared to a brick wall. Many have attributed such overwhelming beneficial effects to the biophilia hypothesis, which proposes that humans have an instinctual attraction to biological and natural elements that support and sustain life.[26]

With respect to the built environment, biophilic design attempts to capture the therapeutic effects of nature by incorporating natural and biological elements directly, indirectly, or symbolically, which reflects the inherent human affinity for nature.[27,28] This includes strategies such as bringing living elements like vegetative facades into buildings and using naturally occurring shapes and patterns such as botanical motifs in building forms or materials. At the neighborhood level, a recent study in an urban setting showed that having a tree density equivalent to 11 more trees in a city block resulted in fewer cardio-metabolic conditions, equivalent to the health status of having an increase in annual personal income of $20,000, or being 1.4 years younger.[29]

Exposure to natural features, such as walks in parks, has been linked with improved performance and restored attention following fatigue.[30,31] Studies have shown that indirect exposure to nature for as little as 6 minutes may provide an attention boost equivalent to caffeine, in young and older adults.[32] Similarly, children diagnosed with attention deficits experienced improved concentration with results similar to those of a common medication for ADD after a 20-minute walk in a nature-like park setting when compared with walks in downtown and residential neighborhoods.[33] Walking in a natural setting versus an urban setting has also been associated with lowered self-reports of rumination and activity in the associated area of the prefrontal cortex.[34] Such findings suggest safe, inexpensive implications for including short nature breaks in daily routines and may serve to benefit myriad user groups.

Unfortunately, according to reports from developed countries around the world, active outdoor play and nature exploration are in decline as a result of factors including children's and parents' fears about the dangers of playing outside, the lure of indoor recreational activities such as television and computer games, and the loss of natural areas.[35,36] This trend is evidenced across rural, suburban, and urban settings as well as across socioeconomic classes. Play in nature is critical to development not only because of the benefits associated with physical activity, but also because it has been associated with increased performance on tests of motor fitness such as balance and agility.[37]

Improvements in quantitative measures of the stress and immune response have also been associated with nature exposure. A review on nature and immune functioning[22] identified several studies with beneficial results from blood tests taken before and after nature walks, compared with urban walks, including an increase in cardioprotective and diabetic factors such as DHEA,[38] adiponectin,[38] and normalized blood glucose.[39] The Japanese practice *Shinrin-yoku*, or taking in the atmosphere of the forest, has been linked with measures of relaxation and reduced stress such as lower blood pressure, lower pulse rate, and lower concentrations of cortisol.[40] Recent studies have established a significant correlation between cortisol levels and self-reports of stress with the quantity of green space in residential areas,[41] which suggests that cortisol can be used as a biomarker to measure short-term environmental effects on stress.

The presence of green space is especially important in economically disadvantaged communities where health disparities and related chronic stress are more severe.[41] Contact with nature has been shown to be an effective pain management strategy for elderly residents and patients in direct and indirect applications such as gardening,[42] natural murals and sounds,[43] window views,[24] and in-room potted plants.[44] Moreover, a meta-analysis of nature and health studies led reviewers to conclude that contact with nature has a positive effect on psychological well-being, including reductions in anger, fatigue, anxiety, and sadness.[45]

Healthcare providers can promote cognitive, physical, and psychological benefits of contact with nature by routinely asking about a patient's exposure to nature in patient interviews and by writing nature prescriptions. Medicine–nature collaborations such as the National Environmental Education Foundation's (NEEF) Rx for Outdoor Activity program have gained momentum in cities such as San Francisco and Washington, DC (DC Parks Rx), by providing a tool that healthcare providers can use to prescribe safe and accessible interactions with nature.

Sensory Environments

Perhaps the greatest advances in scientific understanding on how the built environment affects human health, well-being, and performance fall under the umbrella of sensation and perception. Visual, auditory, and thermal comfort consistently rank high in studies of complaints about workplace characteristics, and these areas of sensation also represent those that are best studied most frequently, particularly research on lighting conditions.

Among the best-established relationship between light and mood comes from the depression literature. It is firmly established that full spectrum light therapy is highly effective in treating symptoms of seasonal affective disorder—a form of depression related to long periods of exposure to low light levels. Yet there are many other relevant applications to different populations. There is evidence that inpatients with bipolar depression staying in hospital rooms exposed to eastern morning light had significantly shorter hospital stays compared to those with western exposure.[46] Patients recovering from elective cervical and lumbar spinal surgery on the more brightly daylit side of another hospital experienced less perceived stress and took less analgesic medication than those in rooms on the more dimly daylit side.[47] Likewise, in yet another hospital, female patient stay post heart attack was also shorter in sunnier rooms compared to less daylit rooms.[48]

Benefits of day-lighting are also seen for nonpatient populations. Residential homes' exposure to sunlight has been found to be negatively associated with mortality from breast, ovarian, prostate, and colon cancer.[49] Likewise, exposing normal, healthy adults to bright light for extended periods of time has been shown to help lower reported levels of anxiety.[50] In an office setting in Finland, exposing employees to brighter light during wintertime boosted subjective vitality and reduced depressive symptoms.[51] Additionally, effects of lighting can be seen in animal studies. For example, rats in a lab setting showed increased growth of human xenograft breast cancer when subjected to electric light at night.[52] This finding contributes to the growing evidence for health and well-being risks in shift workers with artificially compromised circadian rhythms.

Importantly, circadian rhythms are affected by different *types* of light exposure as well. Shorter-wavelength blue light is most effective at triggering our body's internal clock, and is therefore important for circadian shifting when we need to adapt to a new sleep schedule. In one recent study, volunteers were prescribed a shift in their sleeping schedule, but only those who received doses of blue light when they woke up each morning, and orange light when before they went to bed in the evening, showed adaptive circadian phase shifting as measured by melatonin levels.[53] In another study, patients with Alzheimer's disease and related dementia showed improved sleep time and efficiency, improved circadian rhythm, and reduced depression and agitation scores when exposed during the daytime to blue light.[54] Because blue light is often emitted by electronic devices such as computer and smartphone screens, exposure after dark can be problematic for all populations, including adolescents, who may be even more sensitive.[55] Various software products have been recently gaining attention for their ability to filter emitted blue light from computer and smartphone screens.

Often, implementing light manipulation interventions in real-world settings can be difficult because little is known about design factors that contribute to visual discomfort, such as glare. Some evidence suggests that luminance, type of window view, and even the distance of objects in that view all can affect reported discomfort.[56] Workers in one large office building were more annoyed with glare in winter months when there was deeper daylight penetration compared to summer months,[57] while in another study workers experienced less subjective glare for daylit conditions (without a view) compared with electric lighting. Deeper sunlight penetration has been found to be positively correlated with job satisfaction and general well-being,[58] while other research has demonstrated differences in physiological but not subjective out-comes. In one study, workers in renovated areas with increased day-lighting exhibited higher levels of physiological indicators of well-being—heart rate variability and cortisol—at night compared to those in areas with less day-lighting, even though participants' subjective reports did not differ on mood and stress measures.[59] Interestingly, little is known about the immediate effects of light on performance. For example, in one study, light levels were related to frontal activity on an electroencephalogram but not actual performance on a working memory task.[60]

More is understood about the effects both chronic and acute noise have on subjective performance and other psychological and physiological well-being outcomes. Perhaps because noise is a common source for complaints in work environments, much of what we know about the effects of different acoustic environments comes from applied research in real-life work settings and in simulated settings with tasks that represent real work.

Building on previous research showing that different types of noise can be detrimental for cognitive functioning and hospital patient outcomes, one study investigated the impact of shorter, 30-minute exposures of quiet versus prerecorded emergency room sounds on physicians' performance on a set of medical questions.[61] There was not a significant difference in task performance, yet physicians found the noisier conditions more distressing.[61] However, other studies have shown that people can be subjectively unaware of how different noise conditions can affect them both behaviorally and physiologically. In one study, participants were exposed to different conditions of noise, simulating open office noise and a quieter environment, for bouts of 3 hours.[62] Although participants did not perceive differences in stress, those in the noisy condi-tion exhibited elevated urinary epinephrine levels (but not norepinephrine or cortisol), showed lower motivation in attempting to solve a puzzle, and even made fewer ergonomic adjustments to their workstations compared to those in the quiet condition.[62] Interestingly, other research has found that the type of noise to which people are exposed, particularly low-frequency noise, matters a great deal.

In a lab setting, when participants were exposed to low-frequency noise, they exhibited poorer performance on proofreading and grammatical reason-ing tasks and felt more annoyed than when they were exposed to a mixed noise condition of the same intensity.[63] The effects were more pronounced for those who rated themselves as highly sensitive to noise, and the normal cir-cadian cortisol decline during the session was also impaired.[63] Low-frequency noise can have other detrimental effects as well—in fact, very low frequency noise has been found to cause aural pain in many studies.[64] Taken together, these findings indicate that noise, especially low-frequency noise, consistently stimulates the physiological stress response whether or not those who are exposed are subjectively aware of it.

In real-world research settings, even though the effects of single variables on performance, behavior, and physiological and psychological outcomes are difficult to disentangle, they are important to review. In open-office settings there are several contributing factors besides noise (e.g., light, architectural features, social dynamics, air quality, thermal comfort) that may affect observed differences. In one study, workers in an open plan setting were more likely to perceive noise and thermal discomfort, central nervous system symptoms, and mucous membrane irritation compared to workers in more cellular (i.e., enclosed) office settings.[65] In another study, workers in open plan settings also reported more displeasure with noise levels compared to those in more private settings, yet those in the more private offices did not experience the beneficial social aspects those in the open plan enjoyed.[66] Lack of control, personalization, type of work, and perceived privacy are all other important factors in determining the appropriateness of workspace design.

One recent workplace development is the "flex" office, where employees spend a significant portion of their time teleworking, and have no assigned workspaces when they are in the office. Studies of this type of design have reported a lack of control and personalization, but better ratings compared to strict open plan offices on several dimensions including social interaction and privacy.[66] In another study, a switch from private to open plan offices was particularly detrimental for people whose work was less collaborative, as participants felt decreases in privacy, concentration, and performance, and increases in distraction and coping behavior.[67] Interestingly, the noise levels were similar in this study, but the patterns were different; the private offices had noise patterns with more variability over time compared to the open plan office space.[66]

Individual differences clearly matter when determining a design strategy for workspaces. We have seen how individual differences in noise sensitivity can affect reported impacts of environments on health outcome variables. Other research is beginning to uncover interactions between variables like personality, age, and workspace design characteristics. This is important because it may help us understand why significant proportions of building occupants are often not satisfied even when all design standards are met.[68] One study showed the importance of measuring personality variables in the context of work space design. Compared to those low on neuroticism, workers high on neuroticism experienced less perceived control over workspaces that were rated as more exposed, while no differences were found between workspaces rated as more enclosed.[69]

Importantly, other interactions, like those *between* environmental variables typically measured in isolation, may also be important. Advances in wearable sensing technology for environmental and physiological variables make this possible when combined with, and not merely replacing, more common methodologies for collecting subjective measures.

Physical Activity

The health benefits of exercise and regular physical activity have been well documented and have consistently been emphasized in policy interventions at many levels of government. Because the environment plays a dynamic role in the decisions individuals make regarding physical activity, a recent concentration of emphasis on built environment interventions has gained momentum. If fact, the US surgeon general and Department of Health and Human Services recently initiated Step it Up!—a call to action for promoting walking and walkable communities.[70]

Community-scaled design interventions can have lasting public health benefits when the factors of the built environment leading to increased physical activity are better understood. It is well established that higher levels of street connectivity, residential density, and mixed-use land usage (i.e., developments that have a mix of residential and commercial spaces) are associated with higher physical activity.[71] Also, neighborhoods that are low in mixed use and are characterized by curvilinear suburban development are also associated with less walkability.[72] Physical activity is also affected by the availability of the natural environment and view of nature. However, more research is needed to better understand the individual motivating mechanisms that play roles in people's choices to interact with nature. For instance, policies that highlight how the natural environment can motivate physical activity routines may be beneficial.[73]

A current challenge is to develop valid and reliable measures to study the effectiveness of design interventions on physical activity and health. Because there are many types of outcome measurements employed including traditional surveys, geographic information system data, and direct observational measures, there is a large amount of variability in how specific programs aimed at promoting physical activity are evaluated.[74] Policy intervention grading systems with the highest tiers reserved for evaluations that rely on significant positive health outcomes in peer-reviewed studies might be part of the solution going forward.[75]

Characteristics of the built environment that affect physical activity in vulnerable populations, such as children and older adults, are particularly important to understand. Several studies have shown that children's activity levels are linked to publicly provided recreational facilities, sidewalk availability, access to public transportation, and controlled intersections.[76] Interestingly, perceived neighborhood safety appears to be an important predictor for adult activity[72] but less of a clear link for children.[75] For a community to truly be walkable for older adults, specific barriers need to be addressed. Environmental hazards like traffic and fall risks are examples of these barriers and are closely tied to older adults' walking choices.[77]

At the building scale, characteristics of the built environment may play a critical role in physical activity choices that people make on a daily basis. It is known that office workers tend to be more sedentary during certain hours of the workday and at night,[78] but we do not fully understand the features of space that can interact with social dynamics and types of work to encourage nonsedentary behavior and shorter sitting bouts. Two such successful interventions are the adoption of point-of-decision prompts and prominent staircases.

Point-of-decision prompts are those that prompt the occupant to consider a choice they have, such as taking the stairs or the elevator, using signage or other strategies. Several studies of this type of intervention have shown evidence of increased physical activity, but experts caution that the local context is important to understand.[79] For instance, when one office building's staircase was decorated with interactive paintings, maps, and storyboards that the occupants could contribute to, staircase use dramatically increased,[80] but such a tailored intervention may have a different impact depending on each office's culture. Additionally, many forward-thinking companies, organizations, and schools have implemented dynamic, flexible design solutions like standing desks for both individual and team work.

Safety

Optimizing safety features in an environment can positively impact physical and psychological aspects of health and well-being. Accessibility, or how well a room, building, or neighborhood can support the needs of people across cognitive, sensory, physical, and psychological domains, provides a means to gauge the safety, whether real or perceived, of an environment. Increased accessibility benefits not only persons with disabilities but also people across the lifespan with different developmental capabilities and skillsets. Ideally, the demands of the environment should be consistent with the capabilities of the individual using it. For example, lifespan housing designed for aging in place recommends including design features such as zero step entrances and kitchen cabinetry that allows someone to work in a seated position.[81] These practices are increasingly becoming the standard in communities for those 55 years and older. While some aspects of public space design supporting physical accessibility are federally regulated through the American with Disabilities Act standards,[82] most other accessibility dimensions such as cognitive and sensory accessibility are less directed. Emerging research on interactions between the environment and sensation, perception, and cognition should be used to update regulations and improve accessibility.

When an environment is perceived to be unsafe, it is psychologically inaccessible. Both real and perceived safety impact health behaviors including the extent to which people walk to school, play outdoors, and connect with their community. A review on crime, health, and environment concluded that while there are well-established direct links between crime and victim health, effects of crime and fear of crime on the well-being of surrounding populations are less clear and may be better assessed by measures of social cohesion.[83] However, reviewers found that the most promising interventions to lessen fear of crime are small-scale interventions that reduce neglect, including reducing litter and vandalization (graffiti), in public areas such as transportation hubs.[82]

Additional threats to personal physical safety and mobility at the neighborhood level often occur along pedestrian and bike routes with improper separation of vehicular traffic or unsafe intersection crossings, poorly maintained paths due to weather or disrepair, and the absence of signage that enhances navigation through complex environments.[84] In 2007, the World Health Organization published a guide to global age-friendly cities, identifying key environmental barriers to active aging across the life cycle.[85] While this guide can benefit designers to improve the quality of the environment and related safety issues, it is also relevant for clinicians to raise awareness of the types of environmental hazards facing aging populations.

Improving accessibility for persons with sensory differences including low vision, deafness, age-related sensory decline, and sensory-processing disorders increases safety and reduces incidence of injury while promoting increased independence, aging in place, and community engagement. Creative design strategies can be used to prevent falls, such as including elements to boost contrasts in elevation changes, and removing head and body obstacles along paths that can cause injury. Other design interventions can be used to improve wayfinding, such as incorporating salient navigation cues with redundancy across the senses. In combination, such design features can create more accessible environments for all populations. In environments and communities where these strategies are lacking, assistive technology devices are increasingly being used to boost awareness of environmental cues and reduce anxiety for managing complex and novel environments.

Much of the EBD research was originally driven by the goal to improve safety and reduce injury to both patients and staff in healthcare settings. Healthcare administrators are increasingly relying on environmental interventions to reduce medical errors. Examples of such design strategies include improving acoustics and eliminating environmental distractions, reducing healthcare-associated infections (HAIs) by eliminating surface air and water points of infection transmission, reducing patient falls by employing nonslip surfaces, and changing unit configurations to improve clinical staff visibility and monitoring of the patient.[86] Healthcare workers can also benefit from EBD practices: reconfiguring the organization of patient rooms has been able to reduce the amount of walking for nursing staff and increase their visibility of patients, and ceiling lifts in patient rooms have decreased staff injuries from lifting patients. All of these interventions have not only health-related benefits but also economic benefits for the consumer and for the healthcare and insurance industries. Clinicians can participate in the design process through role-playing exercises with designers in mocked-up, stage-like settings to improve communication of their practices and needs, including differences in cultural demographics of patients, to optimize the design of the physical environment before it is completed.

Social Connectedness

Social connectedness is an important factor to consider when evaluating a design at the building or community scale, because it can affect how people's relationships develop with neighbors and levels of social support, both key ingredients to sustaining or improving mental health and even buffering against infectious diseases. At the neighborhood scale, social connectedness can be influenced by densities of both traffic and people. In one study, researchers found that residents on busier streets had lower numbers of both friends and acquaintances on those streets compared with residents on less busy streets.[87] In fact, several studies have shown better social connectedness for residents in low-rise or detached homes compared with residents in high-rise buildings.[88] Safety also seems to be connected to social connectedness. In one study of older adults with chronic health problems, higher neighborhood safety predicted higher levels of social cohesion, which in turn predicted participation in everyday activities.[89] Neighborhood walkability may contribute to social connectedness, as it can facilitate participation in activities with other neighbors. At a smaller scale, from the way entrances to residences are set up to the way furniture is arranged within a shared space, the built environment can also influence social connectedness.

Social interactions have been found to be highest in residential units when their entrances are closer rather than farther away, when they are across from one another, and when they connected to major foot traffic paths or gathering areas.[88] However, at certain densities, crowding can become a problem. Increased numbers of families living in multifamily dwellings tend to have poorer parent–child relationships and exhibit more social withdrawal.[88] Moreover, perceived crowding can happen more easily on long corridors versus short corridors. In one classic study that included an experimental manipulation, dorm residents in long corridors were more likely to experience crowding, had more difficulty in regulating social contact with neighbors, and exhibited higher levels of learned helplessness compared with residents living in dorms with shorter corridors.[90] Inside shared spaces, social interactions can also be influenced by the arrangement of furniture and types of workspaces.

By creating focal points of interaction, placing furniture at socially close distances around tables has been shown to lead to increased social interactions in psychiatric patient populations and in the workplace.[88] In the workplace, lines of sight and visual paths can be beneficial for collaboration and social connectedness, but there are important work-related tradeoffs that have to be considered, such as noise pollution.[91] It is important to consider the type of work being done and the existing culture of a workforce before implementing changes from cellular offices to open plan offices, as there are conflicting effects of social benefits and coworker relations in different populations.[66,67,92]

Summary

Both the outdoor and indoor environment play important roles in affecting human health, well-being, and performance. Many of these effects can be taken advantage of in daily life by informed individuals or through recommendations from their physicians. Poor outdoor air quality can lead to disproportional negative health outcomes for children, the elderly, and populations proximate to pollution sources or environmental hazards. Indoor air quality can similarly affect human health, as limited ventilation and chemical off-gassing from building and furniture materials can be detrimental to both health and cognitive performance. Luckily, the natural environment can offer a reprieve from the myriad elements of fatigue and sedentary behavior often found in the indoor environment. Through strategies of either incorporating natural elements within the indoor environment or promoting interaction with nature in parks or similar settings, people of all populations can benefit, both physiologically and psychologically. One element of the natural environment, daylight, can also promote healthy circadian rhythms through the use of windows and other artificial means. Light can also be filtered for different wavelengths later at night. Chronic noise, particularly low-frequency noise, can be detrimental for cognitive performance in many populations, but less is known about the interactions between different sensory elements of the environment, particularly in real-world settings. At the neighborhood level, walkability and mixed-use land planning are paramount. Physical activity can be encouraged by the removal of hazards and the visibility of neighborhood characteristics like markets and parks. Walkable areas are only truly accessible where safety is not a concern, and they can lead to increases in social connectedness, a protective factor for both mental and physical health.

Much of the current literature on the environment's effects on health and well-being is grounded in decades of work in fields with a varied disciplines and histories. Presently, many of these fields are coming together and being further informed by research methods only recently made possible by new technology. Such quantitative data-gathering methods are not meant to displace but rather to complement methods used previously. It is through this kind of scientific relationship that we can begin to truly understand how the environment we as a species have created and manipulated for ourselves can be now tailored to improve life. Given this depth of evidence for the impact of the built and natural environment on physical health and emotional well-being, it is important for integrative medicine practitioners to include information about optimizing environments in their armamentarium of integrative and preventive care.

References

1. World Health Organization. *Preamble to the Constitution of the World Health Organization as Adopted by the International Health Conference.* Vol 100. New York: Author; 1946.
2. US Department of Health and Human Services. The Secretary's Advisory Committee on National Health Promotion and Disease Prevention Objectives for 2020. *Phase I Report: Recommendations for the Framework and Format of Healthy People 2020.* 2008. https://www.healthypeople.gov/sites/default/files/PhaseI_0.pdf
3. US Department of Health and Human Services. *Healthy People 2020: An Opportunity to Address Societal Determinants of Health in the United States.* 2010. https://www.healthypeople.gov/sites/default/files/SocietalDeterminantsHealth.pdf
4. Bernstein HM. The drive toward healthier buildings: the market drivers and impact of building design and construction on occupant health, well-being and productivity. *McGraw Hill Construction—Smart Market Report.* 2014:100. Bedford, MA.
5. Lewin K. Field theory and experiment in social psychology: concepts and methods. *Am J Sociol* 1939;44(6):868–896.
6. Hebb DO. The effects of early experience on problem solving at maturity. *Am Psychol* 1947;2:306–307.
7. Van Praag H, Kempermann G, Gage FH. Neural consequences of environmental enrichment. *Nat Rev Neurosci* 2000;1(3):191–198.

8. The American Institute of Architects. *Design and Health Topics*, Washington, DC: The American Institute of Architects; 2014:6.

9. Snow J. The cholera near Golden-Square, and at Deptford. *Medical Times and Gazette* 1854;9:321–322.

10. Sternberg EM. *Healing Spaces: The Science of Place and Well-Being*. Cambridge, MA: Belknap Press of Harvard University Press; 2009.

11. King B. Environment and health. *International Encyclopedia of the Social and Behavioral Sciences*. Amsterdam: Elsevier; 2015:815–819.

12. Gruchalla RS, Pongracic J, Plaut M, et al. Inner City Asthma Study: relationships among sensitivity, allergen exposure, and asthma morbidity. *J Allergy Clin Immunol* 2005;115(3):478–485.

13. Suk WA, Murray K, Avakian MD. Environmental hazards to children's health in the modern world. *Mutat Res Rev Mutat Res* 2003;544(2-3):235–242.

14. United States Environmental Protection Agency. *Report to Congress on Indoor Air Quality. Volume II: Assessment and Control of Indoor Air Pollution*. Washington, DC: 1989;244.

15. Mitchell CS, Zhang JJ, Sigsgaard T, et al. Current state of the science: health effects and indoor environmental quality. *Environ Health Perspect* 2007;115(6):958–964.

16. Ilyas S, Emery A, Heerwagen J, Heerwagen D. Occupant perceptions of an indoor thermal environment in a naturally ventilated building. *ASHRAE Trans* 2012;118:114–121.

17. Allen JG, MacNaughton P, Laurent JG, Flanigan SS, Eitland ES, Spengler JD. Green buildings and health. *Curr Environ Health Rep* 2015;2(3):250–258.

18. Allen JG, MacNaughton P, Satish U, Santanam S, Vallarino J, Spengler JD. Associations of cognitive function scores with carbon dioxide, ventilation, and volatile organic compound exposures in office workers: a controlled exposure study of green and conventional office environments. *Environ Health Perspect* 2015:1–32.

19. Coley DA, Greeves R, Saxby BK. The effect of low ventilation rates on the cognitive function of a primary school class. *Int J Vent* 2004;6(2):107–112.

20. Milton DK, Glencross PM, Walters MD. Risk of sick leave associated with outdoor air supply rate, humidification, and occupant complaints. *Indoor Air* 2000;10(4):212–221.

21. Melikov AK, Skwarczynski MA, Kaczmarczyk J, Zabecky J. Use of personalized ventilation for improving health, comfort, and performance at high room temperature and humidity. *Indoor Air* 2013;23(3):250–263.

22. Kuo M. How might contact with nature promote human health? Promising mechanisms and a possible central pathway. *Front Psychol* 2015;6:1093.

23. Chawla L. Benefits of nature contact for children. *J Plan Lit* 2015;30(4):433–452.

24. Ulrich R. View through a window may influence recovery from surgery. *Science* 1984;224(4647):420–421.

25. Taylor AF, Kuo FE, Sullivan WC. Views of nature and self-discipline: evidence from inner city children. *J Environ Psychol* 2002;22(1-2):49–63.

26. Wilson EO. *Biophilia*. Cambridge, MA: Harvard University Press; 1984.

27. Kellert SR, Heerwagen J, Mador M. *Biophilic Design: The Theory, Science and Practice of Bringing Buildings to Life*. Hoboken, NJ: Wiley; 2008.

28. Heerwagen J. Biophilia, health, and well-being. *Restorative Commons: Creating Health and Well-Being Through Urban Landscapes.* US Department of Agriculture, Forest Service, Northern Research Station; Newtown Square, PA; 2009:38–57.
29. Kardan O, Gozdyra P, Misic B, et al. Neighborhood greenspace and health in a large urban center. *Sci Rep* 2015;5:11610.
30. Kaplan S. The restorative benefits of nature: toward an integrative framework. *J Environ Psychol* 1995;15(3):169–182.
31. Berman MG, Jonides J, Kaplan S. The cognitive benefits of interacting with nature. *Psychol Science* 2008;19(12):1207–1212.
32. Gamble KR, Howard JH Jr, Howard DV. Not just scenery: viewing nature pictures improves executive attention in older adults. *Exp Aging Res* 2014;40(5):513–530.
33. Faber Taylor A, Kuo FE. Children with attention deficits concentrate better after walk in the park. *J Atten Disord* 2009;12(5):402–409.
34. Bratman GN, Hamilton JP, Hahn KS, Daily GC, Gross JJ. Nature experience reduces rumination and subgenual prefrontal cortex activation. *Proc Natl Acad Sci U S A* 2015;112(28):8567–8572.
35. Jansson M, Fors H, Lindgren T, Wiström B. Perceived personal safety in relation to urban woodland vegetation—a review. *Urban & Urban Gree* 2013;12(2):127–133.
36. Louv R. *Last Child in the Woods: Saving Our Kids from Nature Deficit Disorder.* Chapel Hill, NC: Algonquin Books of Chapel Hill; 2005.
37. Fjørtoft I. Landscape as playscape: the effects of natural environments on children's play and motor development. *Child Youth Environ* 2004;14(2):21–44.
38. Li Q, Otsuka T, Kobayashi M, et al. Acute effects of walking in forest environments on cardiovascular and metabolic parameters. *Eur J Appl Physiol* 2011;111(11):2845–2853.
39. Ohtsuka Y, Yabunaka N, Takayama S. Shinrin-yoku (forest-air bathing and walking) effectively decreases blood glucose levels in diabetic patients. *Int J Biometeorol* 1998;41(3):125–127.
40. Park BJ, Tsunetsugu Y, Kasetani T, Kagawa T, Miyazaki Y. The physiological effects of Shinrin-yoku (taking in the forest atmosphere or forest bathing): evidence from field experiments in 24 forests across Japan. *Environ Health Prev Med* 2014;15(1):18–26.
41. Ward Thompson C, Roe J, Aspinall P, Mitchell R, Clow A, Miller D. More green space is linked to less stress in deprived communities: evidence from salivary cortisol patterns. *Landscape Urban Plan* 2012;105(3):221–229.
42. Detweiler MB, Sharma T, Detweiler JG, et al. What is the evidence to support the use of therapeutic gardens for the elderly? *Psychiatry Investig* 2012;9(2):100–110.
43. Diette GB, Lechtzin N, Haponik E, Devrotes A, Rubin HR. Distraction therapy with nature sights and sounds reduces pain during flexible bronchoscopy. *Chest* 2003;123(3):941–948.
44. Park S-H. *Randomized Clinical Trials Evaluating Therapeutic Influences of Ornamental Indoor Plants in Hospital Rooms on Health Outcomes of Patients Recovering from Surgery.* Manhattan, KS: Kansas State University; 2006.

45. Bowler DE, Buyung-Ali LM, Knight TM, Pullin AS. A systematic review of evidence for the added benefits to health of exposure to natural environments. *BMC Public Health* 2010;10:456.
46. Benedetti F, Colombo C, Barbini B, Campori E, Smeraldi E. Morning sunlight reduces length of hospitalization in bipolar depression. *J Affect Disord* 2001;62(3):221–223.
47. Walch JM, Rabin BS, Day R, Williams JN, Choi K, Kang JD. The effect of sunlight on postoperative analgesic medication use: a prospective study of patients undergoing spinal surgery. *Psychosom Med* 2005;67(1):156–163.
48. Beauchemin KM, Hays P. Dying in the myocardial in the dark: sunshine, gender and outcomes in infarction. *J R Soc Med* 1998;91(7):352–354.
49. Freedman DM, Dosemeci M, McGlynn K. Sunlight and mortality from breast, ovarian, colon, prostate, and non-melanoma skin cancer: a composite death certificate based case-control study. *Occup Environ Med* 2002;59(4):257–262.
50. Youngstedt SD, Kripke DF. Does bright light have an anxiolytic effect?—An open trial. *BMC Psychiatry* 2007;7:62.
51. Partonen T, Lönnqvist J. Bright light improves vitality and alleviates distress in healthy people. *J Affect Disord* 2000;57(1):55–61.
52. Stevens RG, Brainard GC, Blask DE, Lockley SW, Motta ME. Breast cancer and circadian disruption from electric lighting in the modern world. *CA Cancer J Clin* 2014;64(3):207–218.
53. Appleman K, Figueiro MG, Rea MS. Controlling light-dark exposure patterns rather than sleep schedules determines circadian phase. *Sleep Med* 2013;14(5):456–461.
54. Figueiro MG, Plitnick BA, Lok A, et al. Tailored lighting intervention improves measures of sleep, depression, and agitation in persons with Alzheimer's disease and related dementia living in long-term care facilities. *Clin Interv Aging* 2014;9:1527–1537.
55. Figueiro M, Overington D. Self-luminous devices and melatonin suppression in adolescents. *Light Res Technol* 2015;0:10.
56. Shin JY, Yun GY, Kim JT. View types and luminance effects on discomfort glare assessment from windows. *Energ Buildings* 2012;46:139–145.
57. Hwang T, Kim JT. Effects of indoor lighting on occupants' visual comfort and eye health in a green building. *Indoor Built Environ* 2010;20(1):75–90.
58. Leather P, Pyrgas M, Beale D, Lawrence C. Windows in the workplace: sunlight, view, and occupational stress. *Environ Behav* 1998;30(6):739–762.
59. Thayer JF, Verkuil B, Brosschot JF, et al. Effects of the physical work environment on physiological measures of stress. *Eur J Cardiovasc Prev Rehabil* 2010;17(4):431–439.
60. Park JY, Min BK, Jung YC, Pak H, Jeong YH, Kim E. Illumination influences working memory: an EEG study. *Neuroscience* 2013;247:386–394.
61. Folscher LL, Goldstein LN, Wells M, Rees D. Emergency department noise: mental activation or mental stress? *Emerg Med J* 2014;32(6):468–473.
62. Evans GW, Johnson D. Stress and open-office noise. *J Appl Psychol* 2000;85(5):779–783.

63. Waye KP, Bengtsson J, Rylander R, Hucklebridge F, Evans P, Clow A. Low frequency noise enhances cortisol among noise sensitive subjects during work performance. *Life Sci* 2002;70(7):745–758.

64. Schust M. Effects of low frequency noise up to 100 Hz. *Noise Health* 2004;6(23):73–85.

65. Pejtersen J, Allermann L, Kristensen TS, Poulsen OM. Indoor climate, psychosocial work environment and symptoms in open-plan offices. *Indoor Air* 2006;16(5):392–401.

66. Danielsson CB, Bodin L. Difference in satisfaction with office environment among employees in different office types. *J Archit Plann Res* 2009;26(3):241–257.

67. Kaarlela-Tuomaala A, Helenius R, Keskinen E, Hongisto V. Effects of acoustic environment on work in private office rooms and open-plan offices—longitudinal study during relocation. *Ergonomics* 2009;52(11):1423–1444.

68. Freihoefer K, Guerin D, Martin C, Kim HY, Brigham JK. Occupants' satisfaction with, and physical readings of, thermal, acoustic, and lighting conditions of sustainable office workspaces. *Indoor Built Environ* 2013;24(4):457–472.

69. Lindberg CM, Tran DT, Banasiak MA. Individual differences in the office: personality factors and workspace enclosure. *J Archit Plann Res* 2016;33(2):105–120.

70. US Department of Health and Human Services. *Step It Up! The Surgeon General's Call to Action to Promote Walking and Walkable Communities.* l; 2015:18. Washington, DC.

71. Frank LD, Schmid TL, Sallis JF, Chapman J, Saelens BE. Linking objectively measured physical activity with objectively measured urban form: findings from SMARTRAQ. *Am J Prev Med* 2005;28(2):117–125.

72. Foster S, Giles-Corti B, Knuiman M. Neighbourhood design and fear of crime: a social-ecological examination of the correlates of residents' fear in new suburban housing developments. *Health Place* 2010;16(6):1156–1165.

73. Calogiuri G, Chroni S. The impact of the natural environment on the promotion of active living: an integrative systematic review. *BMC Public Health* 2014;14(1):873.

74. Brownson RC, Hoehner CM, Day K, Forsyth A, Sallis JF. Measuring the built environment for physical activity: state of the science. *Am J Prev Med* 2009;36(4 Suppl):S99–S123 e112.

75. Brennan L, Castro S, Brownson RC, Claus J, Orleans CT. Accelerating evidence reviews and broadening evidence standards to identify effective, promising, and emerging policy and environmental strategies for prevention of childhood obesity. *Annu Rev Public Health* 2011;32:199–223.

76. Davison KK, Lawson CT. Do attributes in the physical environment influence children's physical activity? A review of the literature. *Int J Behav Nutr Phys Act* 2006;3(1):19.

77. Lockett D, Willis A, Edwards N. Through seniors' eyes: an exploratory qualitative study to identify environmental barriers to and facilitators of walking. *Can J Nurs Res* 2005;37(3):48–65.

78. Smith L, Hamer M, Ucci M, et al. Weekday and weekend patterns of objectively measured sitting, standing, and stepping in a sample of office-based workers: the active buildings study. *BMC Public Health* 2014;15:9.

79. Brownson RC, Haire-Joshu D, Luke DA. Shaping the context of health: a review of environmental and policy approaches in the prevention of chronic diseases. *Annu Rev Public Health* 2006;27:341–370.

80. Swenson T, Siegel M. Increasing stair use in an office worksite through an interactive environmental intervention. *Am J Health Promot* 2013;27(5):323–329.

81. Steinfeld E, White J. Levels of access. *Inclusive Housing* 2010:23–36.

82. Department of Justice. *2010 ADA Standards for Accessible Design*. 2010:275.

83. Lorenc T, Petticrew M, Whitehead M, et al. Crime, fear of crime and mental health: synthesis of theory and systematic reviews of interventions and qualitative evidence. *Natl I Health Res* 2014;2(3).

84. O'Donnell E, Athey L, Skolnick G. *Sidewalks and Shared-Use Paths: Improving Mobility and Designing Transit-Ready Communities*. Institute for Public Administration, College of Human Services, Education and Public Policy, Newark, DE: University of Deleware; 2008. http://udspace.udel.edu/bitstream/handle/19716/3933/SidewalksSharedUsePaths2.pdf?sequence=1&isAllowed=y

85. World Health Organization. *Global Age-Friendly Cities: A Guide*. Geneva, Switzerland: WHO Press; 2007:76.

86. Sadler, B, Berry L, Guenther R, Hamilton D, Hessler F, Merritt C, Parker D. *Fable Hospital 2.0: The Business Case for Building Better Health Care Facilities*. In the report: The Hastings Center Report, Garrison, NY; 2001;41(1):13–23.

87. Appleyard D, Lintell M. The environmental quality of city streets: the residents' viewpoint. *J Am Inst Plann* 1972;38(2):84–101.

88. Evans GW. The built environment and mental health. *J Urban Health* 2003;80(4):536–555.

89. Hand C, Law M, Hanna S, Elliott S, McColl MA. Neighbourhood influences on participation in activities among older adults with chronic health conditions. *Health Place* 2012;18(4):869–876.

90. Baum A, Aiello JR, Calesnick LE. Crowding and personal control: social density and the development of learned helplessness. *J Pers Soc Psychol* 1978;36(9):1000–1011.

91. Heerwagen JH, Kampschroer K, Powell KM, Loftness V. Collaborative knowledge work environments. *Build Res Inf* 2004;32(6):510–528.

92. Brennan A, Chugh JS, Kline T. Traditional versus open office design: a longitudinal field study. *Environ Behav* 2002;34(3):279–299.

8

The Role of Spirituality in Integrative Preventive Medicine

The Postmaterialist Paradigm

GARY E. SCHWARTZ, PHD

When asked, "Do you believe in immortality?" he replied,
"No, and one life is enough for me."

Albert Einstein

I regard consciousness as fundamental.
I regard matter as derivative from consciousness.
We cannot get behind consciousness.
Everything that we talk about, everything that we regard
as existing, postulates consciousness.

Max Planck

Introduction

Religion and/or spirituality play important roles in the majority of people's lives worldwide. National and international surveys have historically indicated that approximately 90% of the world's populations believe in some sort of a higher power or intelligence and that this being/entity can sometimes play a role in health and healing.

As summarized by Rayburn,[1] religion can be defined as " 'the service, worship of God or the supernatural'; devotion or commitment to religious observations or faith; a personal set of doctrines or 'institutionalized system of religious attitudes, beliefs, and practices.' "

In contrast, Rayburn and Richard[2] conceive of spirituality as having three factors:

1. Transcendence, involving seeking goodness and truth and valuing peacefulness, cooperation, and forgiveness,
2. Spiritual Growth, involving realizing and attending to hypothesized influences on one's life (e.g., God, Higher Power, nature, trusted guides or teachers, etc.), and
3. Caring for Others, involving people, animals, plants, and ultimately everything in the universe.

Rayburn clarifies the distinction between religion and spirituality in the following ways. I have paraphrased her words for the purpose of clarity and consistency, and have added some comments as well [GES].

Being spiritual is regarded as requiring no adherence to any religious belief. [GES—it should be recognized that people can regularly partici-pate in religious practices or dogma and yet not accept or endorse par-ticular metaphysical/spiritual beliefs of their religions].

A spiritual person might be religious or might be (Rayburn's words) "churched, unchurched, agnostic, or atheistic." [GES—just as there are levels and degrees of religious practice, there are levels and degrees of spirituality.]

Whereas religiousness is typically regarded as doctrinal, holding to specific tenets of a faith system, and usually involving an organized community of believers, spirituality is more concerned with (Rayburn's words) "fervent caring for others, searching for the good and true, and recognizing the guidance of forces outside of oneself that influenced one's life paths." [GES—note that in many instances, religious dogmas may clash with these spiritual factors, especially the honest search for truth and goodness that is the hallmark of responsible and caring science].

Given the scope and spectrum of cognitive, emotional, and social compo-nents inherent in religion and spirituality, it is not surprising that religion and spirituality have been found to play a role in people's physical, psychological, and spiritual health and well-being.

Religion, Spirituality, and Health

The purpose of this chapter is not to review the extensive literature link-ing religion and spirituality to health and wellness. This research has been extensively presented in the *Oxford Handbook of Religion and Health*[3] and Part Six of the *Oxford Handbook of Psychology and Spirituality*,[4] and it is concisely summarized in Koenig.[5] It is also reviewed in a special issue of the journal *Evidence-Based Complementary and Alternative Medicine* devoted to the topic of spirituality and health.

The scope and spectrum of the evidence can be grasped by examining the individual chapter topics in the *Oxford Handbook of Religion and Health*.[3] For effects of religion on mental health (Part III), the chapters include well-being and positive emotions, depression, suicide, anxiety disorders, psychotic disorders, alcohol and drug use, delinquency and crime, marital instability, and personality and personality disorder. For effects of religion on physical health (Part IV), the chapters include heart disease, hypertension, cerebrovascular disease, Alzheimer's disease and dementia, immune functions, endocrine functions, cancer, mortality, physical disability, pain and somatic systems, and health behaviors.

Given the complexity of the cognitive, emotional, and social variables inherently involved in religion and spirituality, it should not be surprising that the comprehensive models proposed for understanding their effects on health are complex.

Figure 8.1 (from Koenig[5]), presents a theoretical model of causal pathways for mental health, based on Western monotheistic religions (Christianity, Judaism, and Islam).

The multivariate complexity of the psychosocial factors involved in religion helps to explain why religion can have such a wide scope and spectrum of effects on mental health. And Koenig's list is not complete. For example, love and caring are not made explicit in this model.

The same applies to physical health. Figure 8.2 (also from Koenig[5]), presents a theoretical model of causal pathways for physical health, again based on Western monotheistic religions.

Koenig's comprehensive models are employed to help explain clinician's observations of the positive effects of mainstream religious practices on health, hardiness, and resilience. They include:

1. Individual prayer,
2. Group prayer,
3. Group singing and chanting,
4. Loving social support received from spiritual leaders and practitioners, and
5. Individual and family psychosocial counseling provided by religious leaders.

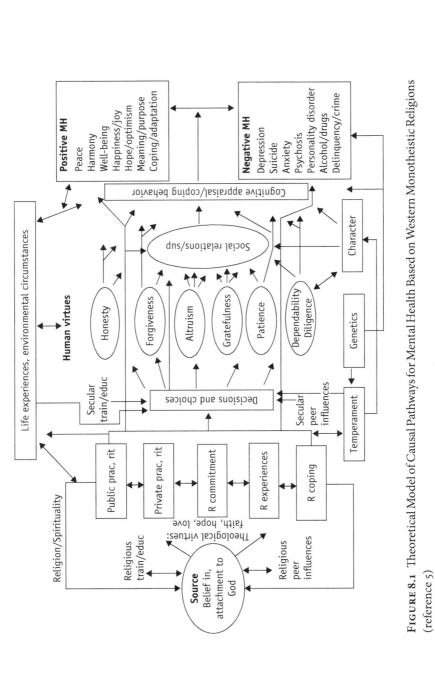

FIGURE 8.1 Theoretical Model of Causal Pathways for Mental Health Based on Western Monotheistic Religions (reference 5)

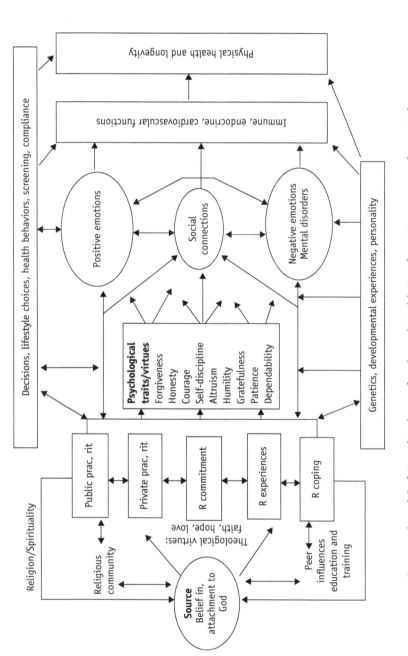

FIGURE 8.2 Theoretical Model of Causal Pathways for Physical Health Based on Western Monotheistic Religions (reference 5)

Koenig's theoretical models are also used to help explain the positive effects of what Jonas et al[6] refer to as "spiritual-body practices." As listed by Jonas et al,[6] these practices include:

1. Shalom Process—a type of "divine healing" involving the development of the "Principles and Skills of Loving." These tenets are said to be the foundation of an integrative approach to healing through "exploration of the energetic blocks created in our bodies by traumas that prevent us from being fully alive and experiencing the fullness of divine love."

2. Transcendental Meditation—a meditative practice derived from the ancient Vedic traditions and popularized in the 1960s and 1970s.

3. Heart Rate Coherence Training—the use of heart rate variability in the psychospiritual training developed by the Heart Math Corporation (http://www.heartmath.com/). In this process, persons are trained to regulate heart rate coherence, usually by cultivating a sense of appreciation and loving kindness.

4. Prayer and Laying On of Hands—including practices of energy and spiritual healing, including touch as well as distant intentionality.

5. Relaxation Response—a coordinate physiological response first described by Benson,[7] which presumably has been elicited by many religious and spiritual traditions throughout the world for thousands of years.

From Materialist to Postmaterialist Models

One might think from the above overview that conventional concepts in neuroscience and psychology would be sufficient to understand and predict the effects of religion and spirituality on health and wellness. However, this is not case. Instead, there is a growing recognition in certain areas of science that the above "materialistic" concepts are insufficient to account for the totality of the observations and evidence linking religion, spirituality, and health.

Scientists from a variety of scientific fields (biology, neuroscience, psychology, medicine, psychiatry) participated in an international summit on postmaterialist science, spirituality, and society. The summit was co-organized by Gary E. Schwartz, PhD, and Mario Beauregard, PhD, the University of Arizona, and Lisa Miller, PhD, Columbia University. The summit was held at Canyon Ranch in Tucson, Arizona, on February 7–9, 2014. The purpose was to discuss the impact of the materialist ideology on science and the emergence of a postmaterialist paradigm for science, spirituality, and society.[7]

Because of its historic significance and deep relevance to understanding religion, spirituality, and health, the text of an editorial written by Beauregard, Schwartz, Miller, et al[8] on the evolution of "post-materialistic science" is included (by permission) here. The following conclusions were reached:

1. The modern scientific worldview is predominantly predicated on assumptions that are closely associated with classical physics. Materialism—the idea that matter is the only reality—is one of these assumptions. A related assumption is reductionism, the notion that complex things can be understood by reducing them to the interactions of their parts, or to simpler or more fundamental things such as tiny material particles.

2. During the 19th century, these assumptions narrowed, turned into dogmas, and coalesced into an ideological belief system that came to be known as "scientific materialism." This belief system implies that the mind is nothing but the physical activity of the brain, and that our thoughts cannot have any effect upon our brains and bodies, our actions, and the physical world.

3. The ideology of scientific materialism became dominant in academia during the 20th century. So dominant that a majority of scientists started to believe that it was based on established empirical evidence, and represented the only rational view of the world.

4. Scientific methods based upon materialistic philosophy have been highly successful in not only increasing our understanding of nature but also in bringing greater control and freedom through advances in technology.

5. However, the nearly absolute dominance of materialism in the academic world has seriously constricted the sciences and hampered the development of the scientific study of mind and spirituality. Faith in this ideology, as an exclusive explanatory framework for reality, has compelled scientists to neglect the subjective dimension of human experience. This has led to a severely distorted and impoverished understanding of ourselves and our place in nature.

6. Science is first and foremost a non-dogmatic, open-minded method of acquiring knowledge about nature through the observation, experimental investigation, and theoretical explanation of phenomena. Its methodology is not synonymous with materialism and should not be committed to any particular beliefs, dogmas, or ideologies.

7. At the end of the 19th century, physicists discovered empirical phenomena that could not be explained by classical physics. This led to the development, during the 1920s and early 1930s, of a *revolutionary*

new branch of physics called quantum mechanics (QM). QM has questioned the material foundations of the world by showing that atoms and subatomic particles are not really solid objects—they do not exist with certainty at definite spatial locations and definite times. Most importantly, QM explicitly introduced the mind into its basic conceptual structure since it was found that particles being observed and the observer—the physicist and the method used for observation— are linked. According to one interpretation of QM, this phenomenon implies that the consciousness of the observer is vital to the existence of the physical events being observed, and that mental events can affect the physical world. The results of recent experiments support this interpretation. These results suggest that the physical world is no longer the primary or sole component of reality, and that it cannot be fully understood without making reference to the mind.

8. Psychological studies have shown that conscious mental activity can causally influence behavior, and that the explanatory and predictive value of agentic factors (e.g., beliefs, goals, desires and expectations) is very high. Moreover, *research* in psychoneuroimmunology indicates that our thoughts and emotions can markedly affect the activity of the physiological systems (e.g., immune, endocrine, cardiovascular) connected to the brain. In other respects, neuroimaging studies of emotional self-regulation, psychotherapy, and the placebo effect demonstrate that mental events significantly influence the activity of the brain.

9. Studies of the so-called "psi phenomena" indicate that we can sometimes receive meaningful information without the use of ordinary senses, and in ways that transcend the habitual space and time constraints. Furthermore, psi research demonstrates that we can mentally influence—at a distance—physical devices and living organisms (including other human beings). Psi research also shows that distant minds may behave in ways that are nonlocally correlated, i.e., the correlations between distant minds are hypothesized to be unmediated (they are not linked to any known energetic signal), unmitigated (they do not degrade with increasing distance), and immediate (they appear to be simultaneous). These events are so common that they cannot be viewed as anomalous nor as exceptions to natural laws, but as indications of the need for a broader explanatory framework that cannot be predicated exclusively on materialism.

10. Conscious mental activity can be experienced in clinical death during a cardiac arrest (this is what has been called a "near-death experience" [NDE]). Some near-death experiencers (NDErs) have reported

veridical out-of-body perceptions (i.e., perceptions that can be proven to coincide with reality) that occurred during cardiac arrest. NDErs also report profound spiritual experiences during NDEs triggered by cardiac arrest. It is noteworthy that the electrical activity of the brain ceases within a few seconds following a cardiac arrest.

11. Controlled laboratory experiments have documented that skilled research mediums (people who claim that they can communicate with the minds of people who have physically died) can sometimes obtain highly accurate information about deceased individuals. This further supports the conclusion that mind can exist separate from the brain.

12. Some materialistically inclined scientists and philosophers refuse to acknowledge these phenomena because they are not consistent with their exclusive conception of the world. Rejection of postmaterialist investigation of nature or refusal to publish strong science findings supporting a post-materialist framework are antithetical to the true spirit of scientific inquiry, which is that empirical data must always be adequately dealt with. Data which do not fit favored theories and beliefs cannot be dismissed a priori. Such dismissal is the realm of ideology, not science.

13. It is important to realize that psi phenomena, NDEs in cardiac arrest, and replicable evidence from credible research mediums, *appear anomalous only when seen through the lens of materialism.*

14. Moreover, materialist theories fail to elucidate how brain could generate the mind, and they are unable to account for the empirical evidence alluded to in this manifesto. This failure tells us that it is now time to *free ourselves from the shackles and blinders of the old materialist ideology*, to enlarge our concept of the natural world, and to embrace a post-materialist paradigm.

15. According to the post-materialist paradigm:
    a. Mind represents an aspect of reality as primordial as the physical world. Mind is fundamental in the universe, i.e., it cannot be derived from matter and reduced to anything more basic.
    b. There is a deep interconnectedness between mind and the physical world.
    c. Mind (will/intention) can influence the state of the physical world, and operate in a nonlocal (or extended) fashion, i.e., it is not confined to specific points in space, such as brains and bodies, nor to specific points in time, such as the present. Since the mind may nonlocally influence the physical world, the intentions, emotions, and desires of an experimenter may not be

completely isolated from experimental outcomes, even in controlled and blinded experimental designs.

    d. Minds are apparently unbounded, and may unite in ways suggesting a unitary, One Mind that includes all individual, single minds.

    e. NDEs in cardiac arrest suggest that the brain acts as a transceiver of mental activity, i.e., the mind can work through the brain, but is not produced by it. NDEs occurring in cardiac arrest, coupled with evidence from research mediums, further suggest the survival of consciousness, following bodily death, and the existence of other levels of reality that are non-physical.

    f. Scientists should not be afraid to investigate spirituality and spiritual experiences since they represent a central aspect of human existence.

16. Post-materialist science does not reject the empirical observations and great value of scientific achievements realized up until now. It seeks to expand the human capacity to better understand the wonders of nature, and in the process rediscover the importance of mind and spirit as being part of the core fabric of the universe. *Post-materialism is inclusive of matter, which is seen as a basic constituent of the universe.*

17. The post-materialist paradigm has far-reaching implications. It fundamentally alters the vision we have of ourselves, giving us back our dignity and power, as humans and as scientists. This paradigm fosters positive values such as compassion, respect, and peace. By emphasizing a deep connection between ourselves and nature at large, the post-materialist paradigm also promotes environmental awareness and the preservation of our biosphere. In addition, it is not new, but only forgotten for four hundred years, that a lived transmaterial understanding may be the cornerstone of health and wellness, as it has been held and preserved in ancient mind-body-spirit practices, religious traditions, and contemplative approaches.

18. The shift from materialist science to post-materialist science may be of vital importance to the evolution of the *human civilization. It may be even more pivotal than the transition from geocentrism to heliocentrism.*

Schwartz[9] has expanded on these points by proposing a heuristic framework for classifying three types of postmaterialist theories:

Type I Postmaterialist Theories: Neophysical theories that are derived from materialist theories, where the materialist theories are seen as primary and are viewed as being fundamentally necessary to create "nonmaterial" (yet physical) phenomena such as consciousness.

Type II Postmaterialist Theories: Postmaterialist theories of consciousness existing alongside materialist theories, where each class of theories is seen as primary and viewed as not being derivable from (i.e., is not reducible to) the other, and

Type III Postmaterialist Theories: Where materialist theories are derived from, and are a subset of, more inclusive postmaterialist theories of consciousness; here postmaterialist theories are seen as primary and are viewed as the ultimate origin of material systems.

Type 1 theories are the least controversial; Type III theories are the most controversial.

The materialist reader may wonder whether established findings from neuroscience allow for a postmaterialist paradigm. As explained below, the answer is a definitive yes.

Does Consciousness Require a Brain?

Though relatively few biomedical scientists and neuroscientists recognize this important fact, it turns out that the three core methods used by neuroscience to come to the conclusion that the brain "creates consciousness" are the *identical core methods used by electrical engineers and computer scientists* to come to the conclusion that radios, televisions, and smart phones are "antenna/receiver/transceivers" for external signals. The logic is explained in Schwartz,[10] and is quoted (by permission, and updated) below.

There are three types of experimental evidence that together seem to point to the conclusion that consciousness is created by the brain. The word "seem" is emphasized here because careful examination of the totality of evidence, when viewed from the perspective of electronics and electrical engineering, reveals how the evidence is actually *as consistent with the explanation that the mind is separate from the brain as it is with the explanation that the mind is created by the brain.* Unfortunately it is not widely appreciated by mainstream scientists that the three experimental approaches used to investigate mind–brain relationships do *not*, by themselves, require a materialistic conclusion—and they are wholly consistent with a nonmaterialistic (postmaterialist) explanation.

The three kinds of evidence are as follows:

1. *Evidence from recordings*—Neuroscientists record brain waves (via electroencephalograms [EEGs]) using sensitive electronic devices. For example, it is well known that occipital alpha waves decrease when people see visual objects or imagine them.

2. *Evidence from stimulation*—Various areas of the brain can be stimulated using electrodes placed inside the head or magnetic coils placed outside the head. For example, stimulation of the occipital cortex is typically associated with people experiencing visual sensations and images.

3. *Evidence from ablation*—Various areas of the brain can be removed with surgical techniques (or areas can be damaged through injury or disease). For example, when areas of the occipital cortex are damaged, people and lower animals lose aspects of vision.

The generally accepted—and seemingly commonsense—neuroscience interpretation of this set of findings is that visual experience is created by the brain.

However, the critical question is whether this *creation of consciousness* explanation is the *only* possible interpretation of this set of findings?

The answer is actually no. The three kinds of evidence are *also consistent with* the brain as being a *receiver of external consciousness information.*

The reasoning is straightforward and is illustrated in electronics and electrical engineering (the same logic applies to computer science). Though it is rare to discuss an electronics example in the context of handbook of preventive medicine (especially in a chapter focused on religion and spirituality), it turns out to be prudent and productive to do so here.

Consider the television (be it analog or digital). It is well known—and generally accepted—that televisions work as *receivers* for processing information carried by *external* electromagnetic fields oscillating in specific frequency bands. Television receivers do *not create* the visual information (i.e., they are *not the source* of the information) —they *detect* the information, *amplify* it, *process* it, and *display* it.

Moreover, today's "smart" televisions (as well as smart phones) can actually function as "transceivers," both receiving and transmitting information.

As mentioned earlier, it is not generally appreciated that electrical engineers conduct the same three kinds of experiments as neuroscientists do. The parallel between the brain and the television is essentially perfect.

1. *Evidence from recordings*—Electrical engineers can monitor signals inside the television set using sensitive electronic devices. For example, electrodes can be placed on particular components in circuits that correlate with the visual images seen on the screen.

2. *Evidence from stimulation*—Electrical engineers can stimulate various components of the television using electrodes placed inside the television set or magnetic coils placed outside the set. For example,

particular circuits can be stimulated with specific patterns of information, and replicable patterns can be observed on the TV screen.

3. *Evidence from ablation*—Electrical engineers can remove various
   components from the television (or areas can be damaged or wear
   out). For example, key components can be removed and the visual
   images on the screen will disappear.

However, do these three kinds of evidence imply that the *source* or *origin*
of the TV signals is *inside* the television—that is, that the television *created*
the signals? The answer is obviously no. Televisions (or smart phones) require
antennas (or cables) to receive signals that are external to the devices/systems.

It should be clear how this basic logic—as applied to television receivers—
can equally be applied to neural network (brain) receivers. The three kinds
of evidence (correlation, stimulation, and ablation) only allow us to conclude
that television sets—as well as brains—play some sort of *role* in visual experience. The truth is that the three kinds of evidence, by themselves, do *not* tell us
whether either television sets or brains:

1. "self-create" the information internally—the materialist assumption, or
2. function as complex receivers of external information—which allows
   for both survival of consciousness after death and a larger spiritual
   reality.

In other words, the three kinds of evidence, by themselves, do not speak
to (and do not enable us to determine) whether the signals—the information
fields—are:

1. coming from *inside* the system (the materialistic interpretation
   applied to brains),

or

2. coming from *outside* the system (the interpretation routinely applied
   to televisions).

It follows that *additional kinds of experiments* are required to distinguish
between the "self-creation" versus "receiver" hypotheses.

Experiments on life after death with skilled research mediums (e.g., Beischel
and Schwartz[11]) provide an important fourth kind of evidence that can neither
be predicted nor explained by the self-creation (i.e., materialism) hypothesis,
but it can be predicted and explained by the receiver/transceiver hypothesis

It should be noted that in physics, external electromagnetic fields are not labeled as being "material" per se. These fields do not have mass (e.g., they do not have weight) and they are invisible; they are described by a set of equations that characterize an as-yet-unexplained property of the "vacuum" of space (which may be empty of "mass" but is actually full of energy and information).

Applications to the Role of Spirituality in Integrative Preventive Medicine

There are many important and innovative applications of postmaterialist science to understanding and applying spiritual concept and practices to integrative medicine treatment and prevention. These examples are not listed in any particular order.

EXAMPLE 1: HIGHER POWER HEALING HYPOTHESIS

Consider various implementations of the Twelve Step Program to the treatment and prevention of addictions (e.g., alcohol, drug, sexual, etc.). Material scientists and practitioners prefer to explain the positive effects observed as being due to conventional psychosocial factors such as group support, catharsis, motivation, expectation, and belief (including placebo). The founder's belief that an addict's accepting and connecting to a "Higher Power" is the central healing component in AA is typically reinterpreted by materialist scientists and practitioners using nonspiritual, psychosocial concepts (e.g., placebo effects).

However, what if a greater spiritual reality exists as predicted by postmaterialist science? If so, then it becomes rationally possible that the mindful acceptance and connection with a Higher Power actually enhances Its capacity to contribute to the person's regulation of their addictive experiences and behaviors.

An *integrative* approach requires that we combine documented psychosocial (materialist) variables and processes with emerging psychoenergetic and psychospiritual (postmaterialist) variables and processes. In fact, as science provides theoretical and empirical support for the Higher Power hypothesis, this provides an added rationale and incentive for addicts and practitioners to foster increased acceptance and connection with a Higher Power.

EXAMPLE 2: SPIRIT-ASSISTED HEALING HYPOTHESIS

Though most mainstream materialist scientists prefer to avoid these facts, the truth is that most energy healers—be they trained in Western practices such as Healing Touch and Reconnection, or Eastern practices such as Reiki and Johrei—believe that their healing powers come from (1) their ability to receive and direct some sort of universal intelligent and loving energy (whose intelligence, wisdom, and healing abilities are far beyond those of the healers—this is another application of the Higher Power healing hypothesis), and (2) the assistance they receive from deceased persons (often deceased physicians and nurses) as well as "higher spiritual beings" such as guides and angels.

When viewed through the paradigm lens of materialism, such beliefs are interpreted as superstitions contributing to placebo effects. However, when viewed through the expanded paradigm lens of postmaterialism, such beliefs become not only plausible but also rational hypotheses capable of being tested scientifically.

Schwartz[12] conducted a proof-of-concept experiment testing claims of spirit-assisted healing professed by a research-oriented clinical psychologist formally trained in healing touch (HT). The psychologist believed that he often received important assistance from his deceased physician father, and that one of the ways he knew that his father was collaborating in healing the patient was that HT's hands would become warm.

After determining that a laboratory-tested, claimant evidential medium (CEM) could accurately receive information from the deceased physician, Schwartz designed the following 10- session experiment:

The night before a given session, the CEM was instructed to contact the hypothesized deceased physician, and the CEM would request that the deceased physician show up at the next healing session either (1) immediately upon beginning the session, or (2) post the middle of the session.

Only the CEM knew which condition (immediate or midway) applied to the next session. Five of the sessions would implement the immediate condition and five the midway condition.

The following day, the HT would conduct a normal energy healing and pay close attention to whether his hands warmed up (1) immediately upon beginning the session, or (2) post the middle of the session. After the 10 sessions were completed, the experimenter compared the CEM and HT records and performed a nonparametric analysis.

The analysis indicated a 100% match (10 out of 10, Yates correct Chi Square $p < .04$). These findings are consistent with the hypothesis that HT was correctly identifying the apparent presence of the purported deceased physician. Future research can test the spirit-assisted healing hypothesis by comparing (1) sessions when specific hypothesized deceased healing individuals are present in healing sessions with (2) sessions when no hypothesized deceased persons are invited to collaborate. Such experiments can be conducted double blinded.

The author has interviewed dozens of gifted research-oriented energy healers who are convinced that the spirit-assisted healing hypothesis is valid.

EXAMPLE 3: DIVINE LOVE MEDITATION HYPOTHESIS

Secular meditation techniques like transcendental meditation and mindfulness meditation, including loving kindness meditation, typically do not encourage the meditators to focus on divine love and caring. However, spiritually oriented meditators in general, and spiritually oriented healers in particular, often focus on spiritual processes, including proposed angels, guides, and the divine.

Beginning in 2010, the author has offered a weekly energy self-care workshop at Canyon Ranch titled "Awakening the Power Within." The workshop teaches guests four skills: (1) how to sense energy with their hands; (2) how to give themselves energy, including healing energy; (3) how to protect themselves against negative energy; and (4) how to send loving energy to others. The author uses the principle "energy flows where the loving mind goes."

One technique has the person putting their left hand over their heart and their right hand over their abdomen. As the person inhales, she is requested to imagine or feel the energy flowing up her left arm into her left hand as she silently thinks to herself "love heart," and as she exhales, she is to imagine or feeling the energy flowing down her right arm into her right hand as she silently thinks to herself "love breath." In over 500 cases, only a handful of persons have *not* reported feelings of relaxation and peacefulness.

However, in approximately 50 cases where the individuals have spontaneously reported that they are spiritual people, I have invited guests to repeat the same procedure only this time substituting the phrase "Divine love heart" and "Divine love breath." Only a few persons have *not* reported feelings of even greater relaxation and peacefulness with the addition of the divine focus. Moreover, I have compared the "love X" versus "Divine love X" energy healing meditations when lecturing to groups of healers and practitioners (e.g., audience sizes of 200 to 300 participants). The vast majority of participants report experiencing the divine love condition as more intense and integrative (i.e., expanding their awareness more fully to their whole body).

Though the Canyon Ranch workshop is taught as a self-care workshop, it ends with a discussion of the value of parents and grandparents teaching such concepts and techniques to their young children and grandchildren for the purpose of physical, emotional, and spiritual health promotion and disease prevention.

EXAMPLE 4: THE SYNCHRONICITY WELLNESS HYPOTHESIS

From a materialist perspective, apparent nonrandom co-occurrences of seemingly meaningful events are typically (1) described as being coincidental events, and (2) interpreted as being due to randomness or chance. However, some combinations of events are so statistically improbable as to be "too coincidental to be accidental," and they potentially serve as empirical evidence of an interactive greater spiritual reality.

In a series of papers, Schwartz has documented multiple cases of what are termed Type III synchronicities (i.e., sequences containing six or move interrelated events in a defined period of time). The totality of the evidence supports the postmaterialist hypothesis that nonrandom synchronicities can sometimes be mediated by spiritual forces, including (1) discarnates (physically deceased persons/spirits), and (2) a Higher Power.

Beginning in 2015, the author has offered a weekly workshop at Canyon Ranch titled "Synchronicity and Spiritual Wellness." The workshop teaches guests how to understand basic methods of science (termed "self-science") and apply these techniques in the "laboratories of our personal lives." As reported in *Synchronicity and the One Mind*,[16] people who believe in synchronicities, pay attention to them, and attempt to interpret their potential meaning(s), tend to experience more hopeful, optimistic, peaceful, grateful, and wonder-filled lives. All of these emotions are associated with positive health and well-being.

EXAMPLE 5: THE SPIRITUAL IMMUNITY HYPOTHESIS

Many religions and cultures believe in the existence of the "evil eye," "negative spirits," "dark forces," and/or "the devil." Materialism treats their ideas as superstitions and myths. In contrast, postmaterialist science recognizes the possibility that "negative forces" can exist and potentially be harmful to unsuspecting individuals.

For example, when principles of electromagnetic and quantum fields are applied to the survival of consciousness hypothesis, predicting how the energy and information of a physical person continues in the vacuum of space after a person has physically died, this hypothesis is not limited to the energy and information of loving, positive people, but it includes the energy and information of hateful, negative people as well. Experiments with research mediums confirm the continued existence of "negative spirits" as well as positive ones.

It is possible that the reason for the existence of the so-called veil between the physical and spiritual worlds is the purpose of protection from negative spirits.

Moreover, just as the human body has a cellular immune system, the mind/psyche might have a spiritual immune system as well. This hypothesis is consistent with reports of healers who claim not only that patients sometimes need to be treated for the presence of "negative entities" but also that various techniques can be applied to strengthen one's spiritual immunity. These techniques span the full range of integrative health practices, including nutrition, exercise, sleep, and stress management. Teaching people about the concept of spiritual immunity could be part of integrative preventive medicine of the future.

It is worth noting that the distinction in physics between energy and information might have a meaningful parallel in semantic differences between the terms "spirit" and "soul." It has been proposed (and I paraphrase slightly) that "spirit is to soul as energy is to information."[17] Together energy and information, spirit and soul, may reflect a core quality of a greater spiritual reality.

Conclusions

As the quotes that introduce this chapter express, distinguished physicists have disagreed about which was primary in nature and the cosmos: (1) matter (e.g., Einstein), or (2) mind (e.g., Max Planck). If one favors the materialist philosophy (and paradigm), one is inclined to interpret the positive effects of religion and spirituality on health in cognitive, emotional, and social (i.e., physical) terms. However, if one favors the emerging postmaterialist philosophy (and paradigm), one is inclined to *add* postmaterialist explanations (including the role of consciousness, discarnates, higher spiritual beings, and the Higher Power/divine) to the materialist explanations.

Integrative medicine in general, and integrative preventive medicine in particular, should strive to integrate not only techniques and practices but also concepts and theories. The emerging postmaterialist science movement is an expression of this expansive, open (e.g., http://www.opensciences.org), integrative framework. If this chapter has helped open the reader's mind to the possible validity and opportunity of a postmaterialist approach to the role of spirituality in integrative preventive medicine, then it has achieved its goal.

References

1. Rayburn CA. Motherhood and female faith development: feminine tapestry of religion, spirituality, creativity, and intuition. In Miller LJ, ed. *The Oxford Handbook of Psychology and Spirituality.* New York, NY: Oxford University Press; 2012:182–196.

2. Rayburn CA, Richard LJ. *Inventory on Religiousness (IR)*. Washington, DC: US Copyright Office; 1997.

3. Koenig HG, King DE, Carson VB, eds. *The Oxford Handbook of Religion and Health*. 2nd ed. New York City, NY: Oxford University Press; 2012.

4. Miller LJ, ed. *The Oxford Handbook of Psychology and Spirituality*. New York, NY: Oxford University Press; 2012.

5. Koenig HG. Religion, spirituality and health: the research and clinical implications. *Int Scholarly Res Network, ISRN Psychiatry* 2012; Article ID 278730, 1–33.

6. Jonas WB, Fritts M, Christopher G, Jonas M, Jonas S. In Miller LJ, ed. *The Oxford Handbook of Psychology and Spirituality*. New York, NY: Oxford University Press; 2012:361–378.

7. Schwartz GE, Miller LJ, Beauregard, M. *International Summit on Post-Materialist Science, Spirituality, and Society: Summary Report*. 2014. http://www.opensciences.org/files/pdfs/ISPMS-Summary-Report.pdf.

8. Beauregard M, Schwartz GE, Miller LJ, et al. Manifesto for a post-materialist science. *Explore* 2014;10(5):272–274.

9. Schwartz GE (2016). What is the nature of a post-materialist paradigm? Three types of theories. *Explore* 2016;12(2):123–127.

10. Schwartz GE. Consciousness, spirituality, and post-materialist science: an empirical and experiential approach. In Miller LJ, ed. *The Oxford Handbook of Psychology and Spirituality*. New York , NY: Oxford University Press; 2012:584–597.

11. Beischel J, Schwartz GE (2007). Anomalous information reception by research mediums demonstrated using a novel triple-blind protocol. *Explore* 2012;3(1):23–27.

12. Schwartz GE. *The Sacred Promise: How Science Is Discovering Spirits Collaboration with Us in Our Daily Lives*. Hillsboro, OR: Beyond Words/Atria Books/Simon & Schuster; 2011.

13. Schwartz GE. God, synchronicity, and post-materialist psychology. I: Proof-of-concept real-life evidence. *Spir Clin Pract* 2014;1(2):153–162.

14. Schwartz GE. God, synchronicity, and post-materialist psychology. II: Replication and extension of real-life evidence. *Spir Clin Pract* 2015;2(1):86–95.

15. Schwartz GE (2014). God, synchronicity, and post-materialist psychology III: Additional real-life evidence and the higher power healing hypothesis. *Spir Clin Pract* 2014;2(4):289–302.

16. Schwartz GE. *Synchronicity and the One Mind: Where Science and Spirit Meet*. Vancouver, BC: Param Media; 2016.

17. Schwartz GE. *The G.O.D. Experiments: How Science Is Discovering God in Everything, Including Us*. New York City, NY: Atria Books; 2007.

9

The Role of Complementary and Alternative Medicine in Integrative Preventive Medicine

FARSHAD FANI MARVASTI, MD, MPH

Key Concepts

- Integrative preventive medicine (IPM) creates a new framework to integrate both conventional and complementary and alternative medicine (CAM) approaches in the practice of preventive medicine.
- Integrative preventive medicine identifies CAM as a key contributor to the shift from acute to chronic disease treatment and prevention with the goal of morbidity compression to extend the period of disease-free high-quality life throughout the lifespan.
- As an integral part of IPM, CAM empowers the patient to take an active role in their health, resulting in a shift away from passive screenings and treatment-centered approaches to prevention-focused care.
- Integrative preventive medicine identifies a broad range of CAM that can be amenable to self-care, is cost-effective, is minimally invasive, and has minimal potential for side effects.
- The role of CAM in IPM is to reemphasize the value of primary prevention as an underused level of prevention in our current approach to healthcare.
- Integrative preventive medicine redefines and expands the levels of prevention to include evidence-based CAM at each level of prevention alongside conventional approaches.
- Key components of CAM have been shown to be effective in treating the major risk factors for morbidity and mortality.

- Integrative preventive medicine affirms the value of evidence-based CAM and thereby contributes to better outcomes by engaging patients to share their CAM usage with their physicians as part of their treatment plan.

Introduction

Complementary and alternative medicine (CAM) has been defined as "a group of diverse medical and health care systems, practices, and products that are not presently considered to be part of conventional medicine."[1] When used in place of conventional treatments, CAM therapies are considered "alternative." When used together with conventional treatments, CAM therapies are considered "complementary."[2] According to the National Center for Complementary and Integrative Health (NCCIH) most people who use CAM use them along with conventional approaches, making them complementary. Integrative health is defined by the NCCIH as bringing conventional and complementary approaches together in a coordinated way. Integrative preventive medicine (IPM) creates a new framework that integrates and brings together both conventional and CAM approaches in the prevention of disease and the promotion of health.

The New Framework of Integrative Preventive Medicine

The new framework created by IPM provides a shift in the focus of our healthcare system from acute disease management to chronic disease prevention. This shift is based on the change in disease epidemiology from acute to chronic disease. Over 100 years ago, acute infectious diseases such as tuberculosis or polio were the major sources of morbidity and mortality.[3] Great success was achieved to eradicate these conditions through advances in public health and the establishment of an acute care model. A hundred years later, the burden of illness has shifted dramatically toward chronic disease. In fact, 7 out of every 10 deaths among Americans are from chronic diseases including cardiovascular disease, cancer, and diabetes.[4] Despite these changes in disease epidemiology mandating a focus on chronic disease prevention, our current healthcare system focuses almost exclusively on acute care.[5] Our acute care model continues to demonstrate success in treating acute conditions as well as acute exacerbations of chronic diseases such as myocardial infarction. However, we have poor success in preventing these episodes in the first place. Focusing on acute care without adequate prevention contributes to the ongoing costs of chronic disease that now account for nearly 75% of healthcare dollars spent each year.[6] In fact, modifiable and preventable factors such as lifestyle choices and behavior account for the majority of premature mortality in the United States.[7]

To address our chronic disease epidemic and maximize the potential of prevention, IPM mandates a new focus on chronic disease prevention and health. In sync with the pathogenesis of chronic disease, IPM focuses on risk factor modification over time. Therefore IPM emphasizes ongoing prevention practices and risk factor modification instead of a narrow focus on episodic treatment and late-stage disease management. Prevention in IPM includes health promotion activities that encourage healthy lifestyles that prevent the progression of chronic disease. The goal of IPM is therefore aligned with the goals of health promotion and prevention. Instead of focusing on treatment and cure, IPM focuses on maintaining health by expanding the period of disease-free high-quality life for as long as possible. Therefore IPM espouses the concept of morbidity compression, first articulated by James Fries as the goal of prevention.[8] In focusing on prevention and health as paramount, IPM seeks to vindicate the quote attributed to Hippocrates, "the function of protecting and developing health must rank even above that of restoring it when it is impaired." The need for this shift in focus also reflects emerging public opinion. Survey data has shown that two-thirds of all adults believe that the US healthcare system should place more emphasis on chronic disease preventive care, with four in five Americans (84%) being in favor of funding for such prevention programs.[9]

CAM Usage and the Goals of IPM

Despite the pressing need and public desire for prevention and health promotion, estimates show that Americans receive only about half the preventive services recommended.[10] Integrative preventive medicine identifies evidence-based CAM therapies as an underused tool in preventive medicine. Although representing a diverse array of modalities with varying levels of evidence, much of CAM inherently focuses on the importance of lifestyle. By emphasizing lifestyle and providing ongoing practices for daily maintenance of health, CAM is a key contributor to the IPM goal of prevention and health promotion. Being cost-effective and amenable to self-care on a large scale, CAM is critical in decreasing morbidity and mortality and controlling costs associated with the chronic diseases of our time. One reason CAM should be considered as a key part of the solution to our chronic disease epidemic is reflected in its continued popularity and widespread usage, which has increased and persisted over time. The 2012 National Health Interview Survey (NHIS) conducted by the National Center for Health Statistics found that 33.2% of adults and 11.6% of children used some form of complementary health approach.[11] This same survey found that 59 million Americans spent over 30 billion dollars a year out-of-pocket on complementary health approaches. The latest 2012 NHIS data has found the following to be the 10 most common complementary health approaches among adults: natural products (dietary supplements other than vitamins and minerals), deep breathing, yoga or tai chi or qi gong, chiropractic or osteopathic manipulation, meditation, massage, special diets, homeopathy, progressive relaxation, and guided imagery.[12]

In sync with the goal of IPM that shifts the focus of our healthcare system to health promotion and wellness, NHIS data has shown the majority of individuals who use CAM do so to maintain wellness, with much smaller numbers using these approaches for treatment.[13] In IPM, CAM provides the cost-effective tools to achieve the goals of health promotion and prevention throughout the lifespan. And CAM can be particularly useful in the modification of personal health behaviors and risk factors for chronic disease. National Health Interview Survey data has shown CAM users to present with risk factors that are a public health priority, making CAM encounters an opportunity to coordinate health promotion and prevention messages with their primary care providers.[14] Furthermore, CAM practitioner visits may be ideal opportunities for behavior change counseling and lifestyle modification.[15]

CAM in IPM Empowers the Patient

In IPM, CAM empowers the patient to actively participate in their health and thereby prevent disease through daily activities and practices that are amenable to self-care, are cost-effective, are minimally invasive, and have limited side effects. One such practice area in CAM is mind body medicine. Mind body therapies are defined as "practices that focus on the interactions of the brain, mind, body and behavior, with the intent to use the mind to affect physical functioning and promote health."[16] Commonly practiced mind body therapies include yoga, tai chi, qi gong, deep breathing, guided imagery, hypnosis, meditation, and progressive relaxation. Several of these therapies are among the top 10 most commonly used CAM therapies. Yoga, for example has grown in popularity. Twice as many US adults were practicing yoga in 2012 as they were in 2002.[17] The latest national health statistics data show that 9.5% or 21 million adults use yoga on a regular basis.[12] Yoga has been shown to have a variety of therapeutic effects. A recent review article found yoga to support muscle strength and flexibility; improve respiratory and cardiovascular function; treat addiction; improve sleep patterns; reduce stress, anxiety, and depression; and enhance overall quality of life.[18] Yoga is a great example of a CAM therapy that is now becoming mainstream. And IPM identifies mind body practices such as yoga to be amenable to self-care, minimally invasive, and cost-effective, with little to no negative side effects. Tai chi, originally practiced as a martial art, is another mind body therapy that is low impact and amenable to self-care. Instead of simply screening elderly populations for osteoporosis and treating osteoarthritis with pain medications, IPM recognizes tai chi as a CAM therapeutic alternative to addressing these conditions. Research on tai chi has shown it to be effective in the treatment of coronary disease, metabolic syndrome, back pain, chronic fatigue, stroke rehabilitation, pain, and osteoporosis.[19,20–25] When considering the conventional care approaches that include addictive and harmful pain medications, the consequences of a pathologic fracture due to poor muscle strength and bone density and the costs associated with these, CAM therapies such as yoga and tai chi provide a safer alternative. In sync with the new framework of CAM in IPM, these therapies provide daily practices for patients to engage in and thereby play an active role in their health. Furthermore, both yoga and tai chi also provide effective ways to expand primary prevention in healthy individuals to maintain health and prevent the onset of disease.

IPM Emphasizes Primary Prevention and Expands the Levels of Prevention to Include Evidence-Based CAM

Integrative preventive medicine emphasizes the value of primary prevention and identifies CAM as a key contributor to this underused aspect of healthcare. Despite the fact that most of our chronic diseases are potentially preventable, most healthcare resources are concentrated on treatment services for advanced disease management and only 2%–3% of all healthcare dollars are spent on prevention.[26] Integrative preventive medicine asserts that this reality is unacceptable and identifies CAM to provide great potential for expanding primordial prevention. Primary prevention is central to the new IPM framework, and CAM provides effective tools to maintain health throughout the lifespan as opposed to episodic, disjointed treatment of symptoms and conditions after they have progressed to higher levels of morbidity. Most people who engage in CAM therapies have health conditions such as hypertension or diabetes and sedentary lifestyles. These patients see their CAM providers as often as two to five times per year.[27] This higher visit rate supports the success of high-intensity behavioral interventions to prevent disease, as these are most effective in settings where there is greater time spent with patients. Therefore,

CAM presents an ideal setting whereby health promotion and primary prevention can take place. Engaging patients in this new paradigm enables physicians to have more support on all levels of prevention to increase access to care for their patients. This increased access and contact has the potential to better prevent disease progression and unnecessary hospitalizations that can lead to higher costs, morbidity, and ultimately death.

Integrative preventive medicine redefines and expands the levels of prevention to include evidence-based CAM at each level of prevention alongside conventional approaches. The concept of prevention in IPM comes from the Latin root *praeventus*, to anticipate.[28] Taken together with this definition of prevention, disease prevention translates to activities intended to forestall or anticipate the development of disease. Prevention has traditionally been conceptualized to occur on three distinct levels: primary, secondary, and tertiary prevention.[29] Prevention can occur in a variety of settings on an individual, community, or societal level. Integrative preventive medicine considers prevention to be a spectrum that encompasses a broader synergy between medicine and public health. In IPM, CAM expands the traditional levels of prevention and reemphasizes the value of primary or primordial prevention as an underused level of prevention in our current healthcare system. As demonstrated in Table 9.1, the levels of prevention in IPM can expand to include CAM and community components at each level. Primary prevention includes activities intended to forestall the development of a disease prior to its clinical diagnosis. As such, daily practices such as tai chi or yoga are a great way to enhance self-efficacy to prevent disease and maintain health.

As seen in Table 9.1, conventional approaches are limited to generic recommendations for healthy diet and exercise. Unfortunately, these recommendations are too vague and generalized. Consequently, most Americans do not meet intake recommendations. For example, fruit and vegetable intake information from the Behavioral Risk Factor Surveillance System (BRFSS) found that 76% of Americans did not meet recommended fruit intake of 1.5–2 cups per day and 87% of Americans did not meet vegetable intake recommended at 2–3 cups per day.[30] Having more sophisticated and personalized dietary advice with CAM in IPM has greater potential for success in achieving dietary goals to maintain health and prevent disease. Dietary practices that are tailored to individual needs are part of many CAM therapies. Alternative health systems such as Ayurveda and traditional Chinese medicine emphasize diet and the use of herbs and spices as a cornerstone in the prevention and treatment of disease.[31,32] A number of herbs in these alternative health systems are taken by healthy individuals as a tonic to maintain health. Emerging evidence has supported the usage of selected herbs for various conditions and more research is needed to validate claims and traditional practices. The new framework of CAM in IPM

Table 9.1 Conventional Approaches to Secondary Prevention

	Primary Prevention	*Secondary Prevention*	*Tertiary Prevention*
Conventional	Generic advice on diet and exercise to maintain weight and glycemic control in patient at risk for type 2 diabetes mellitus	Medication management for early stage diabetes, hypertension, or other diagnosed medical conditions	Treating advanced Diabetes with neuropathy and chronic kidney disease with insulin to prevent renal failure and dialysis, anticoagulants in patients with coronary disease
CAM in IPM	Optimizing physical activity with daily practices such as tai chi or yoga, optimizing diet Mediterranean or anti-inflammatory (AI) diet, meditation for relaxation and stress reduction, tonic herbs and functional foods	evidence-based dietary supplements, diet protocols AI diet, Functional foods for lowering blood glucose like apple cider vinegar, mind body practices such as meditation to lower blood pressure, manual medicine to prevent progression of arthritic disease	Ornish diet and lifestyle protocol to reverse coronary artery disease, tai chi for cardiac rehab, acupuncture for nausea post chemotherapy for better compliance
Community	Addressing the built environment, e.g., safe sidewalks and recreation facilities, addressing food deserts and food policy to make healthy food choices available	Diabetes Prevention Programs in YMCAs and community centers, diabetes educators in communities, public service health education on coronary artery disease	Enhance access to primary and specialty medical care for chronic conditions for all to avoid unnecessary hospitalizations and prevent death

necessitates a new focus on the role of diet in disease prevention and the treatment of chronic disease. Furthermore, nutriceutical dietary supplements are another area requiring further investigation. While challenges remain in regulation of the nutriceuticals, there is mounting evidence of their potential role in maintaining health and preventing disease. Integrative preventive medicine identifies evidence-based dietary supplements as an important tool in the prevention of disease, and more attention is needed on reforming policies to regulate the industry and expand medical research on efficacy and safety. In support of these goals, CAM in IPM advocates for systematic training for current physicians to expand their knowledge of evidence-based nutritional protocols and supplements. Current educational resources for clinicians include a number of ongoing conferences and integrative medicine fellowships.[33,34]

Secondary prevention includes activities intended to forestall the further development of an existing disease while in its early stages before it results in significant morbidity. As shown in Table 9.1, conventional approaches to secondary prevention largely include pharmacological treatments such as medications for blood pressure or blood glucose control. In IPM, CAM expands this to include evidence-based natural products or dietary supplements, specific diet treatment protocols, and lifestyle practices that optimize secondary prevention to forestall disease progression, such as meditation for blood pressure control. Tertiary prevention includes activities intended to forestall end-stage sequelae of symptomatic clinical disease, including significant morbidity leading to functional impairment or death. Tertiary prevention is where the lion's share of conventional medical care is focused. As seen in Table 9.1, CAM in IPM can provide added resources here as well. For example, the intensive lifestyle changes including specific dietary and stress-management protocols of the Ornish plan have been shown to result in regression of coronary atherosclerosis.[35] These and other similar findings for the role of lifestyle and diet expand tertiary prevention to include nonpharmacological, minimally invasive modalities that are amenable to self-care and cost-effective with minimal side effects. These lifestyle interventions can be particularly useful in patients with advanced cardiovascular disease who may not be good candidates for anticoagulant treatment due to fall risk and other comorbidities.

The Evidence for CAM in Treating Chronic Disease and Its Risk Factors

In expanding the levels of prevention, CAM in IPM provides a broader range of options for patients and healthcare providers to consider. These complementary therapeutic options require further research into their efficacy and safety. As research in CAM expands, the principles of preventive medicine can be integrated more fully into CAM encounters to promote health and prevent disease.[36] To date, research in CAM has been supported by the National Center for Complementary and Integrative Health, which has created over 14 research centers through the National Institutes of Health. Key components of CAM have been shown to be effective in treating the major risk factors for morbidity and mortality as well as chronic conditions ranging from cardiovascular disease to chronic pain.[37,38] According to the White House Commission on Complementary and Alternative Medicine Policy, much more evidence for CAM exists than is commonly recognized, as the Cochrane Collaboration lists well over 4,000 randomized studies on CAM therapies.[39] The Cochrane Complementary Medicine website presents a collaboration between the NCCIH and University of Maryland School of Medicine to provide links to summarize the evidence for or against CAM.[40] Additional free resources for physicians and healthcare providers for evidence-based CAM therapies include the Dietary Supplements subset search database in Pub Med, the University of Maryland Medical Center CAM Guide that provides drug-herb interactions and dosage recommendations based on evidence for natural products, and the Dietary Supplements Labels Database at the National Library of Medicine.[41-43] Using these resources for evidence on dietary supplements is increasingly important, as natural products were used by 17.7% of American adults in 2007, making these the most popular form of CAM.[16] Natural products include herbal preparations or botanicals, vitamins or minerals in higher dosages than minimal daily nutritional requirements, and probiotics. The most commonly used natural product in adults is omega 3 fish oil, reported by 37.4% of all adults who said they used a natural product.[16] Omega 3 fish oil is one example of a CAM natural product that has now been well established and incorporated into mainstream treatment of cardiovascular disease and its risk factors such as hypertriglyceridemia.[44] Probiotics and fermented foods are an emerging area of CAM that is gaining increased recognition by conventional medicine, as new research programs are being expanded to understand and define the human microbiome. Evidence for probiotics in certain conditions are already well established. For example, probiotics have been shown to reduce antibiotic-associated diarrhea and effectively aid in the treatment and prevention of recurrence for *Clostridium difficile* infections.[45] Integrative preventive medicine provides a framework and rationale to support the expansion of research in these areas of CAM that have demonstrated potential for better outcomes.

As shown in Table 9.2, CAM in IPM expands therapeutic options in the treatment of the chronic disease and its risk factors. For example, diabetes affects over 29 million people in the United States,[46] and over 57 million American adults are estimated to have prediabetes.[47] Lifestyle interventions

Table 9.2 Therapeutic Options in Treating Chronic Disease

	Conventional Approaches	*CAM in IPM*
Cardiovascular Disease	Statins for hyperlipidemia, antihypertensive medications for hypertension	Omega 3 fish oil for hypertriglyceridemia, anti-Inflammatory diet, integrative lifestyle intervention, e.g., Ornish Tx for coronary artery disease, meditation
Diabetes	Oral hypoglycemic medication, insulin therapy	Lifestyle intervention such as Diabetes Prevention Program, tailored specific dietary intervention such as glycemic index guide, functional foods
Chronic Pain	Nonsteroidal anti-inflammatory drugs (NSAIDs), nerve blocks and interventional pain, steroids	Mind body therapies including tai chi, yoga, acupuncture, anti-inflammatory diet, Omega 3 fish oil, evidence-based supplements

for diabetes such as the Diabetes Prevention Program (DPP) have been shown to be more effective than first-line pharmacotherapy for diabetes.[48] Furthermore, use of DPP has been shown to reduce the risk of developing type 2 diabetes by as much as 58%.[48] Integrative preventive medicine recognizes these lifestyle-based CAM interventions as an integral part of its new framework for healthcare. As noted in the expansion of prevention levels to include CAM, CAM in IPM also recognizes the potential role of diet and micronutrients in the care and prevention of chronic disease. According to a recent epidemiological study by the CDC examining the major risk factors for death and disability-adjusted life-years in the United States, dietary risk factors were found to be associated with the highest percentage of morbidity and mortality.[49] After dietary factors, the other major risk factors identified in the study included tobacco smoking, high blood pressure, high fasting plasma glucose, and physical inactivity and low physical activity. Despite the obvious role that dietary factors play in our current chronic disease epidemic, our current system continues to have inadequate nutrition in medical education, with an average of 19.6 contact hours of nutrition instruction for the entire 4 years of medical school.[50] The new framework of IPM expands primary prevention to include more personalized nutrition and requires expanded nutrition education in medical school curriculum.

In the CDC study identifying the importance of diet, the most important dietary risks included our low intake of vegetables, fruits, nuts, and seeds and high intake of sodium, processed meats, and sources of trans fat.[49] To address these risks, CAM approaches to dietary interventions are much more specific than generic advice and provide a rich source of potential for treating this major risk factor for chronic disease and death. For example, the concept of the glycemic index and glycemic load is more routinely included in CAM approaches to treating diabetes and metabolic syndrome. Additionally, studies on functional foods such as apple cider vinegar and cinnamon have shown promise in improving glycemic control in patients with insulin resistance or type 2 diabetes.[51,52] More research is needed in these areas to validate CAM approaches. By providing a framework to expand this research, CAM in IPM becomes a key part of treating the chronic diseases of our time and should be further supported by insurance reimbursement so as to easily incorporate it into routine medical practice.

Another related area of CAM in IPM is manual medicine. Manipulative and body-based practices focus on the body's systems and structures, including the bones and joints, soft tissues, and circulatory and lymphatic systems.[16] Examples of this type of CAM therapy include spinal or joint manipulation as done by chiropractors, osteopathic physicians, and other practitioners. The latest statistical data show that 8.4% or 19.4 million people use chiropractic or osteopathic manipulation.[12] A systematic review found good evidence for spinal manipulation in the treatment of chronic or subacute low-back pain.[53] Given the preponderance of low-back pain as one of the most common diagnoses and the current burden of opioid addiction that often begins with treating musculoskeletal complaints such as low-back pain, IPM recognizes manual medicine to be a cost-effective, nonpharmacological intervention that is minimally invasive and is associated with minimal side effects. Massage therapy is also one form of manual medicine. References to massage therapy defined as the "the art of rubbing" by Hippocrates have been found in most ancient civilizations.[16] Currently 6.9% or 15.4 million US adults used massage therapy.[12] Massage therapy is another example of a mind body practice that has been shown to play a role in the management of chronic pain, although the evidence is not as strong as it is for manual medicine for chronic low-back pain.[26]

CAM in IPM Engages Patients and Physicians to Openly Discuss and Incorporate CAM in Routine Care Plans

Since the first major national surveys of CAM usage by Eisenberg et al, most patients who use CAM do not inform their physicians.[54] Patients do not discuss CAM usage for a number of reasons. The most common reasons cited by the NCCIH survey on CAM usage include the physician never asked (42%), the patient did not know they should ask (30%), and there was not enough time during the visit (19%).[54,55] These data suggest that simply asking about CAM in a routine visit will enable patients to share their usage with their physicians. IPM recognizes the lack of disclosure of CAM usage to be detrimental to the health of patients. Sharing this information can prevent the potential known side effects of certain CAM therapies and interactions with medications or other conventional treatments. By incorporating CAM into conventional approaches to prevention and chronic disease management, patients will be able to openly discuss their CAM usage with their doctors to optimize their care. Making these discussions a part of routine care will also serve as an opportunity to encourage and support patients' self-efficacy in taking responsibility for their health. This, coupled with the potential of CAM to be incorporated into the activities of daily living, will expand primary prevention and health promotion. By validating the patient's interest in evidence-based CAM as part of routine care, IPM encourages open dialogue with patients. These discussions can promote and reinforce positive behavior change to modify lifestyle to improve health outcomes. Motivational interviewing has been an effective tool for behavior change to modify risk factors for chronic disease. By including CAM in the intake for routine care, physicians have an opportunity to set lifestyle change goals with their patients that engage their CAM usage as part of their health action plan. This can be a more effective approach that will likely lead to better outcomes by enabling patients to be an active part of their treatment plans. This is particularly relevant when considering patients who have or are at risk for chronic disease. Chronic disease requires ongoing effort for management and prevention of progression. IPM provides an important tool to achieve success in chronic disease self-management by empowering patients to discuss CAM and empowering physicians to include it as part of the patient's treatment plan.

Conclusions

"Complementary and alternative medicine" is an antiquated term. More patients are using CAM as an adjunct to their conventional therapies. In redefining our current system to address this reality, IPM creates a new framework where complementary approaches to health are integrated seamlessly into conventional medical practice. The new framework of IPM is focused on prevention and health promotion with the goal of morbidity compression or extending the period of high-quality life that is free of disease throughout the lifespan. The role of CAM in IPM is to provide the needed evidence-based nonpharmacological therapies that are safe, minimally invasive, amenable to self-care, and cost-effective. The inherent focus of CAM on lifestyle and daily practices lends itself well to the new focus in IPM on prevention and health promotion. In IPM, CAM expands the three established levels of prevention to include evidence-based complementary approaches with particular emphasis on empowering patients to engage in more profound primary prevention efforts than are currently afforded to them by a conventional system that relies on passive screening and tertiary prevention. Also CAM brings added value to IPM by providing tools to combat the major risk factors for morbidity and mortality. By actively integrating CAM into a new framework for prevention and treatment of disease, IPM engages patients and physicians to openly discuss and use evidence-based CAM as a routine part of medical practice. This integrative approach will ultimately lead to better outcomes by providing key therapies for primary prevention and health maintenance. Although requiring further outcomes-based research, the new approach of IPM to incorporate CAM into our system provides great potential to effectively address the human and financial costs of our current epidemic of chronic disease.

References

1. US National Library of Medicine. https://www.nlm.nih.gov/tsd/acquisitions/cdm/subjects24.html. Accessed August 21, 2016.
2. The National Center for Complementary and Integrative Health. https://nccih.nih.gov/health/integrative-health. Accessed August 21, 2016.
3. Jones DS, Podolsky SH, Greene JA. The burden of disease and the changing task of medicine. *N Engl J Med* 2012;366:2333–2338.
4. Kung HC, Hoyert DL, Xu JQ, Murphy SL. Deaths: final data for 2005. *National Vital Statistics Reports*. 2008;56(10). http://www.cdc.gov/nchs/data/nvsr/nvsr56/nvsr56_10.pdf. Accessed August 21, 2016.
5. Marvasti FF, Stafford RS. From sick care to health care—reengineering prevention into the U.S. system. *N Engl J Med* 2012;367:889–891.
6. Centers for Disease Control (CDC). *Chronic Diseases: The Power to Prevent, the Call to Control: At a Glance.* 2009. http://www.cdc.gov.laneproxy.stanford.edu/chronicdisease/resources/publications/aag/chronic.htm.
7. Mokdad AH, Marks JS, Stroup DF, Gerberding JL. Actual causes of death in the United States, 2000. *JAMA* 2004;291:1238–1245.
8. Fries JF. Aging, natural death, and the compression of morbidity. *N Engl J Med* 1980;303:130–135.
9. *Two-Thirds of Adult Americans Believe More Money Needs to be Spent on Chronic Disease Prevention Programs, and They're Willing to Pay Higher Taxes to Fund Them, Survey Finds* [press release]. Atlanta, GA: National Association of Chronic Disease Directors; September 3, 2008. http://www.chronicdisease.org/files/public/PressRelease_NACDD_PublicHealthSurvey_August2008.pdf.

10. Koh, HK, Sebelius KG. Promoting prevention through the Affordable Care Act. *N Engl J Med* 2010;363:1296–1299.

11. US Department of Health and Human Services, Centers for Medicare and Medicaid Services. *National Health Expenditure data for 2012.* https://www.cms.gov/Research-Statistics-Data-and-systems/Statistics-Trends-and-reports/NationalHealthExpendData/index.html. Accessed March 31, 2016.

12. Clarke TC, Black LI, Stussman BJ, Barnes PM, Nahin RL. *Trends in the Use of Complementary Health Approaches Among Adults: United States, 2002–2012.* National health statistics reports; no 79. Hyattsville, MD: National Center for Health Statistics; 2015.

13. National Center for Complementary and Integrative Health Strategic Plan. https://nccih.nih.gov/about/strategic-plans/2016/Objective-3-Foster-Health-Promotion-Disease-Prevention#strategy-1. Accessed August 21, 2016.

14. Hawk C, Ndetan H, Evans MW. Potential role of complementary and alternative health care providers in chronic disease prevention and health promotion: an analysis of National Health Interview Survey data. *Prev Med* 2012;54(1):18–22.

15. Davis MA, Whedon JM, Weeks WB. Complementary and alternative medicine practitioners and accountable care organizations: the train is leaving the station. *J Altern Complem Med* 2011;17:669–674.

16. NCCIH. *NCCIH CAM Basics Primer.* https://nccih.nih.gov/sites/nccam.nih.gov/files/D347_05-25-2012.pdf. Accessed August 21, 2016.

17. NCCIH Website. https://nccih.nih.gov/health/integrative-health. Accessed August 21, 2016.

18. Woodyard C. Exploring the therapeutic effects of yoga and its ability to increase quality of life. *Int J Yoga* [serial online]. 2011;4:49–54. http://www.ijoy.org.in/text.asp?2011/4/2/49/85485. Accessed September 5, 2016.

19. Dalusung-Angosta A. The impact of Tai Chi exercise on coronary heart disease: a systematic review. *J Am Acad Nurse Pract* 2011;23(7):376–381.

20. Anderson JG, Taylor AG. The metabolic syndrome and mind-body therapies: a systematic review. *J Nutr Metab* 2011;276419.

21. Hall AM, Maher CG, Lam P, Ferreira M, Latimer J. Tai chi exercise for treatment of pain and disability in people with persistent low back pain: a randomized controlled trial. *Arthritis Care Res (Hoboken)* 2011;63(11):1576–1583.

22. Alraek T, Lee MS, Choi TY, Cao H, Liu J. Complementary and alternative medicine for patients with chronic fatigue syndrome: a systematic review. *BMC Complement Altern Med* 2011;11:87.

23. Taylor-Piliae RE, Coull BM. Community-based Yang-Style Tai Chi is safe and feasible in chronic stroke: a pilot study. *Clin Rehabil* 2012 Feb; 26(2):121–131. PMID:21937523.

24. Dhanani NM, Caruso TJ, Carinci AJ. Complementary and alternative medicine for pain: an evidence-based review. *Curr Pain Headache Rep* 2011;15(1):39–46.

25. Shen CL, Chyu MC, Yeh JK, et al. Effect of green tea and Tai Chi on bone health in postmenopausal osteopenic women: a 6-month randomized placebo-controlled trial. *Osteoporos Int* 2012 May; 23(5):1541–1552. PMID:21766228.

26. Woolf SH. The big answer: rediscovering prevention at a time of crisis in health care. *Harv Health Policy Rev* 2006;7:5–20.

27. Hawk C, Ndetan H, Evans MW Jr. Potential role of complementary and alternative health care providers in chronic disease prevention and health promotion: an analysis of national health interview survey data. *Prev Med* 2012;54:18–22.

28. Merriam-Webster Dictionary. *Prevent*. http://www.merriam-webster.com/dictionary/prevent. Accessed August 21, 2016.

29. Leavell H, Clark E. *Textbook of Preventive Medicine*. 3rd ed. New York, NY: McGraw-Hill; 1953.

30. Moore L, Thompson F. Adults meeting fruit and vegetable intake recommendations—United States, 2013. *MMWR: Morbidity and Mortality Weekly Report* [serial online]. 2015;64(26):709–713. Available from: CINAHL, Ipswich, MA. Accessed September 6, 2016.

31. Kaptchuk, T. *The Web That Has No Weaver: Understanding Chinese Medicine*. 2nd ed. New York, NY: McGraw-Hill; 2000.

32. National Center for Complementary and Integrative Health. *Ayurvedic Medicine: An Introduction*. Bethesda, MD: USDHHS, NIH, National Center for Complementary and Alternative Medicine; 2013.

33. *Nutrition and Health Annual Continuing Medical Education Conference*. http://www.nutritionandhealthconf.org/. Accessed September 4, 2016.

34. *Integrative Medicine Fellowships*. American Board of Physician Specialties. http://www.abpsus.org/integrative-medicine-fellowships. Accessed September 4, 2016.

35. Ornish D, Scherwitz LW, Billings JH, et al. Intensive lifestyle changes for reversal of coronary heart disease. *JAMA*1998;280(23):2001–2007. doi:10.1001/jama.280.23.2001.

36. Ali A, Katz DL. Disease prevention and health promotion how integrative medicine fits. *Am J Prev Med* 2015;49(5 Suppl 3):S230–S240.

37. Hooper L, Summerbell CD, Higgins JPT, et al. Reduced or modified dietary fat for preventing cardiovascular disease. *Cochrane DB Syst Rev* 2000; (2):CD0002137. http://www.update-software.com/cochrane.

38. Van Tulder MW, Cherkin DC, Berman B, et al. The effectiveness of acupuncture in the management of acute and chronic low back pain: a systematic review within the framework of the Cochrane Collaboration Back Review Group. *Spine* 1999;24(11):1113–1123.

39. *The White House Commission on Complementary and Alternative Medicine Policy*. http://www.whccamp.hhs.gov/fr2.html. Accessed September 5, 2016.

40. *Cochrane Complementary Medicine*. http://cam.cochrane.org/. Accessed September 5, 2016.

41. *PubMed Dietary Supplements Subset*. http://ods.od.nih.gov/Research/PubMed_Dietary_ Supplement_Subset.aspx. Accessed September 5, 2016.

42. *University of Maryland Herbal Database*. http://www.umm.edu/altmed/index.htm. Accessed September 5, 2016.

43. *Dietary Supplements Labels Database*. http://dietarysupplements.nlm.nih.gov/dietary. Accessed September 5, 2016.

44. Nies LK, Cymbala AA, Kasten SL, Lamprecht DG, Olson KL. Complementary and alternative therapies for the management of dyslipidemia. *Ann Pharmacother* 2006;40:1984–1992.

45. McFarland LV. Meta-analysis of probiotics for the prevention of antibiotic associated diarrhea and the treatment of *Clostridium difficile* disease. *Am J Gastroenterol* 2006;101:812–822.

46. Centers for Disease Control and Prevention. http://www.cdc.gov/diabetes/basics/index.html. Accessed September 5, 2016.

47. National Center for Chronic Disease Prevention and Health Promotion. *The power of Prevention, Chronic Disease: The Public Health Challenge of the 21st Century.* 2009. http://www.cdc.gov/chronicdisease/pdf/2009-power-of-prevention.pdf. Accessed September 5, 2016.

48. Knowler WC, Barrett-Connor E, Fowler SE, et al. Reduction in the incidence of type 2 diabetes with lifestyle intervention or metformin. *N Engl J Med* 2002;346:393–403.

49. US Burden of Disease Collaborators. The state of US health, 1990–2010: burden of diseases, injuries, and risk factors. *JAMA* 2013;310(6):591–606. doi:10.1001/jama.2013.13805.

50. Adams KM, Kohlmeier M, Zeisel SH. Nutrition education in U.S. medical schools: latest update of a national survey. *Acad Med* 2010;85(9):1537–1542. doi:10.1097/ACM.0b013e3181eab71b.

51. Johnston CS, Kim CM, Buller AJ. Vinegar improves insulin sensitivity to a high-carbohydrate meal in subjects with insulin resistance or type 2 diabetes. *Diabetes Care* 2004;27(1):281–282. doi: 10.2337/diacare.27.1.281.

52. Allen RW, Schwartzman E, Baker WL, Coleman CI, Phung OJ. Cinnamon use in type 2 Diabetes: an updated systematic review and meta-analysis. *Ann Fam Med* 2013;11(5):452–459. doi:10.1370/afm.1517.

53. Chou R, Huffman LH. Nonpharmacologic therapies for acute and chronic low back pain: a review of the evidence for an American Pain Society/American College of Physicians clinical practice guideline. *Ann Intern Med* 2007;147:492–504.

54. Rakel RE, Rakel DP. *Textbook of Family Medicine.* 9th ed. Philadelphia, PA: Elsevier Saunders; 2016.

55. Barnes PM, Bloom B, Nahin RL. *Complementary and Alternative Medicine Use Among Adults and Children: United States, 2007.* Division of Health Interview Statistics, National Center for Health Statistics; National Center for Complementary and Alternative Medicine, National Institutes of Health. Atlanta GA: U.S. Department of Health and Human Services, Centers for Disease Control and Prevention, National Center for Health Statistics online pdf https://www-cdc-gov.laneproxy.stanford.edu.nchs/data/nhsr/nhsr012.pdf

10

The Role of Nutrition in Integrative Preventive Medicine

WALTER C. WILLETT, MD, DRPH

U ntil recently, and still today in low-income countries, undernutrition during pregnancy and the first years of life was a major cause of mortality. However, in recent decades, both in the United States and globally, noncommunicable diseases (NCDs) account for the majority of premature deaths. In analyses of the overall burden of disease, dietary factors were identified as the most important causes in the United States and worldwide.[1] Despite this, physicians and other healthcare providers are taught little about nutrition in medical school or fellowship training.[2] Not surprisingly, in conventional medical practice almost no attention is given to knowing what a patient is eating or providing dietary guidance that has the potential to improve dramatically their long-term health. To counter widespread misinformation and confusion about diet and health, this chapter describes what we know about the elements of a healthy diet and how these elements can be combined into an overall dietary pattern for the prevention of major illness and promotion of well-being. A brief section considers ways that this knowledge can be integrated into preventive healthcare.

Origins of Modern Concepts on Diet and Health

Although diet has been recognized since the time of Hippocrates as an underlying determinant of health, more recent evidence that diet might be important in the prevention of cardiovascular disease and cancer came from studies comparing rates of disease in different countries. Some of the most important evidence emerged from the 7-Countries Study conducted by Dr. Ancel

Keys and colleagues during the 1950s and 1960s.[3] These investigators, for the first time, documented incidence and mortality rates of coronary heart disease (CHD) using standard diagnostic criteria in 14 populations of about 1,000 men in each of 7 different countries. They found an approximately 10-fold difference in rates, with the highest being in Finland and the lowest in Crete. One possible explanation for these huge difference could be genetic factors, but other scientists investigating heart disease among migrants from low-incidence countries to the United States found that the migrants rapidly adopted the rates of heart disease among European Americans,[4] firmly rejecting genetic factors as the explanation for the high rates of heart disease in the United States and northern Europe. This simple but critical finding meant that CHD, the number one cause of death in the United States, was potentially preventable if the causal factors could be identified and modified.

In their quest to identify possible explanations for the large variation in CHD rates, Keys and colleagues noted that these rates correlated strongly with intake of saturated fat but not total fat; those with the highest total fat intake (about 40% of calories) included both Finland, where dairy fat was the dominant source, and Crete, where olive oil was the dominant source.[3] Although these correlations with diet raised important questions, they could have been explained by confounding factors, such as differences in smoking, physical activity, or other aspects of diet, thus indicating the need for more detailed studies. Controlled feeding studies examining changes in blood lipids over a few weeks provided support for saturated fat contributing to heart disease because replacement of carbohydrate intake with saturated fat increased blood total cholesterol. However, these studies did not support total fat being responsible because polyunsaturated fat reduced total blood cholesterol and monounsaturated fat appeared neutral.[5]

During this period, other epidemiologists were investigating rates of breast, colon, prostate, and other cancers around the world. They also found great variation in rates among countries, as much as 8- to 10-fold.[6] Also, like heart disease, the rates in populations migrating from low- to high-risk countries converged with, and sometimes overshot, the rates in European Americans, although for breast cancer the catch-up occurred over several generations.[7] Again, strong correlations were seen between intakes of total or animal fat and rates of these cancers.

Although these crude correlations should have been interpreted cautiously because many potentially confounding factors existed, they were widely interpreted as causal.[8] As a result, beginning in the early 1980s, dietary recommendations in the United States and worldwide emphasized reduction in total fat intake. The cardiovascular prevention world went along with this because reduction in total fat seemed to be a simpler message than advice to replace saturated fat with polyunsaturated fat, which was based primarily on controlled feeding studies.

Because protein intake does not vary greatly across diets, a reduction in total fat implies an increase in carbohydrates, which were widely promoted as healthy choices without any direct evidence. This was epitomized by the original USDA Food Guide Pyramid of 1992, which suggested up to 11 servings a day of grains, along with including potatoes as a vegetable. Because about 80% of the carbohydrates in the US food supply are from refined starch, sugar, and potatoes, the result was that intake of these sources of calories increased by roughly 300 calories per day and the percent of energy from fat decreased from about 40% of energy to about 33% of energy.[9] This corresponded with the huge increase in rates of obesity and diabetes in the United States; as discussed later, this dietary advice was probably contributory. Further, controlled feeding studies conducted in the 1980s and 1990s documented that high intakes of carbohydrate, compared to unsaturated fats or protein, increase triglycerides and blood pressure and reduce HDL cholesterol, and LDL particle size, which would all predict higher rates of heart disease.[5,10]

Randomized Trials and Cohort Studies of Diet and Disease

Motivated by the international correlations between dietary factors and rates of CHD and cancers, more detailed studies were needed to understand the specific dietary factors that might be involved. Ideally, hypotheses about diet and health outcomes would be answered by randomized trials in which many thousands of people are assigned to high intake of a dietary factor and others to low intake. However, such studies are extremely costly, and even when conducted they have often been uninformative because of low adherence to the assigned diets. The Women's Health Initiative low-fat diet trial among 48,000 women provides the most recent example;[11] at no time during the 7 years of follow-up did plasma levels of HDL cholesterol and triglycerides differ between the low-fat and usual diet groups.[12,13] Because these lipids are known to change with low-fat diets, the trial was unfortunately uninformative. Trials of cancer prevention are even more challenging, because the effects of dietary change may not be seen until decades later. For these reasons, prospective cohort studies in which many thousands of persons are followed for many years are likely to be the most useful source of evidence about the relation between diet and major diseases. The Nurses' Health Study (NHS) was among the early cohort investigations of diet and health, and the only one of these to repeatedly update dietary information over time, beginning in 1980. Especially when findings for health outcomes, such as coronary heart disease, are consistent with controlled feeding studies with intermediate outcomes, such as blood lipids or blood pressure, reproducible prospective cohort studies can provide sufficient support for causality to make dietary recommendations and nutrition policy.[14]

Specific Types of Dietary Fats and Heart Disease

Over the last 60 years, findings from controlled feeding studies of blood lipids, prospective cohort studies, and some randomized trials have provided strong evidence that replacing saturated fat with polyunsaturated fat will reduce coronary heart disease.[15,16] Based on this concept, consumption of polyunsaturated fat, until recently mainly as soybean oil and corn oil, approximately doubled in the United States since the 1960s and is almost certainly one of the major contributors to the large decline in coronary heart disease mortality, by more than 60%.

Considerable confusion was caused by a recent meta-analysis by Chowdhury et al[17] concluding that replacement of saturated fat with polyunsaturated fat for reduction of CHD was not supported by evidence. This meta-analysis was deeply flawed in many ways as described in the correspondence, but most fundamentally because it ignored the central concept in nutrition of isocaloric replacement; if we decrease one important source of calories, the effect will depend on what replaces it. In a meta-analysis of published studies, it was not possible to specify the replacement calories because individual studies have not reported their findings in a consistent way. For this reason, Jakobsen et al had earlier conducted an analysis using the original individual data from cohort studies of dietary fats and coronary heart disease.[18] In that analysis, confirming an earlier, detailed analysis of NHS data,[19] higher intake of saturated fat was not significantly associated with risk of coronary heart disease when compared with a similar number of calories from carbohydrate. This is consistent with the metabolic evidence that this replacement reduces both LDL cholesterol and HDL cholesterol and increases triglyceride levels.[20] However, higher intake of saturated fat was associated with greater risk of coronary heart disease when compared with a similar number of calories from polyunsaturated fat, again consistent with well-documented changes in blood lipids. A similar relationship has been seen with total mortality.[16] In controlled feeding studies, monounsaturated fat has effects on blood lipids that are similar to polyunsaturated fat,[20] but cohort studies are complicated by the fact that in Western diets most monounsaturated fats come from meat, dairy products, and partially hydrogenated vegetable oils. In a detailed analysis within the NHS, one of the few studies with details on types of fat, monounsaturated fat was also inversely associated with risk of CHD when compared isocalorically with carbohydrate or saturated fat.[19] The recent PREDIMED randomized trial,[21] in which the addition of nuts or olive oil to a traditional Mediterranean diet reduced the incidence of cardiovascular disease compared to a low-fat diet, is consistent with benefits of monounsaturated fat, although this could not be completely disentangled from other components of the overall Mediterranean diet.

The picture of dietary fat and cardiovascular disease was complicated by recognition of trans-fatty acids, produced by the partial hydrogenation of vegetable oils, as an important element of our food supply. By the mid-1900s the large majority of vegetable oils in the United States were partially hydrogenated because this extended shelf life and produced solid fats that could mimic lard and butter, the traditional fats of northern European diets. However, in the 1970s, we and others became concerned that partial hydrogenation might have serious adverse effects because the oils being hydrogenated were primarily the essential fatty polyunsaturated fatty acids, linoleic and alpha-linolenic acid (ALA), that are critical to the structure of every cell membrane and the precursor molecules for the prostaglandins and other critical molecules. Thus, altering the double bonds of these essential fatty acids from their natural cis to the trans position by partial hydrogenation would almost surely change their functions in ways that were unpredictable and potentially harmful. This issue was of particular concern because intake of trans fat in the form of margarine and vegetable shortening was being strongly promoted for prevention of coronary heart disease because these products were believed to be superior to butter and lard due to a lower saturated fat content. The findings from multiple large cohort studies showing elevated risks of CHD with higher trans fat intake and controlled feeding studies showing that trans fats uniquely increase LDL and reduce HDL cholesterol along with other adverse effects[22] led to compelling conclusions that intake should be as low as possible. Through a combination of education, product reformulation, and banning in restaurants in many cities and states, consumption has greatly decreased,[23] LDL has decreased and HDL has increased in children and adults,[24,25] and the FDA has effectively banned trans fats as of 2018.

Evidence on types of fat and heart disease is summarized in Figure 10.1. If saturated fat were replaced by trans fat, risk of heart disease would increase. However, if saturated fat were replaced by unsaturated fat, especially polyunsaturated fat, risk would decrease. In practice, this means replacing dairy fats and fats from red meat with liquid vegetable oils wherever possible.[26] If saturated fat is replaced with the average carbohydrate in the American diet, there would be little effect on risk of heart disease. However, the average

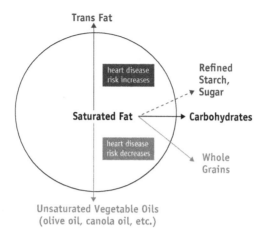

FIGURE 10.1 Evidence on Types of Fat and Heart Disease

carbohydrate in the US diet, about half of total calories, is approximately 80% refined starch, sugar, or potatoes; as discussed later, the quality of carbohydrate also has important impacts on risk of cardiovascular disease, and if saturated fat is replaced by whole grains, risk of heart disease would be lower.[26,27] Given the mix of types of fat and carbohydrate in the United States, total fat intake has not been associated with risks of heart disease;[19] the type of fat and carbohydrate make a major difference.

Although polyunsaturated fat was considered as a homogeneous class of fatty acids in early diet–heart studies, much evidence indicates that the two main families, the N-6 and N-3 fatty acids, have many unique and important roles; both are considered essential fatty acids. A widespread belief has emerged, based on a simplistic interpretation of metabolic pathways, that N-6 fatty acids are proinflammatory and increase risks of heart disease, mental illness, and other conditions, and that the ratio of N-3 to N-6 fatty acids is critical. In fact, both N-6 and N-3 fatty acids are essential and beneficial; thus the ratio is irrelevant;[28,29] in fact, it is possible to have a "perfect" ratio with deficiencies of both types of fatty acids. Linoleic acid, the primary dietary N-6 fatty acid, is a precursor of proinflammatory eicosanoids, but this conversion is highly regulated; and in controlled feeding studies higher intake of dietary linoleic acid does not increase proinflammatory eicosanoids or indicators of inflammation such as C-reactive protein (CRP).[30] Indeed, in about half of the studies, increasing intake of linoleic acids was associated with lower levels of inflammatory factors, probably because it down-regulates NF-kappa B and can increase insulin sensitivity. Most importantly, in the epidemiologic studies and randomized trials described earlier, linoleic acid composed the large majority of the polyunsaturated fat, which is related to lower risk of coronary heart disease. In a recent reanalysis of the Minnesota Heart Study,[31] the role of linoleic acid in the prevention of heart disease was questioned, but the average follow-up was less than 2 years and by the 3rd year approximately 85% of the participants had been lost to follow-up, rendering any conclusions uninterpretable. The relation between linoleic acid and risk of CHD in cohort studies was recently summarized;[29] as shown in Figure 10.1, for total polyunsaturated fat intake, compared to carbohydrate or saturated fat, intake of linoleic acid was related to lower risk of CHD. Intake of total polyunsaturated fat and linoleic acid have also been examined extensively in relation to risk of breast and other cancers, diabetes, and many other conditions without evidence of harm.[32] In a recent large analysis of over 175,000 men and women, higher intake of N-6 polyunsaturated fat intake was strongly related to lower total mortality.[16] Thus, within the range consumed in usual human diets, up to about 9% of calories in the US diet, N-6 fatty acids are both essential and beneficial.

Like N-6 fatty acids, N-3 fatty acids play many essential structural and functional roles, and they have also been hypothesized to have a unique role in preventing cardiac arrhythmias and thus sudden cardiac death.[33] In human diets, fish oils are the major source of extra-long-chain N-3 fatty acids, but ALA, primarily from plants and especially soy and canola oils, is quantitatively the primary source of total N-3 fatty acids. In studies using dietary intake or levels in red blood cells, docosohexaenoic acid (DHA) and eicosapentaenoic acid (EPA) have been inversely associated with fatal coronary heart disease in cohort studies,[15] and reductions in risk of CHD have been seen in some randomized trials.[15] In several recent randomized trials, supplements of EPA/DHA have not reduced cardiac deaths, raising doubts about their benefits. However, randomized trials of dietary supplements are not like trials of new drugs in which the placebo group has no intake of the agent being tested; in the EPA/DHA trials everyone had some intake of N-3 fatty acids at baseline, and if intake was already near optimal for many participants, supplements would have no apparent benefit. This does not exclude a potential benefit among a significant minority in the population or an important overall benefit in other populations, which include major parts of the world with much lower intakes.[34] Studies of ALA and cardiovascular diseases are fewer, but a benefit appears likely where fish intake, and thus EPA/DHA intake, is low.[35] Although the optimal intakes of EPA/DHA and ALA remain to be determined, the AHA recommendation to eat fish at least twice per week is reasonable, and using a variety of plant oils, especially including canola or soybean oil, will provide a source of ALA. Walnuts and flaxseed are other potential sources.

Dietary Fats and Risks of Cancer and Diabetes

Because the presumed relation of total fat intake to risk of breast cancer, based primarily on international correlations, was a key pillar for national dietary recommendations, this was examined in detail at repeated intervals in the Nurses' Health Study; at no time was there any suggestion of a positive relationship.[36] This lack of any important relation has been confirmed in a summary of cohort studies; except for a possible inverse association with monounsaturated fat, specific types of fat have also not been associated importantly with risk of breast cancer.[32,37] The findings for total fat are also consistent with randomized trials,[11,38] although the WHI trial findings are uninformative, as noted earlier.[13] A similar lack of increased risk with total fat has also been seen for cancers of the colon and rectum, and for prostate cancer; indeed, for no cancer examined has total fat intake been found to be a risk factor.

For type 2 diabetes, adiposity is a powerful risk factor, but total dietary fat is not. As for coronary heart disease, trans fat intake is importantly related to increased risk,[39,40] and polyunsaturated fat or the ratio of polyunsaturated to saturated fat is related to lower risk.

Dietary Fat and Body Weight

Perhaps the most deeply embedded belief about the benefits of low-fat/high-carbohydrate diets has been that they are effective in preventing weight gain and treating overweight. This was supported by some early randomized trials,[41] but most of these lasted only a few months and in most trials the low-fat group received intensive intervention and the control group received none. With additional, longer studies, it became apparent that the weight loss in groups assigned to low-fat diets was usually transient, with a nadir at about 6 months, and that the intensity of intervention itself contributes to weight loss. In the most comprehensive meta-analysis of randomized trials with data on dietary fat and body weight that lasted for 1 year or longer, among trials with equal intensity of intervention, persons assigned to low-fat diets lost less weight than the control groups with higher fat intake.[42] Although, low-fat/high-carbohydrate diets are not generally effective for weight control, other characteristics of diet do have important influences. In a comprehensive analysis of specific foods among over 100,000 men and women, potatoes, red meat, soda, and fruit juice were related to more weight gain, and whole grains, fruits, vegetables, and yogurt were related to less weight gain.[43] The foods associated with less weight gain are consistent with a Mediterranean dietary pattern, which was evaluated in a compelling study of diet and weight control, conducted by Shai et al.[44] In that study, employees at a worksite were randomized to a low-fat diet, a high-fat diet, and a Mediterranean diet with fat content just slightly lower than the high-fat diet. By 6 months, weight loss was similar on all diets, but by 2 years, the low-fat group had regained most of their weight. Most notably, after an additional 4 years without intervention, the low-fat group had regained all their weight, the Mediterranean diet group had maintained most of their weight loss and had improved metabolic variables, and the high-fat group was intermediate.[45] The sustained weight loss of the Mediterranean group suggests that the participants had internalized this eating pattern, which is the ultimate goal of an intervention.

Notably, in weight loss trials the primary reported results are average changes in weight, but what has been remarkably consistent is the wide variation in response to changes in dietary fat. On all diets, some persons lose large amounts of weight, but others lose nothing or gain weight. The explanation for this heterogeneity remains unclear but could be related to biological factors or social factors, such as family support. However, this does suggest a role for individual experimentation to find an eating pattern that is effective for them in long-term weight control; an essential criterion is that this must be sufficiently varied, satisfying, and enjoyable so that it can be maintained for years. This likely explains the success of the Mediterranean diet in the study by Shai et al. Of course, a long-term diet must also be compatible with overall good health, which must be evaluated in much larger and longer-term studies.

In summary, despite vast efforts to document a benefit of low-fat diets for prevention of cancer, cardiovascular disease, weight control, and many other health outcomes, such benefits have not emerged. For this reason, the 2015 US Dietary Guidelines removed the earlier upper limits on the percentage of energy from fat, which will allow a wider range of healthy diets.

Carbohydrates

Until recently, intakes of total and specific types of carbohydrates have received much less attention than dietary fat, which is surprising because they are the major source of calories. Because protein intake varies relatively little among persons, the relation of total carbohydrate to health outcomes tends to be the reciprocal of total fat intake; and as for total fat intake, there is insufficient evidence to set limits for carbohydrate intake. Indeed, there is no nutritional requirement for carbohydrate. Similar to fat, the type of carbohydrate has important health implications; unfortunately, there is no single, simple measure of carbohydrate quality, but it can be characterized by its degree of refinement (such as whole grain or fiber content), its glycemic index, and whether in solution or solid form.

The refining of grains has major impacts on their nutritional value because the large majority of fiber, minerals, and vitamins are removed. The remaining starch is simply a chain of glucose molecules with no nutritional value beyond a source of energy and, when broken down into glucose, multiple potential adverse metabolic effects. In contrast, consumption of cereal fiber or whole grains has been consistently associated with lower risks of cardiovascular disease,[46] diabetes,[47] and digestive disorders; evidence for cancer is less consistent.[32,48] As they travel together in whole grains, the contributions of cereal fiber, minerals, and vitamins are difficult to distinguish.

The glycemic index of a carbohydrate, assessed as the incremental increase in blood glucose after fixed amount of carbohydrate is consumed, is influenced by many factors, but the pulverizing of grain into fine flour is particularly important, as this increases the rate of enzymatic conversion of starch to glucose. Because the effect of a food on blood glucose levels will depend on both the amount of carbohydrate and the glycemic index of this carbohydrate, we have developed the glycemic load, which is calculated by multiplying the glycemic index by the amount of the carbohydrate in a food or diet. Along with refined grains, potatoes are also a major source of glycemic load in Western diets because they have large amounts of carbohydrate with a high glycemic index. The concept of glycemic index has been controversial, but in our cohort studies and a meta-analysis, higher glycemic index is importantly associated with higher risks of type 2 diabetes,[49] and glycemic load strongly predicts risk of CHD.[50] This evidence is supported by a large randomized trial of a glucosidase inhibitor,[51] which pharmacologically converts high glycemic index foods to low glycemic index foods within the gastrointestinal tract; incidence of diabetes and cardiovascular disease was reduced.

Liquid carbohydrates, mainly as soda and other sugar-sweetened beverages (SSBs), are particularly problematic, because very large amounts of sugar can be consumed rapidly with minimal induction of satiety. A large body of evidence has documented adverse effects of SSBs on weight gain and risks of diabetes and coronary heart disease.[52] Some have suggested that fructose, half of the sucrose molecule and only slightly more than half of high fructose corn syrup, is substantially more harmful than glucose. Although fructose is metabolized differently than glucose, they both have harmful metabolic effects, and keeping intake of added sugar low, especially in the form of soda and other sugar-sweetened beverages, is a high priority.

Protein Sources

Few foods contain protein as the main form of calories, so the health impacts of dietary protein are best considered as part of the food in which it is packaged, which often includes a substantial amount of fat, which varies greatly in type. Although current US dietary guidelines make little distinction between sources of proteins,[52] the health consequences differ greatly. Red meat stands out as being related to higher risks of CHD, stroke, type 2 diabetes, and some cancers.[53-55] In analyses examining alternatives to red meat, risks of these endpoints are lower with intakes of poultry, fish, low-fat dairy foods, beans, and nuts (see http://www.iarc.fr/en/media-centre/iarcnews/pdf/Monographs-Q&A_Vol114.pdf). Some of these differences are due to a higher proportion of unsaturated fatty acids in most of these alternatives, but the high amounts of heme iron and cholesterol in red meat and other microconstituents may also contribute to the elevated risks. There is no evidence that eating leaner meats mitigates the adverse effects; for example, heme iron and cholesterol are predominately in the lean part of meat.

Apart from the direct health effects of red meat, the impacts of high red meat consumption on environmental sustainability, essential to food security, are a concern. Whether expressed in relation to caloric or protein content, red meat has by far the greatest contribution to greenhouse gas production compared to any other food, and also has disproportionally large water, energy, and land footprints (see http://www.ewg.org/meateatersguide/a-meat-eaters-guide-to-climate-change-health-what-you-eat-matters/climate-and-environmental-impacts/).

Dairy and Vitamin D

High consumption of dairy foods, typically three servings a day, has been promoted, primarily based on expected reductions in osteoporosis and fractures because of its high calcium content. However, the high recommended daily allowances (RDAs) for calcium intake in the United States (e.g., 1,200 mg/day for women over 50 years) are based on studies lasting only 2 weeks, which is far too short to assess long-term calcium needs; the World Health Organization (WHO) has concluded that 500 mg/day is adequate. Further, in a meta-analysis of prospective studies, high intakes of calcium and milk were not associated with lower risk of fractures.[56] Dairy food consumption is not importantly related to weight gain[57] or risk of type 2 diabetes,[58] but is related to higher risk of prostate cancer and lower risk of colorectal cancer.[32] Given these mixed findings, keeping dairy consumption in the range of 0 to 2 servings a day seems sensible; if few or no dairy foods are consumed, taking 500 mg of calcium per day as a safety net is reasonable.

Vitamin D is essential for bone health. Fortification of milk has been an effective public health strategy that almost eliminated rickets in children, and supplements of vitamin D in the range of 700 to 800 mg/day have reduced fractures in older adults.[59] Considerable evidence suggests that low vitamin D levels may be contributing to risks of other diseases including colorectal cancer and multiple sclerosis.[60,61] The natural source of vitamin D is solar exposure, and fish is the only food that contains an appreciable amount of vitamin D. Although vitamin D supplementation remains controversial, taking 1,000 IU per day has been deemed safe[62] and seems reasonable unless someone is routinely exposed to substantial outdoor sunlight. Some people may require substantially more to minimize disease risk, but optimal intakes are not yet clear.

Fruits and Vegetables

Fruits and vegetables contain a wide range of essential nutrients and many other constituents that are hypothesized to reduce risks of many diseases. The strongest evidence is that these foods reduce blood pressure[63] and risk of cardiovascular disease. At least some of the benefit is mediated by their content of potassium[64] and probably folate. These foods have much less impact on cancer risk than had earlier been believed, but reduction in risk of ER-negative breast cancer is likely.[65] The composition of fruits and vegetables varies widely, and it is thus unlikely that they have similar health effects. Potatoes should not be considered a vegetable, but rather a form of starch along with corn.[66-68] In the United States, many consume few green leafy vegetables, which are important to include, and berries appear to be particularly beneficial for prevention of diabetes risk.[69] Although more remains to be learned about specific foods, consuming at least five servings a day of nonstarchy fruits and vegetables is an important goal.

Alcohol, Coffee, and Tea

Heavy alcohol consumption has many adverse health effects and should be avoided; the balance of risks and benefits for low and moderate consumption has been controversial. Very briefly, evidence is strong that moderate alcohol consumption reduces risk of coronary heart disease, and also lower risks of total mortality in middle-aged adults.[70] This benefit appears to be due primarily to ethanol per se rather than other constituents of these beverages. The major counterbalancing health effect at the level of 1–2 drinks per day is an increased risk of breast cancer.[71-76]

Early concerns about possible increases in risks of cancer and cardiovascular disease with coffee consumption have been erased by a large literature showing no increases in risk for any type of cancer, substantial decreases in risk of diabetes, and a likely modestly lower risk of total mortality.[77,78]

Dietary Supplements

Few topics are as controversial as nutritional supplements. If everyone were consuming an ideal diet, a benefit of supplements would likely be small, except for vitamin D, because foods are a poor source. However, fewer than 5% meet the US dietary guidelines recommendations, and we found that none of low-income Americans in a national survey came close to consuming an optimal diet.[79] The fact that multiple vitamins dramatically reduce risk of birth defects and that vitamin D fortification virtually eliminated rickets, demonstrates that diets are not optimal. Some of the controversy over the value of vitamin supplements stems from "negative" randomized trials that were of naively short duration for conditions that develop over decades and/or that likely include many participants who already have adequate intake.[80] For example, the Physician's Health Study was the only trial that lasted for more than a decade, and in that study beta-carotene improved cognitive function relative to placebo[81] and a multiple vitamin reduced total cancer incidence by 8%, which is remarkable because this was an unusually well nourished population.[82] Given available evidence, use of an RDA level multiple vitamin with 800 to 1,000 IU of vitamin D is reasonable for most people. For women of reproductive age, who should already be taking a multiple vitamin with folate for prevention of birth defects, inclusion of an RDA level of iron is also reasonable because approximately 15% of women in the group are iron deficient.

The Overall Impact of a Healthy Diet: Dietary Patterns and Indices

As described earlier, and as shown in Figure 10.2, the key elements of health eating are:

- An abundance of fruits and vegetables, not including potatoes.
- Healthy fats from plant sources, including virtually all liquid vegetable oils.
- Protein from predominantly plant sources, with optionally moderate amounts of fish, poultry, and dairy foods. Red meat to be occasional at most.
- Whole grains, with limited amounts of sugar and refined grains.

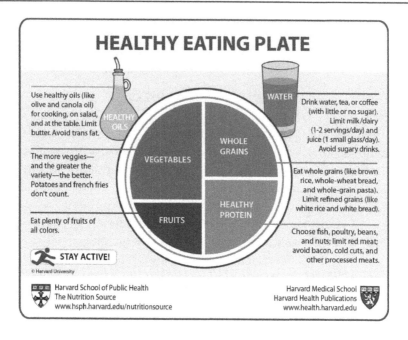

FIGURE 10.2 Healthy Eating Plate

One way of evaluating the healthfulness of an overall diet is to examine an overall dietary pattern in relation to health outcomes. Patterns, such as the traditional Mediterranean dietary pattern,[83] can be defined by using a scoring system, giving points for elements included in a diet or subtracting points for elements not in that diet. Within many countries, adherence to the Mediterranean dietary pattern has been associated with lower risk of cardiovascular disease, diabetes, cognitive decline, and premature mortality. Most of these benefits have been confirmed in the PREDIMED randomized trial conducted in Spain;[21] and in a randomized trial among post-myocardial-infarction patients, a Mediterranean diet reduced recurrence or cardiovascular death by 70%.[84] Another approach has been to define a dietary score or index based on the overall literature regarding the elements of a healthy diet; for example, we created the Alternative Healthy Eating Index (AHEI) because the 2000 USDA Healthy Eating Index (HEI) failed to predict health outcome. With later important changes to the HEI, both indices strongly predict better health outcomes.[85,86] Collectively, these analyses document the importance of a healthy diet across many different outcomes and in many different populations around the world. Our understanding of the elements of a healthy diet allows great flexibility using different foods, flavors, and culinary traditions.

The Potential for Disease Reduction by Diet and Lifestyle

The potential for reduction of major diseases by diet and lifestyle has been examined using data from large cohort studies. Using data from the NHS, the combination of not smoking, being moderately active, eating a healthy diet (defined by a simple five-element score), maintaining a healthy weight, and moderate alcohol consumption was estimated to reduce incidence of coronary heart disease by 82%;[87] the contributions of better diet, physical activity, avoidance of overweight, and not smoking were similar. Similar findings for younger women were recently reported from the Nurses' Health Study II.[88] Using the same approach, 92% of type 2 diabetes and 70% of stroke were estimated to be preventable by a similar set of diet and lifestyle factors.[89]

Encouragingly, through education and policies, dietary quality is gradually improving in the United States, although the room for further improvement is huge. Using the AHEI to score dietary data collected by the NHANES from 1999 through 2012, the score increased from approximately 40 to 50 on a scale of 110.[23] The greatest improvement was due to an approximately 80% reduction in intake of trans fat, and decline in soda consumption of about 25% also contributed importantly. Modest increases were seen for whole grains, fruits, and polyunsaturated fat. Only sodium intake trended in an adverse direction. Although the average changes were encouraging, most of the improvements in dietary quality were among those with higher income and education and among those with healthy weights, thus identifying areas where greater efforts are needed. In this same report, it was estimated that more than 1 million premature deaths were prevented by improvements in diet quality from 1999 through 2012, and that these improvements would reduce incidence of type 2 diabetes by about 12%. Encouragingly, the CDC has recently reported that incidence of type 2 diabetes had decreased by 20% in the United States after years of continuous increases (see http://www.cdc.gov/diabetes/statistics/incidence/fig2.htm).

Putting Knowledge into Practice

Unfortunately, medical schools and postgraduate programs have rarely included more than minimal information about diet and health and how to incorporate this into practice.[2] Although we have learned much about the relation of diet to health over the last several decades, evidence about the most effective ways to integrate this into preventive health care is still rudimentary. This will include basic skills in motivational interviewing that will not be covered here, and a variety of approaches depending on the context and individual patients. Our longer experience in control of smoking provides some guidance, and management of weight is discussed elsewhere in this book (see chapter 18). Some general considerations include:

1. Most importantly, healthcare providers should practice healthy dietary practices themselves. Doing so will make providers more knowledgeable about healthy diets and the benefits they provide as well barriers to healthy eating and ways to overcome these obstacles.

2. Determine a patient's BMI and weight change since age 20 and over the past year or two. Although these are simple and inexpensive to assess, they are often not collected or are ignored, even though they strongly predict many health outcomes and total mortality.[90] Assessment of waist circumference is also desirable, especially as people pass through midlife. Weight gain is important, because increases of more than 5–10 pounds predict adverse outcomes, even though BMI can remain below the standard cutoff of 25 kg/m². Also, this indicates that a person is on a trajectory to gain more weight unless changes are made in diet or physical activity.

3. Assess a patient's diet, even if crudely. If nothing more is possible, add soda consumption to the routine assessment of tobacco and alcohol use. Usual diet can be assessed inexpensively by self-administered food frequency questionnaires used for research purposes; these provide a wealth of information about a person's overall diet and the individual constituents of that diet;[91] as noted above, this information predicts many health outcomes and premature death. Simplified screening questionnaires can capture much of the information provided by more complex dietary assessment.[92] Neither of these approaches has been routinely incorporated into clinical practice, leaving healthcare providers without information about one of the most important determinants of their patient's future and without an informed basis to provide individual counseling. More research is clearly needed on the incorporation of dietary assessment in preventive healthcare.

4. Develop a menu of options for weight control and improvement in diet quality. Some patients are highly motivated and simply need scientifically based evidence to make changes in their diets that can have major benefits. To fill this need, I have written *Eat, Drink and Be Healthy*[93] and, with Molly Katzen, *Eat, Drink, and Weigh Less*.[94] Others will benefit from additional individual counseling or group support. In a recent randomized trial within a clinical setting, impressive weight loss was seen with both individual counseling and a less

expensive intervention that used computer-generated follow-up reminders.[95]

5. Take advantage of teachable moments. Although we would ideally prevent a large proportion of intermediate risk factors—like hypertension, hyperlipidemia, colon adenomas, or metabolic syndrome—by healthy diet and lifestyle, the large majority of people who develop these conditions do not have an optimal diet. The diagnosis of these conditions provides an extra reason to review diet and other lifestyle factors, and potentially additional motivation for the patient. Similarly, the diagnosis of diabetes, cardiovascular disease, or other diet-related condition in a family member can provide a good opportunity to review risk factors, as these people may well be sharing a common diet. Unfortunately, these diagnoses typically are lost opportunities. The reporting of the SPRINT study, showing that a lower target for systolic blood pressure reduced risk of stroke,[96] provides an example. In that study the average BMI of participants was 30 kg/m2, meaning the large majority were overweight, which is the most important cause of hypertension (see http://www8.nationalacademies.org/onpinews/newsitem.aspx?RecordID=12819). Yet the published paper, editorial, and news reports only described the need for further medication (which added to side effects), and did not consider why patients had hypertension (overweight is the primary cause)[64,97] or that blood pressure can be lowered by well-documented changes in diet.[97]

6. Engage directly in enhancement of diets. The role that healthcare providers play in helping patients improve their diet can vary greatly depending on their knowledge, financial and time constraints, and wishes to be deeply involved in this process. At a minimum, a healthcare provider should inform patients of their concern about overweight, a creeping weight gain, excessive soda consumption, or a condition that might be modified by diet. In the case of smoking, just a simple message of concern has a measurable impact on smoking cessation. The next level of engagement would be referral to more information, a group program such as Weight Watchers, a comprehensive lifestyle intervention program,[98] or individual counseling by health coach or dietitian. Some healthcare providers choose to become deeply involved in dietary assessment, nutrition counseling, or hands-on cooking demonstrations, which can be on an individual or group basis.

7. Consider expanding your influence. While healthcare providers can do much to help their patients improve their diets, many powerful

factors influence what we eat, including our family, workplace, schools, food availability in our community, marketing, economic factors, and local, national, and international policies. In *Thinfluence*, Dr. Malissa Wood and I describe ways that individuals can modify or circumvent these external factors to improve their own diets and the well-being of others around them. Healthcare providers can play a special role because of our knowledge and credibility in health-related matters.[99] Hospitals, where many of us work, should be providing the very best example of healthy eating for both patients and staff, but have unfortunately often provided just the opposite. Physicians should be leading the effort to improve this environment, and in places important changes are being made.[100,101] Many other opportunities for leadership exist in our communities, schools, worksites, and other institutions.

8. Avoid nihilism about dietary change. Caring for patients who need to change their diet, or who need to stop smoking, can sometimes be discouraging, and relapses to previous habits are frequent. While some persons make transformational and permanent changes, changes frequently happen slowly, and often after many failed attempts to improve. This is partly because of the many powerful influences on behavior that are beyond our direct control. The best-published smoking interventions have success rates on the order of only 10% to 15% after 1 year, which is hardly detectable by a practicing physician. Yet, over a period of 40 years, smoking rates in men have decreased from about 60% to less than 20%. It is hard to know the specific role that healthcare providers have played in this achievement, but almost certainly their contribution to education, awareness, and motivation has been important. As noted above, as a country we are making progress in improving dietary quality, and some individuals have experienced this directly and profoundly. However, far more needs to be done; we have the knowledge of what should be done, and healthcare providers can do much for their individual patients and our society to make this a reality.

Summary

Optimal diets can play a major role in prevention of the major causes of morbidity and mortality in Western populations; this has been documented by a wealth of data from controlled feeding studies with risk factors as endpoints, long-term prospective studies, and randomized trials. The key elements of a healthy diet are unsaturated sources of fat from plants and plant oils; whole grains; beans, nuts, soy, fish, and poultry as major protein sources; and an abundance of fruits and vegetables. Intake of trans fat, processed meats, and sugar-sweetened beverages should be avoided, and consumption of red meat, dairy fat, refined grains, and fruit juices should be limited. The traditional Mediterranean diet incorporates these elements, and the health benefits of this dietary pattern have been proven. Other combinations of foods and flavors that are based on these elements can be similarly healthy. Physicians and healthcare providers can play an important role in guiding their patients toward healthy eating patterns, and they can also provide leadership in developing a healthier food environment for all.

References

1. Lozano R, Naghavi M, Foreman K, et al. Global and regional mortality from 235 causes of death for 20 age groups in 1990 and 2010: a systematic analysis for the Global Burden of Disease Study 2010. *Lancet* 2012;380:2095–128.
2. Devries S, Dalen JE, Eisenberg DM, et al. A deficiency of nutrition education in medical training. *Am J Med* 2014;127:804–806.
3. Keys A. *Seven Countries: A Multivariate Analysis of Death and Coronary Heart Disease*. Cambridge, MA: Harvard University Press; 1980.
4. Kato H, Tillotson J, Nichaman MZ, Rhoads GG, Hamilton HB. Epidemiologic studies of coronary heart disease and stroke in Japanese men living in Japan, Hawaii and California. *Am J Epidemiol* 1973;97:372–385.
5. Mensink RP, Katan MB. Effect of dietary fatty acids on serum lipids and lipoproteins: a meta-analysis of 27 trials. *Arterioscler Thrombosis* 1992;12:911–919.
6. Armstrong B, Doll R. Environmental factors and cancer incidence and mortality in different countries, with special reference to dietary practices. *Int J Cancer* 1975;15:617–631.
7. Buell P. Changing incidence of breast cancer in Japanese-American women. *J Natl Cancer Inst* 1973;51:1479–1483.
8. National Research Council, Committee on Diet and Health. *Diet and Health: Implications for Reducing Chronic Disease Risk*. Washington, DC: National Academy Press; 1989.
9. Centers for Disease Control and Prevention, National Center for Health Statistics. Daily dietary fat and total food-energy intakes: Third National Health and Nutrition Examination Survey, Phase 1, 1988–91. *MMWR* 1994;43(7):116–117.
10. Appel LJ, Sacks FM, Carey VJ, et al. Effects of protein, monounsaturated fat, and carbohydrate intake on blood pressure and serum lipids: results of the OmniHeart randomized trial. *JAMA* 2005;294:2455–2464.
11. Prentice RL, Caan B, Chlebowski RT, et al. Low-fat dietary pattern and risk of invasive breast cancer: the Women's Health Initiative Randomized Controlled Dietary Modification Trial. *JAMA* 2006;295:629–642.

12. Howard BV, Curb JD, Eaton CB, et al. Low-fat dietary pattern and lipoprotein risk factors: the Women's Health Initiative Dietary Modification Trial. *Am J Clin Nutr* 2010;2010;91(4):860–874.

13. Willett WC. The WHI joins MRFIT: a revealing look beneath the covers. *Am J Clin Nutr* 2010;91(4):829–830.

14. Willett WC. Policy applications. In: Willett WC, ed. *Nutritional Epidemiology*. 3rd ed. New York, NY: Oxford University Press; 2013:357–379.

15. Willett WC, Stampfer MJ. Diet and coronary heart disease. In: Willett WC, ed. *Nutritional Epidemiology*. 3rd ed. New York, NY: Oxford University Press; 2013:426–467.

16. Wang DD, Li Y, Chiuve SE, et al. Association of specific dietary fats with total and cause-specific mortality. *JAMA Intern Med* 2016 Aug 1;176(8):1134–1145.

17. Chowdhury R, Warnakula S, Kunutsor S, et al. Association of dietary, circulating, and supplement fatty acids with coronary risk: a systematic review and meta-analysis. *Ann Intern Med* 2014;160:398–406.

18. Jakobsen MU, O'Reilly EJ, Heitmann BL, et al. Major types of dietary fat and risk of coronary heart disease: a pooled analysis of 11 cohort studies. *Am J Clin Nutr* 2009;89:1425–1432.

19. Hu F, Stampfer MJ, Manson JE, et al. Dietary fat intake and the risk of coronary heart disease in women. *N Engl J Med* 1997;337:1491–1499.

20. Mensink RP, Zock PL, Kester AD, Katan MB. Effects of dietary fatty acids and carbohydrates on the ratio of serum total to HDL cholesterol and on serum lipids and apolipoproteins: a meta-analysis of 60 controlled trials. *Am J Clin Nutr* 2003;77:1146–1155.

21. Estruch R, Ros E, Salas-Salvado J, et al. Primary prevention of cardiovascular disease with a Mediterranean diet. *N Engl J Med* 2013;368:1279–1290.

22. Willett WC, Stampfer MJ, Manson JE, et al. Intake of trans fatty acids and risk of coronary heart disease among women. *Lancet* 1993;341:581–585.

23. Wang DD, Li Y, Chiuve SE, Hu FB, Willett WC. Improvements in US diet helped reduce disease burden and lower premature deaths, 1999–2012; overall diet remains poor. *Health Aff (Millwood)* 2015;34:1916–1922.

24. Kit BK, Carroll MD, Lacher DA, Sorlie PD, DeJesus JM, Ogden C. Trends in serum lipids among US youths aged 6 to 19 years, 1988–2010. *JAMA* 2012;308:591–600.

25. Carroll MD, Kit BK, Lacher DA, Shero ST, Mussolino ME. Trends in lipids and lipoproteins in US adults, 1988–2010. *JAMA* 2012;308:1545–1554.

26. Chen M, Li Y, Sun Q, et al. Dairy fat and risk of cardiovascular disease in 3 cohorts of US adults. *Am J Clin Nutr* 2016 Nov;104(5):1209–1217.

27. Li Y, Hruby A, Bernstein AM, et al. Saturated fats compared with unsaturated fats and sources of carbohydrates in relation to risk of coronary heart disease: a prospective cohort study. *J Am Coll Cardiol* 2015 Oct 6;66(14):1538–1548.

28. Hu FB, Stampfer MJ, Manson JE, et al. Dietary intake of α-linolenic acid and risk of fatal ischemic heart disease among women. *Am J Clin Nutr* 1999;69:890–897.

29. Farvid MS, Ding M, Pan A, et al. Dietary linoleic acid and risk of coronary heart disease: a systematic review and meta-analysis of prospective cohort studies. *Circulation* 2014;130:1568–1578.

30. Fritsche KL. Too much linoleic acid promotes inflammation—doesn't it? *Prostaglandins Leukot Essent Fatty Acids* 2008;79:173–175.

31. Ramsden CE, Zamora D, Majchrzak-Hong S, et al. Re-evaluation of the traditional diet-heart hypothesis: analysis of recovered data from Minnesota Coronary Experiment (1968–73). *BMJ* 2016;353:i1246.

32. World Cancer Research Fund/American Institute for Cancer Research. *Food, Nutrition, Physical Activity, and the Prevention of Cancer: A Global Perspective.* Washington, DC: AICR, 2007.

33. Bang HO, Dyerberg J, Sinclair HM. The composition of the Eskimo food in North Western Greenland. *Am J Clin Nutr* 1980;33:2657–2661.

34. Petrova S, Dimitrov P, Willett WC, Campos H. The global availability of n-3 fatty acids. *Public Health Nutr* 2011;14:1157–1164.

35. Mozaffarian D, Ascherio A, Hu F, et al. Interplay between different polyunsaturated fatty acids and risk of coronary heart disease in men. *Circulation* 2005;111:157–164.

36. Kim EH, Willett WC, Colditz GA, et al. Dietary fat and risk of postmenopausal breast cancer in a 20-year follow-up. *Am J Epidemiol* 2006;164(10):990–997.

37. Smith-Warner SA, Spiegelman D, Adami HO, et al. Types of dietary fat and breast cancer: a pooled analysis of cohort studies. *Int J Cancer* 2001;92:767–774.

38. Martin LJ, Li Q, Melnichouk O, et al. A randomized trial of dietary intervention for breast cancer prevention. *Cancer Res* 2011;71:123–133.

39. Hu FB, Manson JE, Stampfer MJ, et al. Diet, lifestyle, and the risk of type 2 diabetes mellitus in women. *N Engl J Med* 2001;345:790–797.

40. Kavanagh K, Jones KL, Sawyer J, et al. Trans fat diet induces abdominal obesity and changes in insulin sensitivity in monkeys. *Obesity (Silver Spring)* 2007;15:1675–1684.

41. Bray GA, Popkin BM. Dietary fat intake does affect obesity! *Am J Clin Nutr* 1998;68:1157–1173.

42. Tobias DK, Chen M, Manson JE, Ludwig DS, Willett W, Hu FB. Effect of low-fat diet interventions versus other diet interventions on long-term weight change in adults: a systematic review and meta-analysis. *Lancet Diabetes Endocrinol* 2015;3:968–979.

43. Mozaffarian D, Hao T, Rimm EB, Willett WC, Hu FB. Changes in diet and lifestyle and long-term weight gain in women and men. *N Engl J Med* 2011;364:2392–2404.

44. Shai I, Schwarzfuchs D, Henkin Y, et al. Weight loss with a low-carbohydrate, Mediterranean, or low-fat diet. *N Engl J Med* 2008;359:229–241.

45. Schwarzfuchs D, Golan R, Shai I. Four-year follow-up after two-year dietary interventions. *N Engl J Med* 2012;367:1373–1374.

46. Hu FB, Willett WC. Optimal diets for prevention of coronary heart disease. *JAMA* 2002;288:2569–2578.

47. Weickert MO, Pfeiffer AF. Metabolic effects of dietary fiber consumption and prevention of diabetes. *J Nutr* 2008;138:439–442.

48. Park Y, Hunter DJ, Spiegelman D, et al. Dietary fiber intake and risk of colorectal cancer: a pooled analysis of prospective cohort studies. *JAMA* 2005;294:2849–2857.

49. Bhupathiraju SN, Tobias DK, Malik VS, et al. Glycemic index, glycemic load, and risk of type 2 diabetes: results from 3 large US cohorts and an updated meta-analysis. *Am J Clin Nutr* 2014;100:218–232.

50. Augustin LS, Kendall CW, Jenkins DJ, et al. Glycemic index, glycemic load and glycemic response: an International Scientific Consensus Summit from the International Carbohydrate Quality Consortium (ICQC). *Nutr Metab Cardiovasc Dis* 2015;25:795–815.

51. Chiasson JL, Josse RG, Gomis R, et al. Acarbose for prevention of type 2 diabetes mellitus: the STOP-NIDDM randomised trial. *Lancet* 2002;359:2072–2077.

52. US Department of Agriculture, US Department of Health and Human Services. *Scientific Report of the 2015 Dietary Guidelines Advisory Committee.* Washington, DC: US Government Printing Offices; 2015.

53. Bernstein AM, Sun Q, Hu FB, Stampfer MJ, Manson JE, Willett WC. Major dietary protein sources and risk of coronary heart disease in women. *Circulation* 2010;122:876–883.

54. Farvid MS, Cho E, Chen WY, Eliassen AH, Willett WC. Adolescent meat intake and breast cancer risk. *Int J Cancer* 2015;136:1909–1920.

55. Pan A, Sun Q, Bernstein AM, Manson JE, Willett WC, Hu FB. Changes in red meat consumption and subsequent risk of type 2 diabetes mellitus: three cohorts of US men and women. *JAMA Intern Med* 2013;173:1328–1335.

56. Bischoff-Ferrari HA, Dawson-Hughes B, Baron JA, et al. Milk intake and risk of hip fracture in men and women: a meta-analysis of prospective cohort studies. *J Bone Miner Res* 2011;26:833–839.

57. Chen M, Pan A, Malik VS, Hu FB. Effects of dairy intake on body weight and fat: a meta-analysis of randomized controlled trials. *Am J Clin Nutr* 2012;96:735–747.

58. Chen M, Sun Q, Giovannucci E, et al. Dairy consumption and risk of type 2 diabetes: 3 cohorts of US adults and an updated meta-analysis. *BMC Med* 2014;12:215.

59. Bischoff-Ferrari HA, Willett WC, Wong JB, Giovannucci E, Dietrich T, Dawson-Hughes B. Fracture prevention with vitamin D supplementation: a meta-analysis of randomized controlled trials. *JAMA* 2005;293:2257–2264.

60. Dou R, Ng K, Giovannucci EL, Manson JE, Qian ZR, Ogino S. Vitamin D and colorectal cancer: molecular, epidemiological and clinical evidence. *Br J Nutr* 2016;115:1643–1660.

61. Simon KC, Munger KL, Ascherio A. Vitamin D and multiple sclerosis: epidemiology, immunology, and genetics. *Curr Opin Neurol* 2012;25:246–251.

62. Institute of Medicine. *Dietary Reference Intakes for Calcium and Vitamin D.* Washington, DC: National Academy of Sciences; 2010.

63. Moore TJ, Vollmer WM, Appel LJ, et al. Effect of dietary patterns on ambulatory blood pressure: results from the Dietary Approaches to Stop Hypertension (DASH) Trial. DASH Collaborative Research Group. *Hypertension* 1999;34:472–477.

64. Sacks FM, Willett WC, Smith A, Brown LE, Rosner B, Moore TJ. Effect on blood pressure of potassium, calcium, and magnesium in women with low habitual intake. *Hypertension* 1998;31:131–138.

65. Jung S, Spiegelman D, Baglietto L, et al. Fruit and vegetable intake and risk of breast cancer by hormone receptor status. *J Natl Cancer Inst* 2013;105:219–236.
66. Borgi L, Rimm EB, Willett WC, Forman JP. Potato intake and incidence of hypertension: results from three prospective US cohort studies. *BMJ* 2016;353:i2351.
67. Muraki I, Rimm EB, Willett WC, Manson JE, Hu FB, Sun Q. Potato consumption and risk of type 2 diabetes: results from three prospective cohort studies. *Diabetes Care* 2016;39:376–384.
68. Bertoia ML, Mukamal KJ, Cahill LE, et al. Changes in intake of fruits and vegetables and weight change in United States men and women followed for up to 24 years: analysis from three prospective cohort studies. *PLoS Med* 2015;12:e1001878.
69. Muraki I, Imamura F, Manson JE, et al. Fruit consumption and risk of type 2 diabetes: results from three prospective longitudinal cohort studies. *BMJ* 2013;347:f5001.
70. Brien SE, Ronksley PE, Turner BJ, Mukamal KJ, Ghali WA. Effect of alcohol consumption on biological markers associated with risk of coronary heart disease: systematic review and meta-analysis of interventional studies. *BMJ* 2011;342:d636.
71. Rimm EB, Klatsky A, Grobbee D, Stampfer MJ. Review of moderate alcohol consumption and reduced risk of coronary heart disease: is the effect due to beer, wine, or spirits? *Br Med J* 1996;312:731–736.
72. Friedman LA, Kimball AW. Coronary heart disease mortality and alcohol consumption in Framingham. *Am J Epidemiol* 1986;124:481–489.
73. Keil U, Chambless LE, Döring A, Filipiak B, Stieber J. The relation of alcohol intake to coronary heart disease and all-cause mortality in a beer-drinking population. *Epidemiology* 1997;8:150–156.
74. Gaziano JM, Gaziano TA, Glynn RJ, et al. Light-to-moderate alcohol consumption and mortality in the Physicians' Health Study enrollment cohort. *J Am Coll Cardiol* 2000;35:96–105.
75. Thun MJ, Peto R, Lopez AD, et al. Alcohol consumption and mortality among middle-aged and elderly U.S. adults. *N Eng J Med* 1997;337:1705–1714.
76. Chen WY, Rosner B, Hankinson SE, Colditz GA, Willett WC. Moderate alcohol consumption during adult life, drinking patterns, and breast cancer risk. *JAMA* 2011;306:1884–1890.
77. Ding M, Satija A, Bhupathiraju SN, et al. Association of coffee consumption with total and cause-specific mortality in 3 large prospective cohorts. *Circulation* 2015;132:2305–2315.
78. Freedman ND, Park Y, Abnet CC, Hollenbeck AR, Sinha R. Association of coffee drinking with total and cause-specific mortality. *N Engl J Med* 2012;366:1891–1904.
79. Leung CW, Ding EL, Catalano PJ, Villamor E, Rimm EB, Willett WC. Dietary intake and dietary quality of low-income adults in the Supplemental Nutrition Assistance Program. *Am J Clin Nutr* 2012;96:977–988.
80. Morris MC, Tangney CC. A potential design flaw of randomized trials of vitamin supplements. *JAMA* 2011;305:1348–1349.
81. Grodstein F, Kang JH, Glynn RJ, Cook NR, Gaziano JM. A randomized trial of beta carotene supplementation and cognitive function in men: the Physicians' Health Study II. *Arch Intern Med* 2007;167:2184–2190.

82. Gaziano JM, Sesso HD, Christen WG, et al. Multivitamins in the prevention of cancer in men: the Physicians' Health Study II randomized controlled trial. *JAMA* 2012;308:1871–1880.

83. Trichopoulou A, Costacou T, Bamia C, Trichopoulos D. Adherence to a Mediterranean diet and survival in a Greek population. *N Engl J Med* 2003;348:2599–2608.

84. de Lorgeril M, Renaud S, Mamelle N, et al. Mediterranean alpha-linolenic acid-rich diet in secondary prevention of coronary heart disease [Erratum in: *Lancet* 1995;345:738]. *Lancet* 1994;343:1454–1459.

85. McCullough ML, Feskanich D, Stampfer MJ, et al. Diet quality and major chronic disease risk in men and women: moving toward improved dietary guidance. *Am J Clin Nutr* 2002;76:1261–1271.

86. Chiuve SE, Fung TT, Rimm EB, et al. Alternative dietary indices both strongly predict risk of chronic disease. *J Nutr* 2012;142:1009–1018.

87. Stampfer MJ, Hu FB, Manson JE, Rimm EB, Willett WC. Primary prevention of coronary heart disease in women through diet and lifestyle. *N Engl J Med* 2000;343:16–22.

88. Chomistek AK, Chiuve SE, Eliassen AH, Mukamal KJ, Willett WC, Rimm EB. Healthy lifestyle in the primordial prevention of cardiovascular disease among young women. *J Am Coll Cardiol* 2015;65:43–51.

89. Willett WC. Balancing life-style and genomics research for disease prevention. *Science* 2002;296:695–698.

90. Willett WC, Dietz WH, Colditz GA. Guidelines for healthy weight. *N Engl J Med* 1999;341:427–434.

91. Yuan C, Spiegelman D, Rimm EB, et al. Validity of a dietary questionnaire assessed by comparison with multiple weighed dietary records or 24-hour recalls. *Am J Epidemiol*; in press.

92. Rifas-Shiman SL, Willett WC, Lobb R, Kotch J, Dart C, Gillman MW. PrimeScreen, a brief dietary screening tool: reproducibility and comparability with both a longer food frequency questionnaire and biomarkers. *Public Health Nutr* 2001;4:249–254.

93. Willett WC. *Eat, Drink, and Be Healthy.* 2nd ed. New York, NY: Simon & Schuster; 2005.

94. Willett WC, Katzen M. *Eat, Drink, and Weigh Less.* New York, NY: Hyperion; 2006.

95. Appel LJ, Moore TJ, Obarzanek E, et al. A clinical trial of the effects of dietary patterns on blood pressure. DASH Collaborative Research Group. *N Engl J Med* 1997;336:1117–1124.

96. Group SR, Wright JT Jr, Williamson JD, et al. A randomized trial of intensive versus standard blood-pressure control. *N Engl J Med* 2015;373:2103–2116.

97. Sacks FM, Svetkey LP, Vollmer WM, et al. Effects on blood pressure of reduced dietary sodium and the dietary approaches to stop hypertension (DASH) diet. *N Engl J Med* 2001;344:3–10.

98. Ornish D, Scherwitz LW, Billings JH, et al. Intensive lifestyle changes for reversal of coronary heart disease. *JAMA* 1998;280:2001–2007.

99. Willett WC, Wood M, Childs D. *Thinfluence.* New York, NY: Rodale; 2014.

100. Gardner CD, Whitsel LP, Thorndike AN, et al. Food-and-beverage environment and procurement policies for healthier work environments. *Nutr Rev* 2014;72:390–410.

101. Thorndike AN, Riis J, Sonnenberg LM, Levy DE. Traffic-light labels and choice architecture: promoting healthy food choices. *Am J Prev Med* 2014;46:143–149.

11

The Role of Exercise in Integrative Preventive Medicine

MICHAEL F. ROIZEN, MD, FACP, AND
JEFFREY D. ROIZEN, MD, PHD, FAAP

Since the dawn of recorded time, habitual exercise and sport participation were prescribed to promote a healthy body and a healthy mind.[1] Eighty observational association studies (many of which are prospective) and a few controlled trials provide compelling evidence that physical activity makes your body and cells act as if they are many years younger.[2-7] The physiological effect—that is, the effect of physical activity alone (independent of its effects on weight, blood pressure, LDL cholesterol, hs-C-reactive protein, TMAO, and other biomarkers of health and inflammation)—of all four physical activities advocated in the prescription in this chapter makes a 55-year-old woman have a relative risk of death more like someone who is 9 years younger than the typical 55-year-old American woman, and makes a 55-year-old man have a relative risk of death more like someone who is 8.1 years younger than the typical 55 year-old American man.[8-11] (The RealAge metric has been validated by prospective independent analysis by Hobbs and Fowler, 2014.)[8-11] This chapter summarizes the available evidence so that healthcare providers can write a rational prescription for physical activity that allows minimal activity for maximum health benefit.

Prescription of Exercise for Wellness:
Why, How Much, and How Little

In our culture there are two extremes for exercise; most Americans get less than 1 hour of even moderate exercise a week, but, for those who exercise more than this 1 hour, they often get more than 1 hour of the same activity each day 6 or 7 days a week. It turns out that both of these extremes (no exercise and more than an hour a day, 7 days a week of the same exercise) are not optimal for health.[12-16] For optimum health—to maximally prevent morbidity and mortality (for weight control, for longevity, for preventing cancer and arterial diseases, for keeping up sex drive and sex ability, for maintaining brain health, for feeling strong and happy).

Currently, there are no randomized-controlled studies of sufficient duration to precisely identify the ideal amount and kind of exercise with this gold-standard approach. However, the below recommendations to do four kinds of exercise weekly are based on formal and informal meta-analyses of the largest available datasets (Cooper Clinic Studies,[7,19] Cleveland Clinic Studies,[20] Harvard,[21-24] and Penn Alumni Studies,[25] Jerusalem Longevity Studies,[26-28] and others[29-35]).[17-18] Specifically, four different types of exercise—(1) any kind, (2) strength building, (3) bone strengthening (jumping), and (4) stamina building—are needed and are all that are needed for maximize longevity and to minimize morbidity and mortality.[7,19-35] Doing these exercises increases longevity and has multisystem benefits; specifically it increases ability to do daily functions requiring muscular activity like moving to and from a job; it improves metabolic functions and decreases risks of obesity, osteoarthritis, bone fractures, and type 2 diabetes; it increases mental alertness and ability to function in daily activities requiring thinking, it increases hippocampal size[36-37] and improves both short-term and long-term memory; it increases your immune function to ward off cancers and infections and increases disability-free survival if those occur; it even changes the microbiome.[38] Perhaps the most important reason to recommend and stress the importance of exercise to patients is that it can help prevent patients from gaining something unwanted, abdominal fat. Patients increase their risk of heart disease in two ways if seriously overweight (a body mass index [BMI] of above 35—for example, being 5 feet 8 inches and 230 pounds) or if the waist size is greater than 40 inches for men or 37 inches or greater for women (measure around the belly button while you suck in your gut). That waist carries two important risks. First, patients are much more likely to have or develop other risky conditions like high blood pressure, diabetes, lipid disorders like high LDL levels, sleep apnea, or arthritis, which will inhibit their desire to exercise. Second, that extra weight that's carried around the patient's waist places each at an even higher risk, because the fat cells in abdominal fat secrete substances that directly increase inflammation in blood vessels.[39] A weight loss of even 5% of body weight will significantly improve overall and cardiovascular health. Another way exercise can help is by reducing stress, which is one of the greatest agers of your patient's body. And just four types of physical activities have been shown to provide all these benefits. But when recommending that a patient start a new exercise program four questions often arise:

1. Does the patient need an assessment before exercising (and if so, what assessment and why)?
2. What's the specific prescription for minimal effort to get maximal health benefit (and are there limitations in what is advised and for whom)?
3. How does someone who has not been formally exercising start to exercise?
4. What about the other extreme: Can healthy patients do too much exercise?

The answers the literature allows are described in the following sections.

WHAT ASSESSMENTS ARE NEEDED BEFORE A PATIENT STARTS AN EXERCISE PROGRAM?

The conservative caregiver might argue that testing before starting provides an extra measure of safety, but no randomized controlled data supports the point that just starting with activity that is usual and done pain free, for example a slow walk, and increasing gradually, is safer with than without tests first.[40]

Some groups of patients—those with unstable angina (chest pain on walking or at rest, without doing any activity); those with chest heaviness or shortness of breath without doing any activity; or those who are unstable, lose balance, or get dizzy when they walk—should start and advance a physical activity program in a closely supervised environment, such as a cardiac or type 2 diabetes, or kidney or neurologic disease prevention or rehabilitation set of shared medical appointments.

To ensure physical activity is started and done safely by the patient, some tests are needed prior to starting, but others (numbers one to five in the next section) can be delayed until the patient advances from walking to more intense exercise, or before adding resistance exercise (the first 10 in the next section). In the 1960s and prior, the presence of heart disease, whether in the valve structure, muscle structure or force, or arteries and veins of the heart, triggered a prescription of a sedentary lifestyle and recommendation to avoid almost all physical activity and sport. Yet compelling evidence has accumulated that regular and increasing physical activity, even in this group with cardiac disease, reduces all cause mortality and disability rates, and improves quality of life. Even in the face of, and perhaps especially in the presence of, high blood pressure, or type 2 diabetes, or high blood lipid risk, or increased inflammation risk, or prior heart attack or stroke or heart failure, regular and increasing physical activity improves quality of life and reduces disability risk.[41-48] Because doing physical activities decreases risk of disabilities, it could be argued that neither testing nor an assessment is necessary before writing an exercise prescription.

Other rationales for the 16 tests below are they can (1) help judge current status, (2) guide the prescription for speed in advancing, and (3) possibly provide a metric (for the patient) in how far they have come. Engaging in physical activity without a clear starting point may make it more difficult for a patient to maintain motivation; when weight loss is slow or ceases, but healthy benefit is still accruing, having evidence of that benefit will hopefully provide a nonweight motivation. For some patients, seeing improvement in LDL, HDL, blood pressure, or in other areas, and thus in risks for serious and possibly sudden disability or death, is vital to continuing to work (please assume we use "her" to mean "her or him" in each use when appropriate).[41-44]

Ascertaining baseline information about a patient's fitness status, family history, heart, cancer, and brain status can be used to develop a personalized physical activity program that is safe, effective and lets the healthcare provider and the patient evaluate progress.

Many patients on blood pressure medications, cholesterol management medications, and pain medications will likely be able to reduce or stop one or more of their medications, including antidepressants, and in time these may not be needed at all.[41-44] But this should not be rushed. These changes usually start after 90 days and do not progress to full effect to well after 6 months.

WHAT ASSESSMENTS TO GET?

Before the patient starts, or within the first week of starting a walking program:

1. **Blood Pressure:** It should be under 120/80 with or without medications before a patient advances past a walking program.[49]
2. **Resting Heart Rate:** This should be taken when lying down or sitting quietly and not talking for 5 minutes, preferably first thing in the morning. As long as your patient's heart rate is regular or controlled and is between 40 and 96 when resting, beginning a walking program is totally appropriate. (If it is above 96 or below 40, the cause of such abnormal readings should be sought before prescribing an exercise program.)
3. **Height.**

4. **Waist size and weight** (ideally first thing in the morning): Measure the patient's waist size with a tape measure parallel to the floor at the belly button while the patient sucks in the gut.[50]

5. **Recommend that the patient buy a pedometer or use one on a smartphone, have the patient record the steps they walk each day for 3 days:** Average the steps taken in the first 3 days and then advance by 5% of that total every day for the next week. For example, if the patient walked 6,000 steps on average each of the 3 days, then the next week do 5% more per day (6,300 steps a day) and advance by 5% again each day for the next week (6,630 steps per day).

Early in the walking program, take and record the following measurement:

6. **Speed of walking 1 mile (or 6-min walk distance):** This measure is simply how fast can the patient walk a mile.[51-52] All the patient needs for this test is a watch or smartphone with a watch function with a second hand and a level surface on which to walk 1 mile or 8 city blocks, assuming the city is built at 8 blocks to the mile. If not, the patient should find a track at a local high school (the tracks around football fields are usually one-quarter of a mile). Have the patient follow these instructions:

6.1 Warm up by walking at a moderate pace for 5 minutes.

6.2 Walk 1 mile as quickly as possible without causing yourself pain or discomfort. (Do not run on this test, even if you can do so).

6.3 Immediately after completing the walk, take your pulse for 10 seconds. Multiply the number you get by six to obtain your 1-minute heart rate or measure your heart rate with one of the strap-watch monitors. This enables you to obtain your heart rate in the last few seconds of exercise, rather than in the recovery period after exercise. If you do the finger on the pulse method, it is important to do the 10 seconds *immediately* at the end of the exercise, not after 10 or 20 seconds of recovery.

6.4 Record your walk time, and your 1-minute heart rate.

6.5 Cool down by walking at a moderate pace for another 5 minutes.

6.6 Keep track of your progress.

The patient can be her own goal setter for changes in time and heart rate over time. Over the course of several weeks, if her time on the 1-mile walk decreases without a rise in her heart rate, she has become more fit. If her time on the mile walk stays the same but her heart rate drops, she has also improved her fitness level and reduced her risk of some key chronic diseases.

For comparison purposes, if your patient's physiological age (her physiological condition where her relative risk of death is equivalent to that of someone at that age—we call it her RealAge[8-11]) is 40 to 50 years old, she should be able to walk the mile in 20 minutes with a heart rate below 135. If her physiological age is 51 to 60 years old, she should be able to walk the mile in 23 minutes with a heart rate below 140. If her physiological age is 61 to 70 years old, she should be able to walk the mile in 26 minutes with a heart rate below 140. If her physiological age is 71 to 80 years old, she should be able to walk the mile in 29 minutes with a heart rate below 140. If her physiological age is 81 to 90 years old, she should be able to walk the mile in 32 minutes with a heart rate below 140. If her physiological age is 91 to 100 years old, she should be able to walk the mile in 36 minutes with a heart rate below 140. Your patient will see this time shorten (or the heart rate improve, or both) as her health from physical exercise improves.[11]

Do Tests 7–10 Before Recommending That the Patient Advance to Resistance Exercises

There are many tests of maximum exercise capacity for strength and for cardio activity, to help you determine where the patient is (Point A) and help the patient set goals for where she wants to go (Point B).

7. **One Leg Standing Times:** Under supervision (and timing in seconds) and in a room that is padded to protect the patient from injury in case of a fall, and with a person who can catch the patient if the patient starts to fall, have the patient stand on her right leg, close her eyes, and see how long she can stand on one leg. Repeat three times and record the best time of the three attempts. Repeat with other leg. Times less than 15 seconds indicate the patient's balance may be that of a person older than 45.

8. **Grip Strength:** This is measured by a grip strength meter, which most physical rehab offices and many physician offices have. The grip strength correlates with the patient's physiological age (see Figure 11.1).[53-55]

9. **The Push-Up Test (push-ups in 1 minute):** The push-up test evaluates upper-body muscular endurance. Men should perform the test in the standard push-up position, in which *only* the toes and hands have contact with the floor. Women should assume a modified position, in which the knees also rest on the floor.

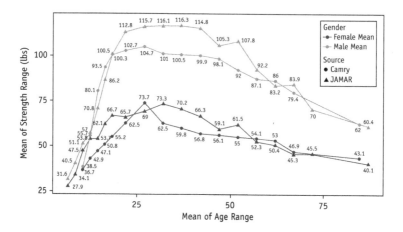

FIGURE 11.1 Grip Strength and Physiological Age
References 53–55.

Whether the patient is male or female, remind each to keep his or her (as earlier, "her" shall refer to "his or her") spine straight and her head in line with her spine and to place her hands directly under her shoulders. Have the patient lower her chest toward the floor until it comes within 3 or 4 inches of the floor, and then push herself back up. She should inhale as she lowers and exhale as she pushes back up.

Have the patient follow these instructions:

9.1 Perform a 5-minute warm-up (i.e., walk at a moderate pace and do a few standing push-ups against the wall).

9.2 Assume the gender-appropriate push-up position.

9.3 Count the number of push-ups you can perform with proper technique. (You may rest during the test but only in the "up" position.)

9.4 Record the number of push-ups completed. This is her score.

The patient's results can be compared to the population norms in Table 11.1[11] (gender adjusted . . . modified knee for women):

10. **Curl-up Test: (curl-ups in 1 minute)** The curl-up test evaluates abdominal muscular endurance. Both men and women perform the exercise in the same manner. Have the patient follow these instructions:

10.1 Warm up for 5 minutes by walking at a moderate pace and tightening your abdominal muscles a few times.

Table 11.1 Push-ups

			Men	Women
If your patient's physiological age is	>20 and <29	your patient can do	>35 or	>18
If your patient's physiological age is	>30 and <39	your patient can do	25-29 or	13-19
If your patient's physiological age is	>40 and <49	your patient can do	20-24 or	11-14
If your patient's physiological age is	>50 and <59	your patient can do	15-19 or	7-10
If your patient's physiological age is	>60 and <69	your patient can do	10-14 or	5-10
If your patient's physiological age is	>70 and <79	your patient can do	6-9 or	4-10
If your patient's physiological age is	>80 and <89	your patient can do	3-5 or	2-6
If your patient's physiological age is	>90	your patient can do	1-3 or	1-4

10.2 Lie on your back with your knees bent 90 degrees and your feet flat on the floor. Place your arms at your sides, palms down.

10.3 Flatten your lower back and curl your head, shoulders, and shoulder blades up off the floor for 4 to 6 inches. Return to the starting position.

10.4 Perform as many curl-ups as possible in a minute.

10.5 Record the number of curl-ups completed.

If the patient has been doing curl-ups for a while, they can take a more advanced test. In order to perform this test, each will need a mat or padded floor, masking tape, a tape measure or ruler, and a metronome. Have the patient follow these instructions:

10.11 Warm up for 5 minutes by walking at a moderate pace and tightening your abdominal muscles a few times.

10.12 Place a line of masking tape width-wise across the mat, about a foot from the end, or on the padded floor. Just beyond that tape, place another line of masking tape parallel to the first. The strips of tape should be 4 inches apart if you are 45 years of age or older and 12 inches apart if you are under 45.

10.13 Lie on your back with your knees bent 90 degrees and your feet flat on the floor. Place your arms at your sides, palms down, with the tips of your fingers touching the first piece of masking tape.

10.14 Set your metronome to a cadence of 40 beats per minute. This will allow for 20 steady curl-ups per minute.

10.15 In time with the metronome, flatten your lower back and curl your head, shoulders, and shoulder blades up off the floor until your fingertips touch the second piece of tape. Return to the starting position. Each complete curl-up should take two beats of the metronome.

10.16 Perform as many curl-ups as possible (75 at the most) until you cannot keep time with the metronome or you can no longer consistently reach the second piece of tape. (Some people naturally slide backward while performing this test. If that is your case, forget the tape and focus instead on lifting your shoulder blades off of the floor.)

10.17 Record the number of curl-ups completed. This is your score.

The patient's results can be compared to the population norms in Table 11.2:[11]

If the patient's usual maximum physical activity fits into a general category like walking or gardening, or if she does not do maximum physical activity like running, jogging, or elliptical training regularly, you should have her do a walk test and the muscular strength tests first.

Table 11.2 Curls

			Men	Women
If your patient's physiological age is	>20 and <29	your patient can do	>45 or	>35
If your patient's physiological age is	>30 and <39	your patient can do	30-34 or	25-29
If your patient's physiological age is	>40 and <49	your patient can do	25-29 or	20-24
If your patient's physiological age is	>50 and <59	your patient can do	20-24 or	15-19
If your patient's physiological age is	>60 and <69	your patient can do	15-19 or	10-14
If your patient's physiological age is	>70 and <79	your patient can do	10-14 or	7-9
If your patient's physiological age is	>80 and <89	your patient can do	6-9 or	4-6
If your patient's physiological age is	>90	your patient can do	2-5 or	1-3

If the patient does a stamina or aerobic activity like running, jogging, elliptical training, squash, or basketball near her maximum capacity, she should do the maximum activity test and the muscular strength tests.

11-13. **Cardio Tests**: What the patient records seems straightforward (see references 7, 10, 19, and 20 to learn how to do these if questions arise):
  11. Maximum Mets with Treadmill or Schwinn Bike or Elliptical
  12. Maximum heart rate you achieve
  13. Two-minute recovery heart rate and the difference in your maximum heart rate and 2-minute recovery heart rate.

14-16. **Flexibility Tests**: Flexibility corresponds to the capacity to move each joint through a full and normal range of motion. Adequate flexibility is essential for optimal functioning, while excessive flexibility can lead to unstable, injury-prone joints. We have selected a few important joints to evaluate in patients (or to have them evaluate with instruction). Before they undertake these tests, have the patient perform an aerobic warm-up, such as a brisk 5-minute walk or ride on a stationary bike.

14. **Trunk Flexion: Low Back**

Have the patient follow these instructions:
  14.1 Sit on the floor with your feet about a foot apart and legs straight out in front of you.[11]
  14.2 Place one hand on top of the other with your fingertips lined up together.
  14.3 Exhale and lean forward, extending your hands between your feet, with your fingertips almost touching the floor. (Keep your knees straight.)

Women: Age 45 and under: She should be able to reach 2 to 4 inches past her feet.
Age 46 and older: She should be able to reach to the soles of her feet.
Men: Age 45 and under: He should be able to reach to the soles of his feet.
Age 46 and older: He should be able to come within three to four inches of the soles of his feet.

If the patient has less than the desired flexibility, recommend that she incorporate low-back stretches into a morning routine.

15. **Trunk Extension:**

Have the patient follow these instructions:
  15.1 Lie on your stomach with your hands in pre-push-up position.

15.2 Trying to maintain contact between your hip bones and the floor, slowly press your chest off the floor. Do not force yourself into any discomfort. Stop pressing upward once the hip bones begin to leave the floor.

The patient should come close to straightening her arms with the hips still in contact with the floor. If the patient has less than the desired flexibility, recommend that she incorporate the abdominal stretches into her routine.

16. **Hip-flexion Test:**

Have the patient follow these instructions:

16.1 Lie flat on your back with your arms down at your sides and your legs straight out on the floor.
16.2 Without moving your hips or pelvis, lift your right leg up toward the ceiling, keeping the knee straight.
16.3 Repeat on the other side.

The patient should be able to lift her leg until it is almost pointing directly toward the ceiling (about 85–90 degrees of hip flexion).[11] If your patient has less than the desired flexibility, incorporate hamstring stretches into her routine.

Ten thousand steps is what we start with.[57] Not many extra tests are needed for that. But other tests you may consider depending on your patient's risk factors, age, and other conditions include an exercise or echo stress test, LDL cholesterol and cholesterol particle size, Lipoprotein A, hsCRP, TMAO, fasting insulin and glucose levels, eye tests, and tests for gene function.[58] These tests may have important implications for your exercise prescription.

WHAT IS THE LEAST EXERCISE TO RECOMMEND TO PATIENTS TO GET THEM MAXIMUM HEALTH BENEFITS? THE EXERCISE PRESCRIPTION

What patients need as the minimum physical activity for maximum health is:

1. 10,000 steps every day
2. 30 minutes of resistance exercise a week, including some for hand and for core strength
3. 20 jumps a day, and
4. 20 minutes of cardio (at a heart rate of 80% or greater than her age adjusted maximum—220 minus calendar age) three times a week.

More physical activity than this will not make patients healthier; yes, they can improve performance, but more exercise than this does not cause any benefit in morbidity and mortality. Let us review these in turn:

1. 10 k a day, every day: 10 k a day gives the patient about half of the total benefit of maximum physical activity for her health, 9 years physiologically younger for a woman and 8.1 years physiologically younger for a man who does the average of all other healthy choices.[8] In addition to the outsize benefit that this recommendation has on health (relative to time investment), it has the added benefit of being a recommendation that people mostly follow through on. That is, when patients are told to do any of a specific exercise they are more likely to consistently do 10,000 steps than almost any other recommendation. Ten thousand steps is approximately 5 miles for most adults. These steps can be done throughout the day and do not need to be in one chunk. In fact, if it takes longer than 2 hours in one chunk to do it, it is better to not do it in one chunk. We do not totally understand the physiology, but 10,000 seems to be the minimum number that provides the most health benefit. For instance, 10 k a day improves insulin resistance much better than 8 k, but 12 k does not help more than 10 k does (yes, she may get more fit, but her health doesn't get better for the long term). Walking those 10,000 steps is the limit at which insulin resistance seems to decrease substantially, allowing you to reverse the *fat accumulation—inflammation—desire to eat more* cycle.[59] Because it is such a simple strategy with such major health benefits, 10 k a day is the first thing I prescribe my patients and the people I coach or am a buddy to—for weight loss; for smoking cessation; for diabetes control; for blood pressure control; for decreasing the risks of heart disease, stroke, and certain cancers; for treating immune-related issues; for better sex; for better kidney, liver, and lung function; for greater resiliency in the face of stress; for better sleep—in fact, for just about everything.

In addition to improving insulin resistance, walking (and exercise in general) increases the size of the brain's memory center, your hippocampus, by up to 2% in a year (the only part of the human body where size really matters).[36-38,60] But stay on the couch, and this key region may shrink 0.5% per year, adding to memory lapses. One reason? Exercise increases levels of brain-derived neurotrophic factor (BDNF), a "brain fertilizer" that helps you grow those new cells and encourages better memory formation. You do not have to be a race walker to get more brainpower, but it helps. The people studied in this research who got their brain's hippocampus measured via a magnetic resonance imaging (MRI) scan started out walking just 10 to 15 minutes at a stretch, building up slowly.[60] And I probably do not need to even tell you what a great stress relief and antidepressant effect walking can have. A big study from Harvard in 2010[61] looked at more than 13,000 women to see who reached or passed age 70 in "super-healthful" condition: no cancer, diabetes, heart attacks, cognitive impairment, or physical or mental health limitations. What these super healthy had in common was physical activity. Those who did the most activity in their 60s (and that was nearly 10 k a day) were roughly twice as likely to be super healthful after age 70 as people who did the least activity.[25-28] If you are not convinced by now, just do this: ask yourself or a patient to make a commitment to try it for 30 days. Every day, do what you can to get in those steps. Will you lose 50 pounds in that time? Of course not. Will you resolve all of your health problems? No, biology does take a little more time than that. But I guarantee that you and your patients will feel better, feel stronger, be more motivated, lose a few pounds, decrease your blood pressure, and create new habits that will provide the foundation to make all of the changes you want in your life.

George Matthew Schilling is said to be the first person to walk around the world—he did it from 1897 to 1904. And according to Guinness World Records, the first verified global transperambulation was by David Kunst from June 20, 1970, to October 5, 1974. He walked 14,450 miles through four continents.[62] But patients do not have to go to all that effort to get the amazing benefits of regular walking.

Getting a pedometer, a walking buddy, and good shoes, and heading out for 10,000 steps a day, 5 to 7 days a week, can dramatically diminish or eliminate the effects of weight-gain promoting genes,[63,64] and can mute the desire for sugary snacks.

If your patient is unable to walk due to a leg issue or balance issue she can substitute other activity for some of the steps. (This is where data tracking becomes especially important.) The general rule is that 1 minute of moderate activity equals a hundred steps (and 1 minute of intense activity can count as 200 steps). If the patient does 20 minutes of moderate swimming, she can count that as 2,000 steps.

2. **Show Some Resistance:** Ignoring resistance training is ignoring the patient's health.

To get optimal benefit from resistance exercise a patient only needs to do it 2 days a week, for about 15 to 20 minutes each session. To get the most benefit, she should aim to do exercises that work her largest muscle groups, such as those in her legs and back, as well as all the muscles in her "core" (abdominal muscles, as well as those in the hips and especially her butt). She can do this with formal weights (e.g., dumbbells), resistance bands or medicine balls or with water or cans of soup, or even with her own body weight (e.g., squats or pushups). Recommend that your patient start with a weight (or suitable substitute) that she can use to do twelve repetitions with no problem. How does she know when she is ready to add weight? If she can do an exercise more than 12 times without feeling fatigued in the muscle area she is working, it is time to graduate to a higher weight. If she cannot perform the move at least eight times, she needs a lighter weight.

Please recommend to patients that they not try to combine resistance exercise with things like walking: carrying weights while walking dramatically increases the risk of rotator cuff injury. When the patient gets tired or starts focusing on dodging potholes, she forgets about proper technique with those weights and increases her odds of meeting someone specializing in rotator-cuff rehabilitation.

There was a time when people thought that training with dumbbells or barbells should be reserved only for bodybuilders and dumbbells; not even football or basketball players were allowed in the weight room. Many people, especially women, shied away from weights because they thought they would beef up to have muscle exploding from every part of their bodies. While weights can certainly help a patient get bigger and stronger in that sense, the tide has turned, and working out with weights is no longer looked at as something that only specific athletes should use. More experts acknowledge that one of the secrets to a healthier body is doing some sort of resistance training, in which you move some kind of weight (even your body) against gravity to put muscles under tension, as opposed to cardiovascular exercises such as running or swimming that are more to work the heart.

To be fair, weight exercises can be cardiovascular, and cardiovascular exercise does involve muscles other than your patient's heart muscles. But moving a weight against gravity is almost always how resistance is separated from cardio—or how they are traditionally distinguished. And by "some," we mean a short routine twice a week to get maximum health benefit. Here is why: when doing resistance training, the patient is breaking down muscle fibers. In the days that follow, the fibers rebuild the muscle stronger. So over time, the patient is adding muscle to her body. Why do people need to add muscle? For one, adding muscle helps protect your joints when you walk or perform other cardiovascular activity. Resistance exercises for the muscles above and below the knee, for example, are the best way to prevent and maybe even quiet the symptoms of knee arthritis. They act as shock absorbers. More muscle means fewer injuries, which means your patient is more likely to stick to her routine and stay healthy.

Second, building muscle burns calories and breaks insulin resistance, just as walking 10,000 steps does. So by improving the process of insulin delivering glucose to her body's cells, the patient is decreasing the potential damage that glucose can do to her genes, her proteins, and her circulatory system, and the chances that she will store fat that causes inflammation.

Best of all, to do resistance exercise, she does not need to join a gym or invest in any fancy equipment. She can use anything. To put her muscles under some type of resistance requires pushing or pulling some weight— that is where the tension is created, and that is where the process of growing muscle begins. But here is the greatest thing: there are a million different ways to do that. She can do it with traditional methods, like barbells, dumb-bells, and exercise machines she would find at the gym. She can do it with medicine balls. She can do it with resistance bands, which are small and light enough to pack so that she can have her own gym-on-the-go. She can do it with household items such as unopened cans of soup, jugs of water, and many other things that can double as equipment. She can also do it with her own body weight. Yes, squatting in place is a form of resistance exercise, as are push-ups. Your patient needs to do it only 2 days a week, for about 15 to 20 minutes each session. To get the most benefit, your patient should aim to do exercises that work her largest muscle groups, such as those in her legs and back, as well as all the muscles in her core. The core consists of the abdominal muscles, as well as those in her hips and especially her butt. Strengthening her core is about providing a sort of anatomical back brace— to improve her posture and prevent injury. A strong core may help keep her safe if she slips on the ice— not because a six-pack of abs can break a fall, but because a strong core may help her keep her balance so that she does not land nose-first on the sidewalk.

Additionally we recommend not ignoring the resistance exercise for the hands. Do not ignore the hands. Building grip strength in midlife can pro-tect patients from inability to do activities of daily living. Several studies[53-55] indicate that grip strength predicts disability risk and death. It is not clear why grip strength is such a good predictor of disability and death, but it is even a better predictor that overall muscle mass, blood pressure, or LDL cholesterol level. However, there are not any studies that show that making your grip stronger in and of itself alters morbidity or mortality. Exercises that you can recommend to your patients to improve her grip strength are to pop bubble wrap, play with clay, squeeze a ball, or even just gently push against a wall (a stretch that can also help prevent carpal tun-nel syndrome).

3. **Buy a Jump Rope:** All your patients need to gain maximum increase in hip bone strength is 40 jumps a day.[67] Using a jump rope and doing more will provide an aerobic exercise. Regarding jumping technique: recommend to the patient that she keep her back straight and her head up and turn the rope from her wrists.

4. **Sweat three times a week:** A major way for your patient to improve her cardiovascular fitness is to do continuous exercise to the point where it makes her sweat and raises her heart rate 80% or more of its age-adjusted maximum (220 minus her age) for an extended period of time.[67] Your patients should aim for a minimum of 60 minutes per week of aerobic activity—ideally in three 20-minute sessions. We recommend low-impact activities like swimming, cycling, or using an elliptical trainer to get her heart rate up without compromising the quality of the joints in the process (and to change activities, so they do not get repetitive use injuries from doing the same activity over and over). We also recommend interval training (alternating periods of maximum effort with periods of recovery)—for the maximum cardiovascular benefit. Even doing 1 minute at the end of every 10 minutes with maximum effort can be beneficial.

Use your best judgment to identify patients who you want to try it in the controlled setting of a stress test first.

HOW DOES SOMEONE WHO HAS NOT BEEN FORMALLY EXERCISING START TO EXERCISE?

Simply get them to walk and e-mail you or a friend (buddy) every day as to how much they have walked. Ask them not to exceed a 10% increase in steps any day of the week but to gradually increase to 10,000 steps a day. (See item #5 in assessments, earlier.) Once the patient hits 10 k a day for 30 days, then add resistance exercise (described earlier).

WHAT ABOUT THE OTHER EXTREME: CAN HEALTHY PATIENTS DO TOO MUCH EXERCISE?

Blood samples from extreme exercisers before and after ultra-exercise reveal deficits in gut barrier integrity.[69] Long-term, excessive endurance exercise (e.g., marathons, ultramarathons, ironman triathlons, etc.), can actually damage the joints, the heart, and arteries. Every time your patient pushes her body to excess it causes transient (but measurable) damage. If she does this once and gives her heart a rest, its function and arterial reactivity returns to normal within a week. Similarly, doing more than 2 hours consecutively of the same exercise predisposes toward overuse injury. Doing more than 1 consecutive hour a day of the same activity 7 days a week predisposes toward overuse injury.

It Is Not Only Exercise: Avoid Too Much Sitting

Several articles showing the harm of too much sitting (that is not mitigated by exercise at other times) have been highlighted in the lay press. One shows a huge benefit of standing, but others show no great benefit of standing. Data is still emerging, but at this point the best data is that walking for 2 minutes to interrupt each hour of sitting mitigates most of the harm from sitting.

Summary

Physical activity is key for the integrative medicine practitioner to prescribe. There is clear evidence that for most diseases and for most individuals, any physical activity is better than none. Walking is the best way to start and can be started safely for most individuals without preactivity tests. The data also are clear that 10,000 steps a day seems to be the minimum for maximum metabolic health. As you advance your patients to greater physical activity for greater benefit, there is greater risk that may be mitigated by assessment of specific tests. We recommend a prescription with the following action steps that you can add to your patient's integrative prescriptions to help her get healthier (you can duplicate the italics below to give the patient):

- *Buy two pedometers (so you'll always have one),*
- *Some great walking shoes,*
- *And find a walking buddy. Just start walking. You can do it.*
- *Start scheduling physical activity into your daily calendar—Do it, and keep doing it!*
- *Start seeing if you are hitting the 10 k a day minimum for maximum health. If not, increase walking by 10 more each week (each day of the week should be 10 minutes or 5% more than the previous week's average) until you get to 10 k.*
- *Buy a jump rope and start learning how to do 20 jumps every morning before you start your car.*
- *Get up from your desk and walk for 2 minutes every hour.*

References

1. Goodyear LJ. The exercise pill—too good to be true? *N Engl J Med* 2008;359(17):1842–1844.

2. Booth FW, Thomason DB. Molecular and cellular adaptation of muscle in response to exercise: perspectives of various models. *Physiol Rev* 1991;71(2):541–585.

3. Fries JF, Bruce B, Chakravarty E. Compression and morbidity 1980–2011: a focused review of paradigms and progress. *J Aging Res* 2011;2011:1–10. doi: 10.4061/2001/261702.

4. Fries JF. The theory and practice of active aging. *Curr Gerontol Geriatr Res* 2012;2012:1–7. doi: 10.1155/2012/420637.

5. McNaughton SA, Crawford D, Ball K, Salmon J. Understanding determinants of nutrition, physical activity and quality of life among older adults: the wellbeing, eating and exercise for a long life (WELL) study. *Health Qual Life Outcomes* 2012;10(109):109–116. doi: 10.1186/1477-7525-10-109.

6. Vina J, Sanchis-Gomar F, Martinez-Bello V, Gomez-Cabrera MC. Exercise acts as a drug; the pharmacological benefits of exercise. *Br J Pharmacol* 2012;167(1):1–12.

7. Blair SN, Kohl HW III, Barlow CE, Paffenbarger RS Jr, Gibbons LW, Macera CA. Changes in physical fitness and all-cause mortality. *JAMA* 1995;273(14):1093–1098.

8. Hobbs WR, Fowler J. Prediction of mortality using on-line self-reported health data: empirical test of the real age score. *PLoS One* 2014;9(1):e86385. doi: 10.1371/journal.pone.0086385.

9. Roizen MF. *RealAge: Are You As Young As You Can Be?* New York, NY: Harper Collins; 1999.

10. Roizen MF. *The RealAge Makeover*. New York, NY: Harper Collins; 2004:296–335.

11. Roizen MF, Hafen T. *The RealAge Workout: Maximum Health, Minimum Work*. New York, NY: Harper Collins; 2006.

12. Lee IM, Paffenbarger RS, Jr. Physical activity and stroke incidence: the Harvard Alumni Health Study. *Stroke* 1998;29(10):2049–2054.

13. Arem H, Moore SC, Patel A, Hartge P, Berrington de Gonzalez A, Vesvanathan K, et al. Leisure time physical activity and mortality: a detailed pooled analysis of the dose-response relationship. *JAMA Intern Med* 2015;175(6):959–967.

14. Mons U, Hahmann H, Brenner H. A reverse j-shaped association of leisure time physical activity with prognosis in patients with stable coronary heart disease: evidence from a large cohort with repeated measurements. *Heart* 2014;100(13):1043–1049.

15. Van Dijk ML, de Groot RH, Savelberg HH, Van Acker F, Kirschner PA. The association between objectively measured physical activity and academic achievement in Dutch adolescents: findings from the GOALS study. *J Sport Exerc Psychol* 2014;36(5):460–473.

16. Lee IM, Djousse L, Sesso HD, Wang L, Buring JE. Physical activity and weight gain prevention. *JAMA* 2010;303(12):1173–1179.

17. Roizen MF. *This Is Your Do-Over: The 7 Secrets to Losing Weight, Living Longer, and Getting a Second Chance at the Life You Want*. New York, NY: Simon & Schuster; 2015.

18. Oz MC, Roizen MF. *You: Staying Young: The Owner's Manual for Looking Good and Feeling Great*. New York, NY: Simon & Schuster; 2015.

19. Blair SN, Kohn HW III, Paffenbarger RS Jr, Clark DG, Cooper KH, Gibbons LW. Physical fitness and all-cause mortality: a prospective study of healthy men and women. *JAMA* 1989;262(17):2395–2401.

20. Gulati M, Black HR, Shaw LJ, et al. The prognostic value of a nomogram for exercise capacity in women. *N Engl J Med* 2005;353(5):468–475.

21. Paffenbarger RS Jr, Hyde RT, Wing AL, Lee IM, Jung DL, Kampert JB. The association of changes in physical-activity level and other lifestyle characteristics with mortality among men. *N Engl J Med* 1993;328(8):538–545.

22. Lee IM, Hsieh C, Paffenbarger RS Jr. Exercise intensity and longevity in men. *JAMA* 1995;273(15):1179–1184.

23. Paffenbarger RS Jr, Lee IM Jr. A natural history of athleticism, health and longevity. *J Sports Sci* 1998;16(Suppl):S31–S45.

24. Lee CD, Folsom AR, Blair SN. Physical activity and stroke risk: a meta-analysis. *Stroke* 2003;34(10):2475–2482.

25. Vita AJ, Terry RB, Hubert HB, Fries JF. Aging, health risks, and cumulative disability. *N Engl J Med* 1998;338(15):1035–1041.

26. Stessman J, Hammerman-Rozenberg R, Cohen A, Ein-Mor E, Jacobs JM. Physical activity, function, and longevity among the very old. *Arch Intern Med* 2009;169(16):1476–1483.

27. Stessman J, Hammerman-Rozenberg R, Maaravi Y, Azoulai D, Cohen A. Strategies to enhance longevity and independent function: the Jerusalem longitudinal study. *Mech Ageing Dev* 2004;126(2):327–331.

28. Jacobs JM, Cohen A, Bursztyn M, Azoulay D, Ein-Mor E, Stessman J. Cohort profile: the Jerusalem longitudinal cohort study. *Int J Epidemiol* 2009;38(6):1464–1469.

29. Eijsvogels TMH, Thompson PD. Exercise is medicine: at any dose? *JAMA* 2015;314(18):1915–1916.

30. Fries JF. Aging, natural death, and the compression of morbidity. *N Engl J Med* 1980;303(3):130–135.

31. Kujala UM, Kaprio J, Sarna S, Koskenvuo M. Relationship of leisure-time physical activity and mortality: the Finnish twin cohort. *JAMA* 1998;279(6):440–444.

32. Sun Q, Townsend MK, Okereke OI, Franco OH, Hu FB, Grodstein F. Physical activity at midlife in relation to successful survival in women at age 70 years or older. *Arch Intern Med* 2010;170(2):194–201.

33. Buchman AS, Yu L, Boyle PA, Shah RC, Bennett DA. Total daily physical activity and longevity in old age. *Arch Intern Med* 2012;172(5):444–446.

34. Thompson PD. Exercise and physical activity in the prevention and treatment of atherosclerotic cardiovascular disease. *Arterioscler Thromb Vasc Biol* 2003;23(8):1319–1321.

35. Erikssen G, Liestol K, Bjornholt J, Thaulow E, Sandvik L, Erikssen J. Changes in physical fitness and changes in mortality. *Lancet* 1998;352(9130):759–762.

36. Voss MW, Vivar C, Kramer AF, van Praag H. Bridging animal and human models of exercise-induced brain plasticity. *Trends Cogn Sci* 2013;17(10):525–544.

37. Erickson KI, Voss MW, Prakas RS, Basak C, Szabo A, Chaddock L, et al. Exercise training increases size of hippocampus and improves memory. *Proc Natl Acad Sci USA* 2011;108(7):3017–3022.

38. Kang SS, Jeraldo PR, Kurti A, Miller ME, Cook MD, Whitlock K, et al. Diet and exercise orthogonally alter the gut microbiome and reveal independent associations with anxiety and cognition. *Mol Neurodegener* 2014;9:36–48.

39. Yang H, Youm Y-H, Vandanmagsar B, Ravussin A, Gimble JM, Greenway F, et al. Obesity increases the production of proinflammatory mediators from adipose tissue T cells and compromises TCR repertoire diversity: implications for systemic inflammation and insulin. *J Immunol* 2010;185:1836–1845.

40. Roizen MF, Oz MC. *You on a Diet: The Owner's Manual for Waist Management*. New York, NY: Simon & Schuster; 2009.

41. Simon HB. Exercise and health: dose and response, considering both ends of the curve. *Am J Med* 2015;128(11):1171–1177.

42. Williams PT, Thompson PD. Walking versus running for hypertension, cholesterol, and diabetes mellitus risk reduction. *Arterioscler Thromb Vasc Biol* 2013;33(5):1085–1091.

43. Willis BL, Gao A, Leonard D, DeFina LF, Berry JD. Midlife fitness and the development of chronic conditions in later life. *Arch Intern Med* 2012;172(17):1333–1340.

44. The Look AHEAD Research Group, Wing RR. Long-term effects of a lifestyle intervention on weight and cardiovascular risk factors in individuals with type 2 diabetes mellitus: four-year results of the Look AHEAD Trial. *Arch Intern Med* 2010;170(17):1566–1575.

45. Nieman DC, Henson DA, Austin MD, Sha W. Upper respiratory tract infections is reduced in physically fit and active adults. *Br J Sports Med* 2011;45(12):987–992.

46. Chakravarty EF, Hubert HB, Lingala VB, Fries JF. Reduced disability and mortality among aging runners: a 21-year longitudinal study. *Arch Intern Med* 2008;168(15):1638–1646.

47. Carter CS, Marzetti E, Leeuwenburgh C, Manini T, Foster TC, Groban L, et al. Usefulness of preclinical models for assessing the efficacy of late-life interventions for sarcopenia. *J Gerontol A Biol Sci Med Sci* 2012;67(1):17–27.

48. Wannamethee SG, Shaper AG, Walker M. Changes in physical activity, mortality, and incidence of coronary heart disease in older men. *Lancet* 1998;351(9116):1603–1608.

49. American Heart Association. *2015 Scientific Sessions: High Risk Hypertensive Patients SPRINT Toward Lower Blood Pressure Target*. 2015.

50. Ladabaum U, Mannalithara A, Myer PA, Singh G. Obesity, abdominal obesity, physical activity, and caloric intake in US adults: 1988 to 2010. *Am J Med* 2014;127(8):717–727.

51. Vestergaard S, Patel KV, Bandinelli S, Ferrucci L, Guralnik JM. Characteristics of 400-meter walk test performance and subsequent mortality in older adults. *Rejuvenation Res* 2009;12(3):177–184.

52. Woo J, Ho SC, Yu ALM. Walking speed and stride length predicts 36 months dependency, mortality, and institutionalization in Chinese aged 70 and older. *J Am Geriatr Soc* 1999;47(10):1257–1260.

53. Sasaki H, Kasagi F, Yamada M, Fujita S. Grip strength predicts cause-specific mortality in middle-aged and elderly persons. *Am J Med* 2007;120(4):337–342.

54. Gale CR, Martyn CN, Cooper C, Sayer AA. Grip strength, body composition, and mortality. *Int J Epidemiol* 2007;36(1):228–235.

55. Leong DP, Teo KK, Rangarajan S, Lopez-Jaramillo P, Avezum A Jr, Orlandini A, et al. Prognostic value of grip strength: findings from the prospective urban rural epidemiology (PURE) study. *Lancet* 2015;386(9990):266–273.

56. Daubenmier JJ, Weidner G, Marlin R, Crutchfield L, Dunn-Emke S, Chi C, et al. Lifestyle and health-related quality of life of men with prostate cancer managed with active surveillance. *Urology* 2006;67(1):125–130.

57. ENCODE Project Consortium. An integrated encyclopedia of DNA elements in the human genome. *Nature* 2012;489(7414):57–74.

58. Ornish D, Lin J, Chan JM, Epel E, Kemp C, Weidner G, et al. Effect of comprehensive lifestyle changes on telomerase activity and telomere length in men with biopsy-proven low-risk prostate cancer: 5-year follow-up of a descriptive pilot study. *Lancet Oncol* 2013;14(11):1112–1120.

59. Ewald B, Attia J, McElduff P. How many steps are enough? Dose-response curves for pedometer steps and multiple health markers in a community-based sample of older Australians. *J Phys Act Health* 2014;11(3):509–518.

60. Varma VR, Chuang YF, Harris GC, Tan EJ, Carlson MC. Low-intensity daily walking activity is associated with hippocampal volume in older adults. *Hippocampus* 2015;25(5):605–615.

61. Hirsch CH, Diehr P, Newman AB, et al. Physical activity and years of healthy life in older adults: results from the cardiovascular health study. *J Aging Phys Act* 2010;18(3):313–334.

62. *First Circumnavigation by Walking*. http://www.guinnessworldrecords.com/world-records/first-circumnavigation-by-walking.

63. *Genes Are Not Destiny*. Harvard T. H. Chan School of Public Health Obesity Prevention Source. http://www.hsph.harvard.edu/obesity-prevention-source/obesity-causes/genes-and-obesity.

64. Ledochowski L, Ruedl G, Taylor AH, Kopp M. Acute effects of brisk walking on sugary snack cravings in overweight people, affect and responses to a manipulated stress situation and to a sugary snack cue: a crossover study. *PLoS One* 2015;10(3). doi: 10.1371/journal.pone.0119278.

65. Hildebrand JS, Gapstur SM, Campbell PT, Gaudet MM, Patel AV. Recreational physical activity and leisure-time sitting in relation to postmenopausal breast cancer risk. *Cancer Epidemiol Biomarkers Prev* 2013;22(10):1906–1912.

66. Nieman DC, Henson DA, Austin MD, Brown VA. Immune response to a 30-minute walk. *Med Sci Sports Exerc* 2005;37(1):57–62.

67. Tucker LA, Strong JE, Lecheminant JD, Bailey BW. Effect of two jumping programs on hip bone mineral density in premenopausal women: a randomized controlled trial. *Am J Health Promot* 2015;29(3):158–116.

68. Gulati M, Shaw LJ, Thisted RA, Black HR, Merz CNB, Arnsdorf MF. Heart rate response to exercise stress testing in asymptomatic women: the St. James women take heart project. *Circulation* 2010;122(2):130–137.

69. Gill S, Hankey J, Wright A, Marczak S, Hemming K, Allerton D, et al. The impact of a 24-h ultra-marathon on circulatory endotoxin and cytokine profile. *International J Sports Medicine* 2015;36(8):688–695.

12

The Role of Supplements in Integrative Preventive Medicine

JOSEPH PIZZORNO, ND

Introduction

Considering the human species has survived solely on the nutrients available in food, a strong case could be made that additional nutritional support is unnecessary. This might be true in an ideal world, composed of healthy humans with uniform biochemistry, living in a clean environment. However, such a world does not exist. Our diet has been mutated to include foods that contain an inherently lower ratio of nutrients in proportion to calories.[1,2] Foods are now produced through modern agricultural methods resulting in decreased nutrient content.[3] Food processing damages and even removes nutrients,[4-6] and the standards used to determine nutrient adequacy are seriously flawed. More importantly, genetic research has revealed huge variations in individual nutrient needs within the general population. Aggravating the situation is the growing body load of environmental toxins that poison enzyme systems. This requires higher than normal levels of nutrients to compete for enzyme activation sites and help prevent oxidative and metabolic damage caused by these toxins. The World Health Organization (WHO) already includes recommendations for several micronutrients including iron + folic acid supplements for pregnancy,[7] high-dose vitamin A supplementation for children <5 years,[8] food fortification, and universal salt iodization.[9,10] However, gaps still exist in micronutrient recommendations for several population groups.[11] Many studies have shown that nutrients in supraphysiological dosages can be very effective therapeutic agents. In this context, maintaining and optimizing health depends on skilled nutritional supplementation.

The Incidence of Nutrient Deficiencies

The measures used to determine deficiency constitute a huge and controversial challenge in determining nutrient status. The NHANES (National Health and Nutrition Examination Survey) regularly assess the health and nutritional status of adults and children in the United States. Comprehensive nutritional reports are provided periodically, the latest of which was published in 2012. Table 12.1 shows the portion of the population deficient in selected nutrients according to the standards used in NHANES (which, as shown later, may be problematic). Note especially that these numbers *include* the use of dietary supplements. In other words, despite the fact that 50% of the population regularly takes nutritional supplements, many deficiencies still exist.[12]

Although the data may suggest nutrient deficiencies are uncommon, the standards for nutrient status have substantial problems. For example, nutrient deficiencies are much more common in patients with chronic disease. A recent review of patients with heart failure found that 75% were deficient in vitamin D and 37% deficient in iron.[14] Researchers also found studies showing supplementation with coenzyme Q10, vitamin D, iron, and L-carnitine improved clinical outcomes. Although unpublished, in a corporate wellness program I helped design and implement laboratory tests (serum levels) assessing several nutritional measures in 4,500 adult Canadian oil field workers showed that 90% were deficient in one or more nutrients.

A disease-by-disease review of nutrient deficiencies is beyond the scope of this chapter. Those interested in more deeply delving into this clinically important topic will find thousands of references in the *Textbook of Natural*

Table 12.1 Percent of US
Adults Deficient in Select
Nutrients

Nutrient	Deficient
Vitamin B6	10.5%
Iron (women)	9.5%
Vitamin D	8.1%
Vitamin C	6.0%
Vitamin B12	2.0%
Vitamin A	<1%
Vitamin E	<1%
Folate	<1%

Source: Reference 13.

Table 12.2 Nutrient Deficiencies in Representative Diseases

Disease	Deficient Vitamins	Deficient Minerals	Deficient Nutrient Factors
Asthma	Vitamin C, omega-3 fatty acids		
ADHD	Omega-3 fatty acids	Iron, magnesium, zinc	
Cervical dysplasia	Folate, vitamin A, vitamin B6, vitamin C	Copper, zinc	Beta-carotene
Diabetes Type I	Vitamin D, omega-3 fatty acids		
Heart failure	Vitamin B1	Magnesium	
Osteoporosis	Vitamin D, vitamin K2	Calcium, magnesium	

Source: Reference 15.

Medicine, which evaluates nutrient status and the efficacy of nutrient supplementation in over 70 of the most common diseases. Table 12.2 provides a brief list of the typical nutrient deficiencies observed in representative diseases.

Foods of Commerce Now Contain Lower Levels of Nutrients

Agriculture precipitated the formation of cities resulting in civilization, and modern agricultural technology allowed growth of the human population. However, the effects on food quality have not all been beneficial. The nutrient content of conventionally grown foods has decreased precipitously. Modern agricultural methods produce food that is bigger and grows faster but is lower in nutrients. One study measured the mineral content of 56 commonly eaten foods—27 vegetables, 17 fruits, 10 meats, and 2 dairy products—from 1940 to 1991. As can be seen in Figure 12.1, every mineral, except phosphorus in fruits and vegetables (from high-phosphate fertilizers) and sodium in dairy (added salt), decreased significantly.[16] Trace minerals showed the worst effects, with copper down a serious 77% in vegetables. The longest study evaluated the trace mineral content of 14 varieties of US wheat over a period of 122 years. Every mineral decreased 20%–33%.[17] Unfortunately, the foods that the average American consumes are truly depleted of nutrients.

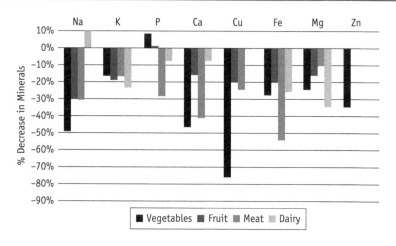

FIGURE 12.1 Content of Trace Minerals Decreased from 1940 to 1991

The cause of this mineral loss appears to be the result of three factors: (1) change in cultivars; (2) depletion of soil mineral content after decades of synthetic fertilizer use; and (3) high-phosphate fertilizers that cause foods to grow bigger but dilute their nutrient content. Figure 12.2 shows the impact of fertilization on the mineral content of raspberries. As can clearly be seen, the use of high-phosphate fertilizers proportionately decreases mineral content.[18] Higher water content in conventionally grown foods leads to nutrient dilution. While the foods still provide calories, the nutrients critical for health are depleted. Several studies have shown the amounts of beneficial constituents are higher in organically grown foods compared to those grown with conventional agriculture practices.[19-21] Speaking subjectively, the raspberries from my garden have dramatically more flavor than those bought at the grocery store. Considering the majority of people consume foods produced by conventional agricultural practices, an argument can easily be made showing the need for nutritional supplementation.

Nutrient Standards Do Not Adequately Address Biochemical Individuality

In 1941, the Food and Nutrition Board, a committee of the National Academy of Sciences, developed recommendations on the amount of essential nutrients that should be provided to the general public. This would come to be known as the recommended dietary allowances (RDAs). The guidelines were developed for the prevention of nutrient deficiency diseases (e.g., scurvy: deficiency of

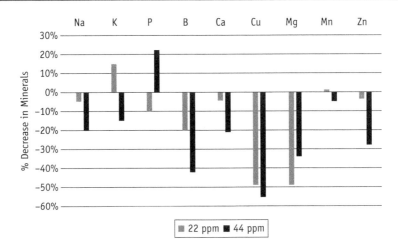

FIGURE 12.2 Increasing Use of High Phosphate Fertilizers Decreases Mineral Content

vitamin C, pellagra: deficiency of niacin, and beri-beri: deficiency of vitamin B1) and to serve as a guide for planning adequate nutrition. The RDAs were designed for the maintenance of good nutrition of *normal healthy* persons under present conditions in the United States.[22] However, considering there is an almost universally sick population, normal may not actually be healthy. It is estimated that over 50% of the US population now suffers from one or more diagnosed chronic diseases, and 25% of the population has two or more chronic conditions. In addition, at least 16% of the population describe themselves as chronically unwell.[23]

Studies have now shown that it is inappropriate to use the RDA to assess the nutrient adequacy of groups.[24] Box 12.1 lists several limitations of the RDAs.

In 1997, the dietary reference intake (DRI) was introduced to expand on the guidelines of the RDAs. The DRI includes several sets of values for nutrient intake: the RDA—(the daily dietary intake level of a nutrient considered sufficient by the Food and Nutrition Board to meet the requirements of 97.5% of healthy individuals); estimated average requirements (EAR—based on a review of scientific literature, these values are expected to satisfy the needs of 50% of the people in an age group); and adequate intake (AI—when an RDA cannot be determined, this is the recommended average daily intake level based on observed or experimentally determined approximations of nutrient intake by apparently healthy people that are assumed to be sufficient for everyone in the demographic group).[25] In addition, the DRI includes a set of values known as tolerable upper intake levels (ULs). The UL is the maximum amount of a nutrient that appears safe for 97.5% of healthy individuals. Although more information is provided, the DRI has similar limitations to the RDA alone.

Box 12.1 Limitations of the RDAs

- They are meant to serve as a guideline for the prevention of nutritional diseases, not the promotion of health.
- The recommendations are based on the nutrient status of large population groups numbering in the millions, not as a guideline to determine individual dietary nutrient requirements.
- The estimates of the RDAs are based only on short-term research that represents less than 1% of the average person's lifespan, so they cannot provide nutrient recommendations that may be of benefit over a lifetime in the prevention or amelioration of diseases associated with aging or certain lifestyles.
- They do not make adjustments for variations in nutrient needs associated with conditions or diseases that affect nutrient requirements.
- They provide no data on compensatory levels of nutrient intake needed to compensate for nutrient-demanding lifestyle factors such as: chronic stress, chronic intense exercise, cigarette smoking, alcoholism, restrictive dieting routines, polluted environments, exposure to chemical carcinogens, etc.

Source: Reference 15.

Neither the DRI nor the RDA addresses biochemical individuality, and neither has the ability to provide specific recommendations for individuals seeking a long and disease-free lifespan. As knowledge of genetic variability in nutrient needs for health promotion and disease prevention arises, a greater case can be made for an individual's need for supplementation of nutrients above the RDAs and RDIs.

Serum levels for several vitamins and minerals may not always be sufficient in assessing vitamin and mineral deficiencies. The latest NHANES report is an improvement from the prior report as a number of biochemical markers of nutrient deficiency were added to the assessment rather than just blood levels of nutrients. As seen in Figure 12.3, an entirely different picture is presented when these markers are included. While only 4% of the older population show deficient levels of vitamin B12 according to serum levels alone, when including the metabolites that increase when vitamin B12 is deficient—such as methylmelonic acid and homocysteine—the number quadruples to 17%–19%.[26]

Now that so many of the human single nucleotide polymorphisms (SNPs) have been mapped, the way genetics affect nutritional needs is much better understood. Three examples out of many that are available—VDR, MTHFR, and COMT polymorphisms—clearly document the need for nutritional supplements.

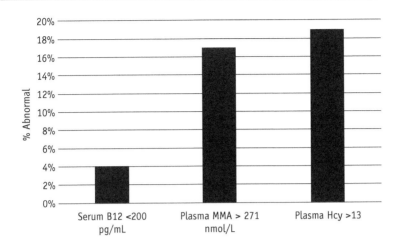

FIGURE 12.3 Incidence of Nutrient Level Deficiency Versus Nutrient Deficiency According to Function

VDR POLYMORPHISMS

The vitamin D receptor site gene has six known polymorphisms with well-researched clinical effects: Apa1 (A/a), Bsml (B/b), Cdx-2, Fok1 (F/f), and Taq1 (T/t). These polymorphisms have multiple effects, most mediated by decreased absorption of vitamin D or impaired ability to bind to and activate cell receptor sites. The clinical impact is huge. In cancer, for example, compared to "wild types":[27]

- Cdx2: 12% increased risk of all cancers
- Taq1: 43% increased risk of colon cancer
- Apa1: increased cancer risk, but only when in combination with other polymorphisms

Many other disease associations with VDR polymorphisms include breast cancer, prostate cancer, pancreatic cancer, cancer metastases, multiple sclerosis, osteoporosis, Parkinson's disease—the list continues to increase as research accumulates.[28,29] For these patients, high-dose vitamin D supplementation is essentially the only solution.[30-32]

A patient example is illustrative. A 50-year-old perimenopausal woman (normal weight) presented with osteopenia. Physical examination was normal. Diet and lifestyle were exemplary. Of particular relevance was a family history of every woman in her family dying from complications of osteoporosis, typically broken hips. Standard treatment with bioidentical estrogen,

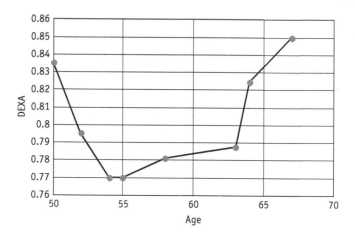

FIGURE 12.4 DEXA Response to High Dose Vitamin D in Patient with Dysfunctional VDR Receptor Site Polymorphisms

vitamin D (1,500 IU/d) and calcium (1,200 mg/d) for 3.5 years was ineffective, with bone loss progressing unabated. An SNP panel revealed she had several of the undesirable VDR polymorphisms. The patient was then given progressively larger dosages of vitamin D, eventually reaching 12,000 IU per day—far beyond RDIs. Other than additional supplementation with vitamin K2, no changes were made in diet, lifestyle, prescriptions, or nutrients. As can be seen in Figure 12.4, her DEXXA results were remarkable. The vitamin D dosage was determined by progressively increasing supplementation until her 25-OH3 was 50 ng/mL.

MTHFR POLYMORPHISMS

Polymorphisms in methylenetetrahydrofolate reductase (MTHFR), the enzyme that converts dietary folate to its active physiological form, have been extensively studied. Several polymorphisms have been shown to increase rates of cancers such as leukemia and squamous cell carcinoma with stronger associations found in cardiovascular disease.[33,34] These polymorphisms are extremely common, affecting 29%–42% of the population, depending on ethnicity.[35] Effective intervention for such polymorphisms requires activated forms of folate that are not possible through food.[36-38] Low folate levels have been found in many patients with depression. In a trial of nearly 3,000 participants, low RBC and/or serum folate was found in patients who met the criteria for major depression.[39] Polymorphisms in the MTHFR gene, in particular the C677T polymorphism, have been reported to influence depression risk.[40-42] Treatment with high-dose L-methylfolate has shown benefit in individuals with depression when used alone and/or in conjunction with SSRI treatment.[43,44]

COMT POLYMORPHISMS

Phase II catechol-O-methyltransferase (COMT) is a key enzyme for detoxifying genotoxic estrogen metabolites and catecholamines. Polymorphisms that decrease activity of this enzyme have been shown to increase risk of breast cancer and post-traumatic stress syndrome.[45,46] The impact of impaired ability to detoxify catecholamines impairs resiliency to stress. Figure 12.5 shows the impact of the COMT SNP polymorphisms for risk of PTSD in soldiers returning from Iraq.

Supplementation with S-adenosyl-methionine (SAM-e) has been shown to increase activity of COMT in patients with genetically lower activity.[47] Administration of SAM-e has also shown benefit in the reduction of aggressive behavior and improvement in overall quality of life in patients with schizophrenia and the low activity COMT polymorphism.[48]

These are just a few examples of the emerging SNP research showing the huge variations in need for nutritional supplementation in dosages and forms unavailable in food. With SNP testing now relatively inexpensive, this tool will over time become key for optimizing and personalizing nutritional therapy. (Note, while complete genetic profiling provides even more clinically relevant measures like deletions and duplications, such testing is 1–2 orders of magnitude more expensive and much less available.)

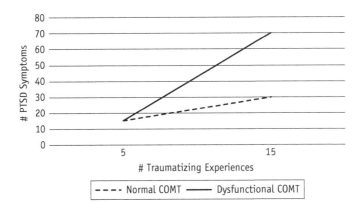

FIGURE 12.5 COMT SNPs Impact Susceptibility to PTSD

Environmental Toxin Load Greatly Changes Nutrient Need

It is estimated that over 60,000 different chemicals are now in use, with 6.5 billion pounds of chemicals released into the air per year in the United States alone. Considering only 20% of disease is genetically influenced and 80% of disease results from diet, lifestyle, and environmental factors, there is mounting evidence that this high level of toxin exposure is responsible for the rising incidence of chronic disease.

Exposure to environmental toxins has a significant impact on nutrient needs. Humans are now exposed to a number of toxins at rates higher than the trace minerals and vitamins they compete with for binding sites. Toxins induce oxidative stress, increasing the need for antioxidant nutrients; displace nutrients from enzyme cofactor binding sites, requiring higher levels for activation; damage DNA, resulting in apoenzymes that are less responsive to nutrient cofactors; replace structure minerals; damage cell membranes, causing fatty acid imbalances; and block insulin receptor sites, requiring increased insulin production and increased amounts of the nutrients needed to produce insulin.[49,50] The combination of nutrient depletion, cofactor displacement, and high toxin-contamination in the food supply may be the main reason the incidence of all chronic disease is increasing.

A few examples:

- Lead aggravates folate, B6, and B12 deficiencies, thus increasing homocysteine. Studies have shown that increasing intake of folate and vitamin B6 may reduce lead-associated increases in homocysteine.[51]
- Cadmium increases production of reactive oxygen species, resulting in increased need for antioxidant nutrients. Antioxidants, such as curcumin, have been shown to protect against cardiovascular dysfunction resulting from oxidative stress associated with cadmium exposure through free radical scavenging, metal chelation, regulation of inflammatory enzymes, and increasing nitric oxide (NO +).[52,53]
- Poison enzyme systems (compete with nutritional cofactors for binding sites).
- Lead poisons delta aminolevulinic acid dehydratase, resulting in impaired utilization of vitamin B12.
- Lead displaces calcium in bones, making them weaker.[54,55]
- Arsenic blocks vitamin A receptor sites. Studies have shown that supplementation with vitamin A may have a protective role toward cells from arsenic-induced injury.[56]

Persistent organic pollutants (POPs) are compounds designed for specific chemical/physical/biological effects as well as resistance to environmental degradation through chemical, biological, and photolytic processes.[57] Examples of these organic pollutants include pesticides, plasticizers, herbicides, and industrial chemicals. The POPs bioaccumulate in human and animal tissue and biomagnify in food chains, thus increasing their concentration and toxicity in the environment. People are exposed to POPs mostly through the diet, with most of exposure coming from the ingestion of animal products.[57] Nine times as many pesticide residues were found in children eating conventionally grown foods compared to those consuming organic foods.[58] This further emphasizes the need for additional supplementation, perhaps beginning as early as childhood.

Several studies show an association between serum concentrations of POPs and prevalence of disease. Individuals with higher concentrations of POPs had a greater occurrence of cardiovascular disease (specifically hypertension), cancer, obesity, and diabetes.[59-63] Neurodegenerative diseases such as Parkinson's, developmental defects, atherosclerosis, and arthritis have also been associated with exposure to persistent organic pollutants.[64,65] Organic, mostly plant-based foods should be consumed when possible. Eating organic foods has been shown to measurably decrease POP levels within 3 days.[66]

Therapeutic Nutrition Works

A key challenge in determining the efficacy of nutritional therapy is that almost all research follows the standard drug trial methodology. Randomized clinical trials (RCTs) are designed to determine statistical efficacy in a generic population with a specific disease. This works for pharmaceuticals, especially those designed to alleviate symptoms by poisoning enzyme systems. The problem with using this model for nutrients is that the supplemented nutrients typically only work where there is a substantial deficiency or an SNP polymorphism requiring above normal dosages. In other words, the supplemented nutrients only work for those who need them and are ineffective for everyone else, while drugs will poison enzymes for virtually everyone. Table 12.3 provides a brief summary of nutritional supplements effective in representative diseases.

Vitamins

Multivitamin/mineral supplements are the most commonly used nutritional supplements in the United States, with many containing nutrients two to

Table 12.3 Nutrients Shown Effective in Representative Diseases

Disease	Vitamins	Minerals	Nutrient Factors
Acne	A, E	Chromium, zinc	
Angina	Pantothene	Magnesium	Arginine, carnitine, coenzyme Q10
Diabetes Type II	B6, biotin, C, E, niacin, omega-3 fatty acids	Chromium, magnesium, manganese, zinc	Fiber
Migraine	B2, omega-3 fatty acids	Magnesium	5-HTP, coenzyme Q10
Osteoarthritis	C, D, pantothenic acid		Glucosamine, niacinamide sulfate, SAMe
Premenstrual Syndrome	B6, E, omega-3 fatty acids	Calcium, magnesium, zinc	

Source: Reference 15.

six times the RDAs.[67] A broad spectrum multivitamin/mineral containing vitamins A, B6, B12, C, D, E, folate, zinc, iron, copper, and selenium is likely to have benefit for innate and adaptive immunity as well as for maintaining the integrity of physical barriers (Table 12.4).[68] Studies have shown that multivitamin/mineral supplements may prevent advanced age-related macular degeneration in high-risk individuals and may prevent cancer in individuals with poor or suboptimal nutritional status.[69,70]

VITAMIN D

It is estimated that only 4% of individuals age 51 or older meet the adequate intake level of vitamin D.[71] Vitamin D has been shown to improve bone density,[72] prevent the progression of osteoarthritis,[73] reduce the risk of hypertension,[74] and prevent osteoporosis.[75]

Considering the relationship between stress symptoms, depression, and low serum levels of 25(OH)-vitamin D, ensuring optimal vitamin D levels is important.[76,77] Studies have shown that supplementation with vitamin D reduces symptoms of depression compared to placebo, and daily supplementation increased positive affect when given to healthy subjects during the winter.[78,79] In individuals diagnosed with major depressive disorder (MDD), vitamin D supplementation has been shown to have beneficial effects

Table 12.4 Sites of Action of Micronutrients on the Immune System

Epithelial Barriers	Cellular Immunity	Antibody Production
Vitamin A	Vitamin A	Vitamin A
Vitamin C	Vitamin B_6	Vitamin B_6
Vitamin E	Vitamin B_{12}	Vitamin B_{12}
Zinc	Vitamin C	Vitamin D
	Vitamin D	Vitamin E
	Vitamin E	Folic acid
	Folic acid	Zinc
	Iron	Copper
	Zinc	Selenium
	Copper	
	Selenium	

Source: Reference 68.

on the Beck Depression Inventory (BDI) and improvements in biomarkers of oxidative stress.[80]

In a trial of over 400 overweight men and women, serum levels of 25(OH)-D were compared with scores on the Beck Depression Inventory. Supplementation of either 20,000 or 40,000 IU per week was associated with improved scores compared to placebo.[81] Additionally, in a small study of patients with fibromyalgia, a deficiency in vitamin D was not only common but also more commonly associated with depression and anxiety.[82]

Vitamin D has been shown to increase innate immunity while modulating adaptive immunity. Researchers have found that in patients with vitamin D deficiency, the normal production of cathelicidin antimicrobial protein (hCAP), which kills invading bacteria, was inhibited without supplemental vitamin D. A direct correlation was found between serum concentration of 25-hydroxyvitamin D_3 and monocyte expression of hCAP following treatment with ligands to pathogen-responsive TLRs. Vitamin D supplementation in patients with vitamin D insufficiency significantly enhanced innate immune responses by rescuing TLR-mediated suppression of hCAP expression suggesting that a key function of vitamin D is to prevent pathogen-induced evasion of innate immunity.[83]

Vitamin D insufficiency is associated with an increased prevalence of many autoimmune diseases, including multiple sclerosis, rheumatoid arthritis, systemic lupus erythematosus (SLE), and inflammatory bowel disease.[84] A 30-year cohort study showed that those who regularly took supplemental vitamin D at a dose of 2,000 IU daily had a nearly 80% lower risk of developing type 1 diabetes compared with those who received less than 2,000 IU per day.[85] Inflammation may also play a role in the development of type I diabetes, as studies have shown an increase in specific TLRs associated with inflammatory markers on monocytes.[86] Supplemental vitamin D modulated some of the monocyte abnormalities in patients with type 1 diabetes and seems to protect against the development of type I diabetes by reducing the activation of TLRs.[87,88]

VITAMIN C

Vitamin C is a water soluble vitamin that is involved in many biological functions including bone metabolism, immune function, and detoxification,[89] and acts as a potent antioxidant.[90] Vitamin C is involved in collagen synthesis and therefore may help in the prevention or treatment of osteoarthritis.[73] Vitamin C was found to reduce the duration of the common cold, and in populations engaging in significant physical exercise or living in cold environments, vitamin C showed a 50% reduction in incidence of the common cold.[91] Taken at the onset of cold and flu symptoms, vitamin C (1,000 mg per hour for 6 hours, followed by 1,000 mg three times per day) demonstrated an 85% decrease in symptoms compared with the control group.[92] Increased intake of vitamin C has been associated with a decreased risk of cervical, stomach, colon, and lung cancers.[93-95] Vitamin C is also beneficial for cardiovascular health and has been shown to inhibit platelet aggregation,[96] increase HDL cholesterol,[97] and lower blood pressure.[98]

VITAMIN E

Vitamin E is a combination of eight different fat-soluble compounds—tocopherols (alpha, beta, gamma, and delta) and tocotrienols. Tocopherols tend to be more biologically active, with alpha-tocopherol being the most active of the group, depending on the measure used. The primary function of vitamin E is to scavenge free radicals, thereby protecting the body from oxidative damage.[99] The typical US diet often provides less than the RDA of alpha-tocopherol. Healthy individuals who consumed a balanced diet that supplied adequate (RDA) vitamin E amounts had decreased oxidative damage when supplemented with vitamin E at 10 times the RDA.[100] Vitamin E supplementation has been shown to enhance immunity,[101] help protect LDL from oxidative damage,[102] repair membranes,[103] and decrease platelet aggregation and blood clot formation.[104] Studies have also shown that supplementation with vitamin

E reduced prostate cancer incidence by 32%, reduced prostate cancer mortality by 41%,[105] and reduced colorectal cancer in heavy smokers by 22%.[106]

Minerals

Minerals are inorganic compounds that are naturally occurring solids found in nature. Minerals have important and wide-ranging actions in the body for both structure and function. Among the most important minerals in the body are magnesium, calcium, selenium, and zinc.

MAGNESIUM

Magnesium deficiency is not uncommon in the West, as magnesium intake has decreased significantly with the increased consumption of processed foods. Magnesium has many critical functions including but not limited to relaxation effects on smooth muscle, regulating heart muscle contractility, regulating calcium absorption, modulating neurotransmitter systems, and reducing HPA axis activity. Magnesium deficiency is associated with increased anxiety-related behavior as well as elevated ACTH levels indicating an up-regulated stress system.[107] Several studies show treatment with magnesium may be beneficial for insomnia, anxiety, depression, seizures, muscle cramping, and fatigue.[108-110]

CALCIUM

Calcium is primarily stored in bones and is associated with multiple functions in the body including energy production, bone formation, nerve transmission, protein and fat digestion, and neuromuscular activity. The average calcium intake in American adults is approximately 761 mg/day which is significantly below the RDA for adults (1,000–1,200 mg/day).[111] Calcium is important in regulating blood pressure and is often recommended for osteoporosis prevention.[112-114] in addition, calcium has shown some benefit in cancer prevention.[115,116]

SELENIUM

Geographical location is significant in determining if there is adequate selenium, as dietary intake depends on the selenium content of the soil. In regions of China where soils are selenium depleted, a cardiomyopathy known as Keshan disease has been attributed to an endemic coxsackievirus. Supplemental selenium not only elevates antiviral immunity but also prevents genetic adaptations in the viral genomic RNA that lead to increased virulence and cardiac pathology. Selenium supplementation also appears to reduce cancer rates,[117,118] induce better host response to viral infections, improve the effects of aging on immunity, and enhance lymphocyte counts and mitogenic responses (Th1).[119] An association exists in areas with increased levels of selenium and lower rates of several cancer types including lung, bladder, colorectal, ovarian, breast, esophageal, pancreatic, and cervical cancers.[120]

ZINC

Zinc has been shown to induce thymic regrowth and activation.[121] Supplementation of zinc significantly improves immune function in those with even a marginal zinc deficiency. The activities of virtually all immune cells of both the adaptive and innate systems are modulated by zinc.[122,123] Additionally, the decline in zinc status with aging is likely a significant contributor to immunosenescence.[124] Zinc (at dosages 10x the RDA) has been shown to be beneficial in treating individuals with intermediate age-related macular degeneration.[70]

OTHER

Antioxidants protect the liver from damage and support detoxification processes. Antioxidants counteract oxidative stress by reducing the formation of free radicals. Dark colored fruits and vegetables are rich sources of antioxidants. Several vitamins, minerals, and nutraceuticals also function as antioxidants.

Glutathione

Glutathione (GSH) is the major endogenous antioxidant produced by cells. It is involved in metabolic and biochemical reactions such as DNA synthesis and repair, protein synthesis, prostaglandin synthesis, amino acid transport, and enzyme activation. Glutathione, therefore, affects every system in the body, especially the nervous system, gastrointestinal system, immune system, and the respiratory system.

Glutathione is made available in three ways: (1) synthesis via a two-step process catalyzed by the enzymes glutamate cysteine ligase (GCL) and glutathione synthetase; (2) regeneration of oxidized glutathione (GSSG) to reduced glutathione (GSH) by glutathione reductase; and (3) recycling of cysteine from conjugated glutathione.[125]

Glutathione can be depleted by oxidative stress, exposure to toxic metals, and alcohol. Glutathione levels decline as conjugation reactions exceed the cells' ability to regenerate GSH. Chemicals such as polychlorinated biphenyls (PCBs) and organochlorine pesticides increase oxidative damage and deplete glutathione levels.[126] If GSH is depleted, de novo synthesis of GSH is upregulated, as is cysteine synthesis.[127] Depleted glutathione has been implicated in several degenerative conditions including neurodegenerative disorders (Alzheimer's, Parkinson's, and Huntington's diseases; amyotrophic lateral sclerosis; Friedreich's ataxia); pulmonary disease (COPD, asthma, and acute respiratory distress syndrome); immune diseases (HIV, autoimmune disease); cardiovascular diseases (hypertension, myocardial infarction, cholesterol oxidation); liver disease; cystic fibrosis; chronic age-related diseases (cataracts, macular degeneration, hearing impairment, and glaucoma); and the aging process itself.[128] There is also an increased risk of cancer and smoking-related heart disease as a result of glutathione conjugation polymorphisms in glutathione transferase.[129]

Considering the significant consequences associated with depleted glutathione, it is essential to maintain adequate glutathione levels. This can be done by decreasing need for glutathione and oxidative stress; increasing production through supplementation with N-acetylcysteine (NAC),[130] whey protein powder,[131] S-adenosyl L-methionine (SAMe rather than methionine to avoid increasing homocysteine),[132] alpha-lipoic-acid,[133] meditation,[134] and exercise;[135] and/or direct administration of GSH via intravenous, nebulized, or intranasal route.[136-140]

Omega-3 Fatty Acids

Omega-3 fatty acid intake has been directly correlated to decreased symptoms of depression and to reduced anger and anxiety levels in substance users.[141] Omega-3 supplementation has been shown to improve white matter integrity, which may explain the positive effects of fish oil in neuropsychiatric conditions.[142] Fish oil has been shown to blunt the increase in cortisol and epinephrine following a stressful exposure.[143] Considering the anti-inflammatory function of fish oil, it is also likely to reduce the inflammatory component of insomnia.[144]

A number of mechanisms may explain the relationship between omega-3 fatty acids and depression risk. The content of omega-3s is known to affect membrane fluidity and the functioning of enzymes, ion channels, and receptor binding affinity and expression. Omega-3 levels have been found to be low in RBC membranes of depressed patients.[145] Omega-3s also affect neuroplasticity and cell survival through their impact on neurotrophins such as BDNF, which has been shown to be associated with depression risk. Omega-3 fatty acids affect gene expression and decrease the production of proinflammatory cytokines such as interleukin-1beta and tumor necrosis factor-alpha, which have been shown to be elevated in depressed patients and inhibited by some antidepressant medications.[146]

Omega-3 fatty acids have well-established anti-inflammatory effects and also improve cellular membrane function, a specific age-related deficit found in neutrophils.[147] A blunting of immunosenescence in aging mice given omega-3 fatty acids has been established, likely the result of an increase in Th1-stimulating cytokines and a lowering of Th2-associated cytokines. In humans, fish oil supplementation also increased interferon gamma production and lymphocyte proliferation.[148]

Conclusion

Nutritional deficiencies in the general population are much more common than generally recognized, and SNP polymorphisms can dramatically impact nutritional requirements. Patients with chronic disease almost certainly benefit from nutritional supplementation. Expert use of nutritional supplements is a critical skill for integrative medicine doctors. The effective integrative medicine clinician is knowledgeable about the signs and symptoms of nutrient deficiencies, recognizes the nutrients most useful for each chronic disease, and is able to prescribe the correct dosages and dosage forms needed by their patients.

Reference

1. Stern D, Ng SW, Popkin BM. The nutrient content of U.S. household food purchases by store type. *Am J Prev Med* 2016;50(2):180–190.
2. Poti JM, Mendez MA, Ng SW, Popkin BM. Is the degree of food processing and convenience linked with the nutritional quality of foods purchased by U.S. households? *Am J Clin Nutr* 2015;101(6):1251–1262.

3. Thomas D. The mineral depletion of foods available to us as a nation (1940–2002)—a review of the 6th edition of McCance and Widdowson. *Nutr Health* 2007;19(1-2):21–55.

4. Moubarac JC, Martins AP, Claro RM, Levy RB, Cannon G, Monteiro CA. Consumption of ultra-processed foods and likely impact on human health. Evidence from Canada. *Public Health Nutr* 2013;16(12):2240–2248.

5. Costa Louzada ML, Martins AP, Canella DS, et al. Ultra-processed foods and the nutritional dietary profile in Brazil. *Rev Saude Publica* 2015;49:38.

6. Louzada ML, Martins AP, Canella DS, Beraldi LG, et al. Impact of ultra-processed foods on micronutrient content in the Brazilian diet. *Rev Saude Publica* 2015;49:45.

7. World Health Organization. *Guideline: Use of Multiple Micronutrient Powders for Point-of-Use Fortification of Foods Consumed by Pregnant Women.* Geneva: World Health Organization; 2016.

8. WHO Global Database on Vitamin A Deficiency. *Global Prevalence of Vitamin A Deficiency in Populations at Risk 1995–2205.* Geneva: World Health Organization; 2009. [24 Sept 2015].

9. *Iodine and Health: A Statement by the World Health Organization.* Geneva: World Health Organization; 1994. [16 Dec 2015].

10. Zimmermann MB, Jooste PL, Pandav CS. Iodine-deficiency disorders. *Lancet* 2008;372:1251–1262.

11. Allen LH. Current information gaps in micronutrient research, programs and policy: how can we fill them? *World Rev Nutr Diet* 2016;115:109–117.

12. http://www.gallup.com/poll/166541/half-americans-vitamins-regularly.aspx. Accessed July 20, 2016.

13. http://www.cdc.gov/nutritionreport/pdf/exesummary_web_032612.pdf. Accessed July 1, 2016.

14. Sciatti E, Lombardi C, Ravera A, et al. Nutritional deficiency in patients with heart failure. *Nutrients* 2016;8:442. doi:10.3390/nu8070442.

15. Pizzorno J, Murray M. *Textbook of Natural Medicine.* St. Louis, MO: Elsevier; 2012.

16. Thomas D. A study on the mineral depletion of the foods available to US as a nation over the period 1940 to 1991. *Nutr Health* 2003;17:85–115.

17. Garvin DF, Welch RM, Finley JW. Historical shifts in the seed mineral micronutrient concentration of US hard red winter wheat germplasm. *J Sci Food Agr* 2006;86:2213–2220.

18. Hughes M, Chaplin MH, Martin LW. Influence of mycorrhiza on the nutrition of red raspberries. *Hort Science* 1979;14:521–523.

19. Asami DK, Hong YJ, Barrett DM, Mitchell AE. Comparison of the total phenolic and ascorbic acid content of freeze-dried and air-dried marionberry, strawberry, and corn grown using conventional, organic, and sustainable agricultural practices. *J Agric Food Chem* 2003;51(5):1237–1241.

20. Worthington V. Effect of agricultural methods on nutritional quality: a comparison of organic with conventional crops. *Altern Ther Health Med* 1998;4(1):58–69.

21. Carbonaro M, Mattera M, Nicoli S, Bergamo P, Cappelloni M. Modulation of antioxidant compounds in organic vs conventional fruit (peach, Prunus persica L., and pear, Pyrus communis L.). *J Agric Food Chem* 2002;50(19):5458–5462.

22. Institute of Medicine (US) Food and Nutrition Board. *How Should the Recommended Dietary Allowances be Revised?* Washington, DC: National Academies Press; 1994.

23. Multiple Chronic Conditions Among Adults Aged 45 and Over: Trends Over the Past 10 Years. http://www.cdc.gov/nchs/data/databriefs/db100.htm. Accessed August 10, 2016.

24. Murphy SP, Poos MI. Dietary reference intakes: summary of applications in dietary assessment. *Public Health Nutr* 2002;5(6A):843–849.

25. https://en.wikipedia.org/wiki/Dietary_Reference_Intake

26. CDC. *Second National Report on Biochemical Indicators of Diet and Nutrition in the U.S. Population.* 2012.

27. Serrano D, Gnagnarella P, Raimondi S, Gandini S. Meta-analysis on vitamin D receptor and cancer risk: focus on the role of TaqI, ApaI, and Cdx2 polymorphisms. *Eur J Cancer Prev* 2016 Jan;25(1):85–96.

28. Köstner K, Denzer N, Müller CS, et al. The relevance of vitamin D receptor (VDR) gene polymorphisms for cancer: a review of the literature. *Anticancer Res* 2009;29(9):3511–3536.

29. Chen L, Davey Smith G, Evans DM, et al. Genetic variants in the vitamin D receptor are associated with advanced prostate cancer at diagnosis: findings from the prostate testing for cancer and treatment study and a systematic review. *Cancer Epidemiol Biomarkers Prev* 2009;18(11):2874–2881.

30. Wei MY, Giovannucci EL. Vitamin D and multiple health outcomes in the Harvard cohorts. *Mol Nutr Food Res* 2010;54(8):1114–1126.

31. de Medeiros Cavalcante IG, Silva AS, Costa MJ, et al. Effect of vitamin D3 supplementation and influence of BsmI polymorphism of the VDR gene of the inflammatory profile and oxidative stress in elderly women with vitamin D insufficiency: vitamin D3 megadose reduces inflammatory markers. *Exp Gerontol* 2015;66:10–16.

32. Suzuki M, Yoshioka M, Hashimoto M, et al. Randomized, double-blind, placebo-controlled trial of vitamin D supplementation in Parkinson disease. *An J Clin Nutr* 2013;97(5):1004–1013.

33. Ojha RP, Gurney JG. Methylenetetrahydrofolate reductase C677T and overall survival in pediatric acute lymphoblastic leukemia: a systematic review. *Leuk Lymphoma* 2014;55(1):67–73.

34. Fang Y, Xiao F, An Z, Hao L. Systematic review on the relationship between genetic polymorphisms of methylenetetrahydrofolate reductase and esophageal squamous cell carcinoma. *Asian Pac J Cancer Prev* 2011;12(7):1861–1866.

35. Bailey LB, Gregory LF. Polymorphisms of methylenetetrahydrofolate reductase and other enzymes: metabolic significance, risks and impact on folate requirement. *J Nutr* 1999;129:919–922.

36. Hekmatdoost A, Vahid F, Yari Z, et al. Methyltetrahydrofolate vs folic acid supplementation in idiopathic recurrent miscarriage with respect to

methylenetetrahydrofolate reductase C677T and A1298C polymorphisms: a randomized controlled trial. *PLoS One* 2015;10(12):e0143569 (note, the abstract does not appear consistent with the actual study results).

37. Lamers Y, Prinz-Langenohl R, Bramswig S, Pietrzik K. Red blood cell folate concentrations increase more after supplementation with [6S]-5-methyltetrahydrofolate than with folic acid in women of childbearing age. *Am J Clin Nutr* 2006;84(1):156–161.

38. Prinz-Langenohl R, Bramswig S, Tobolski O, et al. [6S]-5-methyltetrahydrofolate increases plasma folate more effectively than folic acid in women with the homozygous or wild-type 677C—>T polymorphism of methylenetetrahydrofolate reductase. *Br J Pharmacol* 2009;158(8):2014–2021.

39. Morris MS, Fava M, Jacques PF, et al. Depression and folate status in the US Population. *Psychother Psychosom* 2003;72(2):80–87.

40. Arinami T, Yamada N. Methylenetetrahydrofolate reductase variant and schizophrenia/depression. *Am J Med Genet* 1997;74(5):526–528.

41. Gilbody S, Lewis S, Lightfoot T. Methylenetetrahydrofolate reductase (MTHFR) genetic polymorphisms and psychiatric disorders: a HuGE review. *Am J Epidemiol* 2007;165(1):1–13. Epub 2006 Oct 30.

42. Jiang W, Xu J, Lu XJ, Sun Y. Association between MTHFR C677T polymorphism and depression: a meta-analysis in the Chinese population. *Psychol Health Med* 2016;21(6):675–685.

43. Papakostas GI, Shelton RC, Zajecka JM, Etemad B, et al. Effect of adjunctive L-methylfolate 15mg among inadequate responders to SSRIs in depressed patients who were stratified by biomarker levels and genotype: results from a randomized clinical trial. *J Clin Psychiatry* 2014;75(8):855–863.

44. Papakostas GI, Shelton RC, Zajecka JM, Etemad B, et al. L-methylfolate as adjunctive therapy for SSRI-resistant major depression: results of two randomized, double-blind, parallel-sequential trials. *Am J Psychiatry* 2012;169(12):1267–1274.

45. Yager JD. Catechol-O-methyltransferase: characteristics, polymorphisms and role in breast cancer. *Drug Discov Today Dis Mech* 2012;9(1-2):e41–e46.

46. Clark R, et al. Predicting post-traumatic stress disorder in veterans: interaction of traumatic load with COMT gene variation. *J Psychiatr Res* 2013;47:1849–1856.

47. Graf WD, Unis AS, Yates CM, et al. Catecholamines in patients with 22q11.2 deletion syndrome and the low-activity COMT polymorphism. *Neurology* 2001;57(3):410–416.

48. Strous RD, Ritsner MS, Adler S, Ratner Y, et al. Improvement of aggressive behavior and quality of life impairment following S-adenosyl-methionine (SAM-e) augmentation in schizophrenia. *Eur Neuropsychopharmacol* 2009;19(1):14–22.

49. Flora SJ. Heavy metal induced oxidative stress and its possible reversal by chelation therapy. *Indian J Med Res* 2008 Oct;128(4):501–523.

50. Neel BA, Robert M. Sargis RM. The paradox of progress: environmental disruption of metabolism and the diabetes epidemic. *Diabetes* 2011;60:1838–1848.

51. Bakulski KM, Park SK, Weisskopf MG, Tucker KL, et al. Lead exposure, B vitamins, and plasma homocysteine in men 55 years of age and older: the VA normative aging study. *Environ Health Perspect* 2014;122(10):1066–1074.

52. Kukongviriyapan U, Apaijit K, Kukongviriyapan V. Oxidative stress and cardio-vascular dysfunction associated with cadmium exposure: beneficial effects of cur-cumin and tetrahydrocurcumin. *Tohoku J Exp Med* 2016;239(1):25–38.

53. Kukongviriyapan U, Pannangpetch P, Kukongviriyapan V, et al. Curcumin pro-tects against cadmium-induced vascular dysfunction, hypertension and tissue cadmium accumulation in mice. *Nutrients* 2014;6(3):1194–1208.

54. Theppeang K, Glass TA, Bandeen-Roche K, et al. Associations of bone mineral density and lead levels in blood, tibia, and patella in urban dwelling women. *Environ Health Perspect* 2008;116(6):784–790.

55. Hu H, Payton M, Korrick S, Aro A, et al. Determinants of bone and blood lead lev-els among community exposed middle-aged to elderly men: the normative aging study. *Am J Epidemiol* 1996;144(8):749–759.

56. Avani G, Rao MV. In vitro genotoxicity assays to evaluate the role of vitamin A on arsenic in human lymphocytes. *Ecotoxicol Environ Saf* 2009;72(2):635–638.

57. Ritter L, Solomon KR, Forget J, Stemeroff M, O'Leary C. *Persistent Organic Pollutants (PDF)*. United Nations Environment Programme. Retrieved September 16, 2007.

58. Curl CL, Fenske RA, Elgethun K. Organophosphorous pesticide exposure of urban and suburban preschool children with organic and conventional diets. *Environ Health Perspect* 2003;111(3):377–382.

59. Lee DH. *A Strong Dose-Response Relation Between Serum Concentrations of Persistent Organic Pollutants and Diabetes: Results from the National Health and Examination Survey 1999-2002*. Diabetes Care. 2006 July;29(7):1638–1644.

60. Lee DH, Steffes MW, Sjödin A, et al. Low dose of some persistent organic pollutants predicts type 2 diabetes: a nested case-control study. *Environ Health Perspect* 2010;118(9):1235–1242.

61. Ha MH, et al. Association between serum concentrations of persistent organic pollutants and prevalence of newly diagnosed hypertension: results from the National Health and Nutrition Examination Survey 1999–2002. *J Hum Hypertens* 2009;23(4):274–286.

62. Lee DH, et al. Relationship between serum concentrations of persistent organic pollutants and the prevalence of metabolic syndrome among non-diabetic adults: results from the National Health and Nutrition Examination Survey 1999–2002. *Diabetologia* 2007;50(9):1841–1851.

63. Lim JS, Son HK, Park SK, Jacobs DR Jr, Lee DH. Inverse associations between long-term weight change and serum concentrations of persistent organic pollut-ants. *Int J Obes (Lond)* 2011 May;35(5):744–747.

64. Lee DH, Steffes M, Jacobs DR, et al. Positive associations of serum concentration of polychlorinated biphenyls or organochlorine pesticides with self-reported arthritis, especially rheumatoid type, in women. *Environ Health Perspect*. 2007 June;86(2):122–127.

65. Priyadarshi A, Khuder SA, Schaub EA, Priyadarshi SS. Environmental risk factors and Parkinson's disease: a metaanalysis. *Environ Res*. 2001 June;86(2):122–127.

66. Curl CL, et al. Organophosphorus pesticide exposure of urban and suburban preschool children with organic and conventional diets. *Env Health Perspect* 2003;111:377–382.

67. Radimer K, Bindewald B, Highes J, et al. Dietary supplement use by US adults: data from the National Health and Nutrition Examination Survey, 1999–2000. *Am J Epidemiol* 2004;160(4):339–349.

68. Maggini S, Wintergerst ES, Beveridge S, et al. Selected vitamins and trace elements support immune function by strengthening epithelial barriers and cellular and humoral immune responses. *Br J Nutr* 2007;98(Suppl 1):S29–S35.

69. Hercberg S, Galan P, Preziosi P, et al. The SU.VI.MAX Study: a randomized, placebo-controlled trial of the health effects of antioxidant vitamins and minerals. *Arch Intern Med* 2004;164(21):2335–2342.

70. Age-Related Eye Disease Study Research Group. A randomized, placebo-controlled, clinical trial of high-dose supplementation with vitamins C and E, beta-carotene, and zinc for age-related macular degeneration and vision loss: AREDS report no. 8. *Arch Opthalmol* 2001;119(10):1417–1436.

71. Moore CE, Murphy MM, Holick MF. Vitamin D intakes by children and adults in the United States differ among ethnic groups. *J Nutr* 2005;135(10):2478–2485.

72. Gillespie WJ, Avenell A, Henry DA, et al. Vitamin D and vitamin D analogues for preventing fractures associated with involuntary and postmenopausal osteoporosis. *Cochrane Database Syst Rev* 2001;(1):CD000227.

73. McAlindon T, Felson DT. Nutrition: risk factors for osteoarthritis. *Ann Rheum Dis* 1997;56(7):397–400.

74. Sowers MR, Wallace RB, Lemke JH. The association of intakes of vitamin D and calcium with blood pressure among women. *Am J Clin Nutr* 1985;42(1):135–142.

75. Papadimitropoulos E, Wells G, Shea B, et al. Meta-analyses of therapies for postmenopausal osteoporosis. VIII: Meta-analysis of the efficacy of vitamin D treatment in preventing osteoporosis in postmenopausal women. *Endocr Rev* 2002;23(4):560–569.

76. Ju SY, Lee YJ, Jeong SN. Serum 25-hydroxyvitamin D levels and the risk of depression: a systematic review and meta-analysis. *J Nutr Health Aging* 2013;17(5):447–455.

77. Milaneschi Y, Hoogendijk W, Lips P, et al. The association between low vitamin D and depressive disorders. *Mol Psychiatry* 2014;19(4):444–451.

78. Jorde R, Sneve M, Figenschau Y, et al. Effects of vitamin D supplementation on symptoms of depression in overweight and obese subjects: randomized double blind trial. *J Intern Med* 2008;264(6):599–609. Epub 2008 Sep 10.

79. Smith BW, Shelley BM, Dalen J. A pilot study comparing the effects of mindfulness-based and cognitive-behavioral stress reduction. *J Altern Complement Med* 2008;14(3):251–258.

80. Sepehrmanesh Z, Kolahdooz F, Abedi F, et al. Vitamin D supplementation affects the Beck Depression Inventory, insulin resistance, and biomarkers of oxidative stress in patients with major depressive disorder: a randomized, controlled clinical trial. *J Nutr* 2016;146(2):243–248.

81. Jorde R, Sneve M, Figenschau Y, et al. Effects of vitamin D supplementation on symptoms of depression in overweight and obese subjects: randomized double blind trial. *J Intern Med* 2008;264(6):599–609. Epub 2008 Sep 10.

82. Armstrong DJ, Meenagh GK, et al. Vitamin D deficiency is associated with anxiety and depression in fibromyalgia. *Clin Rheumatol* 2007;26(4):551–554. Epub 2006 Jul 19.

83. Adams JS, Ren S, Liu PT. Vitamin d-directed rheostatic regulation of monocyte antibacterial responses. *J Immunol* 2009;182(7):4289–4295.

84. Adorini L, Penna G. Control of autoimmune diseases by the vitamin D endocrine system. *Nat Clin Pract Rheumatol* 2008;4(8):404–412.

85. Hyppönen E, Läärä E, Reunanen A, et al. Intake of vitamin D and risk of type 1 diabetes: a birth-cohort study. *Lancet* 2001;358(9292):1500–1503.

86. Devaraj S, Dasu MR, Rockwood J, et al. Increased toll-like receptor (TLR) 2 and TLR4 expression in monocytes from patients with type 1 diabetes: further evidence of a proinflammatory state. *J Clin Endocrinol Metab* 2008;93(2):578–583.

87. Du T, Zhou ZG, You S, et al. Regulation by 1, 25-dihydroxy-vitamin D3 on altered TLRs expression and response to ligands of monocyte from autoimmune diabetes. *Clin Chim Acta* 2009;402(1-2):133–138.

88. Adamczak DM, Nowak JK, Frydrychowicz, Kaczmarek M, Sikora J. The roll of Toll-like receptors and vitamin D in diabetes mellitus type 1—a review. *Scand J Immunol* 2014;80(2):75–84.

89. Jakob RA, Kelly DS, Piamalto FS, et al. Immunocompetence and antioxidant defense during ascorbate depletion of healthy men. *Am J Clin Nutr* 1991;54:1302S-1309S.

90. Frei B, England L, Ames BN. Ascorbate is an outstanding antioxidant in human blood plasma. *Proc Natl Acad Sci* 1989;86:6377–6381.

91. Douglas RM, Hemilä H, Chalker E, Treacy B. Vitamin C for preventing and treating the common cold. *Cochrane Database Syst Rev* 2007;(3):CD000980.

92. Gorton HC, Jarvis K. The effectiveness of vitamin C in preventing and relieving the symptoms of virus-induced respiratory infections. *J Manipulative Physiol Ther* 1999;22(8):530–533.

93. Block G. Vitamin C and cancer prevention: the epidemiological evidence. *Am J Clin Nutr* 1991;53:270S–282S.

94. Bjelke E. Epidemiologic studies of cancer of the stomach, colon, and rectum;with special emphasis on diet. *Scand J Gastroenterol* 1974;9:1–235S.

95. Greco AM, Gentile M, DiFilippo O, et al. Study of blood vitamin C in lung and bladder cancer patients before and after treatment with ascorbic acid: a preliminary report. *Acta Vitaminol Enzymol* 1982; 4:155–162.

96. Raghavan SA, Sharma P, Dikshit M. Role of ascorbic acid in the modulation of inhibition of platelet aggregation by polymorphonuclear leukocytes. *Throm Res* 2003;110(2-3):117–126.

97. Hemila H. Vitamin C and plasma cholesterol. *Crit Rev Food Sci Nutr* 1992;32:33–57.

98. Moran JP, Cohen L, Greene JM, et al. Plasma ascorbic acid concentrations relate inversely to blood pressure in human subjects. *Am J Clin Nutr* 1993;57:213–217.

99. Burton GW, Ingold KU. Vitamin E as an in vitro and in vivo antioxidant. In: Diplock AT, Machoin LJ, Parker L, Pryor WA, eds. Vitamin E: biochemistry and health implications. *Ann NY Acad Sci* 1989;570:7–22.

100. Horwilt MK. Supplementation with vitamin E. *Am J Clin Nutr* 1988;47:1088–1089.

101. Prasad JS. Effect of vitamin E supplementation on leukocyte function. *Am J Clin Nutr* 1980; 33:606–608.

102. Kagan VE, Serbinova EA, Forte T, et al. Recycling of vitamin E in low density lipoproteins. *J Lipid Res* 1992;33:385–387.

103. Gonzalez-Flecha BS, Repetto M, Evalson P, Boveris A. Inhibition of microsomal lipid peroxidation by alpha tocopherol and alpha tocopherol acetate. *Xenobiotica* 1991;21:1013–1022.

104. Seiner M. Influences of vitamin E on platelet function in humans. *J Am Col Nutr* 1991;10:466–473.

105. Heinonen OP, Albanes D, Virtamo J, et al. Prostate cancer and supplementation with alpha-tocopherol and beta-carotene: incidence and mortality in a controlled trial. *J Natl Cancer Inst* 1998;90(6):440–446.

106. Malila N, Virtamo J, Virtanen M, et al. The effect of alpha-tocopherol and beta-carotene supplementation on colorectal adenomas in middle-aged male smokers. Cancer Epidemiol. *Biomarkers Prev* 1999;8(6):489–493.

107. Sartori SB, Whittle N, Singewald N, et al. Magnesium deficiency induces anxiety and HPA axis dysregulation: modulation by therapeutic drug treatment. *Neuropharmacology* 2012;62(1):304–312.

108. Murck H. Magnesium and affective disorders. *Nutr Neurosci* 2002; 5(6):375–389.

109. Held K, Antonijevic IA, Kunzel H, Uhr M, Wetter TC, Golly IC, Steiger A, Murck H. Oral Mg(2+) supplementation reverses age-related neuroendocrine and sleep EEG changes in humans. *Pharmacopsychiatry* 2002;35(4):135–143.

110. Murck H, Steiger A. Mg(2+) reduces ACTH secretion and enhances spindle power without changing delta power during sleep in men—possible therapeutic implications. *Psychopharmacology (Berl)* 1998;137(3):247–252.

111. Hajjar IM, Grim CE, Kotchen TA. Dietary calcium lowers the age-related rise in blood pressure in the United States: the NHANES III survey. *J Clin Hypertens* 2003;5(2):122–126.

112. Griffith LE, Guyatt GH, Cook RJ, et al. The influence of dietary and nondietary calcium supplementation on blood pressure: an updated metaanalysis of randomized controlled trials. *Am J Hypertens* 1999;12(1 Pt 1):84–92.

113. Shea B, Wells G, Cranney A, et al. Calcium supplementation on bone loss in postmenopausal women. *Cochrane Database Syst Rev* 2004;(1):CD004526.

114. Arnaud CD, Sanchez SD. The role of calcium in osteoporosis. *Ann Rev Nutr* 1990;10:397–414.

115. Weingarten MA, Zalmanovici A, Yaphe J. Dietary calcium supplementation for preventing colorectal cancer and adenomatous polyps. *Cochrane Database Syst Rev* 2004;(1):CD003548.

116. Baron JA. Calcium. In: Kelloff GJ, Hawk ET, Sigman CC, eds. *Cancer Chemoprevention. Vol 1: Promising Cancer Chemopreventative Agents*. New York, NY: Humana Press; 2004;547–558.

117. Clark LC, Combs GF Jr, Turnbull BW, et al. Effects of selenium supplementation for cancer prevention in patients with carcinoma of the skin. A randomized

controlled trial. Nutritional Prevention of Cancer Study Group. *JAMA* 1996;276(24):1957–1963.

118. Yu SY, Zhu YJ, Li WG, et al. A preliminary report on the intervention trials of primary liver cancer in high-risk populations with nutritional supplementation of selenium in China. *Biol Trace Elem Res* 1991;29(3):289–294.

119. Hoffmann PR, Berry MJ. The influence of selenium on immune responses. *Mol Nutr Food Res* 2008;52(11):1273–1280.

120. Clark LC. The epidemiology of selenium and cancer. *Fed Proc* 1985;44(9):2584–2589.

121. Mocchegiani E, Santarelli L, Costarelli L et al. Plasticity of neuroendocrine-thymus interactions during ontogeny and ageing: role of zinc and arginine. *Ageing Res Rev* 2006;5(3):281–309. Epub 2006 Aug 14.

122. Haase H, Rink L. Functional significance of zinc-related signaling pathways in immune cells. *Annu Rev Nutr* 2009;29:133–152.

123. Maares M, Haase H. Zinc and immunity: An essential interrelation. *Arch Biochem Biophys* 2016. pii: S0003-9861(16)30074-1.

124. Haase H, Mocchegiani E, Rink L. Correlation between zinc status and immune function in the elderly. *Biogerontology* 2006;7(5-6):421–428.

125. Biswas SK, Rahman I. Environmental toxicity, redox signaling and lung inflammation: the role of glutathione. *Mol Aspects Med* 2009;30(1-2):60–76.

126. Ludewig G et al. Mechanisms of toxicity of PCB metabolites: generation of reactive oxygen species and glutathione depletion. *Cent Eur J Public Health* 2000;8(Suppl):15–17.

127. Townsend DM, Tew KD, Tapiero H. The importance of glutathione in human disease. *Biomed Pharmacother* 2003;57(3-4):145–155.

128. Ballatori N, Krance SM, Notenboom S, Shi S, Tieu K, Hammond CL. Glutathione dysregulation and the etiology and progression of human diseases. *Biol Chem* 2009;390(3):191–214.

129. Palma S, Cornetta T, Padua L, Cozzi R, Appolloni M, Ievoli E, Testa A. Influence of glutathione S-transferase polymorphisms on genotoxic effects induced by tobacco smoke. *Mutat Res* 2007 Sep 1;633(1):1–12.

130. Soltan-Sharifi MS, et al. Improvement by N-acetylcysteine of acute respiratory distress syndrome through increasing intracellular glutathione. *Hum Exp Toxicol* 2007;26(9):697–703.

131. Micke P, et al. Oral supplementation with whey proteins increases plasma glutathione levels of HIV-infected patients. *Eur J Clin Invest* 2001;31(2):171–178.

132. Liber CS, Packer L. S-Adenosylmethionine: molecular, biological, and clinical aspects—an introduction. *Am J Clin Nutr* 2002;76(5):1148S–1150S.

133. Jariwalla RJ, et al. Restoration of blood total glutathione status and lymphocyte function following alpha-lipoic acid supplementation in patients with HIV infection. *J Alt Comp Med* 2008;14(2):139–146.

134. Sharma H, et al. Gene expression profiling in practitioners of Sudarshan Kriya. *J Psychosom Res* 2008;64(2):213–218.

135. Rundle AG, et al. Preliminary studies on the effect of moderate physical activity on blood levels of glutathione. *Biomarkers* 2005;10(5):390–400.

136. Mischley LK, et al. Safety survey of intranasal glutathione. *J Altern Complement Med* 2013;19(5):459–463.

137. Bishop C, Hudson VM, Hilton SC, Wilde C. A pilot study of the effect of inhaled buffered reduced glutathione on the clinical status of patients with cystic fibrosis. *Chest* 2005;127(1):308–317.

138. Saitoh T, et al. Intravenous glutathione prevents renal oxidative stress after coronary angiography more effectively than oral N-acetylcysteine. *Heart Vessels* 2011;26(5):465–472.

139. Sechi G, et al. Reduced intravenous glutathione in the treatment of early Parkinson's disease. *Prog Neuropsychopharmacol Biol Psychiatry* 1996;20(7):1159–1170.

140. Hauser RA, et al. Randomized, double-blind, pilot evaluation of intravenous glutathione in Parkinson's disease. *Mov Disord* 2009;24(7):979–983.

141. Buydens-Branchey L, Branchey M, Hibbeln JR. Associations between increases in plasma n-3 polyunsaturated fatty acids following supplementation and decreases in anger and anxiety in substance abusers. *Prog Neuropsychopharmacol Biol Psychiatry* 2008;32(2):568–575. Epub 2007 Nov 1.

142. Chhetry BT, Hezghia A, Miller JM, et al. Omega-3 polyunsaturated fatty acid supplementation and white matter changes in major depression. *J Psychiatr Res* 2016;75:65–74.

143. Delarue J, Marzinger O, Binnert C, et al. Fish oil prevents the adrenal activation elicited by mental stress in healthy men. *Diabetes Metab* 2003;29:289–295.

144. Delarue J, Marzinger O, Binnert C, et al. Fish oil prevents the adrenal activation elicited by mental stress in healthy men. *Diabetes Metab* 2003;29:289–295.

145. Edwards R, Peet M, Shay J, et al. Omega-3 polyunsaturated fatty acid levels in the diet and in red blood cell membranes of depressed patients. *J Affect Disord* 1998;48(2-3):149–155.

146. Owen C, Rees AM, Parker G. The role of fatty acids in the development and treatment of mood disorders. *Curr Opin Psychiatry* 2008;21(1):19–24.

147. Gorjão R, Azevedo-Martins AK, Rodrigues HG, et al. Comparative effects of DHA and EPA on cell function. *Pharmacol Ther* 2009;122(1):56–64.

148. Watson RR, Zibadi S, Vazquez R, Larson D. Nutritional regulation of immunosenescence for heart health. *J Nutr Biochem* 2005;16(2):85–87.

13

Optimizing Integrative and Preventive Medicine

Connecting All the Pieces

CYNTHIA GEYER, MD

iven the powerful impact that integrative and preventive medicine can have on lowering risk of disease, improving health outcomes, and enhancing overall well-being and vitality, coupled with the depth and breadth of possible interventions, how do we connect the pieces with our patients and prioritize recommendations for each individual? The National Academy of Medicine's (NAM's) Vital Directions for Health and Health Care initiative was launched in 2016 in recognition of the strain on the healthcare system due to increased demands and unsustainable cost of care, along with the fact that care decisions do not always align with patient goals. They are mobilizing leading researchers, scientists, and policy makers across the country, and have identified as one of their three goals the ensuring of better health and well-being. The NAM has recognized that shifting emphasis toward prevention, behavioral and social services, and improving physical activity and nutrition while also addressing health disparities will be crucial to advance the health of communities and populations.[1-5] A recent review of NHANEs data showed that only 2.7% of Americans met the four core health behaviors/parameters associated with low risk of disease: eating a healthy diet, being sufficiently active, not smoking, and having a recommended body fat percentage.[6] Clearly there is a critical need to translate evidence into practice for ourselves and for our patients. Integrative and preventive medicine practitioners will continue to play an increasing role in meeting these objectives.

One of the key tenets of integrative and preventive medicine is a reaffirmation of the importance of the therapeutic relationship, with practitioners and patients as partners.[7] The time invested in an initial encounter can be instrumental in establishing a connection in which the clinician develops an understanding of the person seeking care, beyond his or her symptoms: his/ her goals, fears, supports, readiness to change, perceived challenges or barriers, and overall philosophy, level of interest, and understanding related to various modalities and potential therapies. Motivational interviewing, which was initially developed by William R. Miller in the early 1980s as an approach for working with people with alcohol problems,[8] is one model of collaborative communication that is showing evidence of benefit in areas as broad as medication adherence, weight loss, and dietary change.[9-12] It is defined as a "collaborative, person-centered form of guiding to elicit and strengthen motivation for change." The principles taught in motivational interviewing can be helpful in the process of working with patients and include the following:

1. The spirit is collaborative, not confrontational, and seeks to understand the person's frame of reference through reflective listening, acceptance, and nonjudgment.
2. The clinician's role is to draw out the patient's own motivations and skills for change instead of imposing his or her own opinion.
3. Focusing on previous success and highlighting existing skills and strengths supports self-efficacy.

The acronym OARS highlights the type of communication used in motivational interviewing that can facilitate dialogue in an empathetic and non-judgmental way: open-ended questions, affirmation, reflective listening, and summarization.

Although motivational interviewing teaches a nonhierarchical model that may be particularly useful in helping resolve a patient's ambivalence when the focus is on behavior change, it is also important to understand what motivational interviewing is not. As reviewed by Miller in 2009, motivational interviewing is not the transtheoretical model, decisional balance, or client-centered therapy. It is not a way to convince people to do what you want, nor is it a panacea.[13] Positive patient-centered communication,[14] another framework that overlaps with motivational interviewing, has been associated with higher levels of self-efficacy, particularly among people with greater chronic disease burden.[15] Aspects of patient-centered communication include the following:

1. allowing patients to ask questions
2. attending to their emotions
3. involving them in decisions

4. ensuring their understanding
5. helping to deal with uncertainty

Both motivational interviewing and positive patient-centered communication address some of the psychological needs described in self-determination theory that have been found to predict greater adherence to recommended health behaviors.[16,17] Those three needs are autonomy (the feeling of having control over your choices), relatedness (a sense of belonging or connection), and competence (having the skill or knowledge needed). The growing field of integrative health coaching incorporates these tenets in a collaborative relationship that is solution focused, working with factors that can contribute to a person's achieving his or her goals. These factors include accessing resources and support, overcoming internal and external challenges to change, and generating alternatives and backup plans.[18]

One challenge in integrative and preventive medicine is that this type of collaborative approach takes a considerable time investment, especially initially. In addition, the increasing use of electronic medical records can serve to put a physical barrier between the patient and the practitioner. Optimizing time spent between the practitioner and the patient while minimizing distraction that can interfere with the therapeutic relationship is of utmost importance. Having a previsit intake, using a questionnaire and review with a nurse, is one model that can be very effective (CR personal experience). Not only can the nurse ascertain goals, readiness to change, health habits, past and family history, supplement and medication list, and perceived barriers to change prior to the appointment but also he or she can review recommendations, assist with goal setting, and ensure follow-up afterward as a critical member of the integrative healthcare team. The information gathered in advance can be input into the Electronic Health Record (EHR) and help the practitioner and patient prioritize their focus in their subsequent visit. Being present, maintaining eye contact, being able to acknowledge and respond to nonverbal communication—these critical aspects of the therapeutic encounter are at risk of being lost or diminished if the practitioner's focus is on inputting data into the EHR. Having as much done as possible ahead of time creates more time for personal interaction.

In choosing which modalities or therapies to recommend, there are several factors to keep in mind. The concept of "evidence-based practice," introduced by Dr. Sackett in 1996, illustrates the integration of the best research and highest level of evidence in the literature with the expertise and clinical skills of the practitioner and the unique values, concerns, and personal preferences of the patient[19] (see Table 13.1). Dr. Braithwaite wrote an editorial in *JAMA* in 2013 stating that evidence-based medicine's six most dangerous words are "there is no evidence to suggest,"[20] an argument frequently used to reject the

Table 13.1 Clinical Applications of Research Evidence Construct (CARE)

Safety	Efficacy	Science	Other Therapeutic Options	Patient Preference	Cost/Accessibility	Utilization Frequency of Treatment in Question
High	High	Decisive	None that is superior	Prefers recommended approach	Not a concern	Always
Probable	Possible	Unclear	None/few	Anything that will work	Needs consideration	Often
Low	Low	Absent/opposed	Many that are superior	Anything that will work	Prohibitive	Never

Katz D, Ali A. Preventive Medicine, Integrative Medicine, and the Health of the Public. Commissioned paper for IOM Summit on Integrative Medicine and the Health of the Public; February 2009

Source: Reference 24.

use of integrative and preventive approaches to treatment. While "absence of evidence is not the same as evidence of absence,"[21,22] it is equally important for clinicians to look for the best evidence possible and to guard against recommending treatments that might be harmful, expensive, or that might delay a patient's use of more effective treatments. Patients seeking care may be worried, suffering, exploring a multitude of therapies, and receiving conflicting advice from various practitioners; it is incumbent on those of us making treatment recommendations to be as transparent as possible about the level of evidence supporting them, what is not known, and the potential benefits and risks associated with those recommendations. A framework for guiding clinical decision-making, called the Clinical Applications of Research Evidence construct (CARE), has been outlined by Ali and Katz.[23] This guide factors in efficacy, safety, level of evidence, availability of other treatment options, patient preference, and cost in the clinical application of evidence.

A recent Cochrane review found that the use of decision aids, which not only provide evidence-based information about a condition, treatment options, benefits, harms, and uncertainties but also help patients recognize the role of their values in making their decision, showed benefit in several outcome measures. Patients had better knowledge and understanding of risk, were more engaged and decisive in the decision-making process, and felt less decisional conflict related to feeling uninformed or being in conflict with their values, and there was a positive effect on patient–practitioner communication.[25]

Generally speaking, the lowest cost, lowest risk, most effective, and quickest acting option that aligns with the patient's goals will be the highest priority. In the setting of pain, stress, or sleep deprivation, executive function in the frontal lobe is down-regulated and decision-making is more emotionally driven.[26-29] This impacts one's ability to set intentions, think about the long-term impact of lifestyle choices on health and well-being, and engage in behavior change. Someone experiencing physical pain may first need targeted referrals for physical or manual therapies or acupuncture before being in a position to consider dietary change or starting an exercise program. The recent review by the National Institutes of Health (NIH) of nonpharmacologic treatments such as acupuncture and manual therapy for pain[30] is timely in light of the growing opioid epidemic. This along with the broader implications of the benefits of treating pain as an adjunct to supporting people's efforts to adopt and maintain healthier lifestyle habits will hopefully translate toward better insurance coverage for these options. People in emotional distress may need to see a psychologist, social worker, or other qualified mental healthcare specialist to address those concerns first. Working as part of a multidisciplinary integrative and preventive healthcare team can be an effective model for prioritizing treatments and making appropriate referrals. For practitioners who are not working as part of a team in their practice setting, keeping a database of trusted specialists in the community to whom they can refer and having a good understanding of existing community resources and programs that target exercise and nutrition allow the recreation of a team-based approach for their patients.

One important aspect of the therapeutic relationship that is often overlooked, both in traditional and integrative and preventive medicine, is how we use language. Our word choices can have far-reaching impact not only on the establishment of trust but also on a patient's perception of the status of his or her health and sense of self-efficacy. Two areas in particular can have unintentional, and potentially negative, impact: when a practitioner's opinion is stated as fact, and when diagnostic labels are used. An example of the first is illustrated by the story of a woman who came to see me confused about how to manage her significant low mood and vasomotor symptoms that started abruptly after an emergency hysterectomy. Her internist told her she should not take hormones or she would be at risk of a stroke or a heart attack; her gynecologist told her she should take them or she would "dry up and age." Both physicians were undoubtedly interpreting the sometimes conflicting literature about hormone therapy and disease risk. However, by conveying their interpretations as definitive and reaching opposite conclusions, not only was the patient left confused, conflicted, and torn between her two physicians but she was also not asked how she felt about hormone therapy nor offered alternatives to manage her symptoms.[31] An example of the pitfalls of labels is shown in the story of a woman who consulted my colleague for a second opinion after seeing an integrative medicine practitioner who had ordered a battery of tests. When asked how she felt and what was going on related to her health, her answers were primarily repeating the "diagnoses" she was given after her test results: "They told me I was a poor detoxifier and had mercury toxicity that caused adrenal fatigue." In the attempt to find explanations for symptoms, her practitioner had used labels based on testing that is not widely accepted in traditional medicine. The end result was to contribute to her patient's negative and seemingly fixed view of how healthy she was. While both these examples may represent the extremes, it is incumbent on us to be mindful of how we use language. Acknowledging uncertainty in the literature; being clear when our recommendations are based on personal experience/opinion/interpretation of studies versus clear guidelines derived from large clinical trials; and using descriptive language instead of limiting labels when appropriate will guard against the unintentional negative consequences our words may have on our patients' well-being.

What about the role of laboratory testing? It is not necessary to do lab work in order to work with people around strategies to improve dietary habits, incorporate mindfulness or breath-based approaches, or start low-level movement or exercise. Recognizing the potential vulnerability of patients who do not feel well, practitioners have an ethical responsibility to guard against the unnecessary use of expensive laboratory testing that does not add to the clinical picture. Testing may be important to rule out a condition that might need more targeted treatment, such as sleep apnea, hypothyroidism, anemia, or significant ischemia or hypertension in response to exercise. One of my mentors when I was a medical student used to say, "between the laboratory and the diagnosis, you have to stop at the bedside."[32] Those words of wisdom are relevant both in guiding the clinician's choice of testing based on the person's clinical presentation, and in the interpretation of the results. Some types of testing, even in a patient without symptoms, can be motivating for behavior change, aid in the customization of recommendations, and provide a trackable marker of response. No-cost or low-cost anthropometrics, such as height and weight, BMI, waist:hip ratio, validated measures of fitness and strength, and blood pressure are relatively easy to obtain and helpful to track progress for many patients. Questions to consider when ordering tests:

1. Is this necessary to rule out a treatable medical condition?
2. Will the results modify treatment recommendations?
3. Is the patient going to incur significant out-of-pocket cost for testing?

If you are not doing laboratory testing in your practice, know to whom you can refer in the event that someone is not improving or if there are concerning signs or symptoms that warrant more than just a lifestyle or preventive medicine approach.

Whenever possible, an opportunity for experiential learning should be provided.[33,34] This can help someone move from a theoretical or cognitive understanding of a recommended modality or desired behavior toward an embodied connection to how he or she can feel in response to that selected behavior change or treatment option. That also serves to shift motivation for ongoing change away from an external source (provider's recommendation, fear of a disease) to an internal source (feeling better, a sense of self-efficacy), which may be more predictive of long-term success.[35-37] In some instances, for example a guided cooking or exercise class, the experience teaches skills, provides an opportunity for fun, and reinforces confidence in one's ability to embrace change. Options for providing experiential learning range from a destination health resort; to a clinic which might house a teaching kitchen and fitness and yoga classes on site; to a community network in which referrals are made to offsite facilities (such as a local YMCA). Many practices are incorporating group visits as a way to provide these lifestyle-focused experiences and reach more people in a cost-effective way. Groups can also create an additional support structure for patients and an opportunity to share their insights with and learn from others who may have experienced similar symptoms, conditions, or challenges to change.

Providing written recommendations and clearly articulating the rationale behind them, how they align with the patient's goals, describing possible side effects and the expected time frame to see the impact helps set expectations. Allowing time for patients to ask questions and reflect their understanding of recommendations can clarify any potential misunderstandings. Planning follow-up and making sure patients know how to contact the practice (and who the primary contact should be) if questions or concerns arise between visits helps build in accountability and connection. Ongoing coaching between visits can be particularly helpful in supporting behavior change, especially related to nutrition, movement, and smoking cessation.

In summary, it is clear that the practice of integrative and preventive medicine has a critical role to play in improving the health and well-being of people, families, and communities. Key steps to optimize the effective practice of integrative and preventive medicine include the following points.

1. Spend time establishing a collaborative, mutually respectful partnership with your patients; motivational interviewing and patient-centered communication models teach validated approaches to facilitate this process.
2. Align your recommendations with your patient's goals and frame of reference.
3. Recognize when addressing pain, stress, and emotional distress needs to take first priority; in turn, that may support a person's ability to engage in lifestyle changes to support health.
4. Know when and to whom you can refer: create your integrative team of experts in the clinic and in the community.
5. Be clear about whether recommendations are based on personal opinion, clinical experience, or published guidelines.
6. Be mindful of the impact that the use of diagnostic labels may have on a person's sense of well-being and hope.
7. Provide opportunities for experiential learning when possible.
8. Provide a written summary of recommendations and expected/possible outcomes.
9. Ensure understanding of recommendations and allow time for questions.
10. Schedule follow-up at a given interval and provide contact information for questions or concerns.

Engaging patients as partners in their health journey, making appropriate referrals to other members of the integrative medicine team, supporting self-efficacy and health behavior change that is congruent with patients' goals, and ensuring periodic follow-up and reassessment can increase the efficacy of integrative and preventive medicine approaches to improving health outcomes.

References

1. Dzau VJ, McClellan M, McGinnis JM. Vital directions for health and health care. *JAMA* 2016;316(7):711. doi: 10.1001/jama.2016.10692.
2. Dietz WH, Douglas CE, Brownson RC. Chronic disease prevention. *JAMA* 2016;316(16):1645. doi: 10.1001/jama.2016.14370.
3. Goldman LR, Kumanyika SK, Shah NR. Putting the health of communities and populations first. *JAMA* 2016;316(16):1649. doi: 10.1001/jama.2016.14800.
4. McGinnis JM, Diaz A, Halfon N. Systems strategies for health throughout the life course. *JAMA* 2016;316(16):1639. doi: 10.1001/jama.2016.14896.
5. Loprinzi PD, Branscum A, Hanks J, Smit E. Healthy lifestyle characteristics and their joint association with cardiovascular disease biomarkers in US adults. *Mayo Clin Proc* 2016;91(4):432–442. doi: 10.1016/j.mayocp.2016.01.009.
6. Maizes, V, Rakel D, Niemiec C. Integrative medicine and patient-centered care, *Explore (New York, N.Y.)* 2009;5(5):277–289.
7. Miller WR, Rose GS. Toward a theory of motivational interviewing. *Am Psychol* 2009;64(6):527–537. doi: 10.1037/a0016830.
8. Martins R, McNeil D. Review of Motivational interviewing in promoting health behaviors. *Clin Psychol Rev* 2009;29(4):283–293.
9. Bean MK, Biskobing D, Francis GL, Wickham E. Motivational interviewing in health care: results of a brief training in endocrinology. *J Grad Med Ed* 2012;4(3):357–361.
10. Hardcastle S, Taylor A, Bailey M, Harley R, Hagger M. Effectiveness of a motivational interviewing intervention on weight loss, physical activity and cardiovascular disease risk factors: a randomised controlled trial with a 12-month post-intervention follow-up. *Int J Behav Nutr Phy* 2013;10:1–16. doi: 10.1186/1479-5868-10-40
11. Resnicow K, McMaster F, Bocian A, et al. Motivational interviewing and dietary counseling for obesity in primary care: an RCT. *Pediatrics* 2015;135(4):649–657.
12. Miller W, Rollnick S. Ten things that motivational interviewing is not. *Behav Cogn Psychoth* 2009;37(2):129–140.
13. King A, Hoppe RB. Best Practice for patient-centered communication: a narrative review. *J Grad Med Ed* 2013;5(3):385–393.
14. Rutten F, Hesse B, Sauver S, et al. Health self-efficacy among populations with multiple chronic conditions: the value of patient-centered communication. *Adv Ther* 2016;33(8):1440–1451.
15. Eynon M, O'Donnell C, Williams L. Assessing the impact of autonomous motivation and psychological need satisfaction in explaining adherence to an exercise referral scheme. *Psychol Health Med* 2017;22(9):1056–1062.

16. McDavid L, McDonough M, Blankenship B, LeBreton J. A test of basic psychological needs theory in a physical activity-based program for underserved youth. *J Sport Exercise Psy* 2017;39(1):29–42.

17. Simmons LA, Wolever RQ. Integrative health coaching and Motivational interviewing: Synergistic approaches to behavior change in healthcare. *Glob Adv Health Med* 2013;2(4):28–35.

18. Sackett D. *Evidence-Based Practice.* ttp://guides.mclibrary.duke.edu/c.php?g=158201&p=1036021. Accessed December 5, 2016.

19. Braithwaite R. A piece of my mind: EBM's six dangerous words. *JAMA* 2013;310(20):2149–2150.

20. Altman DG, Bland JM () Absence of evidence is not evidence of absence. *BMJ* 1995;311(7003):485.

21. Alderson P. Absence of evidence is not evidence of absence. *BMJ* 2004;328(7438):476–477.

22. Ali A, Katz DL. Disease prevention and health promotion. *Am J Prev Med* 2015;49(5):S230–S240. doi: 10.1016/j.amepre.2015.07.019.

23. Stacey D, Légaré F, Col NF, et al. Decision aids for people facing health treatment or screening decisions. *Cochrane Database Syst Rev* 2014;28(1). doi: 10.1002/14651858. CD001431.pub4.

24. Ali A, Katz DL. Disease prevention and health promotion. *Am J Prev Med* 2015;49(5):S230–S240. doi:10.1016/j.amepre.2015.07.019.

25. Arnsten A. Stress signalling pathways that impair prefrontal cortex structure and function. *Nature* Reviews: *Neuroscience* 2009;10(6):410–422.

26. Arnsten A. Stress weakens prefrontal networks: molecular insults to higher cognition. *Nature Neuroscience* 2015;18(10):1376–1385.

27. Reidy B, Hamann S, Inman C, Johnson K, Brennan P. Decreased sleep duration is associated with increased fMRI responses to emotional faces in children. *Neuropsychologia* 2016;84:54–62.

28. Wang L, Chen Y, Yao Y, Pan Y, Sun Y. Sleep deprivation disturbed regional brain activity in healthy subjects: evidence from a functional magnetic resonance-imaging study. *Neuropsychiatr Dis Treat* 2016;12(1):801–807.

29. Nahin R, Boineau R, Khalsa P, Stussman B, Weber W. Evidence-based evaluation of complementary health approaches for pain management in the United States. *Mayo Clinic Proceedings* 2016;91(9):1292–1306.

30. Becerra-Perez M, Menear M, Turcotte S, Labrecque M, Legare F. More primary care patients regret health decisions if they experienced decisional conflict in the consultation: a secondary analysis of a multicenter descriptive study. *BMC Family Practice* 2016;7(1):156.

31. Middendorf D, faculty at Ohio State University College of Medicine, 1986. Personal communication.

32. Davis JN, Spaniol MR, Somerset S. Sustenance and sustainability: maximizing the impact of school gardens on health outcomes. *Public Health Nutr* 2015;18(13):2358–2367. doi: 10.1017/s1368980015000221.

33. James A, Hess P, Perkins M, Taveras E, Scirica C. Prescribing outdoor play: outdoors Rx. *Clin Pediatr* 2017;56(6):519–524.

34. Teixeira PJ, Carraça EV, Markland D, Silva MN, Ryan RM. Exercise, physical activity, and self-determination theory: a systematic review. *Int J Behav Nutr Phys Act* 2012;9(78). doi: 10.1186/1479-5868-9-78.

35. Teixeira PJ, Silva MN, Mata J, Palmeira AL, Markland D. Motivation, self-determination, and long-term weight control. *Int J Behav Nutr Phys Act* 2012;9. doi: 10.1186/1479-5868-9-22.

36. Schneider ML, Kwan BM. Psychological need satisfaction, intrinsic motivation and affective response to exercise in adolescents. *Psychol Sport Exerc* 2013;14(5):776–785.

37. Schneider ML, Kwan BM. Psychological need satisfaction, intrinsic motivation and affective response to exercise in adolescents. *Psychol Sport Exerc* 2013;14(5):776–785.

14

Reversing Chronic Diseases Using Lifestyle Medicine

BENJAMIN R. BROWN, MD

In memory of the lives and work of our friends and colleagues, James Billings, PhD, Lee Lipsenthal, MD, and Glenn Perelson, who served for many years at the nonprofit Preventive Medicine Research Institute.

* * *

Introduction

Over 86% of the $3.0 trillion in annual healthcare costs in the United States are due to chronic diseases that can often be prevented or even reversed by making comprehensive lifestyle changes.

Lifestyle medicine is an exciting and rapidly growing movement in medicine today in which comprehensive lifestyle changes are used not only to prevent but also often to reverse the progression of many chronic diseases. These include even severe coronary heart disease, type 2 diabetes, hypertension, obesity, hyperlipidemia, and early-stage prostate cancer. Anecdotal evidence exists indicating that these comprehensive lifestyle changes may also beneficially affect the progression of early-stage breast cancer, some autoimmune conditions, multiple sclerosis, and Alzheimer's disease.

Many forces are converging that make this the right idea at the right time. While the limitations of drugs and surgery for treating and preventing chronic diseases are becoming increasingly well documented, the power of comprehensive lifestyle changes are also becoming increasingly well recognized. Changes in how medical care is reimbursed are also paving the way for lifestyle medicine as this approach to chronic illness not only increases quality of life but also saves money.

A guiding principle of lifestyle medicine is that it is usually more powerful to address the underlying *causes* of diseases rather than treating only the symptoms. Imagine a group of doctors busily mopping up the floor around an overflowing sink, yet no one is turning off the faucet.

To a remarkable degree, the faucet—the underlying cause of many chronic diseases—represents the lifestyle choices we make each day. These include:

- a whole foods, plant-based diet (naturally low in fat and refined carbohydrates);
- stress management techniques (including yoga and meditation);
- moderate exercise (such as walking); and
- social support and community (love and intimacy).

In short—eat well, move more, stress less, and love more.

Many people tend to think of advances in medicine as high-tech and expensive, such as a new drug, laser, or surgical procedure. They may have a hard time believing that something as simple as these comprehensive lifestyle changes can make such a powerful difference in our lives—but they often do. Lifestyle medicine is a disruptive technology, akin to an electric car or an iPhone, not just an incremental change.

In our research, we have used high-tech, expensive, state-of-the-art scientific measures to prove the power of these simple, low-tech, and low-cost interventions. These randomized-controlled trials and other studies have been published in leading peer-reviewed medical and scientific journals.

The Paradox of Comprehensive Lifestyle Changes: How Do People Make and Sustain Comprehensive Changes?

We have learned that our bodies often have a remarkable capacity to begin healing—and much more quickly than had once been realized—when we treat these underlying lifestyle causes. And because the underlying biological mechanisms are so dynamic, most people feel so much better, so quickly, it reframes the reason for making lifestyle changes from fear—for example, preventing something bad from happening, such as a heart attack or stroke—to joy and pleasure. Fear is not a sustainable motivator, but joy and pleasure are. What a person has gained is so much more significant than what they have given up.

For example, in all of our studies and demonstration projects, patients with even severe coronary heart disease reported a greater than 90% reduction in angina (chest pain) frequency in just a few weeks. When someone who cannot work, cannot walk across the street before the light changes, cannot make love with their partner, or cannot play with their kids due to chest pain, finds that they can do all of these activities after making these changes for only a few weeks, these choices shift from being a sacrifice to being a gateway to a renewed life and naturally become sustainable.

The paradox here is that we often think of taking a medication as easy and making these lifestyle changes as hard, but when you look at the adherence data it would imply just the opposite. In our studies, adherence was 85%–90% in 3,780 men and women at all 24 sites after 1 year, comparing this with the studies done on statin adherence in adults showing that one-half to two-thirds of patients prescribed statins are not taking them after 1 year. In patients age 65 years or older, adherence to statins for primary prevention after 2 years was 25.4%. Even in patients with documented CAD, Duke University researchers showed that consistent use of all three therapies (aspirin, statins, and beta-blockers) was only 21%.[1]

Selected Clinical Research on Lifestyle Medicine to Prevent Chronic Diseases

Healthcare costs for cardiovascular disease are more than for any other diagnostic group. In 2012, the estimated annual healthcare costs for cardiovascular disease were $316.6 billion, including $193.1 billion in direct costs (hospital services, physicians and other professionals, prescribed medications, home healthcare, and other medical durables) and $123.5 billion in indirect costs from lost future productivity. By comparison, the estimated direct cost of all types of cancer that year was $88.7 billion (50% for outpatient or doctor office visits, 35% for inpatient care, and 11% for prescription drugs).[2]

Despite the prevalence and costs of cardiovascular disease, it is primarily a preventable and even reversible lifestyle illness. Most of the total deaths per year from heart disease and stroke are preventable by lifestyle and medications.[3]

For example, The INTERHEART study followed 30,000 men and women in seven continents and found that nine risk factors modifiable by intensive lifestyle changes accounted for 94% of the risk of a myocardial infarction in women and 90% of the risk in men. Abnormal lipids; smoking; hypertension; diabetes; abdominal obesity; psychosocial factors; consumption of fruits, vegetables, and alcohol; and regular physical activity account for most of the risk of myocardial infarction worldwide in both sexes and at all ages in all regions.[4]

Another study looking prospectively at over 20,000 men found that those who followed a healthy diet, did not smoke, exercised moderately, and did not have excessive belly fat reduced their risk of a heart attack by 80%.[5]

Thus, the disease that accounts for more premature deaths and costs than any other illness is almost completely preventable simply by changing diet and lifestyle. And the same lifestyle changes that can prevent or even reverse heart disease may also help prevent or even reverse many other chronic diseases as well.

In the European Prospective Investigation into Cancer and Nutrition (EPIC) study, patients who adhered to healthy dietary principles (low meat consumption and high intake of fruits, vegetables, and whole-grain bread), never smoked, were not overweight, and had at least 30 minutes a day of physical activity had a 78% lower overall risk of developing a chronic disease. This included a 93% reduced risk of diabetes, an 81% lower risk of heart attacks, a 50% reduction in risk of stroke, and a 36% overall reduction in risk of cancer, compared with participants without these healthy factors.[6]

THE FOUR PARTS OF THE PROGRAM

Our program included intervention across four areas—diet, stress management, exercise, and group support.

The Diet

The approach to nutrition is an abundant low-fat plant-based nutrition plan. This plan emphasizes:

- Whole grains: 6 or more servings a day
- Fresh fruits 2–4 servings a day and vegetables 3 or more servings a day
- Plant protein 3–5 servings a day: Legumes and beans with soy products, egg whites, and meat analogues as options.
- Optional
  - Nonfat dairy 0–2 servings a day.
  - Refined carbohydrates and nonfat sweets 0–2 servings a day.
  - Alcohol 0–1 serving a day.
  - Low-fat foods in limited amounts 0–3 servings a day.

When a person eats this way, without adding oil, the fat content comes out to approximately 10% and cholesterol is 10 mg or less a day. This eating program has been adapted for people following a FODMAPS diet, a gluten-free diet, and a full vegan diet as well as people on dialysis. Modifications can be made if people are losing weight too fast or have increased protein needs for other health reasons.

STRESS MANAGEMENT

The stress management techniques included stretching exercises, breathing techniques, meditation, progressive relaxation, and imagery. The purpose of each technique is to increase the participants' sense of relaxation, concentration, awareness, resiliency, and well-being. Participants were asked to practice these stress management techniques for at least one hour per day.

EXERCISE

Participants were asked to exercise a minimum of 3 hours per week and to spend a minimum of 30 minutes per session exercising within their prescribed target heart rates and/or perceived exertion levels. Two strength training sessions were added later and are now included in the program.

GROUP SUPPORT

Group support sessions were designed to increase social support and a sense of community by creating a safe environment for the expression of feelings and also to help participants adhere to the lifestyle-change program. The methodology of the support group is surprisingly simple, participants learn to listen with empathy and speak their feelings. These simple practices transform relationships, and people often feel understood on a deeper level then they ever have. As they practice this weekly, trust and intimacy develops and participants report no longer feeling isolated and alone.

Selected Clinical Research on Lifestyle Medicine as Treatment to Reverse Chronic Diseases

From 1978 through 1991 we conducted pilot, follow-up and 5-year studies to assess the outcomes of lifestyle medicine in coronary heart disease.

PILOT STUDY

In 1978, we began a series of studies spanning four decades demonstrating the power of a lifestyle medicine intervention, beginning with coronary heart disease.

In the first study, 10 patients with severe coronary artery disease were housed in a hotel for 30 days and asked to make these comprehensive lifestyle changes.

During this time, patients reported a 91% reduction in the frequency of angina, clinically and statistically significant improvements in all modifiable cardiac risk factors, and improved well-being, including enhanced cognitive function and functional status. Eight of these 10 patients showed improvements in myocardial perfusion as measured by exercise thallium scintigraphy.[7] Although there was no randomized control group, it is highly unusual for patients to improve to this degree in such a short time.

FOLLOW-UP STUDY WITH RANDOMIZED CONTROL GROUP

To address this issue, in 1990 we conducted a randomized-controlled trial in which experimental group patients were housed in a residential setting and asked to make these comprehensive lifestyle changes. After 24 days, patients again reported a 91% reduction in frequency of angina, significant improvements in all modifiable cardiac risk factors, and improved well-being, including enhanced cognitive function and functional status.

In addition, there were significant improvements in the ejection fraction response from rest to peak exercise as measured by exercise radionuclide ventriculography. There was also significant improvement in regional wall motion when compared to the randomized control group.[8]

LIFESTYLE HEART TRIAL AND 5-YEAR FOLLOW-UP STUDY

The Lifestyle Heart Trial began in 1986 with 48 subjects randomized to either the intensive lifestyle intervention described earlier or to usual care. Clinical entry criteria included age between 35 and 75 years; no coexisting life-threatening illness; lack of myocardial infarction within 6 weeks of the start of the trial; not currently taking lipid-lowering medication; single, double, or triple vessel coronary disease in nonrevascularized vessels with at least one proximal lesion greater than 75% stenosed; left ventricular ejection fraction greater than 25%.

The original Lifestyle Heart Trial was a 1-year study; based on the results after one year, the National Heart, Lung, and Blood Institute of the National Institutes of Health provided funding to extend the trial for 4 additional years.

Endpoint measurements included: (1) quantitative coronary arteriography at baseline, 1 year, and 5 years to assess the extent of coronary atherosclerosis; (2) cardiac PET scans to measure myocardial perfusion; (3) lipoprotein and apolipoprotein profiles; (4) 3-day diet diaries and other questionnaires designed to measure adherence; (5) psychosocial questionnaires to evaluate change in quality of life; (6) quantitative coronary arteriography and cardiac PET scans blindly read by independent observers; and (7) cardiac events.

After 5 years, experimental patients were exercising an average of 3.6 hours per week, practicing stress management 5.7 hours per week, and consuming an average of 18.6 mg per day of cholesterol and 8.5% of total calories from fat. Control patients were exercising 2.9 hours per week, practicing stress management techniques 0.98 hours per week, and consuming an average of 138.7 mg per day cholesterol and 25% of total calories from fat.

From baseline to 1 year, experimental group patients reported a 91% reduction in frequency of angina, whereas the control group reported a 186% increase in frequency (Table 14.1).

In the experimental group, 82% of the experimental group patients showed overall regression of coronary atherosclerosis after 1 year[9,10] and even more improvement after 5 years than after 1 year.[11] In contrast, the degree of coronary atherosclerosis progressed (worsened) in the control group after 1 year and showed even more progression after 5 years. These differences between groups were statistically significant and clinically significant after 1 year and after 5 years.

The number of cardiac events in the experimental group was less than half that in the control group, including significantly lower rates of angioplasty, bypass surgery, and cardiac-related hospitalizations.

Using an a priori score that took into account all four components of the lifestyle intervention, we found a statistically significant, dose-response

Table 14.1 Results at One Year

Study Group	Control Group
disease regression for 82%	disease progression for 53%
91% decrease in anginal frequency	186% increase in anginal frequency
37% decrease in LDL, without medication	minimal change in LDL
percent diameter stenosis improved	percent diameter stenosis worsened

($p = .001$)

correlation between adherence to the lifestyle intervention and changes in the degree of coronary atherosclerosis (percent diameter stenosis) across both groups after 1 year and also after 5 years.

We also found a statistically significant, dose-response correlation between intake of dietary fat and changes in percent diameter stenosis as well as a statistically significant, dose-response correlation between intake of dietary cholesterol and changes in percent diameter stenosis.[12]

Cardiac PET scans revealed that there was an overall improvement in myocardial perfusion (blood flow to the heart) in the experimental group patients after 5 years, whereas control group patients worsened. The size and severity of perfusion defects in the experimental group improved by 4.2 ± 3.8 units, whereas it worsened by 13.5 ± 3.8 units in the randomized control group—a net differences of 400%.[13]

Lipid-Lowering Medication

None of the experimental group patients in the Lifestyle Heart Trial or the two earlier studies were taking lipid-lowering drugs during these trials. This enabled us to assess the effects of comprehensive lifestyle changes without being confounded by lipid-lowering drug therapy.

Approximately 50% of control group patients began taking lipid-lowering drugs during the study. Progression of coronary atherosclerosis was significantly greater in control group patients who were not talking cholesterol-lowering drugs (40.7% to 59.7%) than those who were (45.7% to 51.7%). There was a 40% average reduction in LDL-cholesterol levels in experimental group patients during the first year even though none of these patients were taking cholesterol-lowering drugs.

Would patients benefit from making comprehensive lifestyle changes *and* taking cholesterol-lowering drugs? On the one hand, if most patients were able to achieve regression of atherosclerosis without drugs, why add the costs and side-effects? On the other hand, would improvement have been even greater by doing both? To answer this question more research is needed.

MULTICENTER LIFESTYLE DEMONSTRATION PROJECT

To determine the scalability and cost-effectiveness of this lifestyle medicine program, we conducted the Multicenter Lifestyle Demonstration Project, sponsored by Mutual of Omaha. We were curious to learn whether patients in community hospitals would do as well as in academic medical centers; if patients could safely avoid revascularization; and if cost savings would occur. The data-coordinating center for this study was directed by Alexander Leaf, MD, who at the time was chair of preventive medicine at Harvard Medical School.

Almost 80% of patients who were recommended to undergo revascularization (bypass surgery or angioplasty) chose this lifestyle medicine intervention as a direct alternative and did not have worse clinical outcomes from doing so. Mutual of Omaha calculated saving almost $30,000 per patient in the first year.[14]

We conducted a second demonstration project in collaboration with Highmark Blue Cross Blue Shield. Through the nonprofit Preventive Medicine Research Institute, we continued to train a total of 53 hospitals and clinics throughout the United States as part of the Multicenter Lifestyle Demonstration Project.[15]

Almost 3,000 men and women from 24 socioeconomically diverse sites in West Virginia, Nebraska, and Pennsylvania participated in this lifestyle medicine program and data was collected at baseline, 12 weeks, and 1 year. Only 46% of these patients had diagnosed coronary artery disease; 34% had type 2 diabetes; 74% had high blood pressure; 79% had hypercholesterolemia; 69% had obesity.

Again, patients made bigger changes in lifestyle and achieved better clinical outcomes and adherence than had ever been shown in an ambulatory group of patients.[16] Overall healthcare costs were reduced by 50% in the first year when compared to a control group matched for age, gender, and disease severity. In the subgroup of these patients who had medical expenses of at least $25,000 in the preceding year, overall healthcare costs were reduced by 400%.

One of the frequent criticisms of preventive medicine from insurance company executives has been that many patients change insurance companies each year. If it takes several years to document cost savings, they may ask, "Why should I pay for a preventive medicine program today when chances are one of my competitors will benefit years later?"

However, since lifestyle medicine is offered as a treatment, not just for prevention, cost savings usually occur during the first year. Thus, lifestyle medicine can be both medically effective and cost-effective, since both clinical outcomes and cost savings occur in the first year.

INTENSIVE CARDIAC REHABILITATION
(A NEW BENEFIT CATEGORY)

One of the lessons we learned is that if a lifestyle medicine program is not reimbursable, it is challenging to make it sustainable.

Because of this, we approached the Centers for Medicare and Medicaid Services (CMS) and asked if they would provide Medicare coverage for this lifestyle medicine program. After 16 years of review, CMS created a new benefit category, "intensive cardiac rehabilitation" (ICR), which provides 72 hours of lifestyle training.

TEAM-BASED CARE

This is a team approach in which the physician is quarterback and works closely with a team of five other healthcare professionals: a registered nurse, exercise physiologist, stress management specialist (certified yoga/meditation teacher), registered dietitian, and psychologist or psychiatrist.

These 72 hours are allocated into 18 sessions of 4 hours—twice/week for 9 weeks;

- one hour of supervised exercise, as seen in traditional cardiac rehabilitation programs;
- one hour of yoga and meditation for stress management;
- one hour of a support group;
- one hour lecture with a group meal.

This allows the physician to leverage his or her time by providing supervisory oversight, but most of the training time is offered by the other five healthcare professionals.

After the 72 hours (9 weeks) of training, patients continue to meet in their support groups on their own.

Physicians report that this is a particularly rewarding way to practice medicine and allows them to return to the roots of what usually attracted them to medicine in the first place: the opportunity to empower patients by helping them address the underlying lifestyle causes of coronary heart disease and many other chronic illnesses.

In short, this is a new paradigm of healthcare. Instead of having to see a new patient every 8 to 10 minutes in a managed care practice—in which there is little time to do more than go through problem list, do a quick physical exam, and write a prescription—the physician can oversee a program in which patients receive 72 hours of training. Most of this time is spent with the other five healthcare professionals, allowing the physician to leverage his or her time most productively. We are actively training individual practitioners and teams from hospitals, physician groups, and clinics in this approach to lifestyle medicine.

OTHER CONDITIONS AND ADDITIONAL BENEFITS

Although there is a lot of interest in personalized medicine, we found that the same lifestyle changes that can reverse the progression of even severe coronary heart disease may also do so for other chronic conditions.

Prostate Cancer

For example, we conducted the first randomized-controlled trial showing that these comprehensive lifestyle changes may slow, stop, or even reverse the progression of early-stage prostate cancer in men. This provides a third alternative to "watchful waiting"—that is, doing nothing—and seeking conventional treatments with surgery, radiation, and drug treatments in which the vast majority of men do not show any benefit from these conventional treatments yet often experience the side-effects of impotence, incontinence, or both.[17]

Gene Expression

Also, we found that this program of comprehensive lifestyle changes changed gene expression in men with early-stage prostate cancer. After three months, 501 genes were beneficially affected: up-regulating 48 genes that are protective and down-regulating 453 genes that promote chronic inflammation, oxidative stress, and RAS oncogenes that promote prostate cancer, breast cancer, and colon cancer.[18]

People often say, "Oh, it's all in my genes, there's not much I can do about it." But knowing that changing lifestyle changes our genes is often very motivating—not to blame, but to empower. Our genes are a predisposition, but our genes are not usually our fate.

Angiogenesis

We also found that comprehensive lifestyle changes inhibit angiogenesis in men with prostate cancer.[19] When tumors grow, they often secrete substances such as VEGF that stimulate blood vessels to feed the tumors, since they grow so quickly they may outstrip the normal blood supply. By interfering with this process, tumors may be killed with fewer side-effects than attacking them directly. Drugs like Avastin may accomplish this, but at very high cost and with significant side-effects.

Telomerase and Telomeres

In addition, we found that this program of comprehensive lifestyle changes increased telomerase by 30% in only 3 months.[20] Telomerase is an enzyme that repairs and lengthens telomeres, the ends of our chromosomes that regulate aging. As our telomeres become shorter, our lives become shorter and the risk of premature death from a wide variety of chronic diseases increases proportionately. Over a 5-year period, we found, for the first time in a controlled study, that these lifestyle changes lengthened telomeres by approximately 10%, whereas telomeres became shorter in the control group.[21] Again, we found a dose-response correlation between adherence to this lifestyle medicine intervention and length of telomeres.

Conclusion

The more mechanisms we study, the greater understanding we have of why comprehensive lifestyle changes can be so beneficial in treating as well as preventing a wide spectrum of chronic diseases and how quickly these benefits can be measured and experienced. And the only side-effects are good ones.

Medical culture and the healthcare system have come a long way since we began doing our research nearly 40 years ago. It is now accepted that heart disease can be reversed with comprehensive lifestyle changes, it is being seen that these same changes have a beneficial effect on many other conditions, a new benefit category called intensive cardiac rehabilitation is now funded by many insurers including the Centers for Medicare and Medicaid Services (CMS), and lifestyle medicine is one of the fastest growing movements in the field of medicine. The increased prevalence of chronic illness has created tremendous financial and social burdens, these positive changes in medicine are creating a new paradigm of healthcare when we need it most.

References

1. Newby LK, LaPointe NM, Chen AY, et al. Long-term adherence to evidence-based secondary prevention therapies in coronary artery disease. *Circulation* 2006;113(2):203–212.
2. Mozaffarian D, Benjamin EJ, Go AS, et al. Heart disease and stroke statistics—2016 update; a report from the American Heart Association. *Circulation* 2015;133:38–360.

3. Centers for Disease Control and Prevention. *Vital Signs: Avoidable Deaths from Heart Disease, Stroke, and Hypertensive Disease—United States, 2001–2010.* Vol 62. 2013. http://www.cdc.gov/mmwr/preview/mmwrhtml/mm6235a6.htm.

4. Yusuf S, Hawken S, Ounpuu S, et al. Effect of potentially modifiable risk factors associated with myocardial infarction in 52 countries (the INTERHEART study). *Lancet* 2004;364(9438):937–952.

5. Åkesson A, Larsson SC, Discacciati A, Wolk A. Low-risk diet and lifestyle habits in the primary prevention of myocardial infarction in men: a population-based prospective cohort study. *J Am Coll Cardiol* 2014;64(13):1299–1306.

6. Ford ES, et al. Healthy living is the best revenge: findings from the European Prospective Investigation Into Cancer and Nutrition-Potsdam study. *Arch Intern Med* 2009;169(15):1355–1362.

7. Ornish DM, Gotto AM, Miller RR, et al. Effects of a vegetarian diet and selected yoga techniques in the treatment of coronary heart disease. *Clin Res* 1979;27:720A.

8. Ornish DM, Scherwitz LW, Doody RS, et al. Effects of stress management training and dietary changes in treating ischemic heart disease. *JAMA* 1983;249:54–59.

9. Ornish DM, Brown SE, Scherwitz LW, et al. Can lifestyle changes reverse coronary atherosclerosis? The Lifestyle Heart Trial. *Lancet* 1990; 336:129–133.

10. Gould KL, Ornish D, Kirkeeide R, Brown S, et al. Improved stenosis geometry by quantitative coronary arteriography after vigorous risk factor modification. *Am J Cardiol* 1992;69:845–853.

11. Ornish D, Scherwitz L, Billings J, et al. Intensive lifestyle changes for reversal of coronary heart disease: five-year follow-up of the Lifestyle Heart Trial. *JAMA* 1998;280:2001–2007.

12. Ornish D, Scherwitz L, Davern M. In press.

13. Gould KL, Ornish D, Scherwitz L, et al. Changes in myocardial perfusion abnormalities by positron emission tomography after long-term, intense risk factor modification. *JAMA* 1995;274:894–901.

14. Ornish D. Avoiding revascularization with lifestyle changes: the Multicenter Lifestyle Demonstration Project. *Am J Cardiol* 1998;82:72T–76T.

15. Koertge J, Weidner G, Elliott-Eller M, et al. Improvement in medical risk factors and quality of life in women and men with coronary artery disease in the Multicenter Lifestyle Demonstration Project. *Am J Cardiol* 2003;91:1316–1322.

16. Silberman A, Banthia R, Estay IS, et al. The effectiveness and efficacy of an intensive cardiac rehabilitation program in 24 sites. *Am J Health Promot* 2010;24(4):260–266.

17. Wilt TJ, Brawer MK, Jones KM, et al., for the Prostate Cancer Intervention versus Observation Trial (PIVOT) Study Group. Radical Prostatectomy versus Observation for Localized Prostate Cancer. *N Engl J Med* 2012;367:203–213.

18. Ornish D, Magbanua MJM, Weidner G, et al. Changes in prostate gene expression in men undergoing an intensive nutrition and lifestyle intervention. *Proc Nat Acad Sci USA* 2008;105:8369–8374.

19. Ornish D, Brown SE, Scherwitz LW, Billings JH, Armstrong WT, Ports TA, McLanahan SM, Kirkeeide RL, Brand RJ, Gould KL. Can lifestyle changes reverse coronary heart disease? *The Lifestyle Heart Trial Lancet* 1990 Jul 21;336(8708):129–133.

20. Ornish D, Lin J, Daubenmier J, et al. Increased telomerase activity and comprehensive lifestyle changes: a pilot study. *Lancet Oncol* 2008;9:1048–1057.
21. Ornish D, Lin J, Chan JM, et al. Effect of comprehensive lifestyle changes on telomerase activity and telomere length in men with biopsy-proven low-risk prostate cancer: 5-year follow-up of a descriptive pilot study. *Lancet Oncol* 2013;14(11):1112–1120.

15

An Integrative Preventive Medicine Approach to Primary Cancer Prevention

HEATHER GREENLEE, KATHLEEN SANDERS, AND ZELDA MORAN

Introduction

There is a growing burden of cancer in the United States and globally, with the majority of new cases and deaths occurring in developing countries. As reported by the American Cancer Society, over the past 20 years, survival rates in the United States for most cancer types have improved and cancer mortality has decreased (Figures 15.1 and 15.2) but the number of new cancer cases worldwide is expected to double from 12.7 million new cases in 2008 to 21.4 million new cases in 2030. The increase in cancer incidence is due not only to aging populations and increased life expectancies but also to unhealthy lifestyle practices, environmental influences, and a lack of effective and accessible prevention strategies. It is estimated that approximately 20% of cancer diagnoses in the United States could be prevented by maintaining a healthy, whole food–based diet, engaging in regular physical activity, and committing to long-term weight management.[1] Further, a large percentage of cancer cases could be prevented by avoiding vaccine-preventable infections, alcohol use, and tobacco use.[1] The proportion of cancers caused by major risk factors differs by level of economic development (Figure 15.3). Overall, knowledge of current cancer prevention strategies is crucial for healthcare providers and patients worldwide. Given the increasing use of integrative medicine both nationally and internationally, it is important to understand the role of an integrative preventive medicine approach and which specific strategies may contribute to cancer prevention.

Primary, Secondary and Tertiary Cancer Prevention

There are three levels of cancer prevention, each of which addresses a different stage of disease. *Primary prevention* seeks to prevent cancer occurrence by reducing an individual's exposure to cancer risk factors. Proven primary cancer prevention strategies include vaccination to prevent viral infections that are known to be carcinogenic, prophylactic removal of at-risk organs among high-risk individuals, reducing environmental and workplace exposures, and promoting healthy lifestyle behaviors. *Secondary cancer prevention* aims to diagnose and treat precancerous and cancerous tissue as early as possible in order to either prevent the progression to cancer or to treat tumors at early stages when they are the most responsive to treatment. The primary form of secondary cancer prevention is screening for disease at regular intervals, such as mammography, colonoscopy, and pap smears. In order to be effective, cancer screening programs need to address geographic, cultural, health literacy and financial barriers to access, along with programs to increase public awareness and use of screening programs as the majority of patients with early-stage tumors are asymptomatic.[2] *Tertiary cancer prevention*, also known as cancer control, emphasizes reducing the risk of recurrence, metastases, and new primary cancers. Tertiary cancer prevention also includes reducing tumor-related complications, managing treatment-related side effects, and improving quality of life.[2]

Cancer Risk Factors

Increasing age is the largest risk factor for developing cancer,[3] and other important risk factors include environmental exposures, health behaviors, genetics, and infectious agents. Risk factors can increase the risk for specific types of cancer and/or for cancer overall. Examples of environmental risk factors include exposure to radiation, sunlight, infectious agents, and dietary contaminants, such as mycotoxins. Common behavioral risk factors associated with increased risk of many types of cancer include tobacco use; being overweight or obese with a body mass index (BMI) over 25 kg/m^2; a diet high in unhealthy fats and low in fruits, vegetables, and fiber; alcohol consumption over 1 drink per day for men and ½ a drink per day for women; and being sedentary with low levels of physical activity. Genetic risk factors specific to certain cancers include genetic mutations such as *BRCA 1* and *BRCA 2*, which dramatically increase a woman's chance of developing breast cancer; other hereditary cancer syndromes, such as Lynch syndrome, also known as hereditary nonpolyposis colorectal cancer, which increases risk of colon cancer as well as endometrial, ovarian, and other cancer in women; and Li

Fraumeni syndrome, which can cause a range of cancers during childhood.[4] There is also now a clear causal link established between specific infectious agents and specific cancers. Human papillomavirus (HPV) is strongly associated with cervical cancer, chronic infection with hepatitis B virus (HBV) or hepatitis C virus (HCV) is the strongest known risk factor for liver cancer, and a growing body of evidence suggests a link between human immunodeficiency virus (HIV) and a number of cancers, particularly cervical cancer, Kaposi sarcoma, and non-Hodgkin's lymphoma.[5,6]

Role of Integrative Preventive Medicine Approaches to Cancer Prevention

A conventional cancer prevention approach begins with assessing cancer risk factors, which often includes age, gender, genetics, personal and family medical history, and occupational and lifestyle exposures. Clinical recommendations for interventions are based on the level of individual risk. In general, the majority of individuals can benefit from a healthful diet, physical activity, and vaccination to prevent infectious disease. Individuals at higher than average risk may receive recommendations for pharmacological chemoprevention and/or surgery to remove the susceptible organ. There is a growing interest by segments of both patients and clinicians to incorporate integrative medicine into cancer prevention strategies. The overarching goal of integrative medicine is to incorporate evidence-based and effective complementary therapies into effective conventional medical therapies in order to provide a more holistic and more effective approach to clinical care.[7] As integrative medicine is an emerging field, especially within cancer prevention and cancer care, it is important to understand what is and is not known about the effectiveness of integrative medicine approaches to cancer prevention. Integrative therapies include biologic therapies and behavioral modifications such as dietary modifications, botanicals (herbs), vitamins and minerals, other dietary supplements, mind/body therapies, acupuncture, energy medicine, and non-Western systems of healing, most of which are not typically used as part of conventional medical practice. Integrative medicine refers to complementary, nonpharmacologic practices that are performed in conjunction with conventional treatments, while alternative medicine refers to practices used in lieu of standard treatments. This chapter focuses on the use of integrative medicine for primary cancer prevention.

Until fairly recently, the concept of primary cancer prevention was not widely accepted because there was limited evidence supporting the concept that carcinogenesis[8] could be reversed or halted by any means. However, over the past few decades, clinical trials have shown that cancers can be prevented or postponed via vaccination, prophylactic surgery, chemoprevention, and behavioral modification such as smoking cessation and dietary change. For example, a trial showed that tamoxifen reduces the risk of developing breast cancer among women at higher than average risk,[9] and that a low-fat diet reduces the likelihood of breast cancer recurrence among women with estrogen receptor-negative breast cancer.[10] We currently have very limited clinical trial data on the effect of integrative approaches to primary cancer prevention, but this is a growing area of interest in basic science and clinical research. In order to understand the role of integrative therapies in cancer prevention, one must first understand the role and strength of evidence of conventional medical approaches to cancer prevention.

Effective Conventional Therapies for Cancer Prevention

We know that even in the absence of known risk factors, cancer is a common occurrence, and better means of primary prevention are needed. The current science also supports prophylactic surgery in some cases. There is an ongoing need for improved methods of early detection and intervention in cancer care.

CHEMOPREVENTION

For some cancers, conventional therapies used for cancer treatment are prescribed to high-risk individuals for cancer risk reduction. The most compelling evidence for this approach is in breast cancer. Among both pre- and postmenopausal women at high risk of breast cancer, 5 years of tamoxifen treatment reduces the risk of breast cancer[11] as does 5 years of raloxifene for postmenopausal women at high risk of breast cancer.[12]

PROPHYLACTIC ORGAN REMOVAL

Prophylactic organ removal has also been shown to be successful at reducing cancer risk, especially for breast and ovarian cancer. For women with a BRCA1 or BRCA2 genetic mutation, mastectomy substantially reduces the risk of breast cancer.[13] Similarly, for women at high risk of ovarian cancer, a salpingo-oophorectomy substantially reduces the risk of both ovarian and breast cancer.[14,15]

VACCINATIONS AND INFECTION CONTROL

Viral infections are estimated to be responsible for 15% of cancers globally,[16] including, but not limited to, liver, stomach, and cervical cancers.[17] There are now effective vaccines to prevent some of these viral infections, with the implication that effective vaccination programs can prevent large numbers of cancer cases worldwide, especially in areas where these infections are common. Hepatitis B and C have been shown to be responsible for the majority of cirrhosis and liver cancer cases globally. While there is no vaccine for HCV, the HBV vaccine has been shown to be effective in preventing chronic hepatitis, which often progresses to liver cancer.[18,19] The HPV vaccine was recently shown to preventing HPV infection with the HPV types that most commonly cause precancerous lesions and cervical, anal, and oropharyngeal cancer. The vaccine prevents infection with HPV 16 and 18, which have been shown to be responsible for 70% of cervical cancer cases worldwide.[20] The HPV vaccine has now been proven as a safe method of risk reduction, and unprecedented in that it may be given to all sexually active females and males, regardless of their risk of transmitting or developing cervical cancer.[21] While the HPV vaccine represents enormous potential for cancer prevention, there are significant public health challenges in implementing large-scale vaccination on a population level, especially for children.[22]

Infection with *Helicobacter pylori*, a bacteria that colonizes the stomach lining, has been identified as a major cause of gastric cancer. It is present in 30%–50% of the population, who are often asymptomatic. Common gastritis is often the first sign of gastric cancer, and cancer risk depends on the specific bacterial strain as well as specific host/microbe interactions, all of which make cost-efficient and effective screening for gastric cancer a major challenge. Gastric cancer is most common in areas with poor sanitation and low socioeconomic resources.[23] Treatment using antibiotics to eradicate *H. pylori* may greatly reduce the risk of gastric cancer, but risk of cancer development depends on bacterial strains as well as certain host pathogen interactions, making effective screening and treatment of *H. pylori* difficult and complex on a large scale.[23,24]

SCREENING

The evidence for efficacy of cancer screening programs to prevent cancer deaths, particularly for breast and prostate, has shown mixed results. Meta-analysis of randomized-controlled trials of mammography screening, for example, has been shown to reduce mortality from breast cancer by 15%–20%.[25] However, the degree of benefit from routine mammography screening is disputed, and there is not agreement among major guideline groups about the age at which routine mammography should begin. For example, the US Preventive Services Task Force (USPSTF) recommends biennial screening mammography for women aged 50 to 74 years,[26] whereas the American Cancer Society recommends annual mammograms beginning at age 45 and biennial mammograms starting at age 55.[27] Both groups state that women outside of these age ranges should be screened based on their individual personal and family history.

Lung cancer is the leading cause of cancer death among both men and women in the United States.[28] Among adults aged 55 to 80 years with a 30-pack-year smoking history who currently smoke or have quit within the past 15 years, the USPSTF recommends annual screening for lung cancer with low-dose computed tomography.[29] The USPSTF recommends that screening be discontinued once a person has not smoked for 15 years, or if the person develops a health problem that substantially limits life expectancy or the ability/willingness to have curative lung surgery.

The advantages and disadvantages of cancer screening programs continue to be researched, monitored, and hotly debated. It is crucial that healthcare providers and clinicians stay current on research findings and recommendations.[30] The USPSTF guidelines are regularly updated and can be located at www.uspreventiveservicestaskforce.org.

Diet

There is a substantial literature based on observational data suggesting that people with healthier diets have a decreased risk of developing cancer.[31] Specific protective dietary behaviors include high intake of fruits, vegetables, and other fiber sources, and low intake of alcohol, red meat, and processed meats. However, there are limited experimental data showing what dose and duration of these behaviors are needed to definitively reduce cancer risk. Thus far, the most compelling research on the use of diet for cancer prevention comes from two separate trials testing dietary change to prevent breast cancer recurrence.[10,32] The trials had conflicting results. The Women's Healthy Eating and Living (WHEL) trial tested a diet high in fruits and vegetables among breast cancer survivors and found no effect of the diet on breast cancer recurrence or survival. However, the Women's Intervention Nutrition Study (WINS) study showed that a low-fat diet was associated with decreased risk of breast cancer recurrence among the subset of breast cancer survivors who had been diagnosed with estrogen receptor-negative tumors. The reason for the different findings in unclear; some researchers have suggested that the reason that the WINS study observed a difference was that the women who effectively lowered their fat intake also lost weight and that perhaps the improvement in survival was actually due to weight loss.

There is considerable research interest in specific bioactive phytochemical components in plant-based foods. Simply speaking, using color as an indicator of specific cancer-fighting phytochemicals has led to the idea of eating "a rainbow" of vegetables and fruits regularly to obtain the anticancer effect. There are a variety of cellular and molecular pathways that phytochemicals have been shown to affect, including immune modulation, growth factors, cancer cell viability, antioxidation, and the inflammatory process.[33,34] Diet may further influence these pathways by altering DNA methylation, histone modification, and noncoding microRNA.[35] For example, several human cohort studies have found association between cruciferous vegetables and decreased cancer risk. Cruciferous vegetables, including cauliflower, kale, cabbage, and broccoli sprouts, contain indole-3-carbinol (I3C), which has been shown to affect uncontrolled cellular growth and the viability of various types of cancer cells.[36,37] In addition, cruciferous vegetables contain isothiocyanates, which have been shown to inhibit cancer development in animal models. Studies are investigating whether it is a specific dietary component that is needed to obtain a cancer prevention effect, or if it is the whole plant that is more effective. For example, in a rat study, neither indole-3 carbinol (I3C) alone nor isothiocyanates alone reduced tumor precursors.[36] However, when rats were fed whole cruciferous vegetables, there was a reduction in colon cancer precursor cells. It is possible that the mix of bioactive compounds in whole cruciferous vegetables is needed to achieve the cancer prevention effects.

Lycopene and resveratrol are two other bioactive food components that have shown strong chemopreventive potential. Tomatoes contain carotenoids and polyphenols, with lycopene being a primary component of interest. Both clinical trials and observational studies have shown that lycopene may be an important active chemopreventive agent, especially for prostate cancer. Similar to the studies on cruciferous vegetables, studies suggest that intake of whole tomatoes may be more effective for cancer prevention compared to isolated lycopene or other bioactive components, and consumption of tomatoes cooked and combined with other foods has been shown to increase the body's absorption of lycopene.[38] Resveratrol is a polyphenol contained in berries, grapes, red wine, and peanuts. A phase I pilot study focused on colon cancer prevention demonstrated that resveratrol in combination with other bioactive components can inhibit the Wnt cellular pathway in vivo.[39]

The impact of dietary fiber on colon and small bowel cancer prevention has long been recognized and demonstrated in many epidemiologic and experimental studies, though there are also conflicting studies. Fiber seems to act both by decreasing the time that a carcinogen rests in the intestines and also by promoting a healthy gut flora. The interactions between dietary fiber, gut health, microbiota, body weight, and fat and protein intake is a very active area of cancer prevention research. Fiber as part of a whole-food approach to cancer prevention continues to be recommended by the American Cancer Society.[40,41]

Dietary fat has been associated with an increased risk of breast, colorectal, ovarian, prostate, and gallbladder cancers. While dietary fat is essential for energy production as well as cell and nervous system function, dietary fat also contributes to inflammation, which promotes carcinogenesis. There is evidence that healthy fats may be an important part of a cancer-preventive diet, distinct from trans fats and saturated animal fats. The balance between omega 6 and omega 3 fatty acids has been shown to be the most important distinction between healthy and unhealthy fats, with a low ratio (close to 1-1) of omega 6 to omega 3 fatty acids being considered ideal, and high ratios contributing to inflammatory and chronic diseases.[42] This is an active area of research, and crucial to understanding both the potential health benefits of certain fatty foods, and in counseling patients on making long-term dietary changes. Examples of healthy fats include olives and olive oils, which contain lignans and peroxidation-resistant lipid oleic acid. It is suggested that high intake of healthy fats could explain why rates of major chronic diseases, such as cancer, are lower in people who follow a Mediterranean diet, which is high in olives and olive oil.[43] Other healthy fat food sources include nuts, avocado, coconut oil, and sunflower oil. Studying the effect of fats on cancer risk has yielded mixed results, but remains an important area of research with many active ongoing cohort studies. The Women's Health Initiative studied the effect of a low-fat diet on cancer risk and did not demonstrate an overall significant change in cancer rates, but women who entered the study with a very high fat diet and then substantially reduced their fat intake did have a reduced rate of subsequent breast cancer.[44]

There is a provocative and growing body of evidence suggesting that a Mediterranean dietary pattern has cancer prevention potential.[45] The traditional Mediterranean diet meets the characteristics of an anticancer diet defined by the World Cancer Research Fund/American Institute for Cancer Research (WCRF/AICR). It is a diet rich in fruits, vegetables, whole grain bread and other cereals, beans, nuts, and seeds; high in olive oil as a key source of monounsaturated fat; low to moderate consumption of dairy, fish, poultry, and eggs; and low alcohol consumption, mainly in the form of wine. Observational study results suggest that high adherence to the Mediterranean diet is significantly associated with a reduced risk of cancer incidence and/or mortality.[46] Provocatively, a recent randomized, clinical trial reported that the Mediterranean diet was effective in decreasing the incidence of primary breast cancer.[47] The number of incident cancer events was small, and study results were planned secondary analyses of a trial testing the effect of the Mediterranean diet on cardiovascular outcome. Nevertheless, the results are provocative enough to warrant follow-up with a future larger trial of a Mediterranean diet examining incident breast cancer as the primary outcome of interest.

Observational studies have shown that vegetarian, vegan, or other diets low in meat or animal products are also associated with lower risk of a variety of cancers, but there are many confounding lifestyle factors among people who follow these diets making it difficult to interpret the observational study results. For example, people who follow these diets often have lower intake of alcohol and saturated fat, are more physically active, and are less likely to smoke. Therefore, given these important confounders, it is difficult to determine which specific factor or combination of factors is the most responsible for decreased cancer risk among vegans and vegetarians.

Food production processes are also considered in cancer prevention strategies. Interest in organically grown foods and animal feeds has increased in recent decades for many reasons, including a belief that these foods may lower the risk of cancer due to the absence of pesticides, herbicides, and other potentially carcinogenic compounds. While it is true that food can be a vehicle for contaminants and possibly harmful substances, whether conventionally grown foods are truly associated with increased cancer risk is unproven.[48] On the other hand, it is well established that foods containing aflatoxins (e.g., grains and peanuts) contribute to the risk of liver cancer, and are most common in tropical countries with poor storage practices where grains are more susceptible to fungal contamination.[49]

Physical Activity

Physical activity has become a cancer prevention strategy of particular interest. Observational studies have also shown exercise to be protective against lung, kidney, endometrial, colon, breast, and possibly prostate cancer.[50-52] To obtain optimal health benefits from physical activity, the *2008 Physical Activity Guidelines for Americans* put forth by the US Surgeon General recommends that adults engage in at least 150 minutes of moderate-intensity aerobic physical activity or 75 minutes of vigorous-intensity physical activity, or an equivalent combination, each week and that children and adolescents be active for at least 60 minutes every day.[5] People who are inactive and those who do not yet meet the guidelines are strongly encouraged to work toward this goal. Adults with disabilities who are unable to meet the guidelines should avoid inactivity and try to engage in regular physical activity according to their abilities.[53]

Possible mechanisms of action of physical activity and cancer risk include improved weight management, lower levels of hormones associated with increased risk of specific cancer (e.g., estrogen, insulin, and insulin-like growth factor), increased immune response, increased metabolism, and reduced gastrointestinal transit time, thereby decreasing the time of exposure to carcinogens in the digestive system. Regardless of the cancer prevention potential, physical activity has been shown to be important in improving quality of life for the general population and improve the prognosis of individuals diagnosed with cancer.[54] Factors leading to sedentary behavior, how to decrease sedentary behavior, and the mechanisms by which sedentary behavior affects cancer risk are all active areas of research. For example, in two trials among colon cancer and prostate cancer survivors, a reduction in sedentary behavior was associated with a change in hormone levels as well in reducing fatigue and improving quality of life.[55-57]

It is important to recognize the need to individualize exercise prescriptions based on an individual's physical ability, access to programs, financial constraints, and access to other resources. Motivational interviewing can be a useful tool for healthcare providers to assist and encourage people to make healthy behavioral changes.[58] However, making simple behavioral changes is only the first step in life-long habit change.[50] The surgeon general's report strongly recognizes the need for community programs that support the ability to achieve and maintain lifelong change in exercise patterns. Public space dedicated for exercise and recreation in local parks or commonly used buildings such as schools, churches, and community centers is crucial to creating an environment where physical activity is feasible and accessible.[59] An increasing amount of research is being conducted on the demand and design of behavioral support for increasing physical activity and other lifestyle behaviors. The use of smartphone apps and wearable devices may be useful for long-term habit change, but research needs to be conducted to identify whether or not these are effective at achieving and maintaining long-term behavior changes.[60] A recent study among young adults with a BMI between 25 and 40 kg/m^2 did not show an improvement in weight loss when the participants used a wearable device that monitors and provides feedback on physical activity.[61] There is a need for larger and more rigorous studies on the potential of using wearable devices to motivate and monitor physical activity.

Weight Management

Obesity has been clearly shown to be a major risk factor for a number of cancers, specifically esophageal, pancreatic, colorectal, breast, endometrial, kidney, thyroid, and gallbladder cancers. There are several biological pathways linking obesity to carcinogenesis.[54] First, fat tissue and fat cells produce excess amounts of hormones, such as estrogens, and adipokines, such as leptin, which stimulate cell proliferation. Both insulin and insulin-like-growth factor (IGF) are readily produced by fat cells, and both have been shown to promote tumor development. In addition, obesity is associated with chronic low levels of inflammation, which is known to promote carcinogenesis.[59] Though genetics and epigenetics may play a role in the development of overweight and obesity, it is well established that a healthy diet and being physical active are both crucial to achieving and maintaining a healthy weight. National cancer prevention organizations have put forth similar recommendations for achieving and maintaining a healthy weight for cancer prevention. The American Cancer Society and the American Institute for Cancer Research both recommend that individuals achieve and maintain a healthy weight throughout life, and be as lean as possible throughout life without being underweight.[62,63]

Individuals often need structural support to effectively manage weight. Behavioral change programs such as Weight Watchers offer healthy diet infor-mation along with group support and a sense of community, and are a very effective way for many people to make and reach weight loss goals.[64,65] When designing and recommending weight loss and weight maintenance programs, perceived benefit, gender, cultural factors, and access to resources need to be considered. Governmental policy on access to weight loss programs and related health insurance coverage affect a patient's ability to make long-term behavioral changes. Recent policy changes related to the Affordable Care Act (ACA) have led to policies that consider obesity as a medically recognized dis-ease and therefore provide coverage for both bariatric surgery and nutritional counseling. As of 2014, the ACA also prohibits the use of surcharges for obese patients as well as any consumer cost-sharing for obesity treatments including obesity screening and counseling.[66]

Dietary Supplements

The use of dietary supplements is very high in the United States, and is especially high among some populations at high risk of cancer.[67] While dietary supplements are used for a wide variety of reasons, it is important to note that in most cases, there is insufficient evidence to conclude that they are protective against cancer, and some have even shown to increase the risk of some cancers.[49,67] For example, large-scale clinical trials have been conducted to determine the effect of beta-carotene dietary supplements to prevent lung cancer in high-risk populations (i.e., smokers and asbestos workers) in the

Alpha-Tocopherol, Beta Carotene Prevention Study (ATBC) and the Beta Carotene and Retinol Efficacy Trial (CARET).[68,69] In contrast to the study hypotheses, both the ATBC and CARET trials[69,70] found increased lung cancer risk among the populations that were expected to be protected. In the SELECT trial, vitamin E and selenium were tested for prostate cancer prevention; there was an increased risk of prostate cancer in participants taking selenium.[71] It is important to note that effects may differ between dietary intake and supplemental intake of vitamins and minerals. Therefore, even if a vitamin in food is shown to be protective against cancer, research must be conducted to confirm that using supplements will also be effective.

At this time, dietary supplements are not recommended for preventing cancer. The US Preventive Services Task Force has stated that supplementation is unlikely to provide clinical benefits and may cause harm to some populations.[72] To date, no dietary supplements have been shown to prevent cancer and a handful of supplements have been shown to increase risk. However, clinical trials are underway for several promising agents such as vitamin D, curcumin, and fish oil, and these important areas of research to monitor. The Natural Medicines database (www.naturalmedicines.therapeuticresearch.com) provides a comprehensive online resource for current information on the evidence on dietary supplements and other natural products.

Mind Body Medicine

There are a wide variety of types of approaches that fall under the rubric of mind body medicine, and while there is no evidence that it is directly effective for cancer prevention, it has been shown to be beneficial to quality of life, and may affect some physiologic pathways related to cancer prevention. Cognitive therapies include mindfulness-based stress reduction (MBSR), meditation, guided imagery, clinical hypnosis, and humor therapy. Sensory therapies include aromatherapy, massage, touch therapy, reiki, healing touch, therapeutic touch, music therapy, and creating a calm and/or beautiful space such as a room with a view or a healing garden. Expressive therapies include writing, journaling, art therapy, support groups, individual counseling, and psychotherapy. Physical therapies include dancing, yoga, and tai chi.[73]

The concept of mindfulness is being actively examined as a tool to promote the development of healthy eating habits, which has shown provocative results in a number of trials.[74,75] Mindfulness-based programs for changing eating habits are an offshoot of the mindfulness-based stress management programs and use similar techniques for slowing down the eating process, improving food choices, and decreasing portion sizes. Mindfulness can also improve enjoyment of food, and programs are often offered in a group setting, which offers the extra social support that may facilitate long-term change.

Studies suggest that the regular practice of mind body medicine techniques affects functions of the neuroendocrine and immune systems in ways that may modify tumor development and/or progression, while also contributing to enhanced general well-being. When practiced regularly, mind body practices have been shown on MRI to positively impact areas of the brain associated with depression,[76] and one cohort study showed that long-term meditation practice had a strong protective effect against high stress levels.[77] For example, breast cancer patients who practiced relaxation and coping methods had lower serum cortisol levels and improved immune function.[78,79] Music intervention programs have shown to improve pain, anxiety, fatigue, and general quality of life in cancer patients.[80] Thus, while to date there is no evidence supporting mind body practices for cancer prevention, these practices are usually safe, often beneficial for mental health and quality of life, and usually low in cost.

Special Populations

Some integrative medicine therapies may have safety issues for special populations, including individuals with comorbidities and/or who are pediatric and geriatric patients. For very elderly or ill populations, physical activity may present risk of injury. Restorative yoga is an example of an exercise form that has been adapted for people who are very ill or physically challenged to move safely. Medications can interact with some natural products with serious side effects. Each patient should be evaluated individually before changes in physical activity, diet, or use of dietary supplements is recommended, and the healthcare provider should counsel the patient on the most effective and safe approach to cancer prevention and/or management.

Conclusion

Identifying and implementing effective cancer prevention strategies on a large population scale, whether they are conventional or integrative, has proven to be challenging. However, there is a growing body of evidence suggesting that there are effective cancer prevention strategies. Vaccinations for HBV and HPV are highly effective. There is a strong body of evidence supporting the role of major lifestyle factors to prevent a range of cancers, including smoking avoidance and cessation; no or reduced use of alcohol; a diet high in fruits and vegetables and low in fat, red meats, and processed meats; regular physical

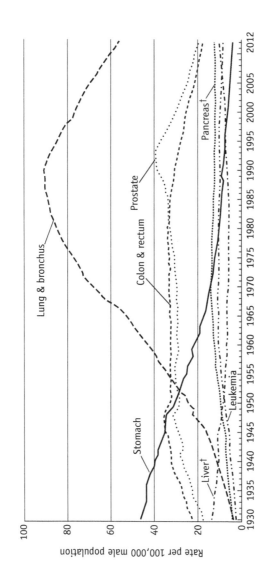

*Per 100,000, age adjusted to the 2000 US standard population. †Mortality rates for pancreatic and liver cancers are increasing.

Note: Due to changes in ICD coding, numerator information has changed over time. Rates for cancers of the liver, lung and bronchus, and colon and rectum are affected by these coding changes.

FIGURE 15.1 Trends in Age-Adjusted Cancer Death Rates* by Site, Males, US, 1930–2012 Reference 1.

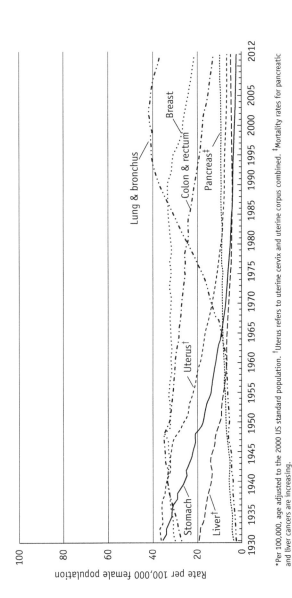

*Per 100,000, age adjusted to the 2000 US standard population. †Uterus refers to uterine cervix and uterine corpus combined. ‡Mortality rates for pancreatic and liver cancers are increasing.

Note: Due to changes in ICD coding, numerator information has changed over time. Rates for cancers of the liver, lung and bronchus, and colon and rectum are affected by these coding changes.

FIGURE 15.2 Trends in Age-Adjusted Cancer Death Rates* by Site, Females, US, 1930–2012 Reference 1.

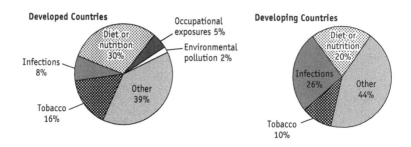

FIGURE 15.3 Proportion of Cancer Causes by Major Risk Factors and Level of Economic Development
Reference 81.

activity; and achieving and maintaining a healthy weight. A nascent but provocative body of literature suggests that stress management and mind body therapies clearly improve quality of life and may have the potential for cancer prevention. Though there is great interest by the general public on the use of dietary supplements for cancer prevention, no dietary supplements have been shown to effectively prevent cancer, while some have shown substantial harm. Therefore, individuals should be advised and coached on how to abstain from tobacco; meet daily recommendations for physical activity; eat a healthy diet high in whole grains, fruits, vegetables, and other sources of fiber, and healthy fats; consume alcohol only in moderation; and maintain a healthy weight. Individuals interested in the use of dietary supplements should be counseled about their known interactions, harms, and effects. And if applicable, individuals can be encouraged to engage in mind body practices that may improve their mood, sleep, and overall well-being, while they also may assist in sustaining lifestyle changes. An optimal preventive healthcare approach includes cancer prevention programs that integrate all evidence-based conventional and integrative treatment approaches and options.

References

1. American Cancer Society. *Cancer Facts and Figures 2016*. Atlanta: American Cancer Society; 2016.
2. Alberts DS, Hess LM. Introduction: to cancer prevention. In: *Fundamentals of Cancer Prevention*. Berlin Heidelberg New York: Springer; 2008:1–12.
3. National Cancer Institute. *Causes and Prevention: Age*. 2015. http://www.cancer.gov/about-cancer/causes-prevention/risk/age. Accessed July 28, 2016.
4. American Cancer Society. *Family Cancer Syndromes*. 2014. http://www.cancer.org/cancer/cancercauses/geneticsandcancer/heredity-and-cancer. Accessed July 28, 2016.

5. National Cancer Institute. *Causes and Prevention*. 2016. http://www.cancer.gov/about-cancer/causes-prevention/. Accessed July 28, 2016.

6. National Cancer Institute. *HIV Infection and Cancer Risk*. 2011. http://www.cancer.gov/about-cancer/causes-prevention/risk/infectious-agents/hiv-fact-sheet - q1. Accessed July 28, 2016.

7. Hughes EF. Overview of complementary, alternative, and integrative medicine. *Clin Obstet Gynocol* 2001;44(4):774.

8. Alberts DS, Hess LM, eds. *Fundamentals of Cancer Prevention*. New York: Springer; 2005.

9. Fisher B, Costantino JP, Wickerham DL, et al. Tamoxifen for prevention of breast cancer: report of the National Surgical Adjuvant Breast and Bowel Project P-1 Study. *J Natl Cancer Inst* 1998;90(18):1371–1388.

10. Chlebowski RT, Blackburn GL, Thomson CA, et al. Dietary fat reduction and breast cancer outcome: interim efficacy results from the Women's Intervention Nutrition Study. *J Natl Cancer Inst* 2006;98(24):1767–1776.

11. Cuzick J, Forbes JF, Sestak I, et al. Long-term results of tamoxifen prophylaxis for breast cancer: 96-month follow-up of the randomized IBIS-I trial. *J Natl Cancer Inst* 2007;99(4):272–282.

12. Freedman AN, Yu B, Gail MH, et al. Benefit/risk assessment for breast cancer chemoprevention with raloxifene or tamoxifen for women age 50 years or older. *J Clin Oncol* 2011;29(17):2327–2333.

13. Domchek SM, Friebel TM, Singer CF, et al. Association of risk-reducing surgery in BRCA1 or BRCA2 mutation carriers with cancer risk and mortality. *JAMA* 2010;304(9):967–975.

14. American Cancer Society. *Medicines to Reduce Breast Cancer Risk*. 2016. http://www.cancer.org/cancer/breastcancer/moreinformation/medicinestoreducebreast-cancer/medicines-to-reduce-breast-cancer-risk-tamoxifen-raloxifene. Accessed June 3, 2016.

15. National Cancer Institute. *Surgery to Reduce the Risk of Breast Cancer*. 2013. http://www.cancer.gov/types/breast/risk-reducing-surgery-fact-sheet. Accessed July 28, 2016.

16. Frazer IH, Lowy DR, Schiller JT. Prevention of cancer through immunization: prospects and challenges for the 21st century. *Eur J Immunol* 2007;37(S1):S148–S155.

17. de Martel C, Ferlay J, Franceschi S, Vignat J, Bray F, Forman D, Plummer M. Global burden of cancers attributable to infections in 2008: a review and synthetic analysis. *Lancet Oncol* 2012 Jun;13(6):607–615.

18. Chang MH. Hepatitis B virus and cancer prevention. *Recent Results Cancer Res* 2011;188:75–84.

19. Perz JF, Armstrong GL, Farrington LA, Hutin YJF, Bell BP. The contributions of hepatitis B virus and hepatitis C virus infections to cirrhosis and primary liver cancer worldwide. *J Hepatol* 45(4):529–538.

20. National Cancer Institute. *Human Papillomavirus (HPV) Vaccines*. 2015. http://www.cancer.gov/about-cancer/causes-prevention/risk/infectious-agents/hpv-vaccine-fact-sheet - q7. Accessed July 28, 2016.

21. Angioli R, Lopez S, Aloisi A, et al. Ten years of HPV vaccines: state of art and controversies. *Crit Rev Oncol Hematol* 2016;102:65–72.

22. Colgrove J. The ethics and politics of compulsory HPV vaccination. *N Engl J Med* 2006;355(23):2389–2391.

23. National Cancer Institute. *Helicobacter pylori and Cancer.* 2013. http://www.cancer.gov/about-cancer/causes-prevention/risk/infectious-agents/h-pylori-fact-sheet - q1. Accessed July 28, 2016.

24. Polk DB, Peek RM Jr. Helicobacter pylori: gastric cancer and beyond. *Nat Rev Cancer* 2010;10(6):403–414.

25. Webb ML, Cady B, Michaelson JS, et al. A failure analysis of invasive breast cancer: most deaths from disease occur in women not regularly screened. *Cancer* 2014;120(18):2839–2846.

26. US Preventive Services Task Force. *Final Update Summary: Breast Cancer: Screening.* 2016. http://www.uspreventiveservicestaskforce.org/Page/Document/UpdateSummaryFinal/breast-cancer-screening. Accessed July 28, 2016.

27. Oeffinger KC, Fontham ET, Etzioni R, et al. Breast cancer screening for women at average risk: 2015 guideline update from the American Cancer Society. *JAMA* 2015;314(15):1599–1614.

28. American Cancer Society. *Cancer Facts and Figures 2013.* Atlanta, GA: Author; 2013.

29. Moyer VA. Screening for lung cancer: U.S. Preventive Services Task Force recommendation statement. *Ann Intern Med* 2014;160(5):330–338.

30. National Cancer Institute. *Breast Cancer Screening (PDQ®)–Health Professional Version.* Bethesda, MD: National Cancer Institute; 2016.

31. World Cancer Research Fund/American Institute for Cancer Research. *Food, Nutrition, Physical Activity, and the Prevention of Cancer: A Global Perspective.* Washington DC: AICR; 2007.

32. Pierce JP, Natarajan L, Caan BJ, et al. Influence of a diet very high in vegetables, fruit, and fiber and low in fat on prognosis following treatment for breast cancer: the Women's Healthy Eating and Living (WHEL) randomized trial. *JAMA* 2007;298(3):289–298.

33. Singh BN, Singh HB, Singh A, Naqvi AH, Singh BR. Dietary phytochemicals alter epigenetic events and signaling pathways for inhibition of metastasis cascade: phytoblockers of metastasis cascade. *Cancer Metastasis Rev* 2014;33(1):41–85.

34. González-Gallego J, García-Mediavilla MV, Sánchez-Campos S, Tuñón MJ. Fruit polyphenols, immunity and inflammation. *Br J Nutr* 2010;104(S3):S15–S27.

35. Bishop KS, Ferguson LR. The interaction between epigenetics, nutrition and the development of cancer. *Nutrients* 2015;7(2):922–947.

36. Arikawa AY, Gallaher DD. Cruciferous vegetables reduce morphological markers of colon cancer risk in dimethylhydrazine-treated rats. *J Nutr* 2008;138(3):526–532.

37. Royston KJ, Tollefsbol TO. The epigenetic impact of cruciferous vegetables on cancer prevention. *Curr Pharmacol Rep* 2015;1(1):46–51.

38. Marti R, Rosello S, Cebolla-Cornejo J. Tomato as a source of carotenoids and polyphenols targeted to cancer prevention. *Cancers (Basel)* 2016;8(6).

39. Nguyen AV, Martinez M, Stamos MJ, et al. Results of a phase I pilot clinical trial examining the effect of plant-derived resveratrol and grape powder on Wnt pathway target gene expression in colonic mucosa and colon cancer. *Cancer Manag Res* 2009;1:25–37.

40. Zeng H, Lazarova DL, Bordonaro M. Mechanisms linking dietary fiber, gut microbiota and colon cancer prevention. *World J Gastrointest Oncol* 2014;6(2):41–51.

41. Schatzkin A, Park Y, Leitzmann MF, Hollenbeck AR, Cross AJ. Prospective study of dietary fiber, whole grain foods, and small intestinal cancer. *Gastroenterology* 2008;135(4):1163–1167.

42. Simopoulos AP. The importance of the ratio of omega-6/omega-3 essential fatty acids. *Biomed Pharmacother* 2002;56(8):365–379.

43. Owen RW, Haubner R, Wurtele G, Hull E, Spiegelhalder B, Bartsch H. Olives and olive oil in cancer prevention. *Eur J Cancer Prev* 2004;13(4):319–326.

44. Prentice RL, Caan B, Chlebowski RT, et al. Low-fat dietary pattern and risk of invasive breast cancer: the Women's Health Initiative Randomized Controlled Dietary Modification Trial. *JAMA* 2006;295(6):629–642.

45. D'Alessandro A, De Pergola G, Silvestris F. Mediterranean diet and cancer risk: an open issue. *Int J Food Sci Nutr* 2016;67(6):593–605.

46. Schwingshackl L, Hoffmann G. Adherence to Mediterranean diet and risk of cancer: a systematic review and meta-analysis of observational studies. *Int J Cancer* 2014;135(8):1884–1897.

47. Toledo E, Salas-Salvado J, Donat-Vargas C, et al. Mediterranean diet and invasive breast cancer risk among women at high cardiovascular risk in the PREDIMED trial: a randomized clinical trial. *JAMA Intern Med* 2015;175(11):1752–1760.

48. American Cancer Society. *Food Additives, Safety, and Organic Foods.* 2016. http://www.cancer.org/healthy/eathealthygetactive/acsguidelinesonnutritionphysicalactivityforcancerprevention/acs-guidelines-on-nutrition-and-physical-activity-for-cancer-prevention-food-additives. Accessed July 28, 2016.

49. Marmot M, Atinmo T, Byers T, et al. *Food, Nutrition, Physical Activity, and the Prevention of Cancer: A Global Perspective.* Washington DC: AICR, 2007.

50. Lemanne D, Cassileth B, Gubili J. The role of physical activity in cancer prevention, treatment, recovery, and survivorship. *Oncology Williston Park* 2013;27(6):580–585.

51. Lynch BM, Neilson HK, Friedenreich CM. Physical activity and breast cancer prevention. *Recent Results Cancer Res* 2011;186:13–42.

52. Holmes MD, Chen WY, Feskanich D, Kroenke CH, Colditz GA. Physical activity and survival after breast cancer diagnosis. *JAMA* 2005;293(20):2479–2486.

53. Physical Activity Guidelines Advisory Committee report, 2008. To the Secretary of Health and Human Services. Part A: executive summary. *Nutr Rev* 2009;67(2):114–120.

54. National Cancer Institute. *Obesity and Cancer Risk.* 2012. http://www.cancer.gov/about-cancer/causes-prevention/risk/obesity/obesity-fact-sheet. Accessed July 28, 2016.

55. Mehta M, Shike M. Diet and physical activity in the prevention of colorectal cancer. *J Natl Compr Canc Netw* 2014;12(12):1721–1726.

56. Bourke L, Gilbert S, Hooper R, et al. Lifestyle changes for improving disease-specific quality of life in sedentary men on long-term androgen-deprivation therapy for advanced prostate cancer: a randomised controlled trial. *Eur Urol* 2014;65(5):865–872.

57. Rock CL, Doyle C, Demark-Wahnefried W, et al. Nutrition and physical activity guidelines for cancer survivors. *CA Cancer J Clin* 2012;62(4):242–274.

58. Lundahl B, Moleni T, Burke BL, et al. Motivational interviewing in medical care settings: a systematic review and meta-analysis of randomized controlled trials. *Patient Educ Couns* 2013;93(2):157–168.

59. Deng T, Lyon CJ, Bergin S, Caligiuri MA, Hsueh WA. Obesity, inflammation, and cancer. *Annu Rev Pathol* 2016;11:421–449.

60. Hermsen S, Frost J, Renes RJ, Kerkhof P. Using feedback through digital technology to disrupt and change habitual behavior: a critical review of current literature. *Comput Human Behav* 2016;57:61–74.

61. Jakicic JM, Davis KK, Rogers RJ, et al. Effect of wearable technology combined with a lifestyle intervention on long-term weight loss: the IDEA randomized clinical trial. *JAMA* 2016;316(11):1161–1171.

62. Kushi LH, Doyle C, McCullough M, et al. American Cancer Society Guidelines on nutrition and physical activity for cancer prevention: reducing the risk of cancer with healthy food choices and physical activity. *CA Cancer J Clin* 2012;62(1):30–67.

63. American Institute for Cancer Research. *Weight—How Much We Weigh*. 2016. http://www.aicr.org/reduce-your-cancer-risk/weight/.

64. Gudzune KA, Doshi RS, Mehta AK, et al. Efficacy of commercial weight-loss programs: an updated systematic review. *Ann Intern Med* 2015;162(7):501–512.

65. Schleper A, Sullivan DK, Thrasher JB, et al. Weight management to reduce prostate cancer risk: a survey of men's needs and interests. *Cancer Clin Oncol* 2016;5(1):43–52.

66. Cauchi R. *Health Reform and Health Mandates for Obesity*. 2016. http://www.ncsl.org/research/health/aca-and-health-mandates-for-obesity.aspx.

67. Greenlee H, Sardo Molmenti CL, Falci L, et al. High use of complementary and alternative medicine among a large cohort of women with a family history of breast cancer: the Sister Study. *Breast Cancer Res Treat* 2016;156(3):527–538.

68. Heinonen OP, Albanes D. The effect of vitamin E and beta carotene on the incidence of lung cancer and other cancers in male smokers. *N Engl J Med* 1994;330(15):1029–1035.

69. Omenn GS, Goodman GE, Thornquist MD, et al. Effects of a combination of beta carotene and vitamin A on lung cancer and cardiovascular disease. *N Engl J Med* 1996;334(18):1150–1155.

70. Heinonen OP, Albanes D, Virtamo J, et al. Prostate cancer and supplementation with alpha-tocopherol and beta-carotene: incidence and mortality in a controlled trial. *J Natl Cancer Inst* 1998;90(6):440–446.

71. Klein EA, Thompson IM Jr., Tangen CM, et al. Vitamin E and the risk of prostate cancer: the Selenium and Vitamin E Cancer Prevention Trial (SELECT). *JAMA* 2011;306(14):1549–1556.

72. Guirguis-Blake J. Routine vitamin supplementation to prevent cancer and cardiovascular disease. *Am Fam Physician* 2004;70(3):559–560.

73. National Center for Complementary and Alternative Medicine. *Mind-Body Medicine Practices in Complementary and Alternative Medicine*. MD: National Institutes of Health; 2013.

74. Mason AE, Epel ES, Kristeller J, et al. Effects of a mindfulness-based intervention on mindful eating, sweets consumption, and fasting glucose levels in obese adults: data from the SHINE randomized controlled trial. *J Behav Med* 2016;39(2):201–213.

75. Katterman SN, Kleinman BM, Hood MM, Nackers LM, Corsica JA. Mindfulness meditation as an intervention for binge eating, emotional eating, and weight loss: a systematic review. *Eat Behav* 2014;15(2):197–204.

76. Chen F, Lv X, Fang J, et al. The effect of body-mind relaxation meditation induction on major depressive disorder: a resting-state fMRI study. *J Affect Disord* 2015;183:75–82.

77. Robb SW, Benson K, Middleton L, Meyers C, Hebert JR. Mindfulness-based stress reduction teachers, practice characteristics, cancer incidence, and health: a nationwide ecological description. *BMC Complement Altern Med* 2015;15:24.

78. Phillips KM, Antoni MH, Lechner SC, et al. Stress management intervention reduces serum cortisol and increases relaxation during treatment for nonmetastatic breast cancer. *Psychosom Med* 2008;70(9):1044–1049.

79. Antoni MH, Lechner S, Diaz A, et al. Cognitive behavioral stress management effects on psychosocial and physiological adaptation in women undergoing treatment for breast cancer. *Brain Behav Immun* 2009;23(5):580–591.

80. Bradt J, Dileo C, Magill L, Teague A. Music interventions for improving psychological and physical outcomes in cancer patients. *Cochrane Database Syst Rev* 2016(8):Cd006911.

81. American Cancer Society. *Global Cancer Facts and Figures*. 2nd ed. Atlanta, GA: American Cancer Society; 2011.

16

Aging, Brain Plasticity, and Integrative Preventive
Medicine

MICHAEL M. MERZENICH, PHD

A large body of evidence has been generated to describe, in elaborate
detail, the physical and functional decline of the brain as we age
beyond the typical human peak performance epoch in the 3rd–4th
decades of life.[1-3] The predominant medical view is that the primary source of
physical and functional deterioration in the brain derives from physical senes-
cence. Those processes often culminate in a catastrophic end-stage expressed
by emergent, progressive neuropathology (Alzheimer's, Parkinson's, etc.) associated with immune response and brain/vascular deterioration, and expressed
by rapid physical dis-elaboration, demyelination, degeneration, and apoptosis. Enormous capital and scientific investment has been predicated on this
view of age-related brain health, with a strong treatment focus directed toward
chemically or electrically manipulating catastrophic end-stage pathologies.

Neuroscience studies now strongly support a compelling alternative perspective.[4,5] By that view, the physical and functional changes described as
brain aging arise, to a large extent, as a product of progressive active "negative" neuroplasticity. Those natural negative-change processes arise as a product of brain-use histories that, by their nature, destructively impact brain
health—with ultimate pathological aging an *expected* end-stage of that long,
degrading negative-plasticity progression. We also now know that there is a
long list of medical vicissitudes that accelerate this negative brain plasticity,
shortening the progression to dementia or to other neuropathological end-
states. With little understanding of the forms of "brain exercise" required to
actually sustain brain health, and with a limited understanding of how medical
vicissitudes that plague our older-age populations contribute to accelerated
decline, average modern citizens—and the medical professionals who care for

them—understandably do a relatively poor job of sustaining the physical and functional integrity of this most important of human organs.

Importantly, while age-related deterioration in the background of life is, of course, an inexorable downhill path, lifestyle-driven physical and functional decline is not. Neuroplasticity science has shown that the negative neuroplasticity–driven changes that are a main source of age-related neurological limitations are, by their nature, reversible.[4-9] By that alternative view, the focus of medicine in older adults should be directed far more strongly toward *strengthening, managing, and sustaining* organic brain health—as opposed to a current strong medical focus on treating substantially irreversible catastrophic end-stage pathology. We envision a transition in neurological health practices in aging akin to the development of modern approaches for monitoring and sustaining cardiovascular health. In that domain, physicians now almost universally apply simple, inexpensive, objective, and reliable indices of general cardiovascular health (measurements of blood pressure and pulse rates; blood oxygenation; blood chemistry including cholesterol titers; EKGs) that provide a primary basis for cardiovascular and cardiorespiratory health management. With ongoing monitoring, and with these elementary diagnostic tools backed up by a hierarchy of more sophisticated assessment strategies, the clinician can effectively prescribe first lifestyle advice then pharmaceutical medicines, and then intervene with surgical procedures to manage and sustain health—all designed to prevent or at least delay cardiovascular catastrophe.

We now have an increasingly clear understanding of how to define risks of progression to senility and end-stage neurodegenerative illness—and measure the risks of onset of many other emergent psychiatric and neurological clinical indications—to similarly inform positive brain-health management strategies, using equivalently simple, reliable, and inexpensive primary assessment strategies backed up by a hierarchy of more-elaborate physical and functional assessment tools. Just as importantly, we have an increasingly clear understanding of how we can restore and sustain organ health, both in the "normally aging" population and in an increasing number of other clinical indications now shown to accelerate the advance to dementia and other later-life catastrophes. Over the next few years, clinicians responsible for brain health management can be expected to widely exploit these new, rapidly emerging diagnostic and treatment approaches.

Our goal here is to review aging and the brain from this important, alternative, still-underappreciated scientific and medical perspective. After a brief description of the history of brain plasticity–related neuroscience, change processes that shape our brains in ways that ultimately distinguish the typical struggling older versus peak-performing younger and more vibrantly functioning brain are described. We then consider how and why processes that contribute to our personal growth at a younger age are commonly (but not always) thrown into reverse at an older age, on the path to cognitive loss, negative physical brain change, infirmity, and ultimately, neuropathological catastrophe. We review the development of new brain science–based tools that appear to throw the "plasticity switch" for brain health back in a corrective and strengthening direction, where change processes again support the growth and the more reliable maintenance of physical and functional brain health. Finally, we summarize how this translational science shall almost certainly evolve to enable a new, neuroscience-directed medical era of brain health management for our older-age populations.

A Brief History of Brain Plasticity-Related Neuroscience

Over an initial long epoch from the time of the historical origins of brain science and neurological medicine, investigators believed that the development of human ability must be a product of physical ("plastic") changes in the brain. In the late 19th century, William James described those changes as being plausibly akin to the creation of a water channel by the continuous passage of water across a dry landscape.[10] With repetition, the channel deepens, as the passage of water becomes more reliable, more predictable, more certain. Many studies in the late 19th and early 20th century appeared to support the view that the brain was continuously physically "plastic"—remodeling itself by use—as abilities were refined or new skills were developed across an animal or human lifespan.[11]

Beginning in the middle of the 20th century, this perspective was challenged by neuroscientists and neurologists who directly studied plasticity across the course of postnatal development using more advanced experimental methods. Those studies were interpreted as showing that neuronal wiring and the functional elements (for example, specific neuron and glial cell populations) of the cerebral cortex were modifiable on a substantial scale in the first weeks to months of mammalian postnatal life—then "froze"—became "hard-wired" into an "adult" form—at the end of an early-life "critical period."[12-14]

This broad conclusion, arising from the mainstream of experimental neurology and neuroscience, had important negative and enduring societal and medical consequences. It led to a failure to understand, in medical practice, that specific forms of brain engagement were a primary determinant of the status of brain health and general physical health. Because almost every brain is continuously plastic, a remarkable capacity for brain change provides a basis for neurological improvement and possible recovery in almost every brain-struggling individual. Medical neurology still predominantly focuses on manipulating the dysfunctional or distorted brain by applying counterbalancing chemical or electrical or surgical interventions, underplaying the remarkable capacity that every brain has to change itself in an improving—and often, completely restorative—direction.

This misunderstanding contributed to the false presumption that the basis of success in school and in life was fundamentally genetically determined—that the abilities of the child determined at the time they entered the schoolhouse door, given their immutable brain hardware, deterministically defined their potential for achievement and success. It led to the still widely held societal belief that as custodians of our health and welfare, while physical exercise clearly matters for us, changes in our neurological abilities are beyond any very significant powers of self-repair.

Almost nothing could be further from the truth.

Importantly, even across the period of the 1950s through the 1980s, when this perspective of the brain as being "hard-wired" in early childhood began to dominate medical and social perspectives, investigators on the periphery of the medical neuroscience mainstream were actively demonstrating that the adult brain was *very* plastic. That counterargument initially came from physiological psychologists who were sharply focused on documenting the changes accounting for Pavlovian ("classical") behavioral conditioning. They repeatedly showed that pairing a stimulus with a following reward or punishment à la Pavlov and his contemporaries resulted in magnified representations of (1) that stimulus, (2) that reward or punishment, and (3) the "conditioned" responses that manifested the expectation of reward or punishment, demonstrating the establishment of neurological association.[15-18] Importantly, investigators showed that these broadly expressed neurological changes could be "reversed" by deconditioning an animal ("extinguishing" the association between the stimulus and the reward/punishment), achieved by repeatedly delivering formerly "conditioned" stimuli without associated rewards or punishments. Plasticity in adult brains, by its nature and at least in this elementary model, appeared to be strongly in play, and by its nature, reversible.

Beginning in the 1980s, we and others began to conduct studies that helped bring these findings into the medical neuroscience mainstream. Specifically, we showed that the brain undergoes large-scale remodeling following the manipulation of inputs associated with peripheral injury and loss,[19-23] studies that were rapidly extended to the human model. We documented large-scale changes achieved via operant conditioning (the predominant behavioral basis of human skill acquisition) that almost certainly account for our improvements and refinements of ability, and for the acquisition of any new skill.[24-29] We showed that the fundamental processing unit of the mammalian cerebral cortex (the cortical minicolumn) was "plastic," subject to large-scale positive or negative revision via specific forms of training, at any age.[25,29,30] We and others showed that plasticity followed (to the level of first approximation) a "Hebbian rule" (coincident input–dependent synaptic strengthening), which defined how changes related to task structures and demands, and with an understanding of the time and space constants involved, revealed to us how we could drive specific bidirectional changes in behavior or in brain machinery operations, at will.[22-23,31-34] We repeatedly showed that both temporal and spatial (or sound-frequency) aspects of stimulus-response selectivity and the refined neurological representations of simple and complex incoming information were plastic.[31,32,35,36] Large-scale remodeling of brain systems was easily achieved in adult primates, by engaging them in simple, progressive natural behaviors. We showed that it was possible to "grow" sequenced behaviors and the expectation or predictions that supported complex "mental" and physical actions, via appropriate forms of rule-based training.[37-39] We showed that we could drive large-scale plasticity that accounted for evident recovery of function in primate models of brain injury and stroke.[40,41] And we showed that *every* tested aspect of change appeared to be "reversible."[42-47] By progressive training, changes could be easily driven in a positive (improving) or negative (degrading) direction— paralleled by corresponding behavioral improvements or losses.

Thus, for example, training an adult monkey on one form of a behavioral task led to the predicted *elaboration, refinement, and expansion* of the cortical machinery supporting (for example) more facile hand use in stimulus identification or manually dexterous digital manipulation.[48,49] Training an adult monkey in a second form of the same task slowly *diselaborated, degraded, and reduced* the hand representation, dramatically shrinking the cortical territory dedicated to hand "representation" in the cerebral cortex, and ultimately catastrophically destroying the functional control of the hand.[29,50-52]

The demonstration that a medical condition like a focal hand dystonia could be induced by training—or more generally, that the cortical machinery that supports refined behaviors are, by their nature, easily driven in either a positive or negative direction—bore the very important implications that neurological and psychiatric disease progressions are (1) actually substantially manifesting natural, negative-plasticity progressions, and (2) are potentially subject to plastic reversal.[3-4,7,48]

On a Path to Developing Computerized Training Strategies to Drive Positive Changes in Neurological Ability

Those observations led us to direct our research efforts toward "harnessing the genie" of postcritical period ("adult") plasticity for the potential benefit of struggling human child and adult populations. In the initial phase of these efforts, we and others investigated the neurological mechanisms that control plastic change, because we knew that optimizing learning-enabling processes would be important for achieving efficient corrective brain remodeling in medical therapeutics. The key plasticity-enabling roles of neuromodulatory neurotransmitters and the operational rules that govern the machinery that controls their release and their cortical and subcortical actions have been richly elucidated by thousands of research studies over the subsequent several decades. We now understand the plasticity-enabling roles of acetylcholine, noradrenaline, serotonin, dopamine, and other modulatory neurotransmitters.[53-61] All have been shown to be expressed by machinery that is itself plastic; and the expression of these neurotransmitters in a learning context has been elucidated in ways that have helped us optimize training effectiveness, by appropriately controlling the timed activation and release of these crucial agents of change. These studies also helped explain one major source of confusion about plasticity in critical-period versus older brains. Scientists studying synaptic plasticity in the older brain had not fully appreciated the fact that the brain positively evolves its *control* of brain change across the early life of the brain. In the post-critical-period brain, changes are modulated as a function of both behavioral state and outcome, by a brain that can now "keep in mind" (hold, in "working memory") and evaluate whether or not it has achieved a training goal.[3,62] In the very young brain, these powerful plasticity-controlling processes are not yet functionally established, and mere exposure to a stimulus is sufficient for plastically modifying brain connections. By contrast, nonattended or behaviorally meaningless stimuli do not drive enduring, large-scale plastic change in the older brain because the older brain *controls* its remodeling, limiting change, in a sense, to those experiential or learning moments that it "judges to be good for it."[4,62]

This "purposeful" plasticity underlying the refinement of brain machinery and acquired skills and abilities, in place from early childhood forward to the end of life, is a *more* (not less) powerful and sophisticated mode of brain remodeling than is the "anything goes," substantially unregulated competitive plastic change processes in play in fetal and infant life.

The Complex Nature of Reversible Brain Plasticity

Plasticity is usually described in positive connection-remodeling terms. Indeed, on the most elementary level, selective synaptogenesis and synaptic strengthening for inputs that provide the basis for skill acquisition and refinement are core achievements of positive plastic remodeling, and the processes underlying these positive connection-change processes have been exhaustively studied.[63-66] At the same time, in brain change processes, nonselected (task-irrelevant) synapses weaken or turn over, as task-relevant synapses strengthen or emerge—and positive and negative changes in synaptic connection strengths represent just one of *many* aspects of experience-induced remodeling that contribute to evolving brain function and organic brain health.

Beginning about a decade ago, we asked, What large-scale physical, chemical, and functional differences distinguish high-performing from struggling brains? [6,7,9] Studies were conducted in the brains of animals in the prime of life, compared with the brains of animals struggling with aging-related deficits near the end of life. In those rat model experiments and in follow-on studies, we (and others) ultimately documented the status of more than 20 major physical, chemical, and functional aspects of brain function and organic brain health. Those indices include (1) receptive field sizes and complex-feature extraction; (2) the orderliness of cortical "maps" (representational topographies); (3) stimulus-evoked excitatory- and inhibitory-response magnitudes; (4) coordination of local neuronal responses underlying controlled, reliable cortical system functioning; (5) excitatory and inhibitory response dynamics; (6) processing speed (cortical "sampling rate"); (7) responses to modulated stimuli; (8) the fidelity and reliability of representation of temporal structure (stimulus durations, intervals, sequences); (9) receptors and receptor subunits controlling specific excitatory and inhibitory responses; (10) intracortical and subcortical tract myelination; (11) numbers and morphologies of parvalbumin inhibitory interneurons; (12) elaboration of dendritic processes of excitatory pyramidal cells;[68] (13) numbers and morphologies of somatostatin interneurons;[69] (14); expression of a brain-derived neurotrophin (BDNF); (15) background neuronal process noise (spontaneous activity; "neuronal chatter"); (16) response adaptation strength, and dynamics; (17) responses to "distractors" in an attended behavioral state; (18) integrity and levels of expression of the neuromodulators of plasticity (acetylcholine; norepinephrine; serotonin; dopamine); and (19) neurotransmitter transporter expression; (20) among other measures.

All of these indices of brain health were shown to substantially differ in aged infirm versus young, vigorous animals. *Every* difference substantially *dis*advantaged the older adult.

In those older animals, we asked, How many of these now-negative indices of physical, functional, and chemical brain function and health are reversible? And how complex would training engagement have to be, with what dosing, to drive changes sharply back in a rejuvenating direction? The answer: *All of them were reversible*. In this animal (rat) model, every physical, chemical, and functional difference that differentiated a struggling older brain from a healthy young adult brain was reversed to a status that approached or equaled that of "young, healthy-adult normalcy" by applying only two simple, specific forms of progressive computer-controlled training over a training epoch of about 1 month (about 25 training hours).[6,7,9]

It might be noted that the intensive, progressive, computer-controlled exercises applied in these rat studies were not conventional "cognitive training tasks." One focused on progressively improving the accuracy of distinguishing elementary incoming signals from increasingly confusable background stimuli, at speed. The second required the animal to first identify (by its behavioral responding) an elementary target stimulus—then hold that stimulus in working memory for long continuously attended epochs, correctly signaling its random recurrence when it was presented in the presence of progressively more confusable background distractors. For us, these training tasks are "brain training" vehicles—as compared with higher-level performance task training usually applied in "cognitive training" programs.

ACCELERATING AGING

The fundamental reversibility of changes generated by natural plasticity processes demonstrated by these studies was further illustrated by an additional experiment in which brain aging was accelerated, simply by maintaining vigorous young adult rats in high-acoustic-noise environments. In that setting, levels of background spontaneous activity—meaningless background "chatter" in the auditory brain—were substantially elevated. Surprisingly rapid *negative* plastic changes were induced, and within a few weeks in these animals, the physical and functional status of their brains again matched, *for all recorded indices*, those documented in physically deteriorated near-end-of-life animals.[67] This is one of several indications that brain noise—meaningless neuronal response chatter— or, from another perspective, the degradation of local response coordination resulting from a continuous bombardment of a brain system by unstructured background activity—has a strong direct or indirect controlling impact on the remarkable changes in gene expression that must underlie this coordinated, multifaceted, reversible plasticity. Initiate the right forms of training in the old rat, and hundreds of genes must change their expression *together*, on the turn of a dime, with all processes changing in a coordinated way to "shift" from the negative ("clastic") progression that characterizes aging, to a positive rejuvenating ("blastic") direction. Bombard a brain system at the peak of a performance growth (blastic) life phase—in this case in healthy, vigorous prime-of-life adulthood—with continuous ongoing meaningless noise, and all of those same genes change their expressions, on the turn of a dime, *to progress in the opposite clastic direction*, again in a remarkably coordinated manner.

These broad, coordinated, bidirectional experience-driven changes in elemental neurology related to brain function *and its organic health* are at the center of any consideration of brain health growth or maintenance—or decline—in human populations.

Physical Brain Changes Recorded in Aging Humans Are Substantially a Product of "Negative" Brain Plasticity

It should be noted that all of the changes recorded above are expressed, of course, by physical brain alterations.[3,4-9] As the brain elaborates its dendrites and axonal arbors and astrocytic processes through intensive engagement, cortical volumes grow. As the brain increases local response coordination and sharpens all of the fast excitatory and inhibitory processes in cortical networks, it grows myelin and positively enables physically more powerful local and system connectivities. Progressive changes in speed of processing and temporal precision necessarily derive from chemical changes in receptors and from physical changes in synapses and networks, neuropil elaboration, and in physical changes that underlie the powers of action of specific excitatory and inhibitory neuron—and astrocyte—populations. Changes in response coordination arising from this physical remodeling directly impact feedforward coincidence-dependent plasticity, thereby generating a cascade of functional and physical changes at every "higher" brain system level.

Coordinated changes in the "negative" direction are expressed as slowly, progressively degrading physical changes that culminate in the physically shrunken and disconnected brain of most near-end-of-life individuals. In this clastic progression, the brain weakens its connections, down-regulates metabolic processes in progressively disengaged forebrain machinery, slowly diselaborates dendritic and axonal arbors, progressively simplifies and shrinks its neuropil, degrades the integrity of the blood-brain barrier and the reactive hyperemia and immune response powers supported by deteriorating astrocyte populations, slowly loses its inhibitory powers, necessarily changes its chemistry to support now-sluggish operations, down-regulates neurotrophins, and slowly disconnects and down-regulates the neuromodulatory machinery that controls plasticity itself—among other documented natural physical neuroclastic changes. The folly of believing that all these changes could be expected to be reversed at a late stage of what is usually a decades-long clastic progression by any singular pharmaceutical redistortion, has been repeatedly borne out by the numerous failed attempts to overcome this grand panoply of negative changes via any simple chemical agency. True restoration of function requires that the plasticity "switch" be thrown back in a blastic direction. From a neuroplasticity perspective, even after that switch is thrown, necessary restorative changes can *only* be achieved through intensive, positive, progressive, natural brain machinery remodeling.

ONSET OF ALZHEIMER'S, PARKINSON'S, AND OTHER NEURODEGENERATIVE DISORDERS AS AN EXPECTED CATASTROPHIC END-STAGE OF PROGRESSIVE NEUROLOGICAL DETERIORATION

As the brain progressively disassembles itself via negative plasticity, the immune-response machinery in brain tissues is challenged both to clear cellular debris and to rise to protect the brain from blood-borne agents that can "invade" it via an increasingly "leaky" blood-brain barrier.[71-73] In parallel, immunoreactive glial cells and the brain machinery that modulates their actions are functionally degraded because their integrity is also almost certainly a product of coordinated negative brain plasticity. In the face of these complex changes, experimental neurologists have posited many theories, expressed via several hundred specific posited variations, about the causes of neuropathological degeneration and collapse defined as Alzheimer's disease. Frequently described causes, not considered in any detail here, include (1) accelerated biological aging; (2) progressive brain system disconnection; (3) cholinergic and other modulation system failures; (4) weakened expression of trophic factors supporting processes of regeneration and renewal; (5) a leaky blood-brain barrier enabling access for infectious and other agents from blood or cerebrospinal fluid compartments; (6) a deterioration in reactive hyperemia supporting brain nutrition and blood-based immune responses; (7) immune system dysfunction for processes intrinsic for brain tissues; (8) environmental factors (head injury, poisons, and many others); (9) genetic factors, for example, resulting in amyloid precursor protein formation, in presenilin, and/ or in allelic variations in apolipoprotein E; (10) oxidative metabolism (mitochrondrial) dysfunction; (11) and others.[74,75]

From a neuroplasticity perspective, in a negative plasticity–driven scenario, *all* of these factors are *expected* to be progressively clastically changing, because declining individuals' environmentally driven experiential activities do not effectively support the positive maintenance of their brain health. As a result, brain systems are progressively disconnecting, acetylcholine expression and the metabolic status of neurons in the basal nucleus of Meynert (and for other modulatory neurotransmitters, in the dorsal raphe nucleus, the locus coeruleus, the ventral tegmental area, and substantia nigra) are down-regulated, the blood-brain barrier is leaky, reactive hyperemia is compromised, and intrinsic immune response actions are degraded because of both negative astrocytic and neuromodulatory changes. Environmental factors add to risks of onset specifically because they add to the brain noise ("chatter") that accelerates negative change. Genetic weaknesses specifically accelerate amyloid poisoning, with resulting differential inhibitory cell apoptosis and disconnection again directly amplifying neuronal "chatter" (reducing the capacity for sustaining local response-coordination powers). In progressively degenerating brain systems, the correlated patterns of action are most difficult to sustain at "highest" system levels. Their deterioration presages later brain-wide disaster.

It is important to understand that in the months, years, or decades preceding this emergent catastrophe, at least most of these negative changes were reversible. The negative expressions and neurological change consequences in what is usually a long, slow progression of *all* of these "causes" can be positively altered by coordinated plastic remodeling driven by simple, intensive forms of brain engagement. As for genetics, because few if any inherited weaknesses confer a certain progression to dementia onset,[76] appropriate intensive training driving blastic changes might be expected to at least delay the onset of emergent neuropathology

Living a Life to the Disadvantage of Your Brain

Why *does* "chatter" grow in the brain as you grow older? The elemental processing of information by the brain is an achievement in the extraction of details against environmental and intrinsic brain activities, from the brain's representation of information delivered from our senses and upstream input sources within cortical systems. We progressively challenge our brain to extract more refined, higher-speed, and more complexly received information in the early phase of our lives, as we slowly advance the machinery that supports our growing neurobehavioral capabilities. "Adult" plasticity contributing to extraction of details with high accuracy at speed is controlled by our capacity for "selective attention" (a neurological process that is often confusedly called "working memory" or "prediction" by cognitive psychologists). As we process information in progressively more complicated ways in our operations in guided behavior and thought, we slowly refine and strengthen this higher-level plasticity-controlling machinery. This progressive refinement is marked by the "completion" of the myelination of cortico-cortical connections to "highest" brain levels at circa age 20.[77,78] Why do the performance characteristics of our neurological processing machinery then usually lead to that slow, progressive decline from the broad neuroblastic peak of young adulthood to the infirmities of an older age?

We have argued that our younger lives are a skill-learning and abilities-refinement epoch, which strongly supports continuous positive plasticity. In the middle years of life, we begin to rely more heavily on well-learned abilities acquired earlier, operating over progressively more hours in the day deploying mastered (automatized) behaviors supported by nondeclarative (habit-supporting) memories. As we operate with greater automaticity and on greater schedules of mental abstraction, we pay progressively less attention to the *details* of our refined neurological operations—for example, to what we hear or feel or see. With that neglect, the encoding of those details—the platform abilities that support all higher-order actions—slowly, inexorably diselaborate. We hypothesize that the basic change in course from a blastic to a clastic phase arises from a slow inexorable growth of process noise (or, expressed in an alternative way, from coherent-response discoordination) in the middle decades of life. Neurons now respond in a progressively less coordinated way; less salient cortical signaling is more prone to error. As error rates grow, negative plastic changes that assure sustained functional control ("getting the answer right") slowly, broadly, negatively impact brain health status.

We have likened these changes to those that occur in a professional musician who has acquired her elaborate, specialized instrumental performance skills through intensive practice.[4] If such an individual attenuates the practicing required to sustain their high-level skills, noise (manifested by imprecision in performance control) slowly grows in their brain and their performance ability necessarily declines—ultimately to a level in which they can no long perform at a professional level. At the same time, any new intense extended practice epoch in just the right forms in such a professional can bring their refined abilities (neuroblastically) all the way back to a high performance level—because the underlying governing plasticity in their (in every) brain is, by its nature, reversible.

Other lifestyle changes that often apply for older lives are especially important to understand. For example, many older people substantially voluntarily withdraw from new-skill learning or experiential challenges. In their stereotypical behavioral realm, little positive plastic change occurs and the unexercised machinery that controls sustained attention and plasticity itself slowly down-regulates. Close attention in a task environment in which an attending brain recognizes performance advances is a prerequisite for positive, health-sustaining plastic change.

A second neurological aspect of "just taking it easy" in a stereotypic life involves the broader engagement on tasks that are errorless. In animal models, errorless tasks have no impact on brain health status.[28,79,80] On the other hand, tasks that continually challenge performance ability while assuring a reasonable level of (but never certain) success strongly enable positive brain-healthy change.

Note that maintaining high functionality in the machinery that *controls* brain change is a key. This modulatory control machinery is up-regulated in a life that is marked by continuous new skill learning and by a rich schedule of positive novel experiences. Predominantly applied skills that were mastered and reduced to automaticity decades before (e.g., reading) have value to the individual in their ongoing personal self-development, but only limited value for the maintenance of brain health. To sustain its physical and functional integrity, the brain requires a life marked by continuous skill learning extending down to the most elemental levels of signal reception and manipulation.

Unfortunately, from the perspective of our plastic brains, modern environments are designed to minimize the necessity of our operating with high input resolution and speed, especially in elementary (platform) skill domains. The average citizen spends the majority of their waking hours in a sitting posture, grossly limiting conditions for natural input refinement, and grossly underexercising the translation of neurological operations into action. Many hours are spent as relatively passive receivers of inputs delivered on screens and audio speakers, again minimizing the translation of neurological operations into actions beyond emotional responding. Our world is paved, and movement through it is largely automatized. In a natural world, every footfall is uncertain. The modern human is thereby deprived of thousands of moments of adjustments in fast vision and in posture that were everyday brain exercise in our human ancestors. In our modern world, we increasingly more often look up answers rather than probe our memories or exercise our reasoning powers to find them. We rely on machines in our navigation, curtailing our practice at closely attending to and recording landmarks mounted on a serial framework of time and place, so important for sustaining organic brain health. Modern humans operate on a higher level of self-directed abstraction, "buried" in their thoughts or in their narrow interactions with their hand-held devices.

All of these modern "advances" advantage our higher-order human operations. At the same time, when carried to excess, they separately and collectively make a substantial contribution to the growth of "chatter" in our neurological machinery.

In addition to lifestyle contributions, there is a very long list of other things that can happen in an adult life that add to brain "noise," accelerating and increasing the risks of a passage to dementia. Brain infections, brain poisoning, antipsychotic and antidepressant drugs, a history of mental illness, numerous historic developmental impairments, historic or concurrent concussive and other traumatic brain injuries, brain bleeds, subdural hematomas, blood-brain barrier compromise associated with ICU delirium, heart failure, multiple sclerosis, diabetes, extended grief, auto-immune disease, loss of mobility, an extended period of high stress, dysregulated sleep, atherosclerosis, multiple sclerosis, and a long list of genetic disorders are just a few of more than a hundred epidemiologically documented examples. Importantly, all of these conditions plausibly result in increased noisiness in cortical processes in the brain that can be expected to result in (and have often been directly shown to result in) associated negative changes in what we view as indices of organic brain health status (for example, processing speed).[4]

Applying This Science to Improve Brain Health in Normal and Struggling Human Populations

We began practical studies for applying this science to help struggling brains by creating programs designed to restore more normal neurological functioning in children that struggled in school because of impairments in speech and language that usually led to reading failure.[4,76,81] We've successfully helped several million children overcome these impairments, through intensive, progressive computerized training. While it is beyond our ability to consider these programs in detail here, that training has been shown to generalize in neurological impact to drive broad, corrective behavioral and neurological changes in the great majority of children who have used it.

With the benefits of this early experience in training child populations, we applied the same science to create the BrainHQ computer training platform[82] to address neurological and psychiatric limitations and distortions in many clinical indications impacting mature individuals. In parallel, a growing number of other scientists have created "cognitive training" tools that have been widely applied in humans. For us, strengthening and sustaining the neurological status of normal older individuals ultimately at risk for dementia onset has been a primary objective. In this respect, our approach differs from that applied by at least most other providers of "cognitive training" tools because our primary goal is to rejuvenate or normalize the neurological assets that support organ function. This approach is predicated on the assumption that with appropriate more-elementary neurological strengthening and recovery of function, more complex behavioral abilities (the primary target of most "cognitive training" tools) and the capacity for new learning can be expected to be broadly positively advanced.

In application, these adaptive, progressive brain-training tools demonstrate that at least most of the rejuvenating changes documented in animal studies of reversible neuroplasticity must also apply for humans. We have engaged tens to hundreds of thousands of individuals on more than 30 elementary training tasks, documenting their performance gains for individuals of all ages. In humans as in rats, performance at every elementary ability rises to a peak across the second into the third decade of life, then systematically and progressively declines out to the end of life. After training, performance abilities in the 8th decade of life (for example) come close to matching—or can exceed—the ability recorded in untrained young peak-performing adults for every elementary neurological ability. These changes in signal resolution, speed of processing, identification and manipulation of rapidly successive inputs, phasic and sustained attention, divided attention, and others, *require* progressive, positive coordinated physical changes in their brain, akin if not identical to the coordinated physical changes recorded in our animal models. Collectively, those presumptive blastic changes manifest a substantial training-driven improvement of organic brain health.

Applying Computerized Brain Training to Strengthen Then Sustain Brain Health-Relevant Neurological Ability in Older-Aged Individuals

Studies of training designed to grow and sustain brain health conducted in animal and human models have evolved into computerized strategies for driving these changes with relatively high efficiency via a game-like software platform. Training exercises at BrainHQ.com are adaptive, adjusting in difficulty as a function of performance ability, and advancing progressively in difficulty as gains are achieved in training. By controlling task difficulty to assure general performance success while sustaining a continuously demanding task level, enduring improvements can be generated with relatively high efficiency. Tasks are organized in an "Angry Birds" format, in which a trainee is asked to progressively improve at an elemental skill or ability within several-minute-long training blocks, at a series of 20–80 progressively more difficult training levels. Most tasks are progressively speed challenged; as each new training "box" (level) is "unlocked," judgments must be made about progressively briefer or more rapidly sequential stimulus events, and responding must be speeded. Note that (1) improvements in accurately identifying successive stimuli at speed engender positive changes in most of the dimensions of brain health described earlier for animal and human studies; (2) the progressive degradation in processing speed is a signature deficit in aging;[83,84] and (3) processing speed is *the* largest single factor contributing to the variance in complex human performance ability—for example, to fluid intelligence.[85,86]

Tasks are also specifically designed to progressively up-regulate elementary processes controlling plasticity itself. With appropriate training, the slower learning rates and the greater number of "false positive responses" again long identified as a signature problem in aging can usually be restored to a substantially more youthful level.[87] Importantly, recovery of the powers of modulatory control provide a basis for strengthening other elemental aspects of brain health: increased up-regulation of norepinephrine, serotonin, acetylcholine, somatostatin, dopamine, and other modulatory neurotransmitters contribute importantly (1) to recovering and sustaining the integrity of the blood-brain barrier, and facile reactive hyperemia; (2) to modulating the brain's immune response; (3) to the regulation of sleep; (4) to baseline levels of brightness/ arousal; and (5) to the regulation of mood.

Task achievements also progress in other dimensions that can only be accounted for by more refined neurological processing. One set of tasks is specifically designed to accelerate input sampling rates in listening and in vision, in the latter case by driving improvements in saccade (fast-eye-movement) rates in active visual exploration. One set is designed to expand an individual's command of the visual horizon, and to sharpen their monitoring of unexpected, changing, and often-subtle visual or auditory events in their local environment. One set is designed to elevate attentiveness, and at the same time magnify the suppression of responses to meaningless distractors—together, keys to sustained attending. One set is designed to clarify the representation of the fast-changing details of what you see or hear, on the path to improving your ability to indelibly record (remember) them. One set is designed to specifically sharpen elemental aspects of your social cognitive ability; another to recover navigation abilities—together, keys for sustaining control of social and physical landscapes.

These Brain Plasticity-Based Strategies Have Been Shown to Be Effective for Improving the Elementary Neurological Abilities of Individuals of All Ages

For every training task, strong, expected improvements in ability are recorded as a rule. Importantly, training is not designed *only* to improve an individual's fundamental neurological machinery. A second equally important goal is to drive *general* improvements in brain health by driving positive changes in the operational characteristics of the processing machinery of the brain that support general, *broad* gains in performance ability. Many studies have now documented generalized ("real life") gains in abilities resulting from this training, in normally aging and in variously neurologically struggling adult populations.

In the Advanced Cognitive Training for Independent and Vital Elderly (ACTIVE) trial,[88] an older-age population of more than 700 subjects (mean age 74) versus 700 controls was trained at a computerized visual task that had many of the core speed, accuracy, attention, and sequence-reconstruction challenges described earlier as important contributors to brain health status. The BrainHQ version of this "useful field of view" (UFOV) task (*Double Decision*) was originally developed by Karlene Ball and Daniel Roenker[89] to address peripheral vision and fast-responding deficits that increased the crash risks for older drivers. In their task, subjects are required to identify brief, confusable stimuli near the center of visual gaze, then report on the location of a second briefly flashed stimulus presented in the visual surround. Task variables were stimulus durations for both central and peripheral stimuli, interstimulus intervals separating central and peripheral stimuli, magnitudes of differences between target and foil stimuli, the confusability of target stimuli with visual backgrounds, and the eccentricity of peripherally flashed stimuli. The reliably achieved goals of this computerized training were (1) an expansion of the "useful field of view" (which progressively contracts in normal aging); (2) the recovery of fast recognition speed and fast responding; and (3) the restoration of attention-based visual monitoring, response amplification, and attention network operations.

In this component of the large, multifaceted ACTIVE trial,[88] subjects who were trained adaptively for 5 hours at this computer-delivered task (following 5 hours of nonadaptive engagement) had a roughly twofold increase in their neurological "speed of processing." Trainees completed timed independent activities of daily living (IADLs) at correspondingly faster rates.[90,91] When subjects completed brief "booster training" sessions at +1 and +3 years, stronger and longer-sustained gains in speed of processing (SOP) and larger and stronger timed IADL gains were recorded; scientists concluded that maintaining full benefits from the initial training epoch would require about 1 hour of additional UFOV "booster training" per annum.[92]

As a result of this limited epoch of computerized training, these (average) 74-year-olds aging to 84-year-olds had about half as many driver-caused traffic accidents over at least the first 6 trial years.[93,94] They were more successful is sustaining their driving mobility, and drove more confidently over longer distances in their more active everyday lives.[95-97] Trainees were significantly less likely to develop "senior depression" following training.[98,99] If depression did arise, it was in a less severe form.[100] The confidence that trainees could manage their own affairs was higher over the initial 5-year post-training epoch.[101] Self-rated health and quality of life were significantly better in trained than in untrained individuals.[102,103] Medical costs savings in the trained cohort were estimated to be about $1,000/subject over the initial 5 years of the study. At a +10-year benchmark (7 years following the completion of the very limited booster "doses" of computerized training) individuals that had completed booster sessions had processing speeds—again, a signature deficit of aging correlated strongly with aged infirmity[83,84]—that were still higher than before training initiation a decade earlier.[104] These speed of processing benefits transferred to timed-IADL scores that still distinguished trainees from controls at the +10-year benchmark.

Given these compelling demonstrations of enduring and generalized neurobehavioral impacts, it was not surprising that these investigators have more recently shown that engaging in this single, simple progressive, attention-demanding, computerized visual task for 10–18 hours (again, with only 5–13 hours of that training delivered in a progressively challenging form, as in *Double Decision* on BrainHQ), resulted in a lower probability of dementia onset over the 10-year period following training initiation.[105,106] Protection against dementia onsets was dose-related. For the entire computer task-trained population, risks were about one-third as high as risks recorded for randomly assigned untrained control cohort. For individuals who had completed brief "booster sessions" at +1-year and +3-year benchmarks risks of dementia onset recorded across this 10-year epoch—in which the average age of trial participants advanced from 74 to 84—were roughly cut in half.[105,106] This is the first randomized controlled trial applying *any* intervention that has been shown to provide apparent protection against dementia onset on this scale.

It is difficult to imagine how time could have been better spent, for these older volunteers, than at this 10 to 18 hours of computerized training at this progressive, elementary inherently neuroblastic exercise. It is almost certain that even modestly higher and more regular dosing could have increased and extended the duration of this apparent intensive-training-provided protection.

It might be noted that two other cohorts that were trained with equal intensity in ACTIVE using noncomputerized classroom strategies to improve memory and reasoning/cognitive skills designed to be habitually deployed in their older lives also very clearly benefited from training—but with no significant benefits with regard to protection from dementia onset over this 10-year epoch.[88,104-106] It should also be noted that positive training impacts have been shown, in other studies, to be substantially independent of age, and independent of whether or not training is self-administered at home on an Internet-connected device or completed in a supervised classroom setting as in ACTIVE.[106-108]

In part because the long-running ACTIVE trial was initiated more than a decade ago, only limited longitudinal brain recording and imaging analyses have been conducted in individuals trained over these durations with this multifaceted (divided attention; speed; reception accuracy; restoration of peripheral vision) elemental visual signal processing task. Those limited studies documented a clear up-regulation of attention modulation and attention network status.[109,110]

Many other randomly assigned, controlled outcomes studies have recorded positive changes in abilities that can be viewed as indices of brain health status, both in normally aging individuals and in subject populations at higher risks for early dementia onset. In the Improvement in Memory with Plasticity-Based Adaptive Cognitive Training (IMPACT) trial, nearly 500 subjects were engaged by either adaptive computerized listening training (BrainHQ) programs or alternative (control) computer games and exercises, over a 40-hour-long training period.[108,111,112] In this elemental listening speed and accuracy training study, gains in trained versus control groups documented strong exercise-driven impacts, and recorded extensive generalization to nontrained abilities extending to general improvements in quality of life. Speed of processing for listening—an elemental ability manifesting necessarily broad neuroblastic remodeling—increased roughly threefold, which translated to a rejuvenation to match the performance level on this assessment of an individual in their 20s or 30s. Gains at higher-level cognitive abilities translated to a reversal in age-related performance on the broader RBANS battery and on memory-for-speech assessments, in an intent-to-treat analysis, that was equivalent to an 11- to 13-year rejuvenation. If a small noncompliant trainee cohort was removed from the analysis, benefits for completers translated to 15- to 18-year "age-performance reversal." At the same time, benefits appeared to fall back toward the baseline more rapidly than in the intensive visual training applied in ACTIVE.[113] This and other studies indicate that sustaining higher-level listening abilities may require a more significant level of ongoing training engagement.

The major behavioral outcomes of these studies were broadly confirmed in other randomly assigned, controlled trials that applied the same multifaceted listening training programs.[114-119] Kraus and colleagues extended these findings by showing that training positively impacted aural speech reception in acoustic noise. With plastic remodeling, auditory brainstem responses representing the spectral and temporal details of speech-related acoustic inputs were renormalized in trained older individuals. These investigators also documented a fall-off in training-generated benefits over time; at a +6-month benchmark, the brainstem still more sharply represented acoustic inputs, but earlier improvements documented for listening in noise were significantly reduced.[120] These studies indicate, again, that more consistent "booster training" may be required to sustain ongoing performance (and brain health?) benefits in the listening modality in humans.

Other randomly assigned, controlled outcomes trials have documented benefits of training that appear to manifest positive neuroclastic change, and that often directly document (in a piecemeal way) evidence of physical remodeling. Those studies have targeted patients with mild cognitive impairment,[121-125] older-age individuals who have endured long-standing HIV-AIDS infections,[126,127] cancer patients who have undergone intensive chemotherapy,[128] stroke patients,[129-133] patients with major depressive disorder[99] or schizophrenia,[134-140] in patients following heart failure[141,142] or multiple sclerosis[143]—among other clinical indications. All studies provide evidence of positive improvements in elemental performance abilities (e.g., gains in processing speed and accuracy) that infer that training is driving positive neuroblastic growth. In most of these studies, the training of more elementary neurological abilities transferred to documented gains in everyday skills indexing these patients' qualities of life.

Beyond Training on a Computer: An Integrated Approach to Sustaining Brain Health

In parallel with our efforts to create neuroscience-inspired brain exercise strategies, other scientists have repeatedly documented the brain-health benefits of other older-age life-style practices. Living your life to the advantage of your brain obviously extends beyond intensive, progressive brain exercises!

For example, there are many hundreds of studies demonstrating the value of adopting a brain-healthy diet[144,145] and for intelligently supplementing or restricting that diet to meet brain health[146] and brain-age-related[147] nutritional needs. Many studies have shown clear benefits of a regular program of physical exercise and balance training extending beyond the support of general health and mobility to reveal specific, positive impacts on neurological health and cognitive (e.g., attention control) ability.[148-153] Social engagement on a level that assures the maintenance of the machinery that supports social cognition and positive mood has also been repeatedly confirmed to contribute to an individual's "cognitive reserve" and to support positive changes and the healthy maintenance of cognitive and action-control abilities.[154-156] Maintaining healthy sleep schedules has also been directly related to sustaining organic brain health.[157,158]

Physical exercises and nutritional supplementation can be of especially high value to the mature brain.[146,148] Sustaining unimpaired mobility, if at all possible, is obviously important for enabling an active brain-healthy experiential engagement with the world. From a neuroplasticity perspective, physical exercise strategies that engage and continuously elaborate the neurological control of actions in a closely attended task setting is an important aspect of any well-ordered older life. Note that progressively exercising the "master movement controller" capabilities of your brain is very different from physical exercise in a typical structured gym environment, or in any conventional form of relatively stereotypical exercise. From the perspective of brain health, the most valuable forms of physical exercise require that you engage in active, progressive, challenging *physical skill learning*. If such exercises are undertaken with appropriate energy and enthusiasm, they can also provide an individual with the additional benefits attributed to aerobics, which by itself is argued to have positive impacts on neuromodulatory and attention-related processes in the brain.[148,149]

For most individuals, all of these goals can be achieved by engaging in physical activities that do not employ stereotypic (e.g., exercise machine–implemented) exercise strategies, that are richly and continuously variable in the action control that they command, that by their nature naturally provide a basis for social interaction, and that provide a basis for progressive motor skill improvement over an extended period of time. Aerobically demanding, fast-responding net games (like tennis, pickle ball, badminton, table tennis), off-road bicycling, off-the-sidewalk walking (hiking, rock climbing, bird-watching, etc.), field games, afoot on the golf course or the trout stream working very hard to improve your skills, ball-room dancing, singing then choir practice—or a hundred other activities—can help fulfill these real-life brain-healthy physical exercise goals.

As we consider the likely scenarios for the medical management of brain health, we envisage a tiered approach beginning with lifestyle adjustments, on the path to assuring that simple behavioral biomarkers are being sustained within safe bounds. While many contemporary practitioners argue for the specific importance of dietary adjustments, or social or physical activities to grow cognitive reserve and sustain brain health, all of these factors can be expected to play a role in integrated brain health management programs. At the same time, it must be remembered that the deterioration and progressive distortion of brain wiring in the aging brain can *only* be restored to normalcy—and ultimately, can only be sustained—via progressive *brain* exercises.

Summary and Conclusions

Scientists have now richly documented the fact and nature of adult brain plasticity, through many thousands of research studies conducted in animal and human models. We now know that almost every aspect of fundamental neurology related to brain performance and organic brain health is plastic, that the processes underlying brain change are remarkably reversible, and that positive growth and negative reductive phases involve broadly coordinated remodeling. Importantly, we understand at a first level how to "throw the switch" to drive changes in a "negative" clastic or a "positive" clastic direction. Broadly expressed changes in elementary functional status and organic brain health status are a product of surprisingly elementary forms of intensive training.

Although data documenting the long-term benefits of these therapeutic strategies are still limited, two large controlled trials have now documented broadly beneficial impacts resulting from limited training doses. Their positive outcomes directly inspire the implementation of new strategies for managing organic brain health. We now know that a determination of processing speed and accuracy, attention control, and distractor suppression powers collectively index the status of a complex array of coordinated physical-chemical processes. Measuring their status can be achieved at low cost, at a first level, in a 20- to 30-minute-long procedure on any smart device, delivered and controlled via the cloud. Those assessment data can be easily conveyed to attending physicians and therapists, to help them manage their patients' brain health. Our research efforts are now directed toward determining what constitutes "safe" performance levels, indexing the status of organic brain health. We envision the use of these simple biomarkers as a primary screening tool for evaluating brain health status.

Brain medicine shall now almost certainly evolve from its focus on the treatment of neurological catastrophe in all of its psychiatric and neuropathological forms to a far stronger emphasis on prophylaxis and prevention, guided by ongoing assessment strategies that both help secure enduring patient safety and continuously document treatment effectiveness. A crucial aspect of this transformation shall be the growing understanding of how lifestyle factors (including dietary supplement and nutritional strategies and physical activities) contribute positively (and negatively) to brain health status, because as in other domains of medicine, the first line of defense for sustaining brain health shall be to ask the patient to live their life to the advantage of the health of this most important of their human organs—because when it dies, now far too often before the body dies, the person that that brain has so magically created is lost to the world.

The adoption of these neuroscience-informed brain health management strategies can be expected to radically transform brain health–related medicine over the next decade.

References

1. Yankner BA, Lu T, Loerch P. The aging brain. *Ann Rev Pathol* 2008;3:41–66.
2. Jagust W, D'Esposito M. *Imaging the Aging Brain*. Oxford: Oxford University Press; 2009.

3. Weiner MW, Veitch DP, Aisen PS, et al. The Alzheimer's Disease Neuroimaging Initiative: a review of papers published since its inception. *Alzheimers Dement* 2012;S1–68. doi: 10.1016/j.jalz.2011.09.172.

4. Merzenich MM. *Soft-Wired*. San Francisco, CA: Parnassus; 2014.

5. Merzenich MM, Van Vleet TM, Nahum M. Brain plasticity-based therapeutics. *Front Hum Neurosci* 2014;8:385. doi: 10.3389/fnhum.2014.00385.

6. de Villers-Sidani E, Alzghoul L, Zhou X, Simpson KL, Lin RC, Merzenich MM. Recovery of functional and structural age-related changes in the rat primary auditory cortex with operant training. *PNAS* 2010;107:13900–13905.

7. De Villers-Sidani E, Merzenich MM. Lifelong plasticity in the rat auditory cortex: basic mechanisms and role of sensory experience. *Prog Brain Res* 2011;191:119–131.

8. Nahum M, Lee H, Merzenich MM. Principles of neuroplasticity-based rehabilitation. *Prog Brain Res* 2013;207:141–171.

9. Mishra J, de Villers-Sidani E, Merzenich M, Gazzaley A. Adaptive training diminishes distractibility in aging across species. *Neuron* 2014;84:1091–1103.

10. James W. *The Principles of Psychology*. New York, NY: Henry Holt; 1890.

11. Boring E. *A History of Experimental Psychology*. New York, NY: Appleton-Century-Crofts; 1929.

12. Hubel DH, Wiesel TN. Ferrier lecture: functional architecture of macaque money visual cortex. *Proc R Soc Lond B Biol Sci* 1977;198:1–59.

13. Kandel E, Schwartz JH. *Principles of Neural Science*. 1st or 2nd ed. New York, NY: McGraw Hill, 1981.

14. Hubel DH, Wiesel TN. *Brain and Visual Perception*. New York, NY: Oxford University Press; 2004.

15. Woody CD, Engel J Jr. Changes in unit activity and thresholds to electrical microstimulation at coronal-pericruciate cortex of cat with classical conditioning of different facial movements. *J Neurophysiol* 1972;35:230:41.

16. Weinberger NM. Physiological memory in primary auditory cortex: characteristics and mechanisms. *Neurobiol Learn Mem* 1998;70:226–251.

17. Thompson RF. In search of memory traces. *Annu Rev Psychol* 2005;56:1–23.

18. Kraus N, Disterhoft JF. Response plasticity of single neurons in rabbit auditory association cortex during tone-signalled learning. *Brain Res* 1982;26:246–257.

19. Merzenich MM, Kaas JH, Wall JT, Sur M, Nelson RJ, Felleman DJ. Progression of change following median nerve section in the cortical representation of the hand in areas 3b and 1 in adult owl and squirrel monkeys. *Neuroscience* 1983;10:639–665.

20. Merzenich MM, Nelson RJ, Stryker MP, Cynader MS, Schoppmann A, Zook JM. Somatosensory cortical map changes following digit amputation in adult monkeys. *J Comp Neurol* 1984;224:591–605.

21. Wall JT, Kaas JH, Sur M, Nelson RJ, Felleman DJ, Merzenich MM. Functional reorganization in somatosensory cortical areas 3b and 1 of adult monkeys after median nerve repair possible relationships to sensory recovery in humans. *J Neurosci* 1986;6:218–233.

22. Clark SA, Allard T, Jenkins WM, Merzenich MM. Receptive fields in the body surface map in adult cortex defined by temporally correlated inputs. *Nature* 1988;332:444–445.

23. Merzenich MM, Jenkins WM. Reorganization of cortical representations of the hand following alterations of skin inputs induced by nerve injury, skin island transfers, and experience. *J Hand Ther* 1993;6:89–104.

24. Jenkins WM, Merzenich MM, Ochs M, Allard TT, Guic E. Functional reorganization of primary somatosensory cortex in adult owl monkeys after behaviorally controlled tactile stimulation. *J Neurophysiol* 1990;63:82–104.

25. Recanzone GH, Merzenich MM, Jenkins WM, Grajski KA, Dinse HA. Topographic reorganization of the hand representational zone in cortical area 3b paralleling improvements in frequency discrimination performance. *J Neurophysiol* 1992;67:1031–1056.

26. Recanzone GH, Merzenich MM, Schreiner CS. Changes in the distributed temporal response properties of SI cortical neurons reflect improvements in performance on a temporally-based tactile discrimination task. *J Neurophysiol* 1992;67:1071–1091.

27. Nudo RJ, Milliken GW, Jenkins WM, Merzenich MM. Use-dependent alterations of movement representations in primary motor cortex of adult squirrel monkeys. *J Neurosci* 1995;16:785–807.

28. Xerri C, Merzenih MM, Peterson BE, Jenkins W. Representational plasticity in cortical area 3b paralleling tactual-motor skill acquisition in adult monkeys. *Cereb Cortex* 1999;9:264–275.

29. Wang X, Merzenich MM, Sameshima K, Jenkins WM. Remodelling of hand representation in adult cortex determined by timing of tactile stimulation. *Nature* 1995;378:71–75.

30. Dinse HR, Recanzone GH, Merzenich MM. Alterations in correlated activity parallel ICMS-induced representational plasticity. *Neuroreport* 1993;5:173–176.

31. Merzenich MM. Development and maintenance of cortical somatosensory representations: functional "maps" and neuroanatomical repertoires. In: Barnard KE, Brazelton TB, eds. *Touch: The Foundation of Experience*. Madison: International University Press; 1990.

32. Merzenich MM, Sameshima K. Cortical plasticity and memory. *Curr Opin Neurobiol* 1993;3:187–196.

33. Grajski KS, Merzenich MM. Neuronal network simulation of somatosensory representational plasticity. In: Touretzky DL, ed. *Neural Information Processing Systems. Vol. 2*. San Mateo, CA: Morgan Kaufman; 1990.

34. Grajski KA, Merzenich MM. Hebb-type dynamics is sufficient to account for the inverse magnification rule in cortical somatotopy. *Neural Comp* 1990;2:74–81.

35. Merzenich MM, Allard T, Jenkins WM. Neural ontogeny of higher brain function; implications of some recent neurophysiological findings. In: Franzén O, Westman P, eds. *Information Processing in the Somatosensory System*. London: Macmillan; 1991.

36. Merzenich MM, Recanzone GH, Jenkins WM, Grajski KA. Adaptive mechanisms in cortical networks underlying cortical contributions to learning and nondeclarative memory. *Cold Spring Harb Symp Quant Biol* 1990;55:863–887.

37. Polley DB, Steinberg EE, Merzenich MM. Perceptual learning directs auditory cortical map reorganization through top-down influences. *J Neurosci* 2006;26:4970–4982.

38. Zhou X, de Villers-Sidani E, Panizzutti R, Merzenich MM. Successive-signal biasing for a learned sound sequence. *PNAS* 2010;107:14839–14844.

39. Gilbert C, Li W, Piech V. Perceptual learning and adult cortical plasticity. *J Physiol* 2009;587:2743–2751.

40. Xerri C, Merzenich MM, Peterson BE, Jenkins W. Plasticity of primary somatosensory cortex paralleling sensorimotor skill recovery from stroke in adult monkeys. *J Neurophysiol* 1998;79:2119–2148.

41. Nudo RJ, Plautz EJ, Frost SB. Role of adaptive plasticity in recovery of function after damage to motor cortex. *Muscle Nerve* 2001;8:1000–1019.

42. Bao S, Chang EF, Davis JD, Gobeske KT, Merzenich MM. Progressive degradation and subsequent refinement of acoustic representations in the adult auditory cortex. *J Neurosci* 2003;23:10765–10775.

43. Bao S, Chang EF, Woods J, Merzenich MM. Temporal plasticity in the primary auditory cortex induced by operant perceptual learning. *Nat Neurosci* 2004;9:974–981.

44. Zhou X, Merzenich MM. Developmentally degraded cortical temporal processing restored by training. *Nature Neurosci* 2009;12:26–28.

45. Zhou X, Merzenich MM. Intensive training in adults refines A1 representations degraded in an early postnatal critical period. *PNAS* 2007;104:15935–15940.

46. Zhou X, Lu JY, Darling RD, et al. Behavioral training reverses global cortical network dysfunction induced by perinatal antidepressant exposure. *PNAS* 2015;112:2233–2238.

47. Zhu X, Liu X, Wei F, et al. Perceptual training restores impaired cortical temporal processing due to lead exposure. *Cereb Cortex* 2014;26:334–345.

48. Xerri C, Merzenich MM, Jenkins W, Santucci S. Representational plasticity in cortical area 3b paralleling tactual motor skill acquisition in adult monkeys. *Cereb Cortex* 1999;9:264–276.

49. Merzenich M, Wright B, Jenkins W, et al. Cortical plasticity underlying perceptual, motor and cognitive skill development: implications for neurorehabilitation. *Cold Spring Harb Symp Quant Biol* 1996;61:1–8.

50. Byl NN, Merzenich MM, Jenkins WM. A primate genesis model of focal dystonia and repetitive strain injury. *Neurology* 1996;47:508–520.

51. Byl NN, Merzenich MM, Cheung S, Bedenbaugh P, Nagarajan SS, Jenkins WM. Primate model for studying focal dystonia and repetitive strain injury: effects on the primary somatosensory cortex. *Phys Ther* 1997;77:269–284.

52. Sanger TD, Merzenich MM. Computational model of the role of sensory disorganization in focal task-specific dystonia. *J Neurophysiol* 2000;84:2458–2464.

53. Kilgard MP, Merzenich MM. Cortical map reorganization enabled by nucleus basalis activity. *Science* 1998;279:1714–1718.

54. Kilgard MP, Merzenich MM. Plasticity of temporal information processing in the primary auditory cortex. *Nature Neurosci* 1998;1:727–731.

55. Kilgard MP, Merzenich MM, Mercado E, et al. Basal forebrain stimulation changes cortical sensitivities to complex sound. *Neuroreport* 2001;12:2283–2287.

56. Bao S, Chan VT, Merzenich MM. Cortical remodeling induced by dopamine-mediated ventral; tegmental activity. *Nature* 2001;412:79–83.

57. Kilgard MP, Merzenich MM. Order-sensitive plasticity in adult primary auditory cortex. *PNAS* 2002;99:3205–3209.

58. Bao S, Chan VT, Zhang LI, Merzenich MM. Suppression of cortical representation through backward conditioning. *PNAS* 2003;100:1405–1408.

59. Froemke R, Merzenich MM, Schreiner CE. A synaptic memory trace for cortical receptive field plasticity. *Nature* 2007;450:425–429.

60. Schultz W. Dopamine reward prediction-error signaling: a two-component response. *Nature Rev Neurosci* 2016;17:183–195.

61. Aston Jones G, Cohen JD. An integrative theory of locus coeruleus-norepinephrine function: adaptive gain and optimum performance. *Ann Rev Neurosci* 2005;28:403–540.

62. Merzenich MM. Cortical plasticity contributing to child development. In: McClelland J, Siegler R, eds. *Mechanisms in Cognitive Development*. Mahwah, NJ: Erlbaum; 2001:67–96.

63. Buonomano DV, Merzenich MM. Cortical plasticity: from synapses to maps. *Annu Rev Neurosci* 1998;21:149–866.

64. Malenka RC, Bear MF. LTP and LTD: an embarrassment of riches. *Neuron* 2004;44:5–21.

65. Cooper LN, Bear MF. The BCM theory of synapse modification at 30: interaction of theory with experiment. *Nat Rev Neurosci* 2012;23:798–810.

66. Huganir RL, Nicoll RA. AMPARs and synaptic plasticity: the last 25 years. *Neuron* 2013;*80*:704–717.

67. Zhou X, Panizzutti R, de Villers-Sidani E, Madeira C, Merzenich MM. Natural restoration of critical period plasticity in the juvenile and adult primary auditory cortex. *J Neurosci* 2011;31:5625–5634.

68. Mohammed AH, Zhu SW, Darmopil S, et al. Environmental enrichment and the brain. *Prog Brain Res* 2002;138:109–133.

69. de Villers-Sidani E, Mishra J, Zhou X, Voss P. Neuroplastic mechanisms underlying perceptual and cognitive enhancement. *Neural Plast* 2016;6238571. doi: 10.11552016/6238571.

70. Ujiie M, Dickstein DL, Carlow DA, Jefferies WA. Blood-brain barrier permeability precedes senile plaque formation in an Alzheimer disease model. *Microcirc* 2003;10:463–470.

71. Zhang X, Tian Y, Zhang C, et al. Near-red fluorescence molecular imaging of amyloid beta species and monitoring therapy in animal models of Alzheimer's disease. *PNAS* 2015;112:943409.

72. Sochocka M, Diniz BS, Leszek J. Inflammatory response in the CNS: friend or foe? *Mol Neurobiol* 2016 [Epub ahead of print]. doi:10.1007/s12035-016-0297.1.

73. Norden DM, Muccigrosso MM, Godbout JP. Microglial priming and enhanced reactivity to secondary insult in aging, and traumatic CNS injury, and neurodegenerative disease. *Neuropharm* 2015;96:29–41.

74. Armstrong RA. What causes Alzheimer's Disease? *Folia Neuropathol* 2013;51:169–188.

75. Vinters HV. Emerging Concepts in Alzheimer's Disease. *Ann Rev Pathol* 2014;10:291–319. doi: 10.1146/annurev-pathol-020712-163927.

76. National Institute on Aging. *Alzheimer's Disease Genetics Fact Sheet.* https://www.nia.nih.gov/alzheimers/publication/alzheimers-disease-genetics-fact-sheet.

77. Flechsig P. *Gehirn und Seele.* Madison: University of Wisconsin library; 1896. https://archive.org/details/gehirnundseeler01flecgoog

78. Sherin JE. Human brain myelination trajectories across the life span. In: *Handbook of the Biology of Aging.* Oxford, UK: Academic Press; 2011:333–346.

79. Merzenich MM, DeCharms RC. Neural representations, experience and change. In: Llinas R and Churchland P, eds. *The Mind-Brain Continuum.* Boston, MA: MIT Press; 1996:61–81.

80. Merzenich, MM, Tallal P, Peterson B, Miller SL, Jenkins WM. Some neurological principles relevant to the origins of—and the cortical plasticity based remediation of—language learning impairments. In: Grafman J, Cristen Y, eds. *Neuroplasticity: Building a Bridge from the Laboratory to the Clinic.* New York, NY: Springer-Verlag; 1998:169–187. Also see http://www.scilearn.com.

81. Tallal P. Improving language and literacy is a matter of time. *Nat Rev Neurosci* 2004;5:721–728.

82. See http://www.BrainHQ.com.

83. Salthouse TA. Aging and measures of processing speed. *Bil Psychol* 2000;54:35–54.

84. Finkel D, Reynolds CA, McArdle JJ, Pedersen NL. Age changes in processing speed as a leading indicator of cognitive aging. *Psychol Aging* 2007;22:558–568.

85. Fry AF, Hale S. Processing speed, working memory, and fluid intelligence: evidence for a developmental cascade. *Psychol Sci* 1996;7:237–241.

86. Salthouse TA, Pink JE, Tucker-Drob EM. Contextual analysis of fluid intelligence. *Intelligence* 2008;35(6):464–486.

87. Van Vleet TM, DeGutis JM, Merzenich MM, Simpson GV, Zomet A, Dabit S. Targeting alertness to improve cognition in older adults: a preliminary report of benefits in executive function and skill acquisition. *Cortex* 2016;82:100–118.

88. Jobe JB, Smith DM, Ball K, et al. ACTIVE: A cognitive intervention trial to promote independence in older adults. *Control Clin Trials* 2001;22:453–479.

89. Ball KK, Beard BL, Roenker DL, Miller RL, Griggs DS. Age and visual search: expanding the useful field of view. *J Opt Soc Am A* 1988;5:2210–2219.

90. Edwards J, Wadley V, Myers R, Roenker DL, Cissell G, Ball KK. Transfer of a speed of processing intervention to near and far cognitive functions. *Gerontology* 2002;48:329–340.

91. Edwards JD, Wadley VG, Vance DE, Wood K, Roenker DL, Ball KK. The impact of speed of processing training on cognitive and everyday performance. *Aging Mental Health* 2005;9:362–371.

92. Ball KK, Ross LA, Roth DL, Edwards JD. Speed of processing training in the ACTIVE study: how much is needed and who benefits? *J Aging Health* 2013;25:S65–S84.

93. Ball KK, Edwards JD, Ross LA, McGwin G Jr. Cognitive training decreases motor vehicle collision involvement in older drivers. *J Am Geriat Soc* 2010;58:210–213.

94. Roenker DL, Cissell GM, Ball KK, Wadley VG, Edwards JD. Speed of processing and driving simulator training result in improved driving performance. *Hum Factors* 2003;45:218–233.

95. Ross LA, Edwards JD, O'Connor ML, Ball KK, Wadley VG, Vance DE. The transfer of cognitive speed of processing training to older adults driving mobility across 5 years. *J Gerontol B Psychol Sci Soc Sci* 2016;71:87–97.

96. Edwards JD, Delahunt PB, Mahncke HW. Cognitive speed of processing training delays driving cessation. *J Gerontol A Biol Sci Med Sci* 2009;64:1262–1267.

97. Edwards JD, Myers et al. 2009.

98. Wollinsky FD, Mahncke HW, Vander Weg MW, et al. The ACTIVE cognitive training interventions and the onset of and recovery of suspected clinical depression. *J Gerontol B Psychol Sci Soc Sci* 2009;64:577–585.

99. Morimoto S, Wexler BE, Alexopoulos GS. Neuroplasticity-based computerized cognitive remediation for treatment-resistant geriatric depression. *Int J Geriatr Psychiatry* 2012;27:1239–1247.

100. Wolinsky FD, Vander Weg MW, Martin R, et al. The effect of speed-of-processing training on depressive symptoms in ACTIVE. *J Gerontol A Biol Sci Med Sci* 2009;64:478–472.

101. Wolinsky FD, Vander Weg MW, Martin R, et al. Does cognitive training improve internal locus of control among older adults? *J Gerontol B Psychol Sci Soc Sci* 2010;65:591–598.

102. Wolinsky FD, Mahncke H, Vander Weg MW, et al. Speed of processing training protects self-rated health in older adults enduring effects observed in the multisite ACTIVE randomized controlled trial. *Int Psychogeratr* 2010;22:470–478.

103. Wolinsky FD, Unverzagt FW, Smith DM, Jones R, Stoddard A, Tennstedt SL. The ACTIVE cognitive training trial and health-related quality of life: protection that lasts for 5 years. *J Gerontol A Biol Sci Med Sci* 2006;61:1324–1329.

104. Rebok GW, Ball K, Guey LT, et al. Ten-year effects of the advanced cognitive training for independent and vital elderly cognitive training trial on cognition and everyday functioning in older adults. *J Am Geriatr Soc* 2014;2:16–24.

105. Edwards JD. *Cognitive Training Reduces Incident Dementia Across Ten Years*. AAIC abstract; 2016. (Manuscript in review.)

106. Wolinsky FD, Vaner Weg MW, Howren MB, Jones MP, Dotson MM. A randomized controlled trial for cognitive training using a visual speed of processing intervention in middle aged and older adults. *PLoS One* 2013;8:361624. doi: 10.1371/journal.pone.0061624.

107. Wolinsky FD, Vander Weg MW, Howren MB, Jones MP, Dotson MM. Effects of cognitive speed of processing training on a composite neuropsychological outcome: results at one-year from the IHAMS randomized controlled trial. *Int Psychogeriatr* 2016;28:817–830.

108. Mahncke HW, Bronstone A, Merzenich MM. Memory enhancement in healthy older adults using a brain plasticity-based training program: a randomized, controlled study. *Proc Natl Acad Sci* 2006;103:12523–12528.

109. Scalf PE, Colcombe SJ, McCarley JS, et al. The neural correlates of an expanded functional field of view. *J Gerontol B Psych Sci Soc Sci* 2007;62:32–44.

110. O'Brien JL, Edwards JD, Maxfield ND, Peronto CL, Williams VA, Lister JJ. Cognitive training and selective attention in the aging brain: an electrophysiological study. *Clin Neurophysiol* 2013;124:2198.

111. Smith GE, Housen P, Yaffe K, et al. A cognitive training program based on principles of brain plasticity: results from the improvement in memory with plasticity-based adaptive cognitive training (IMPACT) study. *J Am Geriatr Soc* 2009;57:594–603.

112. Mahncke HW, Bronstone A, Merzenich MM. Brain plasticity and functional losses in the aged: scientific bases for a novel intervention. *Prog Brain Res* 2006;157:81–109.

113. Zelinski EM, Spina LM, Yaffe K, et al. Improvement in memory with plasticity-based adaptive cognitive training: results of the 3-month follow-up. *J Am Geriatr Soc* 2011;59:258–265.

114. Frantzidis CA, Ladas AK, Vivas AB, Ssolaki M, Bamidis PD. Cognitive and physical training for the elderly: evaluating outcome efficacy by means of neurophysiological synchronization. *Int J Psychophys* 2014;93:1–11.

115. Klados M, Styliadis C, Frantzidis CA, Paraskevopoulos E, Bamidis PD. Beta-band functional connectivity is reorganized in mild cognitive impairment after combined computerized physical and cognitive training. *Front Neurosci* 2016;10:55. doi: 10.3389/fnins.2016.00055.

116. Jacobs HL, Radua J, Luckmann HC, Sack AT. Meta-analysis of functional network alterations in Alzheimer's disease: toward a network biomarker. *Neurosci Biobehav Rev* 2013;37:753–765.

117. Anderson S, White-Schwoch T, Parbery-Clark A, Kraus N. Reversal of age-related neural timing delays with training. *PNAS* 2013;110:4357–4362.

118. Anderson S, White-Schwoch T, Choi HJ, Kraus N. Training changes processing of speech cues in older adults with hearing loss. *Front Syst Neurosci* 2013;7:97. doi: 10.3389/fnsys.2013.00097.eCollection2013.

119. Anderson S, Kraus N. Auditory training: evidence for neural plasticity in older adults. *Perspec Hear Hear Disord Res Res Diagn* 2013;17:37–57.

120. Anderson S, White-Schwoch T, Choi HJ, Kraus N. Partial maintenance of auditory-based cognitive training benefits in older adults. *Neuropsychologia* 2014;62:286–296.

121. Strenziok M, Parasuraman R, Clarke E, Cisler DS, Thompson JC, Greenwood PM. Neurocognitive enhancement in older adults: comparison of three cognitive training tasks to test a hypothesis of training transfer in brain connectivity. *Neuroimage* 2014;85:1027–1039.

122. Barnes DE, Yaffe K, Belfor N, Jagust WJ, DeCarli C, Reed BR, Kramer JH. Computer-based cognitive training for mild cognitive impairment: results from a pilot randomized, controlled trial. *Alzheimer Dis Assoc Disord* 2009;23:205–210.

123. Valdez EG, O'Connor ML, Edwards JD. The effects of cognitive speed of processing training among older adults with psychometrically-defined mild cognitive impairment. *Curr Alzheimer Res* 2012;9:999–1009.

124. Lin F, Heffner KL, Ren P, et al. Cognitive and neural effects of vision-based speed-of-processing training in older adults with amnestic mild cognitive impairment. *J Am Geriatr Soc* 2016;64:2293–2298.

125. Rosen AC, Sugiura L, Kreamer JH, Whitfield-Gabrieli S, Gabrieli JD. Cognitive training changes hippocampal function in mild cognitive impairment: a pilot study. *J Alzheimers Dis* 2011;26:349–357.

126. Vance DE, Cody SL, Moneyham L. Remediating HIV-associated neurocognitive disorders via cognitive training: a perspective on neurocognitive aging. *Interdiscip Top Gerontol Geriatr* 2017;41:173–186.

127. Cody SL, Vance DE. The neurobiology of HIV and its impact on cognitive reserve: a review of cognitive interventions for an aging population. *Neurobiol Dis* 2016;92:144–156.

128. Von Ah D, Carpenter JS, Sayki A, et al. Advanced cognitive training for breast cancer survivors: a randomized controlled trial. *Breast Cancer Res Treat* 2012;135:799–809.

129. Mazer BL, Sofer S, Korner-Bitensky N, Gelinas I, Hanley J, Wood-Dauphine S. Effectiveness of a visual attention retraining program on the driving performance of clients with stroke. *Arch Phys Med Rehabil* 2003;84:541–550.

130. DeGutis JM, Van Vleet TM. Tonic and phasic alertness training: a novel behavioral therapy to improve spatial and non-spatial attention in patients with hemispatial neglect. *Front Hum Neurosci* 2010;24:4. doi:10.3389/fnhum.2010.00060. PMID: 20838474.

131. Van Vleet TM, Degutis JM. Cross-training in hemispatial neglect: auditory sustained attention training ameliorates visual attention deficits. *Cortex* 2013;49:679–690.

132. Van Vleet TM, DeGutis JM. The nonspatial side of spatial neglect and related approaches to treatment. *Prog Brain Res* 2013;207:327–349.

133. Chen CX. Effect of visual training on cognitive function in stroke patients. *Int J Nursing Sciences* 2015. doi: org/10.1016/j.ijnss.2015.11.002.

134. Fisher M, Holland C, Merzenich MM, Vinogradov S. Using neuroplasticity-based auditory training to improve verbal memory in schizophrenia. *Am J Psychiatry* 2009;166:805–811.

135. Fisher M, Loewy R, Hardy K, Schlosser D, Vinogradov S. Cognitive interventions targeting brain plasticity in the prodromal and early phases of schizophrenia. *Annu Rev Clin Psychol* 2013;9:435–463.

136. Popov T, Jordanov T, Rockstroh B, Elbert T, Merzenich MM, Miller GA. Specific cognitive training renormalizes auditory sensory gating in schizophrenia: a randomized trial. *Biol Psychiatry* 2011;69:465–471.

137. Popov T, Rockstroh B, Weisz N, Elbert T, Miller GA. Adjusting brain dynamics in schizophrenia by means of perceptual and cognitive training. *PloS One* 2012;7:e39051. doi: 10.1002/hbm.22064.

138. Subramaniam K, Luks TL, Fihser M, Simpson GV, Nagarajan S, Vionogradov S. Computerized cognitive training restores neural activity within the reality monitoring network in schizophrenia. *Neuron* 2012;73:842–853.

139. Subramaniam K, Luks TL, Garrett C, Chung C, Fisher M, Nagarajan S, Vinogradov S. Intensive cognitive training in schizophrenia enhances working memory and associated prefrontal cortical efficiency in a manner that drives long-term functional gains. *NeuroImage* 2014;99:281–292.

140. Popov TG, et al. A randomized study of cognitive remediation for forensic and mental health patients with schizophrenia. *NeuroImage: Clin* 2015;7:807–814.

141. Ellis ML, Edwards JD, Peterson L, Roker R, Athilngam P. Effects of cognitive speed of processing training among older adults with heart failure. *J Aging Health* 2014;26(4):600–615.

142. Pressler SJ, Titler M, Koelling TM, et al. Nurse-enhanced computerized cognitive training increases serum brain-derived neurotropic factor levels and improves working memory in heart failure. *J Cardiac Failure* 2015;21:630–641.

143. Hancock LM, Bruce JM, Bruce AS, Lynch SG. Processing speed and working memory training in multiple sclerosis: a double-blind randomized controlled pilot study. *J Clin Exp Neuropsychol* 2015;37:113–127.

144. *Nutrition Across the Lifespan for Healthy Aging*. National Academies Press. Leslie Pray, Rapporteur: Washington, DC. 2016. https://www.ncbi.nim.nih.gov/books/NBK409023/.

145. Otaegui-Arrazola A, Amiano P, Elbusto A, Urdaneta E, Martínez-Lage P. Diet, cognition, and Alzheimer's disease: food for thought. *Eur J Nutr* 2014;53:1–23.

146. Bredesen DE, Amos EC, Canick J, et al. Reversal of cognitive decline in Alzheimer's disease. *Aging* 2016;8:1250–1258.

147. Mattson MP. Lifelong brain health is a lifelong challenge: from evolutionary principles to empirical evidence. *Ageing Res Rev* 2015;20:37–45.

148. Hillman CH, Erickson KI, Kramer AF. Be smart, exercise your heart: exercise effects on brain and cognition. *Nat Rev Neurosci* 2008;9:58–65.

149. Voss MW, Vivar C, Kramer AF, van Praag H. Bridging animal and human models of exercise-induced brain plasticity. *Trends Cogn Sci* 2013;17:525–544.

150. Scherder E, Scherder R, Verburgh L, et al. Executive functions of sedentary elderly may benefit from walking: a systematic review and meta-analysis. *Am J Geriatr Psychiatry* 2014;22:782–791.

151. Van Uffelen JG, Chin A, Paw MJ, Hopman-Rock M, van Mechelen W. The effects of exercise on cognition in older adults with and without cognitive decline: a systematic review. *Clin J Sports Med* 2008;18:486–500.

152. Mansfield A, Wong JS, Bryce J, Knorr S, Patterson KK. Does perturbation-based balance training prevent falls? Systematic review and meta-analysis of preliminary randomized controlled trials. *Phys Ther* 2015;95:700–709.

153. Gillespie LD, Robertson MC, Gillespie WJ, et al. Interventions for preventing falls in older people living in the community. *Cochrane Database Syst Rev* 2012;9:CD007146.

154. McFadden SH, Basting AD. Healthy aging persons and their brains: promoting resilience through creative engagement. *Clin Geriatr Med* 2010;26:149–161.

155. Scarmeas N, Stern Y. Cognitive reserve and lifestyle. *J Clin Exp Neuropsychol* 2003;25:625–633.

156. Fried LP, Carlson MC, Freedman M, et al. A social model for health promotion for an aging population: initial evidence on the Experience Corps model. *J Urban Health* 2004;81:64–78.

157. Lo JC, Loh KK, Zheng H, Sim SKY, Chee MWL. Sleep duration and age-related changes in brain structure and cognitive performance. *Sleep* 2014 Jul 1;37(7):1171–1178. doi: 10.5665/sleep.3832.

158. Miller MA, Wright H, Ji C, Cappaccio FP. Cross-sectional study of sleep quantity and quality and amnestic and non-amnestic cognitive function in an ageing population: the English Longitudinal Study of Ageing (ELSA). *PLoS One* 2014;9:e100991 doi: 10.1371/journal.pone.0100991.

17

An Integrative Approach to the Assessment and Treatment of Inflammatory Conditions

MARK LIPONIS, MD, AND BETTINA MARTIN, MD

Introduction

The past two decades could easily be considered the golden age of recognizing the importance of inflammation in medicine. Research has pointed to the presence of inflammation in some of the most serious human illnesses, including cardiovascular disease, diabetes, cancer, Alzheimer's disease and other dementia, and infectious and autoimmune diseases.[1-8]

Advances in the clinical measurement of inflammation and the immune response have ushered in a new era of thinking about ways that immunomodulation might affect chronic diseases and outcomes.[9] The benefits of integrative approaches for managing inflammation can be measured, and treatment can be better targeted and quality of life improved.

There is a long history of drug development directed at inflammation; these drugs have advanced from steroid therapy to nonsteroidal anti-inflammatories, to broad-spectrum immunosuppressives to targeted anticytokine agents, offering new and powerful options for intervening in inflammatory conditions.[10]

This explosion in the number of drugs targeting various parts of the inflammatory process is testament to the complexity of inflammatory pathways. It has also led to a growing understanding of the many ways that integrative and preventive approaches might be used for better control and outcomes in inflammatory disorders. Food, fitness, physical activity, sleep, supplements, and stress have all been shown to affect levels of inflammation and can be used as complementary approaches to help reduce inflammation.[11-16]

But first, what is inflammation and why is it so common?

Simply defined, *inflammation is a stress response of the immune system intended to promote healing.*

The most common triggers of inflammation are infection and injury; both require a response of the immune system to invoke healing. That immune response produces the classic clinical signs of inflammation, often described as rubor, calor, tumor, and dolor—redness, heat, swelling, and pain. Redness and warmth result from the increase in blood flow triggered by cytokines that cause both vasodilation and growth of new capillaries (angiogenesis). Increased permeability of capillaries leads to accumulation of fluid (swelling) and the release of pain mediators like prostaglandins, substance P, histamine, and bradykinin contribute to causing pain (dolor). The accumulation of these numerous inflammatory mediators has been coined the "inflammatory soup."[17]

These clinical features are the hallmarks of inflammation and in most cases are essential to the healing process. Increase in blood flow helps to dilute the number of pathogens, while bringing more leukocytes and macrophages to the area to help control infection. Pain and swelling are likely a protective response to help immobilize the site and reduce the damaging effects of trauma to the healing process.

The intricate deployment of the inflammatory response is a complex and dynamic process, and there are a variety of possible responses from minor, local reactions to full-blown and life-threatening systemic reactions in anaphylaxis, sepsis, or multisystem organ failure. The wide range of immune response means that control of the inflammatory cascade is also critical; it is possible that the immune response might be inadequate, or at times excessive. The response of our immune system should match the perceived threat, as both inadequate and excessive responses carry serious risks.[18]

Excessive or inappropriate immune responses, themselves, are known to cause disease or complications in such conditions as influenza and other viral syndromes, allergy and hypersensitivity, and in autoimmune diseases.[19] More recently, inflammation has been found to play a role in acute coronary syndromes,[1] stroke,[20] type 2 diabetes,[3] Alzheimer's disease,[5] obesity,[21,22] macular degeneration,[7] atrial fibrillation,[23,24] aneurysms,[25-27] and many other noninfectious conditions.[28-33] These may represent instances in which inappropriate or dysregulated immune responses can cause serious problems.

Like so many processes in the body, the inflammatory response—the healing stress response of our immune system—needs to be appropriate for the actual threat. It is a Goldilocks situation—the immune response cannot be too little or too big; it needs to be "just right." Regulation of the immune response is as important as its speed and capabilities.

Inflammatory Pathways—The Process of Inflammation

The immune system comprises a wide range of cells, tissues, and organs, each with specific functions in immunity and inflammation. The immune system has both built-in (innate) and learned (adaptive) immune responses. Immune responses can be both cellular, for example macrophages and cytotoxic cells, and humoral, conveyed by chemical structures such as antibodies, complement cascade, and cytokines (Box 17.1).

Inflammation is usually set into motion by local factors that trigger release of proinflammatory cytokines by tissue macrophages, neutrophils, or lymphocytes responding to local infection, injury, or ischemia, most often. These proinflammatory cytokines include interleukin 1-beta, TNF-α (tumor necrosis factor alpha), and interleukin-6, which are produced after the activation of nuclear factor kappa B (NF-kB).

The NF-kB family of transcription factors plays a crucial role in regulation of the inflammatory response. Normally, NF-kB is held in an inactive state in the cytosol, and translocates to the nucleus of the cell when triggered to initiate cytokine transcription.[34,35] Regulation of nuclear factors in the NF-kB family and its movement from nuclear DNA back to the cytosol is also

---

Box 17.1 Components of the Humoral Immune System

Antibodies—IgM, IgA, IgG, IgE
Complement cascade
Eicosanoids
  • Prostaglandins PGE2, PGI2, PGD2, PF2a
  • Leukotrienes
  • Thromboxanes
  • Lipoxins
  • Eoxins
Kinin-kallikrein system
Cytokines
C-reactive protein
TNF family—TNF-α and 18 others
Interleukins—IL 1 through 36
Interferons—a group of ~17 antiviral proteins
VEGF (vascular endothelial growth factor)
Colony stimulating factors
Chemokines

involved in down-regulation of the inflammatory response. NF-kB has been found in almost all cells and can bind to many genes involved in a broad range of cellular, immune, and inflammatory processes. Along with eicosanoids, ROI (reactive oxygen intermediates), TNF-α, and NF-kB can not only escalate inflammation but also contribute to its resolution and are pivotal in the overall regulation of the immune response.

Other important mediators of inflammation include prostaglandins, leukotrienes, and lipoxins; histamine; the complement system; the kinin-kallikrein system; nitric oxide (NO); and the clotting system. Key regulatory cytokines include Transforming Growth Factor (TGF)-beta and interleukin-10.

Prostaglandins are also key regulators of the immune response. The four principal prostaglandins, derived from cyclooxygenase (COX) and arachidonic acid are PGE2, PGI2, PGD2, and PGF2a.[36] The COX inhibitors, targeting the two isoforms of COX are an effective class of nonsteroidal anti-inflammatory agents.

Nearly all cells in the body produce prostaglandins, and at least 10 types of receptors are identified, controlling a wide range of effects in different tissues.

Prostaglandin E2 is the most widely produced prostaglandin and it is involved in the vasodilation, swelling, and pain—rubor, tumor, and dolor—of inflammation. It is a small molecule that exerts control over macrophages, granulocytes, mast cells, dendritic cells, and natural killer cells as well as B-cells.[37]

Prostaglandin I2 is produced mainly in the cells of the cardiovascular system, endothelial cells, vascular smooth muscle cells, and endothelial progenitor cells. It is a vasodilator and inhibitor of platelet aggregation and leukocyte adhesion. Prostaglandin D2 is found in the central nervous system involved in pain perception, and in peripheral tissues, primarily mast cells.[37]

Cellular components used in the inflammatory response (Table 17.1) can also be regulated in many ways, for example the Treg CD4 T-cells responsible for controlling the immune effects of Th helper cells.[38] T-helper cells include Th1 and Th2 cells, which release different cytokines; Th1 produce interferon-gamma, IL-2, TNF-beta, and Th2 produce IL-4, IL-5, IL-10, and IL-13.[39]

If regulatory measures are insufficient or there is inappropriate or excessive reaction of the immune system, the result is hypersensitivity or autoimmunity. Four types of hypersensitivity reactions are characterized based on their clinical patterns. Type I is acute IgE-mediated and includes anaphylaxis, asthma, eczema, and urticaria, and the basis for skin prick allergy testing. Type 2 is IgG-mediated cytotoxic cell-mediated immunity, for example in transfusion reactions. Type 3 immune complex–mediated hypersensitivity for example in glomerulonephritis, and Type 4 delayed cell-mediated hypersensitivity from sensitized Th1 cells, for example in the PPD skin reaction.

Table 17.1 Components of the Cellular
Immune System

T-lymphocytes	B-lymphocytes
Cytotoxic T cells	Plasma cells
Th1	Natural killer cells
Th2	
CD4 + helper	
Treg suppressor	
Granulocytes	**Monocytes**
Neutrophils	Dendritic cells
Eosinophils	Macrophages
Basophils	
Mast cells	

Measuring Inflammation

Measuring inflammation is helpful in several ways. It allows for monitoring disease activity and clinical response, can help identify when a remission has been achieved, and can help guide duration of therapy.[42-44] It can also confirm the effectiveness or ineffectiveness of drug therapy.[41]

Since inflammation precedes symptoms, measuring inflammation might provide some predictive value, which could help to improve prevention. An example is the JUPITER trial, in which C-RP (C-reactive protein) levels predicted the risk of subsequent heart attack and stroke, and successful lowering of C-RP reduced heart attack and strokes.[40]

In Rome between 30 and 45 AD, Aulus Celsus first described the four cardinal signs of redness, warmth, swelling and pain.[45] Ever since, we have been finding new ways of describing and measuring inflammation. And to this day, healthcare providers rely on these physical signs for diagnosis. But visible redness, warmth, swelling, and pain are often later signs of an underlying infection or inflammatory process. Inflammation can often be detected before symptoms develop by measuring inflammatory markers in the blood.

The most basic and often requested is the WBC, or white blood count. Peripheral blood white blood counts (usually expressed in thousands per microliter) have long been used to assess the severity of infections and the response to therapy. Surgical decisions, antibiotic therapy, transplant rejection, transfusion reactions, and cancer care all rely on the white blood count for critical decision-making.

White blood counts have even been shown predictive of cardiovascular events[46,47] as well as noncardiac deaths in coronary disease patients.[48]

In 1897 the Polish doctor Edmund Biernacki discovered that red blood cells dropped or sedimented more quickly in the presence of inflammation, leading to the erythrocyte sedimentation rate test, aka ESR or "sed rate."[49] The ESR is useful in the diagnosis and monitoring of rheumatic diseases rheumatoid arthritis, polymyalgia rheumatic, temporal arteritis, and inflammatory bowel disease, among others. The ESR has in many cases been supplanted by widerspread use of the C-RP test because of its increased sensitivity.

Discovered in 1930 by Tillett and Francis, C-RP was named initially as a substance reacting with the "C" carbohydrate antigen of *Pneumococcus*. More sensitive assays using nephelometry became available around 2000 measuring levels as low as 0.04 mg/L, leading to numerous studies of low-level inflammation and cardiovascular disease. These studies have popularized the notion of "cardiac" C-RP, though the term is misleading, since C-RP is not specific to the cardiovascular system. The "highly sensitive C-RP" refers to the same assay, providing sensitivity as low as 0.04 mg/L.

Since 1995, numerous studies have linked the presence of low-level inflammation as measured by C-RP with a variety of disorders, the list of which includes:

- Unstable coronary syndromes[1,8,9]
- Stroke[20]
- Aortic aneurysm size and rupture[25-27]
- Hypertension[50]
- Type 2 diabetes[7]
- Macular degeneration[7]
- Alzheimer's disease and other forms of dementia[5]
- Atrial fibrillation[23,24]
- Colon cancer[51]
- Lung cancer[52-54]

Some large-scale studies have also supported the idea that therapeutic intervention with treatment designed to lower C-RP also produced improved clinical outcomes, as shown in the JUPITER study involving almost 18,000 participants.[40] The study results supported the idea of lowering C-RP as a form of primary prevention for men and women over age 50. These studies have reframed the target ranges for C-RP levels, which now are generally accepted as:

Optimal: <1.0 mg/L
Average: 1–3 mg/L

High: Above 3 mg/L*

*Clinicians reviewing results from laboratories reporting units in mg/dL will need to multiply results by *10* for comparisons with *mg/L* results.

Beyond WBC, ESR, and C-RP, there are also other laboratory measures and findings with inflammation. Myeloperoxidase (MPO) is an enzyme found predominantly in granulocytes, where it is used in bacterial defenses. Similar to C-RP, elevated levels of MPO have also been shown to predict future acute coronary syndromes.[55]

CYTOKINES

Deriving their name from the origins of the root for "cell" and "movement," cytokines are chemicals that were initially found to direct the movement of cells. Cytokines are "trophic" for mobile cells, meaning they act as a homing signal for macrophages, neutrophils, and the like. Some cytokines are also growth factors for certain cell lines, or for regulating the immune response. Cytokines can be produced in virtually any cell, and are primarily used for communication—cell signaling for cells to "speak" to one another.

Cytokines include chemicals such as the interferons, interleukins, the TNF-α family, mesenchymal growth factors, stem cell factors, adipokines, and neurotrophic factors.[56] At least a hundred cytokines have been identified, and most cells have the ability to produce and react in some way to cytokines. That is different from the more specialized hormones, for example, which are produced by only a few cells specialized for that purpose.

Cytokines are primarily involved in inflammation and the immune response, but cytokines have also been found to play a role in embryogenesis. Cytokines can be chemokines (chemical attractants), interleukins (targeting leukocytes), interferons (targeting viruses), proinflammatory (e.g., TNF-α family), or growth factors (e.g., hematopoietic growth factors G-CSF, erythropoietin, and others).

Cytokines that increase the inflammatory process include the TNF-α, IL-6 and IL-1beta among others. There are also anti-inflammatory cytokines like IL-1 receptor antagonist, IL-4, IL-10, IL-11, and IL-13.[57]

Measurement of cytokines is becoming an increasingly useful tool in the assessment and management of inflammatory disorders. Multiplex cytokine panels have been developed to aid in clinical assessment of rheumatic disorders, for example, the Vectra-DA panel and others.[58,59]

In addition to these markers, which are thought to be somewhat specific for inflammation, there are also a number of elevated markers that are less specific, and these could be lumped together as "acute phase reactants." Acute phase reactants are proteins that increase at least 25% in the blood in response to inflammation, but they have other primary functions in the body. An example would be ferritin, which goes up during acute inflammation, but is normally involved with iron storage. Another example would be fibrinogen (clotting), ceruloplasmin (copper transport), serum amyloid A (cholesterol transport), or alpha-2-macroglobulin (enzyme regulation).

It is worth reinforcing that any markers of inflammation are nonspecific, in that none identify the cause of inflammation, nor its location, nor do they identify a specific treatment. They are signs *of* a problem, but they are not specific for any *particular* problem. They can provide some predictive value, but the timeline of endpoints and symptoms is not easily discerned. Unless the specific cause of inflammation is known, measurement of inflammation can cause undue anxiety and fear about risk without having specific preventive strategies in place; so how can assessment of inflammation be more helpful?

Imaging Inflammation

There are several ways that imaging inflammation can be used clinically, where it can help to diagnose its source or determine the best treatment. In some conditions, imaging inflammation is being used for early diagnosis, for example the use of FDG PET-CT imaging in neurologic disease including Alzheimer's disease, cardiovascular disease, cancer, and inflammatory disorders.[60] Improved tracers and markers could help to better understand different disease processes and pathways.

Traditional forms of imaging, such as X-ray, CT, MRI, and ultrasound, all show typical and pathologic signs of inflammation and are widely used in the diagnosis of inflammatory conditions such as abscesses, diverticulitis, arthritis, tendonitis, fractures, cancer, or appendicitis.

Some integrative practitioners have championed the use of thermography for noninvasive screening for breast cancer, for example.[61] By detecting the increased heat from localized inflammation and blood flow, thermography uses the calor feature of inflammation to detect tumors. It is unknown how thermography screening compares with mammography,[62] although recent concerns about the increasing oversensitivity of mammography should lead to a deeper investigation of alternative screening in breast cancer.

Blood measures combined with selective imaging in certain conditions might give the most insight. Understanding the possible causes of inflammation should help inform decisions about whether to consider imaging.

Causes of Inflammation

In order to address the specific cause of inflammation most successfully, it is helpful to know as best we can, what the source, the site, and the mechanism of inflammation might be. That way, we can make better decisions about treatment and understand how to monitor therapy. Causes of inflammation could be categorized as follows:

1. Well-recognized causes:
   a. Infection
   b. Injury
   c. Ischemia and hypoxia
   d. Allergy/hypersensitivity
   e. Cancer[4,78,79]
   f. Autoimmunity
2. Other less-recognized causes:
   a. Sleep deprivation[63-65]
   b. Obesity and overeating[22,66-68]
   c. Stress and mood disorders including depression, anxiety, hostility[69-72]
   d. Drug/medication effect[73,74]
   e. Smoking and air pollution exposure[75-77]

Regardless of the cause of inflammation, it can be either acute or become chronic. The immune and healing responses are different in their early and late manifestations.

Inflammation and Cancer

The connection between inflammation and cancer is complex. Chronic inflammation is one known risk of cancer, which is seen not uncommonly in chronic inflammatory bowel disease (IBD) or the development of mesothelioma lung cancer years after asbestos exposure. Levels of inflammation have been found to be elevated prior to the development of colon cancer, suggesting a role for inflammation in colon carcinogenesis.[4] But levels of inflammation are also increased in people with advanced cancer, presumably representing the immune response to cancer itself.

To make matters more confusing, the immune response may in some ways contribute to the growth and spread of cancer through the production and release of angiogenic substances such as VEGF that unintentionally increase blood and nutrient flow into tumors.[80,81]

In these ways, inflammation can contribute to the initiation, propagation, and spread of cancer. Knowing the level of inflammation does not necessarily predict the presence of cancer, or necessarily its stage or grade.

Treating Inflammation

The treatment of inflammation offers great opportunities because of the many locations to impact the inflammatory cascade. Successful treatment requires targeting the cause of inflammation; antibiotics will not cure cancer, and a baby aspirin will not treat obstructive sleep apnea.

On the other hand, regardless of the source of inflammation, it is often imperative to protect against the complications of having it. If you cannot immediately resolve the obesity issue, it is crucial to guard against heart attack and stroke in the meantime.

So there are specific ways of targeting the cause of inflammation, and more general ways of reducing the overall level of inflammation that would both improve symptoms and outcomes.

Since its synthesis in 1853 and commercialization as "Aspirin" by Bayer, acetylsalicylic acid is still in widespread use primarily in prophylaxis against cardiovascular events.[82] Prophylactic benefits of low-dose aspirin appear to be working through its COX-1 inhibition and antiplatelet effects rather than lowering C-RP.[83]

Corticosteroid medications have long been the mainstay of managing chronic inflammatory disorders from asthma to rheumatic and other autoimmune diseases. Corticosteroids have broad immunosuppressive effects that affect cell-mediated immunity as well as working by suppressing transcription of genes involved in the inflammatory process.[84] Unfortunately, side effects and long-term adverse effects severely compromise the value of corticosteroids in the management of chronic inflammation.

More targeted therapies offer the potential of controlling inflammation potentially with fewer adverse effects. Discovery of cytokines and understanding their role has led to more targeted anti-inflammatory therapies that are now becoming the mainstay for many challenging inflammatory conditions.

In 1998, Enbrel (etanercept) was the first biologic anticytokine drug released for commercial use in the treatment of rheumatoid arthritis. Designed as a decoy TNF-α receptor, etanercept bound and inactivated TNF-α. Since the successful release of Enbrel, there has been an explosion in biologic drugs targeting cytokines or other components of the inflammatory pathway. Approved indications for the use of Enbrel have broadened to include psoriatic arthritis, ankylosing spondylitis, and plaque psoriasis.

A second TNF-α-blocking biologic, Remicade (infliximab) was FDA-approved and released in 2001 for the treatment of rheumatoid arthritis, and subsequently broadened its indications for use in inflammatory bowel diseases (Crohn's disease and ulcerative colitis), ankylosing spondylitis, and severe plaque psoriasis.

Growth in the immunomodulating biologic drugs has accelerated, and biologics now account for 17% of the total global pharmaceutical revenues.[85] Anti-TNF-α-blocking biologics now include Enbrel, Remicade, Humira, Cimzia, Inflectra, Ridaura, and Simponi. Specific anticytokine therapy now also includes specific IL-6-blocking agents (e.g., Actemra, released in July 2014, for treatment of rheumatoid arthritis in the United States). Newer biologics are now also targeting IL-1 (e.g., Kineret), and cell-mediated immunity (Orencia). Consentyx was designed to block IL-17A in psoriasis and uveitis. Xeljanz is approved as an inhibitor of JAK1 and JAK3 signaling pathway enzymes. The availability of biologics for specific cancers is also growing rapidly; for example, Rituxan in the treatment of lymphomas as well as some autoimmune diseases.

Indications for the use of targeted biologic drugs has grown from the prototype of rheumatoid arthritis to include a wide range of autoimmune and neoplastic disorders including psoriatic arthritis, ankylosing spondylitis, psoriasis, inflammatory bowel disease, systemic lupus erythematosus, scleroderma and progressive systemic sclerosis, vasculitis, and giant-cell arteritis.[86]

Herbal and OTC products have also been shown to have some activity in inhibiting TNF-α or other inflammatory cytokines.

Turmeric (*Curcuma longa*) has a long history of use as a spice as well as a medicinal herb. Curcumin is the extract of turmeric, and has a number of potential mechanisms to explain its anti-inflammatory effect. Curcumin may act by blocking or interfering with TNF-α[60] or other proinflammatory cytokines such as IL-1B and IL-6[87] or by blocking NF-kB activation.[88] Clinical studies of curcumin in humans have shown promising results. Curcumin seems to be a beneficial adjunct in the treatment of osteoarthritis[89,90] as well as possibly rheumatoid arthritis.[91]

Curcumin may also have an effect in reducing levels of some inflammatory cytokines—IL-1β, IL-4, and VEGF, at doses of 1 gram daily, in obese individuals.[92]

In patients undergoing chemotherapy for solid tumors, "boosted bioavailable" curcumin supplements in doses of 180 mg per day improved levels of inflammatory cytokines TNF-α, TGFβ, IL-6, and substance P, and improved quality of life scores.[93]

It is recognized that bioavailability of oral curcumin is quite poor,[94] but processing methods might improve its bioavailability and effectiveness.[95,96]

There may also be gender differences in absorption of curcumin, with women absorbing relatively more.[97]

Curcumin supplements reduce skin complications of radiotherapy for breast cancer[98] and reduce symptoms in autoimmune oral lichen planus.[99]

Curcumin has also been shown to have benefits in preventing the onset of type 2 diabetes,[100] which is suggested to have an inflammatory origin.[3]

Curcumin supplements dramatically reduce the chance of myocardial infarction in patients undergoing coronary artery bypass surgery (CABG) and significantly reduce C-RP and markers of oxidative stress postoperatively.[101]

Milk thistle (silymarin), resveratrol, epigallocatechin gallate (green tea extract), mangostin, other polyphenols have displayed inhibitory activity of TNF-α,[102] however there are few controlled clinical trials examining anti-inflammatory effects in humans.

Silymarin may help reduce levels of C-RP in patients with type 2 diabetes[103] and in one study significantly improved survival in cirrhosis[104] but did not seem to help normalize liver enzymes in some hepatitis C patients.[105]

Herbal products have some evidence for inhibiting other proinflammatory cytokines. Herbal IL-6 inhibitors include green tea extract (epigallocatechin gallate)[106] and andrographolide (*Andrographis paniculata*).[107,108]

Andrographis extract supplements have shown salutatory effects in ulcerative colitis[109] and may reduce symptoms in children with upper respiratory tract infections.[110]

Quercetin is another flavonol compound that has IL-6 inhibitory activity.[110,111] Quercetin supplements have shown anti-inflammatory effects in vitro, though human clinical trials are lacking.

There has been much recent interest in cannabinoids and their immune and anti-inflammatory properties, with particular interest in their use in chronic pain and inflammatory conditions. Cannabinoids are a family of compounds mediating their effects via the cannabinoid receptor. Two receptors, CB1 and CB2, have been identified in the brain and the immune system, respectively. Cannabinoids work in part by down-regulating T-cells, but also by reducing cytokine and chemokine production.[112] Preliminary studies show some benefits in inflammatory bowel disease,[113] however a consistent anti-inflammatory effect has not been demonstrated.

Integrative Approaches to Reducing Inflammation

While medications and supplements can be important tools in the management of inflammatory conditions, there are also a number of successful integrative and lifestyle methods of achieving similar benefits.

EXERCISE

Perhaps one of the most important ways that exercise exerts its pleomorphic benefits is through its anti-inflammatory effects. Moderate aerobic exercise has been shown to consistently reduce inflammation over time.[114,115] Short-term exercise produces a transient increase in inflammation, which over time results in lower levels of systemic inflammation.[116] There is some conflict in the literature as to whether exercise has an independent effect on reducing inflammation, or only has the effect if weight loss occurs. Some studies suggest that exercise improves inflammation even without weight loss[117,118] (the so-called fat but fit), while others suggest that exercise without weight loss does not lower C-RP.[119]

Short-term responses to high-intensity exercise consistently show increases in inflammation and C-RP. Following intense exercise, like a marathon, C-RP levels have been found to rise 266% before returning to baseline by 48 hours.[120] Long-term responses to moderate exercise consistently produce a drop in levels of C-RP.[116]

WEIGHT LOSS AND DIET

Weight loss is a strong lifestyle approach for controlling inflammation. Several studies have linked obesity and overweight with increased inflammatory markers,[21,121] and weight loss has also been shown to help reduce them.[115,122] Inflammation may represent a mechanism where obesity accelerates cardiovascular disease, or cancer. Obesity as a chronic inflammatory disease may help explain the many complications of obesity, from type 2 diabetes to hypertension, cancer, asthma, stroke, and heart attack.[123]

Weight loss has been shown to help reduce the risk of those same conditions. The adverse effects of obesity are numerous, and there are numerous mechanisms by which obesity contributes to the acceleration of illness. Inflammation is but one of these mechanisms, but is perhaps one we have more control of.

One of the dietary measures often found to be most helpful and successful with weight loss includes increasing intake of dietary fiber.[124,125] Increasing dietary fiber intake has also been found to help reduce inflammatory markers.[126-128] Both insoluble and soluble fiber are helpful, although supplements of predominantly soluble fiber may not be sufficient as foods such as legumes, fruits, and berries that have both soluble and insoluble fiber.[129,130]

Another common piece of advice for healthy eating and weight loss is to eat more fish and omega-3 fish oils. Consumption of essential omega-3 fish oils

EPA (eicosapentaenoic acid) and DHA (docosahexaenoic acid) either through consumption of fish[131,132] or fish oil supplements[133] appear to have a beneficial effect in lowering C-RP. Clinically, fish oil supplements have shown benefits in rheumatoid arthritis,[134] with significant improvement in symptoms and additive effects with standard therapies.[135]

Surprising news perhaps is the effect of moderate alcohol consumption on inflammatory markers. Unlike smoking, which raises C-RP, moderate alcohol consumption lowers it.[136,137] The problem is that it seems to take at least moderate alcohol consumption to significantly impact C-RP; a 5-ounce glass of red wine daily may not be enough.[138] Unfortunately, at the intakes needed to effectively lower C-RP, secondary problems of alcohol excess may occur, including dependency, addiction, accidents, and the increased rates of cancer found especially for reproductive cancers.[139] For these reasons, and because of the common tendency to imbibe more than the recommended amount, it is not prudent to recommend alcohol use for controlling inflammation or lowering C-RP.

SLEEP, STRESS, MOOD, MEDITATION, AND MASSAGE

Sleep deprivation increases inflammation, whether it results from a medical sleep disorder such as obstructive sleep apnea, or from menopause, or simply from self-imposed sleep restriction.[14,31] The human body needs a certain amount of sleep, and getting less than it needs is stressful. Stress from almost any source produces the stress response of the immune system—inflammation. Emotional stress has a physical reaction, also, and that is inflammation. Techniques used to help relieve stress, to improve the quality of sleep, and to relieve anxiety, anger, and despair also help to lower inflammation.

Some of the most helpful techniques in relieving stress are yoga, breathing exercises, meditation, and massage and other bodywork. Yoga has a long tradition with millions of practitioners, and there are many different techniques and styles of yoga practice, from hot Bikram yoga to strenuous Ashtanga or calming restorative yoga. While the forms of yoga may be quite different, the elements of breathing, focus, and mindfulness extend across all of them. Extensive trials of different yoga techniques have not been done, but research suggests yoga and breathing techniques have a beneficial effect on reducing inflammation.

A trial of 218 volunteers studied baseline levels of cytokines TNF-α and IL-6 levels in a group of regular yoga practitioners (at least an hour daily for over 5 years) and found lower baseline inflammatory cytokine levels compared with age and gender-matched controls.[140] Yoga was also found to be beneficial in a group of women breast cancer survivors, who displayed lower inflammatory markers over 3 months than similar survivors who were not practicing yoga.[141] A recent innovative trial looked at salivary cytokine and suggested a benefit of yogic breathing practices in reducing inflammation.[142]

Mindfulness-based meditation practices are another nonpharmacologic way of reducing inflammation. In a recent small study comparing mindfulness-based meditation with relaxation, lower levels of proinflammatory IL-6 were found in meditators.[143] A meta-analysis of mindfulness meditation and the immune system found possible but heterogeneous effects on reducing inflammatory markers.[144] A novel study of the effects of mindfulness meditation on the stress response showed that meditators had lower levels of inflammatory TNF-α and IL-8 in blister fluid evoked by capsaicin application. The study suggested that mindfulness-based meditation might help dampen the inflammatory response to emotional and physical stress and inflammation.[145]

Massage is a modality often recommended for treating pain and inflammation, and yet studies on its physiologic effects are limited. A bold study in 2012 actually took muscle biopsies in 11 volunteers immediately after massage and 2.5 hours later. Findings suggested an anti-inflammatory effect of massage that was felt to be mediated by NF-kB and down-regulation of TNF-α, IL-6, and heat shock protein 27. This preliminary study suggested a mechanism by which massage might exert its anti-inflammatory effects.[146]

Acupuncture is another commonly recommended modality for addressing pain and inflammatory conditions. Despite a long history of clinical use around the world, mechanisms for the effects of acupuncture on pain and inflammation are still largely theoretical.[147-149] There are a large number and variety of clinical trials of acupuncture. A 2012 meta-analysis of 29 randomized-controlled trials of acupuncture in chronic pain showed acupuncture to be superior to sham treatment or no-acupuncture control conditions.[150] Results of these trials have raised some questions, however, because of the partial responses to "sham" acupuncture in controlled trials. Clearly more work is needed to explain the clinical effects of acupuncture, its mechanism, and for what conditions it provides clear benefits.

Perhaps the most underappreciated effect on inflammation is the effect of social relationships. Humans are social creatures, and we know that relationships are important for both the quality and quantity of human life. One of the ways that social relationships might improve health could be through reducing inflammation. A comprehensive review of the interplay between relationships and inflammation reveals close parallels between the quality of important relationships and levels of inflammatory cytokines, especially IL-6, TNF-α and C-RP.[151]

The authors concluded: "Close relationships matter. Not only do close relationships shape people's emotions, they affect the very physiological processes that underlie disease. Close relationships across the lifespan contribute to elevated inflammation—now a well-regarded risk factor for disease."

Summary

The awareness, assessment, and management of inflammation has finally come of age—both for prevention and as a focus of treatment it has improved outcomes and quality of life in chronic diseases. Science has improved our understanding of the many causes of inflammation and how it affects health. Great progress has been made with therapeutic options for treating inflammation, and those options are becoming more targeted and more powerful as we learn how to impact different points on the inflammatory cascade. Many questions remain for future investigation: Can the immune response be guided to improve outcomes in infectious and inflammatory diseases without adverse effects or contributing to cancer growth? What are the negative effects of reducing inflammation? What are the best lifestyle strategies for controlling inflammation and extending healthy lifespan? Are there benefits to mild immunosuppression in the aging population to improve age-related disorders and inflammatory diseases? Is lifestyle superior to medications or are they complementary? Do anti-inflammatory therapies extend life or reduce morbidity?

Hopefully with advances in the understanding and measurement of inflammation, these answers will be forthcoming soon!

References

1. Pai JK, Pischon T, Ma J, et al. Inflammatory markers and the risk of coronary heart disease in men and women. *N Engl J Med* 2004;351:2599–2610.
2. Eltzschig HK, Carmeliet P. Hypoxia and inflammation. *N Engl J Med* 2011;364:656–665.
3. Pradhan AD, Manson JE, Rifai N. C-Reactive protein, interleukin 6, and risk of developing type 2 diabetes mellitus. *JAMA* 2001;286(3):327–334.
4. Erlinger TP, Platz EA, Rifai N. C-reactive protein and the risk of incident colorectal cancer. *JAMA* 2004;291(5):585–590.
5. Engelhart MJ, Geerlings MI, Meijer J, et al. Inflammatory proteins in plasma and the risk of dementia: the Rotterdam Study. *Arch Neurol* 2004;61(5):668–672.
6. Coussens LM, Werb Z. Inflammation and cancer. *Nature* 2002;420(6917): 860–867.

7. Seddon JM, Gensler G, Milton RC. Association between C-reactive protein and age-related macular degeneration. *JAMA* 2004;291(6):704–710.

8. Ridker PM, Buring JE, Cook NR, Rifai N. C-reactive protein, the metabolic syndrome, and risk of incident cardiovascular events. *Circulation* 2003;107:391–397.

9. Ridker PM. High-sensitivity C-reactive protein: potential adjunct for global risk assessment in the primary prevention of cardiovascular disease. *Circulation* 2001;103:1813–1818.

10. Rider P, Carmi Y, Cohen I. Biologics for targeting inflammatory cytokines, clinical uses, and limitations. *Int J Cell Biology* 2016;2016:Article ID 9259646.

11. Ma Y, Griffith JA, Chasan-Taber L, et al. Association between dietary fiber and serum C-reactive protein. *Am J Clin Nutr* 2006; 83(4):760–766.

12. Sadeghipour HR, Rahnama A, Salesi M, Rahnama N, Mojtahedi H. Relationship between C-reactive protein and physical fitness, physical activity, obesity and selected cardiovascular risk factors in schoolchildren. *Int J Prev Med* 2010;1(4):242–246.

13. Kasapis C, Thompson PD. The effects of physical activity on serum C-reactive protein and inflammatory markers: a systematic review. *J Am Coll Cardiol* 2005;45(10):1563–1569.

14. Meier-Ewert HK, Ridker PM, Rifai N, et al. Effect of sleep loss on C-reactive protein, an inflammatory marker of cardiovascular risk. *J Am Coll Cardiol* 2004;43(4):678–683.

15. Carroll MF, Schade DS. Timing of antioxidant vitamin ingestion alters postprandial proatherogenic serum markers. *Circulation* 2003;108(1):24–31.

16. Wium-Andersen MK, Ørsted DD, Nielsen SF, Nordestgaard BG. Elevated C-reactive protein levels, psychological distress, and depression in 73,131 individuals. *JAMA Psychiatry* 2013;70(2):176–184.

17. Basbaum AI, Bautista DM, Scherrer G, Julius D. Cellular and molecular mechanisms of pain. *Cell* 2009;139(2):267–284.

18. Rittirsch D, Flierl MA, Ward PA. Harmful molecular mechanisms in sepsis. *Nat Rev Immunol* 2008;8(10):776–787.

19. Iwasaki A, Pillai PS. Innate immunity to influenza virus infection. *Nat Rev Immunol* 2014;14(5):315–328.

20. Cao JJ, Thach C, Manolio TA, et al. C-reactive protein, carotid intima-media thickness, and incidence of ischemic stroke in the elderly: the Cardiovascular Health Study. *Circulation* 2003;108:166–170.

21. Visser M, Bouter LM, McQuillan GM, Wener MH, Harris TB, Elevated C-reactive protein levels in overweight and obese adults. *JAMA* 1999;282(22):2131–2135.

22. Aronson D, Bartha P, Zinder O, et al. Obesity is the major determinant of elevated C-reactive protein in subjects with the metabolic syndrome. *Int J Obes Relat Metab Disord* 2004;28(5):674–679.

23. Chung MK, Martin DO, Sprecher D, et al. C-reactive protein elevation in patients with atrial arrhythmias. inflammatory mechanisms and persistence of atrial fibrillation. *Circulation* 2001;104:2886–2891.

24. Galea R, Cardillo MT, Caroli A, et al. Inflammation and C-reactive protein in atrial fibrillation: cause or effect? *Tex Heart Inst J* 2014;41(5):461–468.

25. Norman P, Spencer CA, Lawrence-Brown MM, Jamrozik K. C-Reactive Protein Levels and the expansion of screen-detected abdominal aortic aneurysms in men. *Circulation* 2004;110:862–866.

26. C-reactive protein (CRP) elevation in patients with abdominal aortic aneurysm is independent of the most important CRP genetic polymorphism. *J Vasc Surg* 2009;49(1):178–184.

27. De Haro J, Bleda S, Acin F. C-reactive protein predicts aortic aneurysmal disease progression after endovascular repair. *Int J Cardiol* 2016;202:701–706.

28. Gosling P, Dickson GR. Serum C-reactive protein in patients with serious trauma. *Injury* 1992;23(7):483–486.

29. Mok CC, Birmingham DJ, Ho LY, Hebert LA, Rovin BH. High-sensitivity C-reactive protein, disease activity, and cardiovascular risk factors in systemic lupus erythematosus. *Arthritis Care Res* 2013;65:441–447.

30. Ma Y, Chiriboga DE, Pagoto SL, et al. Association between depression and C-reactive protein. *Cardiol Res Pract* 2011;2011:286509.

31. Shamsuzzaman AS, Winnicki M, Lanfranchi P, Wolk R, Kara T, Accurso V, Somers VK. Elevated C-reactive protein in patients with obstructive sleep apnea. *Circulation* 2002;105(21):2462–2464.

32. Galez D, Dodig S, Raos M, Nogalo B. C-reactive protein in children with asthma and allergic rhinitis. *Biochemia Medica* 2006;16(2):163–169.

33. Aleem S, Masood Q, Hassan I. Correlation of C-reactive protein levels with severity of chronic urticaria. *Indian J Dermatol* 2014;59(6):636.

34. Oeckinghaus A, Ghosh S. The NF-κB family of transcription factors and its regulation. *CSH Perspect Biol* 2009;1(4):a000034.

35. Shih R-H, Wang C-Y, Yang C-M. NF-kappaB signaling pathways in neurological inflammation: a mini review. *Front Mol Neurosci* 2015;8:77.

36. Ricciotti E, FitzGerald GA. Prostaglandins and inflammation. *Arterioscl Throm Vas* 2011;31(5):986–1000.

37. Kalinski P. Regulation of immune responses by prostaglandin E2. *J Immunol (Baltimore, Md.: 1950)* 2012;188(1):21–28.

38. Corthay A. How do regulatory T cells work? *Scand J Immunol* 2009;70(4): 326–336.

39. Romagnani S. Th1/Th2 cells. *Inflamm Bowel Dis* 1999;5(4):285–294. Review.

40. Ridker PM, Danielson E, Fonseca FAH, et al., for the JUPITER Study Group. Rosuvastatin to prevent vascular events in men and women with elevated C-reactive protein. *N Engl J Med* 2008;359:2195–2207.

41. Heiro M, Helenius H, Sundell J, et al. Utility of serum C-reactive protein in assessing the outcome of infective endocarditis. *Eur Heart J* 2005;26:1873–1881.

42. Shrotriya S, Walsh D, Bennani-Baiti N, Thomas S, Lorton C. C-reactive protein is an important biomarker for prognosis tumor recurrence and treatment response in adult solid tumors: a systematic review. *PLoS One* 2015;10(12):e0143080.

43. Leuzzi G, Galeone C, Gisabella M, et al. Baseline C-reactive protein level predicts survival of early-stage lung cancer: evidence from a systematic review and meta-analysis. *Tumori* 2016;102(5):441–449.

44. Køstner AH, Kersten C, Löwenmark T, et al. The prognostic role of systemic inflammation in patients undergoing resection of colorectal liver metastases: C-reactive protein (CRP) is a strong negative prognostic biomarker. *J Surg Oncol* 2016;114(7):895–899.

45. Granger DN, Senchenkova E. *Inflammation and the Microcirculation*. San Rafael, CA: Morgan & Claypool Life Sciences; 2010.

46. Margolis KL, Manson JE, Greenland P, et al; Women's Health Initiative Research Group. Leukocyte count as a predictor of cardiovascular events and mortality in postmenopausal women: the Women's Health Initiative Observational Study. *Arch Intern Med* 2005;165(5):500–508.

47. Madjid M, Awan I, Willerson JT, Casscells SW. Leukocyte count and coronary heart disease. *J Am Coll Cardiol* 2004;44(10):1945–1956.

48. Haim M, Boyko V, Goldbourt U, Battler A, Behar S. Predictive value of elevated white blood cell count in patients with preexisting coronary heart disease: the Bezafibrate Infarction Prevention Study. *Arch Intern Med* 2004;164(4):433–439.

49. Grzybowski A, Sak J. Edmund Biernacki (1866–1911): discoverer of the erythrocyte sedimentation rate; on the 100th anniversary of his death. *Clin Dermatol* 2011;29(6):697–703.

50. Sesso HD, Buring JE, Rifai N, Blake GJ, Gaziano JM, Ridker PM. C-reactive protein and the risk of developing hypertension. *JAMA* 2003;290(22):2945–2951.

51. Erlinger TP, Platz EA, Rifai N, Helzlsouer KJ. C-reactive protein and the risk of incident colorectal cancer. *JAMA* 2004;291(5):585–590.

52. Aref H, Refaat S. CRP evaluation in non-small cell lung cancer. *Egypt J Chest Diseases and Tuberculosis* 2014;63(3):717–722.

53. Vagulienė N, Žemaitis M, Miliauskas S, Urbonienė D, Šitkauskienė B, Sakalauskas R. Comparison of C-reactive protein levels in patients with lung cancer and chronic obstructive pulmonary disease. *Medicina (Kaunas)* 2011;47(8):421–427. Epub 2011 Nov 18.

54. Alifano M, Falcoz PE, Seegers V, et al. Preresection serum C-reactive protein measurement and survival among patients with resectable non-small cell lung cancer. *J Thorac Cardiovasc Surg* 2011;142(5):1161–1167.

55. Meuwese MC, Stroes ES, Hazen SL, et al. Serum myeloperoxidase levels are associated with the future risk of coronary artery disease in apparently healthy individuals: the EPIC-Norfolk Prospective Population Study. *J Am Coll Cardiol* 2007;50(2):159–165. Epub 2007 Jun 21.

56. Dinarello CA. Historical review of cytokines. *Eur J Immunol* 2007;37(Suppl 1):S34–S45.

57. Zhang J-M, An J. Cytokines, inflammation and pain. *Int Anesthesiol Clin* 2007;45(2):27–37.

58. Centola M, Cavet G, Shen Y, et al. Development of a multi-biomarker disease activity test for rheumatoid arthritis. *PLoS One* 2013;8(4):e60635.

59. Curtis JR, van der Helm-van Mil AH, Knevel R, et al. Validation of a novel multibiomarker test to assess rheumatoid arthritis disease activity. *Arthritis Care Res* 2012;64(12):1794–1803.

60. Wu C, Li F, Niu G, Chen X. PET imaging of inflammation biomarkers. *Theranostics* 2013;3(7):448–466.

61. Fitzgerald A, Berentson-Shaw J. Thermography as a screening and diagnostic tool: a systematic review. *N Z Med J* 2012;125(1351):80–91.

62. Mainiero MB, Lourenco A, Mahoney MC, et al. ACR appropriateness criteria breast cancer screening. *J Am Coll Radiol* 2013;10(1):11–14.

63. Meier-Ewert HK, Ridker PM, Rifai N, et al. Effect of sleep loss on C-reactive protein, an inflammatory marker of cardiovascular risk. *J Am Coll Cardiol* 2004;43(4):678–683.

64. Wu SQ, Liao QC, Xu XX, Sun L, Wang J, Chen R. Effect of CPAP therapy on C-reactive protein and cognitive impairment in patients with obstructive sleep apnea hypopnea syndrome. *Sleep Breath* 2016;20(4):1185–1192.

65. Wu WT, Tsai SS, Shih TS, et al. The impact of obstructive sleep apnea on high-sensitivity C-reactive protein in subjects with or without metabolic syndrome. *Sleep Breath* 2015;19(4):1449–1457.

66. Visser M, Bouter LM, McQuillan GM, Wener MH, Harris TB. Elevated C-reactive protein levels in overweight and obese adults. *JAMA* 1999;282(22):2131–2135.

67. Raz O, Steinvil A, Berliner S, Rosenzweig T, Justo D, Shapira I. The effect of two iso-caloric meals containing equal amounts of fats with a different fat composition on the inflammatory and metabolic markers in apparently healthy volunteers. *J Inflamm (London, England)* 2013;10:3.

68. Carroll MF, Schade DS. Timing of antioxidant vitamin ingestion alters postprandial proatherogenic serum markers. *Circulation* 2003;108(1):24–31.

69. Kobrosly R, van Wijngaarden E. Associations between immunologic, inflammatory, and oxidative stress markers with severity of depressive symptoms: an analysis of the 2005–2006 National Health and Nutrition Examination Survey. *Neurotoxicology* 2010;31(1):126–133. doi: 10.1016/j.neuro.2009.10.005.

70. Silić A, Karlović D, Serretti A. Increased inflammation and lower platelet 5-HT in depression with metabolic syndrome. *J Affect Disord* 2012;141(1):72–78. doi: 10.1016/j.jad.2012.02.019.

71. Bremmer MA, Beekman AT, Deeg DJ, et al. Inflammatory markers in late-life depression: results from a population-based study. *J Affect Disord* 2008;106(3):249–255.

72. Valkanova V, Ebmeier KP, Allan CL. CRP, IL-6 and depression: a systematic review and meta-analysis of longitudinal studies. *J Affect Disord* 2013;150(3):736–744. doi: 10.1016/j.jad.2013.06.004. Review.

73. Decensi A, Omodei U, Robertson C, et al. Effect of transdermal estradiol and oral conjugated estrogen on C-reactive protein in retinoid-placebo trial in healthy women. *Circulation* 2002;106(10):1224–1228.

74. Costello EJ, Copeland WE, Shanahan L, Worthman CM, Angold A. C-reactive protein and substance use disorders in adolescence and early adulthood: a prospective analysis. *Drug Alcohol Depen* 2013;133(2):712–717.

75. Dietrich T, Garcia RI, de Pablo P, Schulze PC, Hoffmann K. The effects of cigarette smoking on C-reactive protein concentrations in men and women and

its modification by exogenous oral hormones in women. *Eur J Cardiovasc Prev Rehabil* 2007;14(5):694–700.

76. Li Y, Rittenhouse-Olson K, Scheider WL, Mu L. Effect of particulate matter air pollution on C-reactive protein: a review of epidemiologic studies. *Rev Environ Health* 2012;27(2-3):133–149.

77. Lee PC, Talbott EO, Roberts JM, Catov JM, Sharma RK, Ritz B. Particulate air pollution exposure and C-reactive protein during early pregnancy. *Epidemiology* 2011;22(4):524–531. doi: 10.1097/EDE.0b013e31821c6c58. Erratum in: *Epidemiology* 2011;22(5):752.

78. Allin KH, Nordestgaard BG. Elevated C-reactive protein in the diagnosis, prognosis, and cause of cancer. *Crit Rev Clin Lab Sci* 2011;48(4):155–170.

79. Mazhar D, Ngan S. C-reactive protein and colorectal cancer. *QJM* 2006;99(8):555–559.

80. Williams CB, Yeh ES, Soloff AC. Tumor-associated macrophages: unwitting accomplices in breast cancer malignancy. *NPJ Breast Cancer* 2016;2. pii: 15025.

81. Chanmee T, Ontong P, Konno K, Itano N. Tumor-associated macrophages as major players in the tumor microenvironment. *Cancer* 2014;6(3):1670–1690.

82. Ittaman SV, VanWormer JJ, Rezkalla SH. The role of aspirin in the prevention of cardiovascular disease. *Clin Med Res* 2014;12(3-4):147–154.

83. Feldman M, Jialal I, Devaraj S, Cryer B. Effects of low-dose aspirin on serum C-reactive protein and thromboxane B2 concentrations: a placebo-controlled study using a highly sensitive C-reactive protein assay. *J Am Coll Cardiol* 2001;37(8):2036–2041.

84. Barnes PJ. How corticosteroids control inflammation: Quintiles Prize Lecture 2005. *Brit J Pharmacol* 2006;148(3):245–254.

85. Van Arnum P. Tracking growth in biologics: the share of biologic-based drugs in the global pharmaceutical market is on the rise. *Pharm Tech* 2013;37(2).

86. Catanoso M, Pipitone N, Magnani L, Boiardi L, Salvarani C. New indications for biological therapies. *Intern Emerg Med* 2011;6(Suppl 1):1–9.

87. Aggarwal BB, Gupta SC, Sung B. Curcumin: an orally bioavailable blocker of TNF and other pro-inflammatory biomarkers. *Br J Pharmacol* 2013;169(8):1672–1692.

88. Sun J, Zhao Y, Hu J. Curcumin inhibits imiquimod-induced psoriasis-like inflammation by inhibiting IL-1beta and IL-6 production in mice. *PLoS One* 2013;8(6):e67078.

89. Wang SL, Li Y, Wen Y, et al. Curcumin, a potential inhibitor of up-regulation of TNF-alpha and IL-6 induced by palmitate in 3T3-L1 adipocytes through NF-kappaB and JNK pathway. *Biomed Environ Sci* 2009;22(1):32–39.

90. Panahi Y, Rahimnia AR, Sharafi M, Alishiri G, Saburi A, Sahebkar A. Curcuminoid treatment for knee osteoarthritis: a randomized double-blind placebo-controlled trial. *Phytother Res* 2014;28(11):1625–1631.

91. Rahimnia AR, Panahi Y, Alishiri G, Sharafi M, Sahebkar A. Impact of supplementation with curcuminoids on systemic inflammation in patients with knee osteoarthritis: findings from a randomized double-blind placebo-controlled trial. *Drug Res (Stuttg)* 2015;65(10):521–525.

92. Chandran B, Goel A. A randomized, pilot study to assess the efficacy and safety of curcumin in patients with active rheumatoid arthritis. *Phytother Res* 2012;26(11):1719–1725.

93. Ganjali S, Sahebkar A, Mahdipour E, et al. Investigation of the effects of curcumin on serum cytokines in obese individuals: a randomized controlled trial. *Sci World J* 2014;2014:898361.

94. Panahi Y, Saadat A, Beiraghdar F, Sahebkar A. Adjuvant therapy with bioavailability-boosted curcuminoids suppresses systemic inflammation and improves quality of life in patients with solid tumors: a randomized double-blind placebo-controlled trial. *Phytother Res* 2014;28(10):1461–1467.

95. Klickovic U, Doberer D, Gouya G, et al. Human pharmacokinetics of high dose oral curcumin and its effect on heme oxygenase-1 expression in healthy male subjects. *Biomed Res Int* 2014;2014:458592.

96. Schiborr C, Kocher A, Behnam D, Jandasek J, Toelstede S, Frank J. The oral bioavailability of curcumin from micronized powder and liquid micelles is significantly increased in healthy humans and differs between sexes. *Mol NutrFood Res* 2014;58(3):516–527.

97. Ryan JL, Heckler CE, Ling M, et al. Curcumin for radiation dermatitis: a randomized, double-blind, placebo-controlled clinical trial of thirty breast cancer patients. *Radiat Res* 2013 Jul;180(1):34–43.

98. Chainani-Wu N, Madden E, Lozada-Nur F, Silverman S Jr. High-dose curcuminoids are efficacious in the reduction in symptoms and signs of oral lichen planus. *J Am Acad Dermatol* 2012 May;66(5):752–760.

99. Chuengsamarn S, Rattanamongkolgul S, Luechapudiporn R, Phisalaphong C, Jirawatnotai S. Curcumin extract for prevention of type 2 diabetes. *Diabetes Care* 2012;35(11):2121–2127.

100. Wongcharoen W, Jai-Aue S, Phrommintikul A, et al. Effects of curcuminoids on frequency of acute myocardial infarction after coronary artery bypass grafting. *Am J Cardiol* 2012;110(1):40–44.

101. Gupta SC, Tyagi AK, Deshmukh-Taskar P, Hinojosa M, Prasad S, Aggarwal BB. Downregulation of tumor necrosis factor and other proinflammatory biomarkers by polyphenols. *Arch Biochem Biophys* 2014;559:91–99.

102. Ebrahimpour Koujan S, Gargari BP, Mobasseri M, Valizadeh H, Asghari-Jafarabadi M. Effects of Silybum marianum (L.) Gaertn. (silymarin) extract supplementation on antioxidant status and hs-CRP in patients with type 2 diabetes mellitus: a randomized, triple-blind, placebo-controlled clinical trial. *Phytomedicine* 2015;22(2):290–296.

103. Ferenci P, Dragosics B, Dittrich H, et al. Randomized controlled trial of silymarin treatment in patients with cirrhosis of the liver. *J Hepatol* 1989;9(1):105–113. PubMed PMID: 2671116.

104. Fried MW, Navarro VJ, Afdhal N, et al; Silymarin in NASH and C Hepatitis (SyNCH) Study Group. Effect of silymarin (milk thistle) on liver disease in patients with chronic hepatitis C unsuccessfully treated with interferon therapy: a randomized controlled trial. *JAMA* 2012;308(3):274–282.

105. Li M, Liu JT, Pang XM, Han CJ, Mao JJ. Epigallocatechin-3-gallate inhibits angiotensin II and interleukin-6-induced C-reactive protein production in macrophages. *Pharmacol Rep* 2012;64(4):912–918.

106. Kou W, Sun R, Wei P, et al. Andrographolide suppresses IL-6/Stat3 signaling in peripheral blood mononuclear cells from patients with chronic rhinosinusitis with nasal polyps. *Inflammation* 2014;37(5):1738–1743.

107. Chun JY, Tummala R, Nadiminty N, et al. Andrographolide, an herbal medicine, inhibits interleukin-6 expression and suppresses prostate cancer cell growth. *Genes Cancer* 2010;1(8):868–876.

108. Sandborn WJ, Targan SR, Byers VS, et al. Andrographis paniculata extract (HMPL-004) for active ulcerative colitis. *Am J Gastroenterol* 2013;108(1):90–98.

109. Saxena RC, Singh R, Kumar P, et al. A randomized double blind placebo controlled clinical evaluation of extract of Andrographis paniculata (KalmCold) in patients with uncomplicated upper respiratory tract infection. *Phytomedicine* 2010;17(3-4):178–185.

110. Chen W, Padilla MT, Xu X, et al. Quercetin inhibits multiple pathways involved in interleukin 6 secretion from human lung fibroblasts and activity in bronchial epithelial cell transformation induced by benzo[a]pyrene diol epoxide. *Mol Carcinog* 2016;55(11):1858–1866.

111. Kim BH, Lee IJ, Lee HY, et al. Quercetin 3-O-beta-(2"-galloyl)-glucopyranoside inhibits endotoxin LPS-induced IL-6 expression and NF-kappa B activation in macrophages. *Cytokine* 2007;39(3):207–215.

112. Nagarkatti P, Pandey R, Rieder SA, Hegde VL, Nagarkatti M. Cannabinoids as novel anti-inflammatory drugs. *Future Med Chem* 2009;1(7):1333–1349.

113. Naftali T, Bar-Lev Schleider L, Dotan I, Lansky EP, Sklerovsky Benjaminov F, Konikoff FM. Cannabis induces a clinical response in patients with Crohn's disease: a prospective placebo-controlled study. *Clin Gastroenterol Hepatol* 2013;11(10):1276–1280.e1.

114. Kasapis C, Thompson PD. The effects of physical activity on serum C-reactive protein and inflammatory markers: a systematic review. *J Am Coll Cardiol* 2005;45(10):1563–1569.

115. Ryan AS, Ge S, Blumenthal JB, Serra MC, Prior SJ, Goldberg AP. Aerobic exercise and weight loss reduce vascular markers of inflammation and improve insulin sensitivity in obese women. *J Am Geriatr Soc* 2014;62(4):607–614.

116. Kasapis C, Thompson PD. The effects of physical activity on serum C-reactive protein and inflammatory markers: a systematic review. *J Am Coll Cardiol* 2005;45(10):1563–1569.

117. Arikawa AY, Thomas W, Schmitz KH, Kurzer MS. Sixteen weeks of exercise reduces C-reactive protein levels in young women. *Med Sci Sports Exerc* 2011;43(6):1002–1009.

118. Beavers KM, Brinkley TE, Nicklas BJ. Effect of exercise training on chronic inflammation. *Clin Chim Acta* 2010;411:785–793.

119. Church TS, Earnest CP, Thompson AM, et al. Exercise without weight loss does not reduce C-reactive protein: the INFLAME study. *Med Sci Sports Exerc* 2010;42(4):708–716.

120. Taylor C, Rogers G, Goodman C. Hematologic, iron-related, and acute-phase protein responses to sustained strenuous exercise. *J Appl Physiol* 1987;62:464–469.

121. Rodríguez-Hernández H, Simental-Mendía LE, Rodríguez-Ramírez G, Reyes-Romero MA. Obesity and inflammation: epidemiology, risk factors, and markers of inflammation. *Int J Endocrinol* 2013;2013:Article ID 678159.

122. Forsythe LK, Wallace JM, Livingstone MB. Obesity and inflammation: the effects of weight loss. *Nutr Res Rev* 2008;21(2):117–133.

123. Deng T, Lyon CJ, Bergin S, Caligiuri MA, Hsueh WA. Obesity, inflammation, and cancer. *Annu Rev Pathol* 2016;11:1–644.

124. Slavin JL. Dietary fiber and body weight. *Nutrition* 2005;21(3):411–418. Review.

125. Champagne CM, Broyles ST, Moran LD, et al. Dietary intakes associated with successful weight loss and maintenance during the Weight Loss Maintenance Trial. *J Am Diet Assoc* 2011;111(12):1826–1835.

126. Jiao J, Xu JY, Zhang W, Han S, Qin LQ. Effect of dietary fiber on circulating C-reactive protein in overweight and obese adults: a meta-analysis of randomized controlled trials. *Int J Food Sci Nutr* 2015;66(1):114–119.

127. Ning H, Van Horn L, Shay CM, Lloyd-Jones DM. Associations of dietary fiber intake with long-term predicted cardiovascular disease risk and C-reactive protein levels (from the National Health and Nutrition Examination Survey Data [2005–2010]). *Am J Cardiol* 2014;113(2):287–291.

128. Ma Y, Griffith JA, Chasan-Taber L, et al. Association between dietary fiber and serum C-reactive protein. *Am J Clin Nutr* 2006;83(4):760–766.

129. King DE, Mainous AG, Egan BM, Woolson RF, Geesey ME. Effect of psyllium fiber supplementation on C-reactive protein: the Trial to Reduce Inflammatory Markers (TRIM). *Ann Fam Med* 2008;6(2):100–106.

130. North CJ, Venter CS, Jerling JC. The effects of dietary fibre on C-reactive protein, an inflammation marker predicting cardiovascular disease. *Eur J Clin Nutr* 2009;63(8):921–933. doi: 10.1038/ejcn.2009.8. Review.

131. Zampelas A, Panagiotakos DB, Pitsavos C, et al. Fish consumption among healthy adults is associated with decreased levels of inflammatory markers related to cardiovascular disease: the ATTICA study. *J Am Coll Cardiol* 2005;46(1):120–124.

132. Pot GK, Geelen A, Majsak-Newman G, et al. Increased consumption of fatty and lean fish reduces serum C-reactive protein concentrations but not inflammation markers in feces and in colonic biopsies. *J Nutr* 2010;140(2):371–376.

133. Bowden RG, Wilson RL, Deike E, Gentile M. Fish oil supplementation lowers C-reactive protein levels independent of triglyceride reduction in patients with end-stage renal disease. *Nutr Clin Pract* 2009;24(4):508–512.

134. Kremer JM, Jubiz W, Michalek A, et al. Fish-oil fatty acid supplementation in active rheumatoid arthritis: a double-blinded, controlled, crossover study. *Ann Intern Med* 1987;106(4):497–503.

135. Proudman SM, James MJ, Spargo LD, et al. Fish oil in recent onset rheumatoid arthritis: a randomised, double-blind controlled trial within algorithm-based drug use. *Ann Rheum Dis* 2015;74(1):89–95.

136. Roseman C, Truedsson L, Kapetanovic MC. The effect of smoking and alcohol consumption on markers of systemic inflammation, immunoglobulin levels and immune response following pneumococcal vaccination in patients with arthritis. *Arthritis Res Ther* 2012;14(4):R170.

137. Sacanella E, Vázquez-Agell M, Mena MP, et al. Down-regulation of adhesion molecules and other inflammatory biomarkers after moderate wine consumption in healthy women: a randomized trial. *Am J Clin Nutr* 2007;86(5):1463–1469.

138. Retterstol L, Berge KE, Braaten Ø, Eikvar L, Pedersen TR, Sandvik L. A daily glass of red wine: does it affect markers of inflammation? *Alcohol Alcohol* 2005;40(2):102–105.

139. McDonald JA, Goyal A, Terry MB. Alcohol intake and breast cancer risk: weighing the overall evidence. *Curr Breast Cancer Rep* 2013;5(3):10.1007/s12609-013-0114-z.

140. Vijayaraghava A, Doreswamy V, Narasipur OS, Kunnavil R, Srinivasamurthy N. Effect of yoga practice on levels of inflammatory markers after moderate and strenuous exercise. *J Clin Diagn Res* 2015;9(6):CC08–CC12.

141. Kiecolt-Glaser JK, Bennett JM, Andridge R, et al. Yoga's impact on inflammation, mood, and fatigue in breast cancer survivors: a randomized controlled trial. *J Clin Oncol* 2014;32(10):1040–1049.

142. Twal WO, Wahlquist AE, Balasubramanian S. Yogic breathing when compared to attention control reduces the levels of pro-inflammatory biomarkers in saliva: a pilot randomized controlled trial. *BMC Complement Altern Med* 2016;16:294.

143. Creswell JD, et al. Alterations in resting-state functional connectivity link mindfulness meditation with reduced interleukin-6: a randomized controlled trial. *Biol Psychiat* 2016 July;80(1):53–61.

144. Black DS, Slavich GM. Mindfulness meditation and the immune system: a systematic review of randomized controlled trials. *Ann N Y Acad Sci* 2016;1373(1):13–24.

145. Rosenkranz MA, Davidson RJ, Maccoon DG, Sheridan JF, Kalin NH, Lutz A. A comparison of mindfulness-based stress reduction and an active control in modulation of neurogenic inflammation. *Brain Behav Immun* 2013;27(1):174–184.

146. Crane JD, Ogborn DI, Cupido C, et al. Massage therapy attenuates inflammatory signaling after exercise-induced muscle damage. *Sci Transl Med* 2012;4(119):119ra13.

147. Zijlstra FJ, van den Berg-de Lange I, Huygen FJ, Klein J. Anti-inflammatory actions of acupuncture. *Mediators Inflamm* 2003;12(2):59–69. Review.

148. Kavoussi B, Ross BE. The neuroimmune basis of anti-inflammatory acupuncture. *Integr Cancer Ther* 2007;6(3):251–257. Review.

149. McDonald JL, Cripps AW, Smith PK, Smith CA, Xue CC, Golianu B. The anti-inflammatory effects of acupuncture and their relevance to allergic rhinitis: a

narrative review and proposed model. *Evid Based Complement Alternat Med* 2013;2013:591796.

150. Vickers AJ, Cronin AM, Maschino AC, et al; Acupuncture Trialists' Collaboration. Acupuncture for chronic pain: individual patient data meta-analysis. *Arch Intern Med* 2012;172(19):1444–1453.

151. Fagundes CP, Bennett JM, Derry HM, Kiecolt-Glaser JK. Relationships and inflammation across the lifespan: social developmental pathways to disease. *Social and Personality Psychology Compass* 2011;5(11):891–903.

18

The Integrative Preventive Medicine Approach to Obesity and Diabetes

DAVID L. KATZ, MD, MPH, FACPM, FACP, FACLM

Origins and Pathogenesis

The global prevalence of obesity has engendered understandable frustration among policy makers, public health practitioners, and health-care providers alike. Attendant on this frustration has been a tendency to see obesity as complex. However, while resolving the modern obesity pandemic may indeed prove as complex as it is challenging, explaining it is easy. People who gain excess weight over time are in a state of positive energy balance. The longer that state persists, and the greater the imbalance, the more weight is gained.

There is a strong genetic contribution to obesity, mediated along several important pathways. Genes influence resting energy expenditure, thermogenesis, lean body mass, and appetite. There is, thus, an important potential genetic influence on both energy intake and expenditure. Overall, genetic factors are thought to explain roughly 40% of the variation in BMI. Adoption studies demonstrating an association between obesity in a child and the biological parents, despite rearing by surrogate parents, and twin studies showing anthropometric correspondence between identical twins reared apart are particularly useful sources of insight in this area[1-4]—genetic factors are of clinical importance as they help explain individual vulnerability to weight gain and its sequelae. Minimally, an appreciation for genetic factors in energy balance should foster insight and compassion relevant to clinical counseling. Maximally, elucidation of genetic contributions to obesity may illuminate novel therapeutic options over time.

Dozens of genes have been implicated as candidates for explaining, at least partly, susceptibility to obesity in different individuals; gene–gene interactions are highly probable in most cases.[5-9] Only in rare instances is a monogenic explanation invoked. A variety of mutations may interfere with leptin signaling, and some of these may prove to be monogenic causes of obesity. In the most recent update from the Human Obesity Gene Map, 127 candidate genes for obesity-related traits were listed.[10] Leptin, produced in adipose tissue, binds to receptors in the hypothalamus, providing information about the state of energy storage and affecting satiety.[11,12] Binding of leptin inhibits secretion of neuropeptide Y, which is a potent stimulator of appetite.

The Ob gene was originally identified in mice, and Ob/Ob mice are deficient in leptin and obese.[13] The administration of leptin to Ob/Ob mice results in weight loss. In humans, obesity is associated with elevated leptin levels.[14] Nonetheless, the administration of leptin to obese humans has been associated with modest weight loss,[15] suggesting that leptin resistance rather than deficiency may be an etiologic factor in some cases of human obesity.[16] Leptin is the primary chemical messenger that signals adipocyte repletion to the hypothalamus; leptin resistance thus has the potential to delay or preclude satiety. The importance of leptin to the epidemiology of obesity has recently been reviewed.[17-20] Much of the genetic influence on weight regulation may be mediated by variation in resting energy expenditure[21] and appetite/satiety.

While the contribution of genes to obesity deserves both recognition and respect, it should not distract from the ultimate hegemony of environmental influences. Genes help explain varied susceptibility to, and expression of, obesity under any given set of environmental conditions. Stated another way, genes help explain the expanse of the "bell curve" characterizing the distribution of weight in a given population at a given time. Isolating the effects of genes on obesity from obesigenic elements in the environment is a considerable challenge;[22] thinking of obesity as a product of gene–environment interaction in most cases may be the best means of meeting this challenge.[23,24]

Environmental factors better explain the position of that entire bell curve relative to a range of potential distributions. The genetic profile of US residents today, for example, may be quite similar to the profile 60 years ago, while the weight distributions for those two populations differ dramatically. The explanation for this divergence over time has much more to do with environmental change than with genetic change. This is true globally as well.

Initial research done in mouse models,[25-27] followed by subsequent studies in humans,[28-30] demonstrated distinct gut microbiota in obese as compared to lean individuals. Moreover, studies suggest that these differences in gut microbiota may influence energy balance and thus obesity.[24] Interestingly, the effects of the microbiome on obesity seems to be transmissible. In mouse models, "transplantation" of gut microbes from obese mice to normal mice results in greater increases in total body fat as compared to those receiving microbes from lean mice.[31] Although more research needs to be conducted before this becomes a mainstay of treatment, alterations of the gut microbiome through probiotics, antibiotics, and fecal transplantation open intriguing new pathways for the treatment of obesity.[32,33]

The balance referred to in "energy balance" is between energy units (typically, but not necessarily, measured in kilocalories or kilojoules) taken into the body and energy units expended by the body. Because the relationship between energy and matter is governed by fundamental laws of physics, the implications of energy balance are substantially self-evident. When more energy is taken into the body than is consumed by all energy-expending processes, the surplus is converted into matter. When energy expenditure exceeds energy intake, matter must be converted into energy to make up the deficit. Thus, positive energy balance increases a body's matter, and negative energy balance decreases it. When energy intake and output are matched, matter—body mass in this case— remains stable.

Several details of clinical interest complicate this otherwise simple construct. The first is that while energy intake is limited to a single activity, eating, energy output is expressed in several ways, including thermogenesis, physical activity, basal metabolism, and growth. The second is that while excess energy intake is convertible into matter, the nature of that matter can vary. Namely, and in simple terms, excess calories can build lean body tissue, fat, or a combination of the two.

The calorie is a measure of food energy and represents the heat required to raise the temperature of 1 g, or cm^3, of water by 1°C at sea level. A kilocalorie, the measure applied to foods, is the heat required to raise the temperature of 1 kg or L of water by the same extent, under the same conditions.[34] The joule is an alternative measure of energy used preferentially in most applications other than food. The joule, and the corresponding kilojoule, is 4.184 times smaller than the calorie and kilocalorie, respectively.

There has been some recent controversy around the question "Is a calorie, a calorie?"[35] A calorie is simply a unit of energy, and as such, 1 cal will always equal 1 cal (just as 1 mL will always equal 1 mL). Where the difference truly lies is that some foods are better for us than others, and one of the many virtues of better-for-us foods is that they tend to help us feel full on fewer calories and thus can tip the balance in the calories in, calories out equation.[36] Calories consumed ("in") is at least conceptually relatively simple: food. As noted, calories expended ("out") is the more complicated combination of resting energy expenditure (REE), basal metabolic rate (BMR), physical activity, and thermogenesis. The formula includes energy dedicated to linear growth in children, which contributes to basal requirements. There is a limited literature to suggest an association between relatively greater protein intake and relatively higher REE at a given body mass than that associated with other macronutrient classes. Thermogenesis is influenced by sympathetic tone and leptin, which in turn may be influenced by insulin and, therefore, to some degree, by macronutrient distribution. A comparable number of calories from different macronutrient sources almost certainly will not be comparably satiating, so macronutrient distribution may influence satiety and, thereby, subsequent energy intake.

If an individual is genetically predisposed to insulin resistance, high levels of postprandial insulin may contribute to weight gain, all else being equal. If that individual restricts calories sufficiently, however, weight gain will not occur. But given the difficulty people with access to abundant and tasty food have restricting calories, the likelihood is that the individual will not do so effectively. High insulin levels may result in more efficient conversion of food energy to body fat, given adequate energy intake for fat deposition to occur. Body fat deposition will lead, in predisposed individuals, to the accumulation of visceral fat and thereby to more insulin resistance, raised insulin levels, and potentially more fat deposition. Thus, while the predominant dietary determinant of weight regulation is clearly total energy intake, macronutrient distribution, endocrine factors, and diverse genetic predispositions may contribute important mitigating influences at any given level of calorie consumption.

In essence, then, the pathogenesis of obesity involves the complex details of a very simple energy balance formula: When calories in exceed calories out, weight rises, and vice versa.

> Theoretically, a pound of fat stores 4,086 kcal (9 kcal per g of fat, multiplied by the 454 g in a pound). However, a pound of living tissue is not actually just fat but must also contain the various structures and fluids required for the viability of that fat, such as blood, blood vessels, neurons, etc. By convention, an excess of 3,500 kcal is used to approximate the energy requirement for a pound of weight gain. By the same convention, a deficit of 3,500 kcal relative to expenditure will translate into a pound of body fat lost.

This thinking has evolved, however, informed by both theory and empirical evidence of neglected nuance. For one thing, as body mass increases, energy requirements for weight maintenance rise; and they fall as body mass declines. A more sophisticated view of the dynamic relationship between energy balance and weight change is fast supplanting the overly simplistic, static view that formerly prevailed.[37,38]

The complexity underlying the energy balance formula is reflected in a wide range of genetic, physiologic, psychological, and sociologic factors implicated in weight gain. Efforts to control weight, prevent gain, or facilitate loss must address energy balance to be successful. Control of body weight relies on achieving a stable balance between energy input and energy consumption at a desired level of energy storage.

Working against this goal is the natural tendency of the body to accumulate fat. The storage of energy in the form of adipose tissue is adaptive in all species with variable and unpredictable access to food. In humans, only about 1,200 kcal of energy is stored as glycogen in the prototypical 70 kg adult, enough to support a fast of 12 to 18 hours at most. A human's ability to survive a more protracted fast depends on energy reserves in body fat, which average 120,000 kcal in a 70 kg adult. The natural tendency to store available energy as body fat persists, although the constant availability of nutrient energy has rendered this tendency maladaptive, whereas it once was, and occasionally still is, vital for survival.

The development of obesity appears to be related to an increase in both the size and number of adipocytes. Excess energy intake in early childhood and adolescence leads more readily to increases in fat cell number. In adults, excess energy consumption leads initially to increases in adipocyte size and only with more extreme imbalance to increased number. Childhood obesity does not lead invariably to adult obesity, as the total number of adipocytes in a lean adult generally exceeds the number in an obese child. Thus, correction for early energy imbalance can restore the number of adipocytes to the normal range. However, childhood obesity is a strong predictor of obesity, and its complications, in adulthood.[39]

In general, lesser degrees of obesity are more likely to be due to increased fat cell size, whereas more severe obesity often suggests increased fat cell number as well. Obesity due exclusively to increased adipocyte size is hypertrophic, whereas that due to increased fat cell number is hyperplastic. Weight loss apparently is more difficult to maintain in hyperplastic as compared to hypertrophic obesity because it requires reducing an abnormally high number of total adipocytes down to an abnormally low size. Adipocytes may actively regulate their size so that it is maintained within the normal range. Such signaling involves various chemical messengers released from adipose tissue, including angiotensinogen, tissue necrosis factor, and others, along with leptin. Adipocytes also produce lipoprotein lipase, which acts on circulating lipoprotein particles, especially very-low-density lipoprotein, to extract free fatty acids, which then are stored in the adipocyte as triglyceride.

The imbalance between energy consumption and expenditure that leads to excess weight gain can be mediated by either and generally is mediated by both. Relative inactivity and abundantly available calories both contribute.

On average, resting energy expenditure accounts for up to 70% of total energy expenditure, thermogenesis approximately 15%, and physical activity approximately 15%. The contribution of physical activity to energy expenditure is, of course, quite variable.

Resting energy expenditure can be measured by various methods, with the doubly labeled water method representing the prevailing standard in research settings.[34,40] In clinical settings, basal energy requirements for weight maintenance can be estimated by use of the Harris-Benedict equation. A rough estimate of calories needed to maintain weight at an average level of activity is derived by multiplying the ideal weight of a woman (in pounds) by 12 to 14 and that of a man by 14 to 16. The REE is lower in women than in men when matched for height and weight due to the higher body fat content in women; muscle imposes a higher metabolic demand than fat at equal mass. A strong genetic component to the REE results in familial clustering as well as clustering within ethnic groups predisposed to obesity.[41-45]

The REE may fall by as much as 30% with dieting, although sustained reductions tend to be smaller, which explains why the maintenance of weight loss becomes increasingly difficult over time after initial success. The phenomenon of the "weight-loss plateau" is attributable in part to the equilibration of lower caloric intake with lower energy requirements resulting from reduced body mass. Weight-management counseling should anticipate and address this universal tendency.

Reductions in BMR may contribute as well to increasing difficulty in losing weight after successive attempts,[46] although this concept is debated.[47-49] A plausible mechanism is that both fat mass and lean body mass are reduced when calories are restricted, whereas weight regain due to caloric excess will result in an increase in fat mass preferentially. Thus, cycles of weight loss and regain have the potential to increase the percentage of body fat and thereby lower calorie requirements for maintenance at any given weight.

When exercise is used as a mainstay in weight loss or maintenance efforts, this mechanism is forestalled. Resistance training that builds muscle can increase BMR, both by increasing total body mass and/or by increasing the percentage of lean body mass. As muscle is more metabolically active than fat, the conversion of body mass from fat to muscle at a stable weight will increase BMR. This pattern may frustrate patients who rely on a scale to gauge weight loss success, but in fact a reduction in fat mass and an increase in lean body mass clearly is a weight management success and should be regarded as such, despite the unmoving dial on a bathroom scale. There is consensus among authorities that in those experiencing cardiometabolic complications of obesity, a weight reduction of 10% is often conducive to clinically important risk reduction. Less well described, but certainly plausible, is similar improvement in those who lower weight less but redistribute weight from fat to lean.

Energy expenditure per unit body mass peaks in early childhood due to the metabolic demands of growth. Total energy expenditure generally peaks in the second decade, and energy intake often does as well. Thereafter, energy requirements decline with age, as does energy consumption. Energy expenditure tends to decline more than energy intake, so that weight gain and, increasingly, adiposity are characteristic of aging.

It is of interest that the capacity of the body to store excess calories in an energy reserve composed of adipose tissue is adaptive in any environment imposing cyclical caloric deprivation. This tendency becomes maladaptive only when an excess of calories is continuously available. Also of note, the adaptive capacity for weight gain is generally variable among individuals and populations, and it is somewhat systematically variable between men and women.

Men are far more prone than premenopausal women to accumulate excess fat at the belly and within the abdominal viscera, rendering them more susceptible to cardiometabolic sequelae of obesity. The central pattern of obesity, known colorfully as the "apple" pattern, is referred to as android. In contrast, the "pear," or peripheral, pattern of obesity is gynoid. There is a potential explanation for the tendency of women of reproductive age to store body fat more innocuously than men in evolutionary biology. Namely, reproduction depends on a woman's ability to meet both her own caloric needs and those of a developing fetus. The capacity to create a large enough energy reserve to help ensure a successful pregnancy may be a critical, and of course uniquely female, adaptation. A final contribution to this admittedly speculative construct is made by the effects in women of reducing body fat content below a critical threshold. Menses ceases, and a state of infertility ensues. This effect is most commonly observed in young female athletes as well as girls with eating disorders, in whom it represents a threat of irreversible osteopenia.

Some ethnic groups are prone to the deposition of fat around the middle, and more importantly within the viscera, the liver in particular, with even minimal weight gain. This has led to the recognition of so-called lean obesity, in which the BMI is well below cutoffs for obesity or even overweight, but the metabolic complications of excess adiposity ensue nonetheless. These manifest generally as insulin resistance, with a high rate of progression to type 2 diabetes. Thus, the spectrum from obesity to diabetes, or "diabesity," is not limited to obesity per se, but can be propagated by excess visceral adiposity in the absence of it.

Food ingestion increases sympathetic tone, raising levels of catecholamines as well as insulin. Brown adipose tissue, concentrated in the abdomen and present in varying amounts, functions principally in the regulation of energy storage and wastage by inducing heat generation in response to stimulation by catecholamines, insulin, and thyroid hormone. The increase in sympathetic tone postprandially results in thermogenesis (heat generation), which may consume up to 15% of ingested calories. Some researchers even suggest targeting thermogenesis for antiobesity efforts.[50,51] A reduced thermic effect of food may contribute to the development of obesity, although this is controversial.[52,53] Approximately 7% to 8% of total energy expenditure is accounted for by obligatory thermogenesis, but up to an additional 7% to 8% is facultative and may vary between the lean and obese.

Insulin resistance may be associated with reduced postprandial thermogenesis. However, obesity apparently precedes reduced thermogenesis, suggesting that impaired thermogenesis is unlikely as an explanation for susceptibility to obesity. Thermogenesis is related to the action of b_3-adrenergic receptors, the density of which varies substantially. Reduced thermogenesis may contribute to weight gain with aging, as thermogenesis apparently declines with age, at least in men.[54,55]

Energy consumption generally has risen in industrialized countries over recent decades as both the energy density of the diet and portion sizes have increased. During the same period, energy expenditure generally has fallen, largely due to changes in the environment and the patterns of work and leisure activity. According to the most recent data from the CDC, a majority of Americans do not meet the physical activity recommendations of 30 minutes of moderate-intensity activities at least 5 days per week.[56] A reduction in exercise-related energy expenditure contributes to energy imbalance and weight gain. The attribution of weight gain to physical inactivity is compounded by the associations between sedentary behavior and poor diet.[57,58]

Although there is consensus that physical activity is essential to long-term weight maintenance, the mechanisms of benefit remain controversial. Evidence that physical activity reduces food intake or results in extended periods of increased oxygen consumption is lacking, and there is evidence to the contrary. Exercise has the potential to increase the REE by increasing muscle mass. Energy consumption during exercise can help maintain energy balance.

Although the utility of physical activity per se in promoting weight loss is uncertain, lifetime physical activity apparently mitigates age-related weight gain and clearly is associated with important health benefits.[59-62] Moreover, the argument that physical activity does not promote weight loss is flawed. Physical activity can indeed promote weight loss and burn fat but only if we engage in enough of it and do not then overeat. The problem is that even those of us who exercise daily are relatively sedentary by historical standards. In the obesigenic environment of the modern world, we are more prone to excessive energy intake and inadequate energy expenditure than any previous generation.[63,64]

The issue of whether physical activity and attendant fitness are more important to health than weight control has generated some controversy. Some authors have argued that fitness is more important than fatness, while others have defended the alternative view.[65-86]

This dispute may be more distracting than helpful. At the population level, most fit people are at least relatively lean, while relative fatness and lack of fitness similarly correlate. While "fit" might trump "fat" in terms of health effects, only an estimated 9% of the population resides in this category of both fit and fat.[87] Evidence from large cohort studies suggests that fitness and fatness are independent predictors of health outcomes. The combination of fit and lean is clearly preferable over all others. Of the two, it appears that weight may influence outcomes slightly more strongly than fitness level.[70]

Evidence from the National Weight Control Registry suggests that regular physical activity may be an important element in lasting weight control.[88,89] Physical activity is among the best predictors of long-term weight maintenance.[90-95] It has been estimated that the expenditure of approximately 12 kcal per kg body weight per day in physical activity is the minimum protective against increasing body fat over time.[93] The contribution of physical activity to weight maintenance may vary among individuals on the basis of genetic factors that are as yet poorly understood.[96,97]

Over recent years, there has been accumulating and encouraging evidence that lifestyle activity, as opposed to structured aerobic exercise, may be helpful in both achieving and maintaining weight loss.[98] Such unobtrusive physical activity may be more readily accepted by exercise-averse patients.

Type 2 Diabetes Mellitus

The development of type 2 diabetes results from the interplay of genetic susceptibility and environmental factors.[99] The responsible genes have not been identified with certainty, although multiple alleles are almost certainly involved, and certain candidate mutations have been under study for some time.[100] The clustering of type 2 diabetes in families is well established. Interest in genetic susceptibility to type 2 diabetes dates at least to the early 1960s, when James Neel,[101,102] who went on to head the human genome project, speculated that expression of diabetes was due to the confrontation of a thrifty metabolism designed for dietary subsistence with a world of nutritional abundance. The theory of metabolic thriftiness essentially posits that a brisk insulin release in response to ingestion is advantageous in the utilization and storage of food energy when such energy is only sporadically available. The same brisk response in the context of abundantly available nutrient energy leads to hyperinsulinemia, obesity, insulin resistance, and ultimately, with the advent of b-cell failure, diabetes. The thrifty genotype theory is supported by certain lines of evidence but is far from universally accepted and continues to generate considerable interest and debate.[103-108]

Factors associated with expression of the disease include excessive nutrient energy intake with resultant obesity, physical inactivity, and advancing age. These factors contribute to the development of insulin resistance at the receptor, an often key element in the development of type 2 diabetes mellitus. Physical activity appears to protect against the advent of type 2 diabetes mellitus both independently and by preventing and mitigating weight gain and obesity.[109] As with type 1 diabetes, the role of the microbiome is currently of intense interest.

Insulin resistance generally precedes, by an uncertain and probably variable period of time, the development of diabetes, although type 2 diabetes can develop in the absence of insulin resistance.[110-112] Diabetes generally occurs when receptor-mediated resistance is compounded by b-cell dysfunction and reduced insulin secretion. Basal insulin production in a healthy, lean adult is roughly 20 to 30 units per 24-hour period. In insulin resistance, that output may be as much as quadrupled to maintain euglycemia. Type 2 diabetes following insulin resistance indicates the failure of b-cells to sustain supraphysiologic output of insulin, a decline of insulin output to below normal levels, and the consequent advent of hyperglycemia.[113,114] Whereas type 1 diabetes is associated with nearly absent insulin release (0 to 4 units daily), type 2 diabetes is generally thought to emerge in lean individuals when production falls to approximately 14 units per day.

An association between weight gain and the development of diabetes is supported by prospective cohort studies,[115-117] although insulin resistance may contribute to the development of obesity as well, so that causality may be bidirectional.[118] Data from such sources suggest that weight loss is protective against the development of diabetes. The currently worsening epidemic of obesity in the United States suggests that the prevalence of diabetes will likely rise and that efforts to combat obesity, if ultimately successful, will translate into reduced rates of diabetes as well.

The incidence of type 2 diabetes in the pediatric population parallels the increase in pediatric obesity.[119] A generation ago, type 2 diabetes was called "adult-onset" diabetes to distinguish it from "juvenile-onset" diabetes. What was a chronic disease of midlife has become an increasingly routine pediatric diagnosis.[120-122]

The Adult Treatment Panel of the National Cholesterol Education Program has essentially equated diabetes with established coronary disease in its guidance for cardiac risk factor management.[123] With adult-onset diabetes now seen in children younger than age 10, we may anticipate the emergence of cardiovascular disease (CVD) in ever younger individuals.[124,125]

The development and manifestations of insulin resistance relate to the principal actions of insulin. In the liver, insulin inhibits gluconeogenesis, inhibits glycogenolysis, and promotes glycogen production.[126] In muscle and adipose tissue, insulin facilitates the uptake of glucose as well as its use and storage. Insulin exerts important influences on protein and lipid metabolism as well. The fundamental role of insulin is to coordinate the use and storage of food energy. This requires regulation of both carbohydrate and fat metabolism, as total body glycogen and glucose stores in a healthy adult approximate 300 g. At 4 kcal per g, this represents an energy reserve of 1,200 kcal, enough to support a fast of approximately 12 to 18 hours. Energy stored as triglyceride in adipose tissue in a lean adult totals nearly 120,000 kcal, or 100 times the carbohydrate reserve. Thus, release of energy stores from adipose tissue can protect vital organs during a protracted fast.

In the fed state, the entry of amino acids and monosaccharides into the portal circulation stimulates release of proinsulin from pancreatic b-cells. Insulin is cleaved from the connecting ("C") protein to generate active insulin. Insulin transports both amino acids and glucose into the liver, where it stimulates glycogen synthesis, protein synthesis, and fatty acid synthesis, while suppressing glycogenolysis and gluconeogenesis as well as proteolysis and lipolysis. Insulin carries both glucose and amino acids into skeletal muscle, and it carries glucose into adipose tissue. Insulin facilitates glycogen synthesis and glycolysis in muscle, and it facilitates fatty acid synthesis in adipose tissue. Insulin also stimulates the synthesis of lipoprotein lipase in capillaries, facilitating the extraction of fatty acids from circulation, and promotes hepatic very-low-density lipoprotein (VLDL) synthesis.

During a fast, insulin levels decline, as levels of glucagon, a product of the pancreatic a-cells, rise. Falling insulin levels promote glycogenolysis, followed by gluconeogenesis, in the liver. In adipose tissue, low insulin levels stimulate lipolysis, releasing fatty acids for use as fuel; ketones are generated in the process of hepatic fatty acid oxidation. High levels of circulating fatty acids inhibit insulin action. Reduced insulin action at skeletal muscle stimulates proteolysis.

In the insulin-resistant state, insulin levels are high, but receptors, particularly those on skeletal muscle, are relatively insensitive to insulin action.[127,128] High levels of insulin presumably compensate for receptor-mediated resistance. High insulin levels promote fatty acid synthesis in the liver. The accumulation and circulation of free fatty acids and triglycerides packaged in VLDL aggravate insulin resistance, driving insulin levels higher. Thus, the metabolic derangements are self-perpetuating, generating in the process the manifestations of the insulin-resistance syndrome associated with cardiovascular risk, until the *b*-cells fail and diabetes develops.

With *b*-cell failure, the resultant low levels of circulating insulin mimic conditions during a fast. The metabolic derangements that distinguish diabetes from fasting include pathologically low insulin levels and, of course, high levels of circulating glucose. Hepatic gluconeogenesis compounds the hyperglycemia, with excess glucose leading to tissue damage through glycosylation. Glycosylation of hemoglobin is routinely used as a measure of the extent of prevailing glycemia (i.e., HgbA1c). High ambient levels of glucose lead to the production of sugar alcohols (e.g., sorbitol, fructose) in many tissues, which in turn can cause cellular distention. The accumulation of such polyols in the lens is causally implicated in the blurred vision that often occurs with poorly controlled diabetes.

In studies of the Pima Indians, a tribe of Native Americans particularly subject to the development of obesity and diabetes mellitus, Lillioja et al[129] showed that insulin resistance is an antecedent of diabetes. During the phase of insulin resistance, serum glucose is normal but insulin levels are abnormally elevated, both in the fasting and postprandial states. The development of obesity appears to be of particular importance in the development of IGT secondary to insulin resistance. A modest degree of hyperglycemia may occur during the period of insulin resistance, acting as a signal to the endocrine pancreas that insulin action is impaired and stimulating more insulin release. Ultimately, both protracted hypersecretion and hyperglycemia may contribute to *b*-cell dysfunction and overt diabetes.

The development of type 2 diabetes often is preceded by a protracted period of insulin resistance manifested as the "metabolic syndrome" of obesity, dyslipidemia, and hypertension. Abdominal obesity and hypertriglyceridemia may be particularly early markers of the syndrome and represent a readily detectable indicator of risk for diabetes.[130] Of note, the defining features of the insulin-resistance syndrome, and the nomenclature applied, have been matters of contention. The American Heart Association supports diagnostic criteria for the metabolic syndrome,[131] while the American Diabetes Association has questioned the utility of defining a syndrome at all.[132]

Regardless of the terminology applied to the various manifestations of the insulin-resistant state, interventions to treat the condition, particularly supervised weight loss, may both mitigate associated cardiovascular risk and prevent the evolution of diabetes. The Diabetes Prevention Program has provided definitive evidence that intervention with either lifestyle modification or pharmacotherapy can prevent type 2 diabetes in a significant proportion of at-risk individuals.[133] In individuals with diagnosed type 2 diabetes, the Look AHEAD trial has demonstrated that intensive lifestyle intervention can improve glucose control and reduce CVD risk factors and medication use.[134,135]

Epidemiology

In the United States, obesity is among the gravest and most poorly controlled public health threats of our time.[136-138] Over two-thirds of the adults in the United States are overweight or obese. Recent data suggest that the prevalence of obesity may have plateaued for some age groups over the past few years.[139,140] While this may offer a glimmer of hope, there are less sanguine interpretations of the data. A plateau in any trend is inevitable as the limits of its range are approximated. Further, the prevalence of overweight and obesity does not adequately reflect the distribution of actual weights in the population.

There is evidence that the more extreme degrees of obesity are increasing in prevalence faster than overweight.[141] This suggests that the minority in the population that has resisted the tendency toward excessive weight gain thus far may remain resistant and not contribute to the ranks of the overweight and obese. Those, however, who have already succumbed to obesity trends may remain vulnerable to increasing weight gain over time, thus transitioning through overweight to progressively severe degrees of obesity. This implies that even if the cumulative prevalence of overweight and obesity were to stabilize at current levels, the health effects of obesity may well continue to worsen. Compounding such concerns, the most recent trend data indicate continued, significant increases in obesity prevalence for women and for children and adolescents in the United States; insignificant increases for men; and increases in severe obesity for all groups.[142,143]

The rate of childhood obesity has tripled in the past two decades.[144] Over 30% of children in the US population at large are considered overweight or obese. In some ethnic minority groups, this figure rises to 40%.[140]

Recent studies indicate that obesity is occurring at ever-younger ages. A marked rise in the prevalence of overweight among infants and toddlers has been documented both in the United States and globally.[145,146] As in adults, BMI is a crude indicator of adiposity and fat distribution in children. Data indicate that waist circumference has been rising in tandem with BMI in children, which is of concern since abdominal adiposity has worse health implications.[147]

The increasingly global economy has rendered obesity an increasingly global problem, with the United States the putative epicenter of an obesity pandemic.[148-150] Worldwide, an estimated 1.4 billion adults are overweight or obese.[151] Rates of obesity are already high and rising in most developed countries, and they are lower but rising faster in countries undergoing a cultural transition.[152] In China, India, and Russia, the constellation of enormous population, inadequate control of historical public health threats such as infectious disease, and the advent of epidemic obesity and attendant chronic disease represent an unprecedented challenge.[153-155] In countries undergoing a time of even more rapid cultural transition and development, the effects on obesity and chronic disease are astonishing. For example, in Qatar, the rates of obesity and diabetes are even higher than those in the United States, with 75% of adults overweight or obese and 17% of adults with type 2 diabetes.[156]

Obesity control is among the current priorities the World Health Organization. Universal dietary preferences evidently predominate over cultural patterns as nutrient-dilute, energy-dense foods become available.[157,158] At the 10th International Congress on Obesity held in Sydney, Australia, in September 2006, World Health Organization data were reported, indicating that for the first time in history, there were more overweight than hungry people on the planet.

The fundamental health implications of obesity appear to be universal. Appropriate threshold values for the definition of overweight and obesity, however, should likely vary with ethnicity and associated anthropometry. Certain Asian populations appear to have a predilection for central, and visceral, fat deposition and thus a vulnerability to insulin resistance at a BMI deemed normal and innocuous for most occidental populations. There are noteworthy variations in BMI, waist circumference, and lean body mass among diverse ethnic groups. Genetic variability in the susceptibility to obesity and its metabolic sequelae is quite pronounced.

In the United States, there are some 25.8 million diabetics, of whom roughly 18.8 million are diagnosed and the remainder undiagnosed.[159,160] The ratio of diagnosed to undiagnosed diabetes has declined slightly over recent years among the overweight, apparently in response to heightened awareness of diabetes risk in this group.[160] More than 90% of the diagnosed cases and virtually all of the undiagnosed cases of diabetes are type 2. Prediabetes, encompassing both IGT (a blood sugar level of 140 to 199 mg per dL after a 2-hour oral glucose tolerance test) and IFG (blood sugar level of 100 to 125 mg per dL after an overnight fast), affects some 79 million.[159] The metabolic or insulin-resistance syndrome now affects nearly one-fourth of US adults, and some 80 million or more are insulin resistant.[161,162]

The World Health Organization estimates that there were approximately 347 million diabetics worldwide as of 2012, and it projects that diabetes deaths will increase by two-thirds between 2008 and 2030.[163] Projections in the United States suggest that nearly 1 in 3 individuals born in the year 2000 or after will develop diabetes in their lifetime, and for Hispanics, the figure is nearly 1 in 2.[164-166] Some more recent projections are more dire still, pointing to diabetes in 40% of the general population and 50% or more in certain ethnic groups.[167] Other data indicating modest improvement in recent trends support somewhat less ominous projections.[168]

Sequelae

The health consequences of obesity are in general well characterized, as is the economic toll.[169-177] The toll of the epidemic is most starkly conveyed by the impact on children. The claim has been made that due to epidemic obesity, we are now raising the first generation of children with a shorter projected life expectancy than that of their parents.[169,178] This view has been contested, however, with claims that life expectancy will continue to rise into the future despite a rising burden of chronic disease.

Obesity, at least when distributed centrally, engenders a plethora of cardiac risk factors and is thus an important contributor to cardiovascular disease. An observational cohort study conducted by the American Cancer Society[179] representing more than 15 million person years of observation has demonstrated a link between obesity and most cancers. Obesity is associated with asthma, sleep apnea, osteoarthritis, and gastrointestinal disorders as well.

Obesity in children has been linked to increased risk of developing hypertension,[180-183] hypercholesterolemia,[184,185] hyperinsulinemia,[184] insulin resistance,[186,187] hyperandrogenemia,[186,187] gallstones,[65,188,189] hepatitis and fatty liver,[190-193] sleep apnea,[194-198] orthopedic abnormalities (e.g., slipped capital epiphyses),[199-203] and increased intracranial hypertension.[204-209] Obesity during adolescence increases rates of cardiovascular disease[210-214] and diabetes[211,215] in adulthood, in both men and women. In women, adolescent obesity is associated with completion of fewer years of education, higher rates of poverty, and lower rates of marriage and household income. In men, obesity in adolescence is associated with increased all-cause mortality and mortality from cardiovascular disease and colon cancer.[211,216] Adults who were obese as children have increased mortality and morbidity, independent of adult weight.[39,211,217-219] Childhood obesity appears to be accelerating the onset of puberty in girls and may delay puberty in boys.[220]

Reports that weight cycling may be associated with morbidity or mortality, independently of obesity, are of uncertain significance.[219,221-223] There is evidence that when other risk factors are adequately controlled in the analysis, weight cycling does not predict mortality independently of obesity.[224-226] There is also evidence that cardiovascular risk factors are dependent on the degree of obesity and fat accumulation over time rather than weight regain follow-ing loss.[227,228] The benefits of weight loss are thought to override any potential hazards of weight regain;[229] therefore, efforts at weight loss generally should be encouraged even in obese individuals with a prior history of weight cycling.[230] However, repeated cycles of weight loss and regain may render subsequent weight loss more difficult by affecting body composition and metabolic rate, although this is an area of some controversy. For this reason, among others, weight-loss efforts should be predicated on sustainable adjustments to diet and lifestyle, whenever possible, rather than extreme modifications over the short term.

Often overlooked but of clear relevance to office-based dietary counseling is the relationship between obesity and mental health. Body image, adversely affected and even distorted by obesity, is important to self-esteem.[231,232] Thus, poor self-esteem is a common consequence of obesity (the converse often also being true, with poor self-esteem adversely affecting diet).[233] This has impor-tant implications for dietary modification efforts. Repeated cycles of weight loss and regain may have particularly adverse effects on psychological well-being, although research in this area is limited.[221,234,235]

Evidence consistently and clearly indicates that obesity engenders antipa-thy, resulting in stigma, social bias, and discrimination.[231,236,237] Obese children suffer from poor self-esteem[233,238,239] and are subjected to teasing, discrimina-tion, and victimization.[217,240,241] Bullying and weight status can develop into a vicious cycle in which the stress of being teased may make the child more likely to seek out comfort food, thus further hindering the chance of achiev-ing a healthy weight. The topic of weight bias is of ever-increasing concern as the worsening epidemic of obesity directs increasing societal attention to the topic.

The severity of prejudice against obesity is startling. Studies among school-children consistently indicate a strong and nearly universal distaste for obesity as compared to other and equally noticeable variations in physiognomy.

In addition to its obvious implications for the overall well-being of obese persons, weight bias has implications for public policy. There is some evidence to suggest that the routine measurement of student BMI by schools, with reports home to parents, may enhance awareness of, and responses to, child-hood obesity. This intervention was implemented successfully in Arkansas and is thought to have contributed to an apparent turnaround in childhood obesity trends in the state.[242] Nonetheless, there is considerable opposition to this strategy, due largely to its potential for stigmatizing obese children and vilifying their parents.[243] The solution to weight bias, however, cannot be to deny the problem of obesity. Rather, obesity and prejudice must both be con-fronted. And when the problem of obesity is attacked, it must be consistently and abundantly clear that the attack is against the condition and its causes, not its victims. All clinicians share in the responsibility for highlighting this distinction. As is true of the metabolic effects of obesity, psychosocial sequelae of the condition tend to vary with its severity.[244]

Type 2 diabetes is often, although not always, a complication of obesity. It, in turn, may be complicated by all of the end-organ injuries associated with type 1 diabetes, from the heart and vasculature, to the eyes, nerves, limbs, and kidneys.

Obesity and Mortality

One of the most contentious and controversial aspects of the obesity epidemic has been a reliable accounting of the mortality toll. In 1993, McGinnis and Foege[245] identified the combination of dietary pattern and sedentary lifestyle as the second leading cause of preventable, premature death in the United States, accounting for some 350,000 deaths per year. Obesity contributes to the majority of these deaths and was considered to be directly or indirectly responsible for approximately 300,000 annual deaths.[246]

Calle et al[247] reported a linear relationship between BMI and mortality risk, based on an observational cohort of more than 1 million subjects followed for 14 years. In this cohort, high BMI was less predictive of mortality risk in blacks than in whites. Manson et al[248] found a linear relationship between BMI and mortality risk in women from the Nurses' Health Study; the lowest risk of all-cause mortality occurred in women with a BMI 15% below average with stable weight over time.

In a study of over half a million adults by Adams et al,[249] after controlling for smoking status and initial health, both overweight and obesity was associated with an increased risk of death. More recently, a highly publicized meta-analysis by Flegal et al[250] found that while obesity was associated with a higher all-cause mortality relative to normal weight, overweight was associated with a significantly *lower* all-cause mortality rate.

There is now a rich litany of arguments on both sides of the obesity/mortality divide, with arguments for and against a high mortality toll now[178,251-253] and in the future. The CDC has officially addressed the controversy on more than one occasion, with much of the debate spilling over into the popular press.[246,254-282]

Masters et al, adjusting for birth cohort, demonstrated a high and rising contribution of obesity to mortality moving through the past toward the present.[283] Other important considerations are that some obesity is metabolically innocuous, while metabolically significant "obesity" can occur in the context of a normal BMI; both of these bias the BMI/mortality association toward the null. In addition, studies showing null or inverse associations between BMI and mortality have often failed to exclude those with cachexia related to ill health at baseline.

Fortunately, there is no need to reach absolute consensus on the death toll of obesity to appreciate the threat it represents. It may be that obesity is killing fewer people than projected because of advances in tertiary care. Certainly the means of compensating for chronic diseases in advanced states improve with each passing year. But compensation for chronic disease by such means as endovascular procedures, polypharmacy, and/or surgery is not nearly as good as, and is vastly more expensive than, preserving good health. That obesity accounts for an enormous burden of chronic disease is beyond dispute; it lies on the well-established causal pathway toward virtually all of the leading causes of premature death and disability in industrialized countries, including diabetes, cardiovascular disease, cancer, degenerative arthritis, dementia, stroke, and, to a lesser extent, obstructive pulmonary disease. Thus, while the number of years obesity may be taking out of life is debatable, there is no argument that it is taking life out of years.

There is, finally, a simple logic about the association between obesity and mortality. Obesity contributes mightily to the prevalence of diabetes, cancer, heart disease, and, to a lesser extent, stroke. These, in turn, are the leading proximal causes of death in the United States. It would seem far-fetched that a condition contributing to all the leading causes of death is entirely unimplicated itself.

Economic Toll of Obesity

Overweight and obesity are thought to add an estimated $113 billion to national health-related expenditures in the United States each year or fully 5% to 10% of the nation's medical bill.[284] Obesity has been a major driver of increased Medicare expenditures over the past decade.[285] Compared to medical spending on healthy weight adults, medical spending on obese adults may be as much as 100% higher.[171] Additionally, if the current childhood obesity epidemic is not halted, researchers forecast that from 2030 to 2050, there will be an additional $254 billion of obesity-related costs from both direct medical costs and loss of productivity.[286]

There is also evidence to suggest that obesity results in personal financial disadvantage; poverty is predictive of obesity, and obesity is also predictive of less upward financial mobility.[287-289] Thorpe et al[285] have attributed to obesity alone 12% of the increase in healthcare spending in the United States over recent years.[290,291] Obesity-related expenditures by private insurers purportedly increased 10-fold between 1987 and 2002.

A report in the *American Journal of Health Promotion*[292] indicates that obesity increases healthcare- and absenteeism-related costs by $460 to $2,500 per worker per year. Roughly one-third of this cost is induced by higher rates of absenteeism, and two-thirds are induced by healthcare expenditures. These costs are distributed to lean workers as well, who pay higher healthcare premiums as a result, and to the employer, who experiences higher operating costs.

But some may actually profit from obesity, notably those in businesses responsible for selling the excess calories that make weight gain possible. In a provocative piece in the *Washington Post*, Michael Rosenwald[293] suggested that obesity is an integral aspect of the American economy, influencing industries as diverse as food, fitness, and healthcare. The trade-off between obesity-related profits and losses has been considered elsewhere.[294] Costs and benefits are often a matter of perspective, and what is good finance for the seller may be bad for the buyer.

Close and Schoeller[295] have pointed out that bargain pricing on oversized fast-food meals and related products actually increases net cost to the consumer, largely as a consequence of weight gain. The higher costs over time relate to adverse health effects of obesity as well as increased food intake by larger persons. Note the paradox here: In order to sustain the market for the excess calories that contribute to obesity, obesity is necessary, as it drives up the calories required just to maintain weight; obesity depends on an excess of calories, and the effective peddling of that excess of calories depends on obesity.

Another cost of obesity is reduced fuel efficiency when driving and carrying more weight. Stated bluntly, the "all-you-can- eat" buffet is not much of a bargain both because excess calories resulting in excess weight lead to increased costs of living and because most beneficiaries of discounted dietary indulgences wind up willing to spend a fortune to lose weight they gained at no extra charge. There may be some utility in pointing this out to patients.

The Integrative Preventive Medicine Approaches to Clinical Treatment

Bariatric surgery of varying types is well established as efficacious treatment for severe or complicated obesity. Pharmacotherapy for obesity per se is rather less convincingly supported in the literature, but the mere existence of FDA-approved drugs for weight loss and management bespeaks a relevant body of evidence. Pharmacotherapy for type 2 diabetes is, of course, the standard of practice, and an area of bountiful and ever-evolving evidence.

Relative inattention to these topics here is not indicative of their unimportance; rather the contrary. These approaches are promoted by the prevailing forces and profit centers of modern medicine, and thus predominate. Consequently, the attendant literature is vast, continuously refreshed, and readily accessible to all, including excellent, current reviews on each of these topics. For that reason, then, this chapter will focus preferentially on those aspects of treatment rooted in lifestyle, and generally relegated to lesser, supporting roles.

Evidence that sustainable weight loss is enhanced by means other than caloric restriction is lacking. Whereas short-term weight loss is consistently achieved by any dietary approach to the restriction of choice and thereby calories, lasting weight control is not. Competing dietary claims imply that fundamental knowledge of dietary pattern and human health is lacking; an extensive literature belies this notion. The same dietary and lifestyle pattern conducive to health promotion is consistently associated with weight control. A bird's-eye view of the literature on diet and weight reveals a forest otherwise difficult to discern through the trees. Competing diet claims are diverting attention and resources from what is actually and urgently needed: a dedicated and concerted effort to make the basic dietary pattern known to support both health and weight control more accessible to all.

Against the backdrop of this increasingly acute need, the identification of practical and generalizable solutions to the obesity crisis has proved elusive. From research interventions, to commercial weight loss programs, to supplements, potions, and devices, innumerable approaches to weight loss have been devised. That none of these has yet met the need of the population is clearly reflected in the stubborn epidemiology of obesity.

Obesity is as relevant to prevailing views on beauty, fashion, and body image as it is to public health, and thus it engenders unique preoccupations.[296-302] Individuals reluctant to take antihypertensive or lipid-lowering medication for fear of side effects may aggressively pursue pharmacotherapy, or even surgery, for weight control.[303-305] The visibility of obesity, the stigma associated with it[306-308] (it is often said that antiobesity sentiment is the last bastion of socially acceptable prejudice), and the difficulty most people experience in their efforts to resist it contribute to its novel influences on attitude and behavior. This widespread state of volatile frustration renders the public susceptible to almost any persuasive sales pitch for a weight-loss lotion, potion, or program.

The natural consequence of acute and substantially unmet need is frustration. This public frustration has created a seemingly limitless market for weight-loss approaches. This same frustration has engendered a prevailing gullibility so that virtually any weight-loss claim is accepted at face value. Dual aphorisms might be considered for characterizing the obesity epidemic. Until recently, organized responses to this degenerating crisis have been tepid at best, suggesting that among public health professionals, familiarity breeds complacency, if not outright contempt. Among members of the general public, desperation breeds gullibility.

It is thus a seller's market for weight-loss wares. The litany of competing claims for effective weight loss is producing increasing confusion among both the public at large and healthcare professionals.[309] In the mix is everything from science to snake oil, with no assurances that science is the more popular choice.

The concept of the "ideal" body weight and efforts to reach it may be both unrealistic and harmful for most overweight patients. The benefits of moderate weight loss are sufficiently clear to justify efforts to induce a loss of 5% to 10% of total weight, which is apt to be much more readily achievable. Perhaps better still is an emphasis on the means of achieving weight loss—namely changes in diet and activity pattern rather than weight per se, as the patient has control over the former but can only indirectly influence the latter. Most adult patients concerned about weight regulation will have made multiple attempts at weight control, with at best transient success. Above all, clinicians must not submit to "blame the victim" temptations in this setting.

Temporary weight loss is no more a definitive resolution of the metabolic factors that promote obesity than transient euglycemia is a resolution of diabetes. Therefore, diets designed for short-term weight loss offer no convincing benefit either in terms of sustained weight loss or health outcomes. Because dietary and lifestyle management of weight must be permanent, it is essential that the dietary patterns applied be compatible with recommendations for health promotion in general. Fad diets promoted for purposes of rapid weight loss are unsubstantiated in the peer-reviewed literature. Even if conducive to weight management over time, such diets would be ill advised unless shown to promote health and prevent disease.

Several general modifications of the overall dietary pattern are likely to facilitate weight control. Some benefit may derive from frequent, small meals or snacks rather than the conventional three meals a day. One study examining snacking habits in overweight women enrolled in a weight- loss study found that mid-morning snackers lost more weight than afternoon or evening snackers.[310] Physiologically, there is some evidence that distributing the same number of calories in small snacks ("nibbling") rather than larger meals ("gorging") may reduce 24-hour insulin production, at least in insulin-resistant individuals.[311] Speechly et al[312] reported evidence that snacking attenuates appetite relative to larger meals spaced farther apart. A group of seven obese men was provided an ad libitum lunch following a morning "preload" provided as a single meal or multiple snacks with the same total nutrient and energy composition. Subjects ate significantly (27%) less following multiple small meals than after a single larger one. Insulin peaked at higher levels following the single meal and was sustained above baseline for longer with the multiple small meals. Total area under the insulin curves was similar in both groups.

Evidence in support of "snacking" as a means of controlling weight or improving insulin metabolism is preliminary and not undisputed.[313,314] However, there is generally a profound psychological component to disturbances of weight regulation, and the distribution of meals and calories may be germane. Most patients trying to control their weight are both tempted by and afraid of preferred foods. Consequently, many such patients resist eating for protracted periods during the day, only to overindulge in a late-day or evening binge. This pattern perpetuates a dysfunctional and tense relationship between the patient and his or her diet.

Patients caught up in this pattern may benefit from advice to bring nutrient dense, wholesome, satiating foods with them every day and systematically to resist foods made available by others. Patients should be encouraged to eat whenever they want, but only those foods chosen in advance. By having free access to such foods (e.g., fresh fruits, fresh vegetables, nuts, etc.), patients may overcome their fear of needing to "go hungry" for extended periods each day. In addition, frequent snacking during the day obviates the need and desire for a compulsive and binge-like meal at the end of the day. Finally, for many patients, the ideal time for exercise is after work. Overweight patients who have avoided food much of the day may simply be too hungry after work to exercise. A meal at such a time often is prepared impulsively and eaten not only to satisfy energy needs but also to assuage the pent-up frustrations of the day. On questioning, many overweight patients acknowledge that they often eat, and overeat, for reasons having nothing to do with hunger.

Exercise is an effective means of moderating psychological stress[315] and may attenuate the need to resolve such stress with food. In addition, exercise may temporarily suppress appetite and generally enhance self-esteem, both of which are conducive to more thoughtful choices as the evening meal is prepared. Finally, and most evident, is the additional caloric expenditure resulting from the added activity. A meta-analysis of weight-loss studies published in 1997 reveals important limitations in the field of obesity management but suggests that best results to date have been achieved by combining energy-restricted diets with aerobic exercise.[316]

The primary clinical intervention for weight management is lifestyle counseling. The case for universal weight-management counseling in clinical care has not yet been made on the basis of evidence. The US Preventive Services

Task Force recommends intensive dietary counseling for patients with overt cardiovascular risk factors and routine screening for obesity, but it concludes that evidence is insufficient to support routine dietary or weight-management counseling for adults without known hypertension, hyperlipidemia, cardiovascular disease, or diabetes.[317-319]

For the most part, effective and practical methods of obesity prevention in clinical context are as yet not reliably established.

Relatively few interventions have been conducted that aim to introduce such counseling into the native environments of clinical practice, and even fewer have demonstrated efficacy of low-intensity interventions, such as brief counseling sessions with the primary care clinician.[320] There are exceptions, however,[321] with more attention thus far to physical activity than to diet.[322-326]

There is suggestive evidence that physician counseling of overweight patients is supportive of weight loss and of the use of appropriate methods to achieve such weight loss.[327] Overall, evidence in support of counseling is limited, largely because such counseling is limited;[328] the only effective interventions appear to be those of medium- and high-intensity behavioral counseling.[318]

Worth noting in societies such as the United States, which has both highly prevalent obesity and preoccupation with slimness, is a tendency for even normal-weight individuals to "diet." In addition, such injudicious practices as smoking may be used as a means to maintain body weight.[329] The clinician should be equally prepared to discourage ill-advised weight control practices as to encourage salutary ones. There is some evidence that patients who discuss weight control with their healthcare providers are more apt to pursue weight loss and control by healthful and prudent means.[327,330] Also noteworthy is increasing recognition of the need to reform clinical practice patterns on the basis of both available evidence and professional judgment.

Encouraging patients to eat well for the promotion of health and the prevention and/or amelioration of disease should be approached in the context of well-established principles of behavior modification. Some patients need to be motivated before they are willing to consider change, others need help strategizing to maintain change currently under way, and still others need help overcoming the sequelae of prior failed attempts. This latter group, perhaps predominant, may be harmed by counseling efforts focusing only on motivation. Much effort at dietary modification fails due to the diverse and challenging obstacles to a healthy diet in the modern "toxic" nutritional environment. The clinician committed to promoting the nutritional health of patients must commit to devising strategies, tailored to individual patients, over and around such obstacles.

Relevant models of behavior modification encompass motivational interviewing; the transtheoretical model; adaptations of these specific to the primary care setting; and the social ecological model.

Several salient principles warrant particular emphasis here. First, given the prevalence of obesity, counseling for weight control should be universal. Second, given the popularity of weight-loss approaches that diverge from well-established practice for health promotion, the principal focus of weight control efforts should, in fact, be health. The best available evidence links dietary and activity patterns conducive to health with long-term maintenance of weight. Third, given that obesity is epidemic in both adults and children, the unit to which counseling should be aimed is the family or household rather than the individual patient. Adult patients have a responsibility to engage their children in healthful lifestyle practices, and they will find lifestyle change easier and more sustainable for themselves when the effort involves household-wide solidarity. Finally, weight control efforts should be directed toward long-term sustainability rather than the fast start that seems perennially tantalizing to patients.

A final, important consideration is that clinical approaches to the obesity/diabetes spectrum invite, if they do not require, attention to holism. All too often a platitude, holistic care can and should be approached as a practicable, replicable, and testable method. As such, its relevance to weight management is particularly salient.

Consider a woman of roughly 70, who comes to the clinic ostensibly to get dietary advice because she wants to lose weight. She is, indeed, obese—with a body mass index of 32. She has high blood pressure and type 2 diabetes, and is on medication for these. Her husband passed away 4 years ago, and she lives alone. She is lonely, tends toward sadness, and is always tired. She sleeps poorly.

She eats in part because she is often hungry, in part to get gratification she does not get from other sources. She does not exercise because she has arthritis that makes even walking painful. Her arthritis has worsened as her weight has gone up, putting more strain on already taxed hips and knees. Medication for her joint pains irritates her stomach, and worsens her hypertension. And so on.

Such a patient, likely familiar to all clinician readers, is, in the coarse vernacular of medicine, *circling the drain*. A complex array of medical, emotional, and social problems really can resemble a cascade in which each malady worsens another, and the net effect is a downward spiral into despondent disability. "Circling the drain" is crude, but apt.

The term actually has hidden utility. If one can descend one degenerating spiral at a time, there is reason to think treatment can reverse engineer the process, allowing for ascent in much the same fashion. This is what holistic care—in its practical details—needs to be; both when practiced by a healthcare professional and in the context of self-care by patients. There are no magical means by which a complex array of interconnected problems can be fixed in one fell swoop. But this array can be appreciated, deconstructed, and addressed in a logical sequence that is respectful of the whole, even while managing it in parts.

For the hypothetical case in question, and innumerable real people like her, reversing a descent begins with one well-prioritized move in the other direction. So, for instance, it is likely that this woman has markedly impaired sleep, due perhaps to sleep apnea. A test and intervention to address this effectively may be the best first move for a number of reasons.

Poor sleep can cause, and/or compound depression; poor sleep invariably lowers pain thresholds, making things hurt that otherwise might not, and things that would hurt anyway, hurt more; poor sleep leads to unrestrained and emotional eating; poor sleep leads to hormonal imbalances that foster hypertension, insulin resistance, and weight gain; and poor sleep saps energy that might otherwise be used for everything from social interactions, to exercise.

Whether a focus on sleep is the right first step will vary with the patient, of course. If it is, as soon as sleep does improve, the benefits start to accrue. Our patient has a bit less pain, a bit more energy, and a slightly more hopeful outlook. So now that she has some more resources, we ask more of her. We are devoted to her, and on her team, but that only means we will hold her hand—not carry her. So, we now need her to invest these benefits back into herself.

The energy available now but not before allows for the start of a gentle exercise regimen (water-based if need be to avoid joint strain). Mobility in turn allows for social activity of interest to get some stimulation and purpose reintroduced into her life. Now, or soon, the process of dietary improvements to address the weight loss goals initially espoused can begin.

We might also start a course of massage therapy or acupuncture to further alleviate joint pain, now that our patient believes feeling better is possible, and is thus motivated to try new things.

A little exercise further improves energy, and sleep, and self-esteem, and actually helps ease joint pain. Less pain further improves energy, sleep, and the willingness, maybe even eagerness, to exercise. Social engagement—perhaps in a church or civic group—confers gratification that no longer needs to come from food. Hormonal rebalancing that occurs with restoration of circadian rhythms alleviates constant hunger. Diet improves. Medication doses are dialed down. Helpful supplements may be started.

Weight loss starts. Energy goes up. Joint pain improves some more. Physical activity becomes less and less problematic, and increases incrementally. Energy and sleep improve further, weight loss picks up. With more hope, and more opportunity to get out, our patient establishes, or reestablishes, social contacts that restore friendship and love to their rightful place in her life. Her spirit rises, and with it, the energy she has to invest back into her own vitality.

And so on, with many details left out, of course, and unique to any given patient. This may sound like wishful thinking—but it is a rewarding reality seen routinely in the context of holistic clinical approaches to the seemingly isolated challenge of weight management, and its associated morbidities.

A Role for Technology in the Integrated Preventive Medicine Remedy

By supplanting physical activity, technology, notably "screen time," has long been implicated among the causes of obesity. There is now rapid development in the use of technology-based solutions, spanning both innovative hardware and software, the latter most commonly in the form of applications, or "apps," for smartphones. This area is evolving so rapidly that any summary verdict is sure to be obsolete by the time it is read. Readers are encouraged to monitor developments in this area. For now, what may be said is that there is a literature to support at least the promise of technology-based contributions to the prevention and management of both obesity and diabetes.[331,332]

Culture, in Integrated Preventive Medicine Context

Clinicians will, in fact, not be *the* solution to the problem of epidemic obesity, as many components of a comprehensive weight-management campaign that would satisfy population needs fall outside the clinical purview. But clinicians have a vital role to play, as both educators and advocates. And given the magnitude and urgency of this crisis, to do otherwise is simply no longer acceptable. We have a choice of being part of the solution or, failing that, being part of a status quo that propagates the problem. As the IOM outlines in its recent report on obesity prevention, we need healthcare providers to adopt standards of practice for prevention, screening, diagnosis, and treatment of overweight and obesity; emphasize pre-pregnancy counseling on maintenance of a healthy weight before, during, and after pregnancy; and advocate publically for healthy communities that support healthy eating and active living.[333]

In the weight-loss literature, interventions achieve caloric restriction by various means, ranging from direct provision of food,[334] systems of incentive/disincentive,[335] cognitive-behavioral therapy,[336] fat restriction,[337] and the color-coding of food choices based on nutrient density.[338] In general, those interventions achieving the most extreme degrees of caloric restriction also produce the greatest initial weight loss. However, a rebound weight gain is typically observed; in general, the more rapid the initial weight loss, the greater and more rapid the subsequent weight gain.[339,340] This observation appears to be of generalizable significance, likely due to the fact that the extreme caloric restriction necessary for very rapid weight loss is intrinsically unsustainable. When the means used to achieve initial weight loss are unsustainable, weight regain is consistently observed.

Where the spectrum from obesity to type 2 diabetes is most reliably prevented, and where that is done in the context of the true "prize" at which all healthcare is ostensibly directed, the combination of vitality and longevity, the principal means to such ends are not clinical. Nor are they a matter of the triumph of personal will and responsibility over adverse elements in the social and cultural environment. Rather, they are a product of culture itself.

This is epitomized by the world's so-called Blue Zones, representing the populations identified to date with the highest concentrations of healthy centenarians.

Related work attributes such advantages to lifestyle, but not to medicine. Clinical counseling does not figure among the explanations for Blue Zone blessings; rather, the explanations all reside at the level of culture.[341]

If anything, our culture is prone to "overmedicalization,"[342] for reasons we might readily suppose. Even the currently massive societal preoccupation with so-called healthcare reform[343] is principally about access to care for the treatment of illness, and much less about building health at its origins in daily living.

We have long had indications of this societal bias. Nearly two decades of effort were required before clear evidence supporting a lifestyle intervention as an alternative to coronary bypass surgery resulted in comparable reimbursement.[344] Our society readily accepts the bill for bariatric surgery in obese adolescents, while neglecting potentially better, less medical remedies.[345] To the extent that we medicalize obesity, we may divert both attention and resources away from cultural and environmental responses to it.[346]

The importance of the built environment[347] and public polices[348] in the epidemiology of obesity and chronic disease are well established. There is evidence as well of the favorable impact of community-wide interventions that treat a population, rather than an individual, as the patient.[349] And, of course, there is the flagrant if uncontrolled evidence of our recent cultural history. Obesity and its metabolic sequelae were relatively rare before the advent of highly obesigenic environmental and cultural conditions, and became prevalent in tandem with their proliferation. During this time, genes and metabolic pathways changed not at all, while prevailing dietary and activity patterns changed substantially. Purists might fuss over the want of randomized clinical trials to establish true causality here, but there are no clinical trials to substantiate the link between striking a match and starting a fire either.

The role of clinicians in lifestyle medicine varies with circumstance. In the case of advanced metabolic complications, it is inevitably a large role. In the case of lifestyle and weight management counseling, it is a supporting role, but an important one nonetheless. We can and should cultivate widespread competency in constructive, compassionate, and streamlined counseling.[350] We can, and should, design programs for finding health and losing weight that involve clinicians strategically, while sparing them excessive burdens of time and effort.[351]

There is a strong case for better application of lifestyle in medicine, and the engagement of clinicians in the delivery of effective programming and constructive counseling. There is, perhaps, particular promise here in efforts to control, curtail, and reverse both obesity and type 2 diabetes. But populations around the world enjoying the longest, happiest, most vital lives do not attribute such blessings preferentially to clinical care, but rather to culture. Lifestyle in medicine, laudable though it may be, and preferable as it is to the omission of lifestyle from medical practice, raises the prospect of overmedicalization if we stop there. If we stop there, we fail to concede that lifestyle actually happens not in hospitals and clinics, but in the places people live and learn, work and play, eat and pray, and love. We are thus duty bound to exert a collective, salutary influence beyond the halls of medicine where disease care is concentrated, propagating the practice of "health" care throughout culture itself.

Source

Katz DL, with Friedman RSC, Lucan S. *Nutrition in Clinical Practice*. 3rd ed. Philadelphia, PA: Lippincott Williams & Wilkins/Wolters Kluwer; 2014.

References

1. Rasmussen F, Kark M, Tholin S, et al. The Swedish Young Male Twins Study: a resource for longitudinal research on risk factors for obesity and cardiovascular diseases. *Twin Res Hum Genet* 2006;9(6):883–839.
2. Hakala P, Rissanen A, Koskenvuo M, et al. Environmental factors in the development of obesity in identical twins. *Int J Obes Relat Metab Disord* 1999;23(7):746–753.
3. Koeppen-Schomerus G, Wardle J, Plomin R. A genetic analysis of weight and overweight in 4-year-old twin pairs. *Int J Obes Relat Metab Disord* 2001;25(6):838–844.

4. Echwald S. Genetics of human obesity: lessons from mouse models and candidate genes. *J Intern Med* 1999;245:653–666.

5. Perusse L, Bouchard C. Genotype-environment interaction in human obesity. *Nutr Rev* 1999;57(5 pt 2):s31–s37.

6. Bell CG, Walley AJ, Froguel P. The genetics of human obesity. *Nat Rev Genet* 2005;6(3):221–234.

7. Walley AJ, Asher JE, Froguel P. The genetics contribution to non-syndromic human obesity. *Nat Rev Genet* 2009;10(7):431–442.

8. Cheung WW, Mao P. Recent Advances in obesity: genetics and beyond. *ISRN Endocrinol* 2012;2012:1–11.

9. Rankinen T, Zuberi A, Chagnon YC, et al. The human obesity gene map: the 2005 update. *Obesity* 2006;14(4):529–644.

10. Clement K. Leptin and the genetics of obesity. Leptin and the genetics of obesity. *Acta Paedietr Suppl* 1999;88:51–57.

11. Marti A, Berraondo B, Martinez J. Leptin: physiological actions. *J Physiol Biochem* 1999;55:43–49.

12. Lonnquist F, Nordfors L, Schalling M. Leptin and its potential role in human obesity. *J Intern Med* 1999;245:643–652.

13. Ronnemaa T, Karonen S-L, Rissanen A, et al. Relation between plasma leptin levels and measures of body fat in identical twins discordant for obesity. *Ann Intern Med* 1997;126:26–31.

14. Heymsfield S, Greenberg A, Fujioka K, et al. Recombinant leptin for weight loss in obese and lean adults: a randomized, controlled, dose-escalation trial. *JAMA* 1999;282:1568–1575.

15. Hamann A, Matthaei S. Regulation of energy balance by leptin. *Exp Clin Endocrinol Diabetes* 1996;104:293–300.

16. Enriori PJ, Evans AE, Sinnayah P, et al. Leptin resistance and obesity. *Obesity (Silver Spring)* 2006;14(Suppl 5):254S–258S.

17. Zhang Y, Scarpace PJ. The role of leptin in leptin resistance and obesity. *Physiol Behav* 2006;88(3):249–256.

18. Paracchini V, Pedotti P, Taioli E. Genetics of leptin and obesity: a HuGE review. *Am J Epidemiol* 2005;162(2):101–114.

19. Oswal A, Yeo G. Leptin and the control of body weight: a review of its diverse central targets, signaling mechanisms, and role in the pathogenesis of obesity. *Obesity* 2010;18(2):221–229.

20. Ravussin E. Energy metabolism in obesity: studies in the Pima Indians. *Diabetes Care* 1993;16(1):232–238.

21. Konturek SJ, Konturek JW, Pawlik T, et al. Brain-gut axis and its role in the control of food intake. *J Physiol Pharmacol* 2004;55(1 Pt 2):137–154.

22. Bouchard C. Gene-environment interactions in the etiology of obesity: defining the fundamentals. *Obesity* 2008;16(S3):S5–S10.

23. Qi L, Cho YA. Gene-environment interaction and obesity. *Nutr Rev* 2008;66(12):684–694.

24. Turnbaugh PJ, Ley RE, Mahowald MA, et al. An obesity- associated gut microbiome with increased capacity for energy harvest. *Nature* 2006; 7122(444):1027–1031.

25. Turnbaugh PJ, Bäckhed F, Fulton L, et al. Diet-induced obesity is linked to marked but reversible alterations in the mouse distal gut microbiome. *Cell Host Microbe* 2008;3(4):213–223.

26. Bäckhed F, Ding H, Wang T, et al. The gut microbiota as an environmental factor that regulates fat storage. *Proc Natl Acad Sci U S A* 2004;101(44):15718–15723.

27. Turnbaugh PJ, Gordon JI. The core gut microbiome, energy balance and obesity. *J Physiol (Lond)* 2009;587(pt 17):4153–4158.

28. Turnbaugh PJ, Hamady M, Yatsunenko T, et al. A core gut microbiome in obese and lean twins. *Nature* 2009;457(7228):480–484.

29. Ley RE. Obesity and the human microbiome. *Curr Opin Gastroenterol* 2010;26(1):5–11.

30. Schwiertz A, Taras D, Schafer K, et al. Microbiota and SCFA in lean and overweight healthy subjects. *Obesity (Silver Spring)* 2010;18:190–195.

31. Kootte RS, Vrieze A, Holleman F, et al. The therapeutic potential of manipulating gut microbiota in obesity and type 2 diabetes mellitus. *Diabetes Obes Metab* 2012;14(2):112–120.

32. Vrieze A, Holleman F, Serlie MJ et al. Metabolic effects of transplanting gut microbiota from lean donors to subjects with metabolic syndrome. *Diabetologia* 2010;53:S44–S44.

33. Holt SH, Miller JC, Petocz P, et al. A satiety index of common foods. *Eur J Clin Nutr* 1995;49(9):675–690.

34. Schoeller, D., Recent advances from application of doubly labeled water to measurement of human energy expenditure. *J Nutr* 1999;129:1765–1768.

35. *Is-a-Calorie-a-Calorie?* 2012. http://opinionator.blogs.nytimes.com.

36. *Calories.* http://www.huffingtonpost.com/david-katz-md/calories_b_1369749.html.

37. Chow CC, Hall KD. Short and long-term energy intake patterns and their implications for human body weight regulation. *Physiol Behav* 2014;134:60–65.

38. Hall KD. Modeling metabolic adaptations and energy regulation in humans. *Annu Rev Nutr* 2012;32:35–54.

39. Reilly JJ, Kelly J. Long-term impact of overweight and obesity in childhood and adolescence on morbitdity and premature mortality in adulthood: systematic review. *Int J Obes* 2005 2011;35(7):891–898.

40. Schoeller DA. Insights into energy balance from doubly labeled water. *Int J Obes (Lond)* 2008;32(suppl 7):S72–S75.

41. Rush E, Plank L, Robinson S. Resting metabolic rate in young Polynesian and Caucasian women. *Int J Obes Relat Metab Disord* 1997;21:1071–1075.

42. Ravussin E, Gautier J. Metabolic predictors of weight gain. *Int J Obes Relat Metab Disord* 1999;23(Suppl 1):37–41.

43. Luke A, Dugas L, Kramer H. Ethnicity, energy expenditure and obesity: are the observed black/white diferences meaningful? *Curr Opin Endocrinol Diabetes Obes* 2007;14(5):370–373.

44. Gannon B, DiPietro L, Poehlman ET. Do African Americans have lower energy expenditure than Caucasians? *Int J Obes Relat Metab Disord* 2000;24(1):4–13.

45. Sun M, Gower BA, Bartolucci AA, et al. A longitudinal study of resting energy expenditure relative to body composition during puberty in African American and white children. *Am J Clin Nutr* 2001;73(2):308–315.

46. Astrup A, Gotzsche P, Werken KD, et al. Meta-analysis of resting metabolic rate in formerly obese subjects. *Am J Clin Nutr* 1999;69:1117–1122.

47. Weinsier RL, Nagy TR, Hunter GR, et al. Do adaptive changes in metabolic rate favor weight gain in weight- reducing individuals? An examination of the set point theory. *Am J Nutr* 2007;72(5):1088–1094.

48. Byrne NM, Wood RE, Schutz Y, et al. Does metabolic compensation explain the majority off less-than-expected weight loss in obese adults during a short-term severe diet and exercise intervention? *Int J Obes (Lond)* 2012;36(11):1472–1478.

49. Maclean PS, Bergouignan A, Cornier M-A, et al. Biology's response to dieting: the impetus for weight regain. *Am J Physiol Regul Integr Comp Physiol* 2011;301(3):R581–R600.

50. Wijers SL, Saris WH, Van Marken Lichtenbelt WD. Recent advances in adaptive thermogenesis: potential implications for the treatment of obesity. *Obes Rev* 2009;10(2):218–226.

51. Clapham JC, Arch JRS. Targeting thermogenesis and related pathways in anti-obesity drug discovery. *Pharmacol Ther* 2011;131(3):295–308.

52. Stock M. Gluttony and thermogenesis revisited. *Int J Obes Relat Metab Disord* 1999;23:1105–1117.

53. Lowell BB, Bachman ES. β-Adrenergic receptors, diet-induced thermogenesis, and obesity. *J Biol Chem* 2003;278(32):29385–29388.

54. Kerckhoffs D, Blaak E, Baak MV, et al. Effect of aging on beta-adrenergically mediated thermogenesis in men. *Am J Physiol* 1998;274:E1075–E1079.

55. Saely CH, Geiger K, Drexel H. Brown versus white adipose tissue: a mini-review. *Gerontology* 2012;58(1):15–23.

56. Centers for Disease Control and Prevention. *US Physical Activity Statistics*. 2010.

57. Gillman MW, Pinto BM, Tennstedt S, et al. Relationships of physical activity with dietary behaviors among adults. *Prev Med* 2001;32(3):295–301.

58. Simoes E, Byers T, Coates R, et al. The association between leisure-time physical activity and dietary fat in American adults. *Am J Public Health* 1995;85:240–244.

59. Dipietro L. Physical activity in the prevention of obesity: current evidence and research issues. *Med Sci Sports Exerc* 1999;31(11 suppl):s542–s546.

60. Goldberg JH, King AC. Physical activity and weight management across the lifespan. *Annu Rev Public Health* 2007;28:145–170.

61. Jakicic JM, Davis KK. Obesity and physical activity. *Psychiatr Clin North Am* 2011;34(4): 829–840.

62. Catenacci VA, Wyatt HR. The role of physical activity in producing and maintaining weight loss. *Nat Clin Pract Endocrinol Metab* 2007;3(7):518–529.

63. *Exercise-of-Math-and-Myth*. 2012. http://health.usnews.com/health-news/blogs/eat-run/.

64. Katz DL. Unfattening our children: forks over feet. *Int J Obes (Lond)* 2011;35(1):33–37.

65. Holcomb GW Jr, O'Neill JA Jr, Holcomb GW. Cholecystitis, cholelithiasis and common duct stenosis in children and adolescents. *Ann Surg* 1980;191(5):626–635.

66. Christou DD, Gentile CL, DeSouza CA, et al. Fatness is a better predictor of cardiovascular disease risk factor profile than aerobic fitness in healthy men. *Circulation* 2005;111(15):1904–1914.

67. Eisenmann JC, Wickel EE, Welk GJ, et al. Relationship between adolescent fitness and fatness and cardiovascular disease risk factors in adulthood: the Aerobics Center Longitudinal Study (ACLS). *Am Heart J* 2005;149(1):46–53.

68. Norman AC, Drinkard B, McDuffie JR, et al. Influence of excess adiposity on exercise fitness and performance in overweight children and adolescents. *Pediatrics* 2005;115(6):e690–e696.

69. Coakley EH, Kawachi I, Manson JE, et al. Lower levels of physical functioning are associated with higher body weight among middle-aged and older women. *Int J Obes Relat Metab Disord* 1998;22(10):958–965.

70. Hu FB, Willett WC, Li T, et al. Adiposity as compared with physical activity in predicting mortality among women. *N Engl J Med* 2004;351(26):2694–2703.

71. Weinstein AR, Sesso HD, Lee IM, et al. Relationship of physical activity vs body mass index with type 2 diabetes in women. *JAMA* 2004;292(10):1188–1194.

72. Fang J, Wylie-Rosett J, Cohen HW, et al. Exercise, body mass index, caloric intake, and cardiovascular mortality. *Am J Prev Med* 2003;25(4):283–289.

73. Haapanen-Niemi N, Miilunpalo S, Pasanen M, et al. Body mass index, physical inactivity and low level of physical fitness as determinants of all-cause and cardiovascular disease mortality—16 y follow-up of middle-aged and elderly men and women. *Int J Obes Relat Metab Disord* 2000;24(11):1465–1474.

74. Martinez ME, Giovannucci E, Spiegelman D, et al. Leisure-time physical activity, body size, and colon cancer in women. Nurses' Health Study Research Group. *J Natl Cancer Inst* 1997;89(13):948–955.

75. Giovannucci E, Ascherio A, Rimm E, et al. Physical activity, obesity, and risk for colon Cancer and Adenoma in Men. *Ann Intern Med* 1995;122:327–334.

76. Patel AV, Rodriguez C, Bernstein L, et al. Obesity, recreational physical activity, and risk of pancreatic cancer in a large U.S. Cohort. *Cancer Epidemiol Biomarkers Prev* 2005;14(2):459–466.

77. Wei M, Kampert JB, Barlow CE, et al. Relationship between low cardiorespiratory fitness and mortality in normal-weight, overweight, and obese men. *JAMA* 1999;282(16):1547–1553.

78. Katzmarzyk PT, Janssen I, Ardern CI. Physical inactivity, excess adiposity and premature mortality. *Obes Rev* 2003;4(4):257–290.

79. Wessel TR, Arant CB, Olson MB, et al. Relationship of physical fitness vs body mass index with coronary artery disease and cardiovascular events in women. *JAMA* 2004;292(10):1179–1187.

80. Lee DC, Sui X, Blair SN. Does physical activity ameliorate the health hazards of obesity? *Br J Sports Med* 2009;43(1):49–51.

81. Fogelholm M. Physical activity, fitness and fatness: relations to mortality, morbidity and disease risk factors: a systematic review. *Obes Rev* 2010;11(3):202–221.

82. Kwon S, Burns TL, Janz K. Associations of cardiorespiratory fitness and fatness with cardiovascular risk factors among adolescents: the NHANES 1999–2002. *J Phys Act Health* 2010;7(6):746–753.

83. Woo J, Yu R, Yau F. Fitness, fatness and survival in elderly populations. *Age (Dordrecht, Netherlands)* 2013;35(3):973–984.

84. Hainer V, Toplak H, Stich V. Fat or fit: what is more important? *Diabetes Care* 2009;32(Suppl 2):S392–S397.

85. Suriano K, Curran J, Byrne SM, et al. Fatness, fitness, and increased cardiovascular risk in young children. *J Pediatr* 2010;157(4):552–558.

86. McAuley P, Pittsley J, Myers J, et al. Fitness and fatness as mortality predictors in healthy older men: the veterans exercise testing study. *J Gerontol A Biol Sci Med Sci* 2009;64A(6):695–699.

87. Duncan GE. The "fit but fat" concept revisited: population-based estimates using NHANES. *Int J Behav Nutr Phys Act* 2010;7:47.

88. Phelan S, Wyatt HR, Hill JO, et al. Are the eating and exercise habits of successful weight losers changing? *Obesity (Silver Spring)* 2006;14(4):710–716.

89. Wing RR, Hill JO. Successful weight loss maintenance. *Annu Rev Nutr* 2001;21:323–341.

90. Zachwieja JJ. Exercise as a treatment for obesity. *Endocrinol Metab Clin North Am* 1996;25(4):965–988.

91. Doucet E, Imbeault P, Almeras N, et al. Physical activity and low-fat diet: is it enough to maintain weight stability in the reduced-obese individual following weight loss by drug therapy and energy restriction? *Obes Res* 1999;7:323–333.

92. Rippe JM, Hess S. The role of physical activity in the prevention and management of obesity. *J Am Diet Assoc* 1998;98(10 Suppl 2):S31–S38.

93. Saris W. Exercise with or without dietary restriction and obesity treatment. *Int J Obes Relat Metab Disord* 1995;1995(Suppl 4): S113–S116.

94. Mekary RA, Feskanich D, Hu FB, et al. Physical activity in relation to long-term weight maintenance after intentional weight loss in premenopausal women. *Obesity* 2010;18(1):167–174.

95. Lee I, Djousse L, Sesso HD, et al. Physical activity and weight gain prevention. *JAMA* 2010;303(12):1173–1179.

96. Heitmann B, Kaprio J, Harris J, et al. Are genetic determinants of weight gain modified by leisure-time physical activity? A prospective study of Finnish twins. *Am J Clin Nutr* 1997;66:672–678.

97. Andersen R, Wadden T, Bartlett S, et al. Effects of lifestyle activity vs structured aerobic exercise in obese women: a randomized trial. *JAMA* 1999;281(4):335–340.

98. Eaton S, Eaton SB 3rd, Konner M. Paleolithic nutrition revisited: a twelve-year retrospective on its nature and implications. *Eur J Clinical Nutrition* 1997;51:207–216.

99. Lebovitz H. Type 2 diabetes: an overview. *Clin Chem* 1999;45:1339–1345.

100. Drong AW, Lindgren CM, McCarthy MI. The genetic and epigenetic basis of type 2 diabetes and obesity. *Clin Pharmacol Ther* 2012;92(6):707–715.

101. Resnicow K. *Cancer Prevention and Comprehensive School Health Education: The Role of the American Cancer Society.* Paper presented at the American Cancer Society National Conference, Atlanta, GA. May 28–30, 1991.
102. Neel, J. Diabetes mellitus: a "thrifty" genotype rendered detrimental by "progress"? *Am J Human Genetics* 1962;14:353–362.
103. Benyshek DC, Watson JT. Exploring the thrifty genotype's food-shortage assumptions: a cross-cultural comparison of ethnographic accounts of food security among foraging and agricultural societies. *Am J Phys Anthropol* 2006;131:120–126.
104. Prentice AM. Early influences on human energy regulation: thrifty genotypes and thrifty phenotypes. *Physiol Behav* 2005;86:640–645.
105. Prentice AM, Rayco-Solon P, Moore SE. Insights from the developing world: thrifty genotypes and thrifty pheno-types. *Proc Nutr Soc* 2005;64:153–161.
106. Chakravarthy MV, Booth FW. Eating, exercise, and "thrifty" genotypes: connecting the dots toward an evolutionary understanding of modern chronic diseases. *J Appl Physiol* 2004;96(1):3–10.
107. Speakman JR. Thrifty genes for obesity and the metabolic syndrome—time to call off the search? *Diab Vasc Dis Res* 2006;3:7–11.
108. Dulloo AG, Jacquet J, Seydoux J, et al. The thrifty "catch-up fat" phenotype: its impact on insulin sensitivity during growth trajectories to obesity and metabolic syndrome. *Int J Obes (Lond)* 2006;30:S23–S35.
109. Allen DB, Nemeth BA, Clark RR, et al. Fitness is a stronger predictor of fasting insulin levels than fatness in overweight male middle-school children. *J Pediatr* 2007;150:383–387.
110. Goldfine AB, Bouche C, Parker RA, et al. Insulin resistance is a poor predictor of type 2 diabetes in individuals with no family history of disease. *Proc Natl Acad Sci USA* 2003;100:2724–2729.
111. Kadowaki T. Insights into insulin resistance and type 2 diabetes from knockout mouse models. *J Clin Invest* 2000;106:459–465.
112. Cavaghan MK, Ehrmann DA, Polonsky KS. Interactions between insulin resistance and insulin secretion in the development of glucose intolerance. *J Clin Invest* 2000;106:329–333.
113. Leahy JL. Pathogenesis of type 2 diabetes mellitus. *Arch Med Res* 2005 May–June; 36(3):197–209.
114. Meece J. Pancreatic islet dysfunction in type 2 diabetes: a rational target for incretin-based therapies. *Curr Med Res Opin* 2007;23:933–944.
115. Colditz GA, Willett WC, Rotnitzky A, et al. Weight gain as a risk factor for clinical diabetes mellitus in women [see comments]. *Ann Intern Med* 1995;122(7):481–486.
116. Ford E, Williamson D, Liu S. Weight change and diabetes incidence: findings from a national cohort of US adults. *Am J Epidemiol* 1997;146:214.
117. Biggs ML, Mukamal KJ, Luchsinger JA, et al. Association between adiposity in midlife and older age and risk of diabetes in older adults. *JAMA* 2010;303(24):2504–2512.

118. Lazarus R, Sparrow D, Weiss S. Temporal relations between obesity and insulin: longitudinal data from the normative aging study. *Am J Epidemiol* 1998;147:173–179.

119. Aye T, Levitsky LL. Type 2 diabetes: an epidemic disease in childhood. *Curr Opin Pediatr* 2003;15:411–415.

120. Fagot-Campagna A, Pettitt DJ, et al. Type 2 diabetes among North American children and adolescents: an epidemiologic review and a public health perspective. *J Pediatr* 2000;136(5):664–672.

121. Pontiroli AE. Type 2 diabetes mellitus is becoming the most common type of diabetes in school children. *Acta Diabetol* 2004;41(3):85–90.

122. Wiegand S, Maikowski U, Blankenstein O, et al. Type 2 diabetes and impaired glucose tolerance in European children and adolescents with obesity—a problem that is no longer restricted to minority groups. *Eur J Endocrinol* 2004;151(2):199–206.

123. Expert Panel on Detection, Evaluation, and Treatment of High Blood Cholesterol in Adults. Executive Summary of the Third Report of the National Cholesterol Education Program (NCEP) Expert Panel on Detection, Evaluation, and Treatment of High Blood Cholesterol in Adults (Adult Treatment Panel III). *JAMA* 2001;285(19):2486–2497.

124. Apedo MT, Sowers JR, Banerji MA. Cardiovascular disease in adolescents with type 2 diabetes mellitus. *J Pediatr Endocrinol Metab* 2002;15(Suppl 1):519–523.

125. Steinberger J, Daniels SR. Obesity, insulin resistance, diabetes, and cardiovascular risk in children: an American Heart Association scientific statement from the Artherosclerosis, Hypertension, and Obesity in the Young Committee (Council on Nutrition, Physical Activity, and Metabolism). *Circulation* 2003;107:1448–1453.

126. Moller D, Flier J. Insulin resistance-mechanisms, syndromes, and implications. *N Engl J Med* 1991;325:938–948.

127. Ye J. Role of insulin in the pathogenesis of free fatty acid-induced insulin resistance in skeletal muscle. *Endocr Metab Immune Disord Drug Targets* 2007;7: 65–74.

128. Sesti G. Pathophysiology of insulin resistance. *Best Pract Res Clin Endocrinol Metab* 2006;20:665–679.

129. Lillioja S, Mott D, Spraul M, et al. Impaired glucose tolerance as a disorder of insulin action. *N Engl J Med* 1988;318:1217–1225.

130. Grundy S. Hypertriglyceridemia, insulin resistance, and the metabolic syndrome. *Am J Cardiol* 1999;83(9B):25F–29F.

131. American Heart Association. *Metabolic Syndrome.* http://www.americanheart. org/presenter.jhtml?identifier= 4756; accessed3/20/13.

132. Kahn R, Buse J, Ferrannini E, et al; for the American Diabetes Association and the European Association for the Study of Diabetes. The metabolic syndrome: time for a critical appraisal (ADA statement). *Diabetes Care* 2005;28:2289–2304.

133. Knowler WC, Barrett-Connor E, Fowler SE, et al. Reduction in the incidence of type 2 diabetes with lifestyle intervention or metformin. *N Engl J Med* 2002;346(6): 393–403.

134. Look AHEAD Research Group, Pi-Sunyer X, Blackburn G, et al. Reduction in weight and cardiovascular disease risk factors in individuals with

type 2 diabetes: one-year results of the look AHEAD trial. *Diabetes Care* 2007;30(6):1374–1383.

135. Look AHEAD Research Group, Wing RR. Long-term effects of a lifestyle intervention on weight and cardiovascular risk factors in individuals with type 2 diabetes mellitus: four-year results of the Look AHEAD trial. *Arch Intern Med* 2010;170(17):1566–1575.

136. Mascie-Taylor CG, Karim E. The burden of chronic disease. *Science* 2003;302:1921–1922.

137. Tillotson JE. Pandemic obesity: what is the solution? *Nutr Today* 2004;39(1):6–9.

138. Jeffery RW, Utter J. The changing environment and population obesity in the United States. *Obes Res* 2003;11:12S–22S.

139. Flegal KM, Carroll MD, Kit BK, et al. Prevalence of obesity and trends in the distribution of body mass index among US adults, 1999–2010. *JAMA* 2012;307(5):491–497.

140. Ogden CL, Carroll MD, Kit BK, et al. Prevalence of obesity and trends in body mass index among US children and adolescents, 1999–2010. *JAMA* 2012;307(5):483–490.

141. Sturm R, Hattori A. Morbid obesity rates continue to rise rapidly in the United States. *Int J Obes* 2013;37(6):889–891.

142. Flegal KM, Kruszon-Moran D, Carroll MD, Fryar CD, Ogden CL. Trends in obesity among adults in the United States, 2005 to 2014. *JAMA* 2016;315(21):2284–2291.

143. Ogden CL, Carroll MD, Lawman HG, et al. Trends in Obesity Prevalence Among Children and Adolescents in the United States, 1988–1994 through 2013–2014. *JAMA* 2016;315(21):2292–2299.

144. Ogden CL, Carroll MD, Flegal KM. Epidemiologic trends in overweight and obesity. *Endocrinol Metab Clin North Am* 2003;32:741–760.

145. Kim J, Peterson KE, Scanlon KS, et al. Trends in overweight from 1980 through 2001 among preschool-aged children enrolled in a health maintenance organization. *Obesity (Silver Spring)* 2006;14(7):1107–1112.

146. de Onis M, Blössner M, Borghi E. Global prevalence and trends of overweight and obesity among preschool children. *Am J Clin Nutr* 2010;92(5):1257–1264.

147. Li C, Ford ES, Mokdad AH, et al. Recent trends in waist circumference and waist-height ratio among US children and adolescents. *Pediatrics* 2006;118(5):e1390–e1398.

148. Chopra M, Galbraith S, Darnton-Hill I. A global response to a global problem: the epidemic of overnutrition. *Bull World Health Organ* 2002;80:952–958.

149. Damcott CM, Sack P, Shuldiner AR. The genetics of obesity. *Endocrinol Metab Clin North Am* 2003;32:761–786.

150. Katz DL. Pandemic obesity and the contagion of nutritional nonsense. *Public Health Rev* 2003;31:33–44.

151. World Health Organization. *Cardiovascular Diseases—Fact sheet N°317.* 2011. http://www.who.int/mediacentre/factsheets/fs317/en/index.html.

152. Drewnowski A. Nutrition transition and global dietary trends. *Nutrition* 2000;16:486–487.

153. Silventoinen K, Sans S, Tolonen H, et al. WHO MONICA Project. Trends in obesity and energy supply in the WHO MONICA Project. *Int J Obes Relat Metab Disord* 2004;28:710–718.
154. Misra A, Vikram NK. Insulin resistance syndrome (metabolic syndrome) and obesity in Asian Indians: evidence and implications. *Nutrition* 2004;20:482–491.
155. Jahns L, Baturin A, Popkin BM. Obesity, diet, and poverty: trends in the Russian transition to market economy. *Eur J Clin Nutr* 2003;57:1295–1302.
156. Wisdom, and Opportunity. http://www.linkedin.com/today/post/article/20130315152612-23027997-qatar-s-cultural-crisis-wealth-health-wisdom-and-opportunity?trk=mp-author-card.
157. Lands W, Hamazaki T, Yamazaki K, et al. Changing dietary patterns. *Am J Clin Nutr* 1990;51:991–993.
158. Drewnowski A, Popkin BM. The nutrition transition: new trends in the global diet. *Nutrition Reviews* 1997;55(2):31–43.
159. Centers for Disease Control and Prevention. *National Diabetes Fact Sheet: National Estimates and General Information on Diabetes and Prediabetes in the United States.* 2011. http://www.cdc.gov/diabetes/pubs/pdf/ndfs_2011.pdf. Accessed March 18, 2013.
160. Gregg EW, Cadwell BL, Cheng YJ, et al. Trends in the prevalence and ratio of diagnosed to undiagnosed diabetes according to obesity levels in the U.S. *Diabetes Care* 2004;27(12):2806–2812.
161. Ford ES, Giles WH, Mokdad AH. Increasing prevalence of the metabolic syndrome among U.S. Adults. *Diabetes Care* 2004;27(10):2444–2449.
162. Reaven G, Abbasi F, McLaughlin T. Obesity, insulin resistance, and cardiovascular disease. *Recent Prog Horm Res* 2004;59:207–223.
163. World Health Organization. *Diabetes Programme: Diabetes Fact Sheet.* http://www.who.int/mediacentre/ factsheets/fs312/en/index.html. Accessed February 28, 2013.
164. Engelgau MM, Geiss LS, Saaddine JB, et al. The evolving diabetes burden in the United States. *Ann Intern Med* 2004;140:945–950.
165. Narayan KM, Boyle JP, Thompson TJ, et al. Lifetime risk for diabetes mellitus in the United States. *JAMA* 2003;290(14):1884–1890.
166. Honeycutt AA, Boyle JP, Broglio KR, et al. A dynamic Markov model for forecasting diabetes prevalence in the United States through 2050. *Health Care Manag Sci* 2003;6:155–164.
167. Centers for Disease Control and Prevention. *Diabetes Report Card, 2014.* http://www.cdc.gov/diabetes/pdfs/library/diabetesreportcard2014.pdf.
168. Geiss LS, Wang J, Cheng YJ, et al. Prevalence and incidence trends for diagnosed diabetes among adults aged 20 to 79 years, United States, 1980–2012. *JAMA* 2014;312(12):1218–1226.
169. Thompson D, Wolf AM. The medical-care cost burden of obesity. *Obes Rev* 2001;2:189–197.
170. Thompson D, Edelsberg J, Colditz GA, et al. Lifetime health and economic consequences of obesity. *Arch Intern Med* 1999;159(18):2177–2183.

171. Hammond RA, Levine R. The economic impact of obesity in the United States. *Diabetes Metab Syndr Obes* 2010;3:285–295.

172. Finkelstein EA, Ruhm CJ, Kosa KM. Economic causes and consequences of obesity. *Annu Rev Public Health* 2005;26(1):239–257.

173. Finkelstein EA, Trogdon JG, Brown DS, et al. The lifetime medical cost burden of overweight and obesity: implications for obesity prevention. *Obesity (Silver Spring)* 2008;16(8):1843–1848.

174. Shamseddeen H, Getty JZ, Hamdallah IN, et al. Epidemiology and economic impact of obesity and type 2 diabetes. *Surg Clin North Am* 2011;91(6):1163.

175. Trasande L, Elbel B. The economic burden placed on healthcare systems by childhood obesity. *Expert Rev Pharmacoecon Outcomes Res* 2012;12(1):39–45.

176. Wang Y, Beydoun MA, Liang L, et al. Will all Americans become overweight or obese? estimating the progression and cost of the US obesity epidemic. *Obesity* 2008;16(10):2323–2330.

177. Withrow D, Alter DA. The economic burden of obesity worldwide: a systematic review of the direct costs of obesity. *Obes Rev* 2011;12(2):131–141.

178. Olshansky SJ, Passaro DJ, Hershow RC, et al. A potential decline in life expectancy in the United States in the 21st century. *N Engl J Med* 2005;352(11):1138–1145.

179. Calle EE, Thun MJ. Obesity and cancer. *Oncogene* 2004;23(38):6365–6378.

180. Rames LK, Clarke WR, Connor WE, et al. Normal blood pressure and the evaluation of sustained blood pressure elevation in childhood: the Muscatine study. *Pediatrics* 1978;61(2):245–251.

181. Figueroa-Colon R, Franklin FA, Lee JY, et al. Prevalence of obesity with increased blood pressure in elementary school-aged children. *South Med J* 1997;90(8): 806–813.

182. Urrutia-Rojas X, Egbuchunam CU, Bae S, et al. High blood pressure in school children: prevalence and risk factors. *BMC Pediatr* 2006;6:32.

183. Sorof J, Daniels S. Obesity hypertension in children: a problem of epidemic proportions. *Hypertension* 2002;40(4):441–447.

184. Falkner B, Michel S. Obesity and other risk factors in children. *Ethn Dis* 1999;9(2):284–289.

185. Friedland O, Nemet D, Gorodnitsky N, et al. Obesity and lipid profiles in children and adolescents. *J Pediatr Endocrinol Metab* 2002;15(7):1011–1016.

186. Richards GE, Cavallo A, Meyer WJ, et al. Obesity, acanthosis nigricans, insulin resistance, and hyperandrogenemia: pediatric perspective and natural history. *J Pediatr* 1985;107(6):893–897.

187. Viner RM, Segal TY, Lichtarowicz-Krynska E, et al. Prevalence of the insulin resistance syndrome in obesity. *Arch Dis Child* 2005;90(1):10–14.

188. Friesen CA, Roberts CC. Cholelithiasis: clinical characteristics in children; case analysis and literature review. *Clin Pediatr (Phila)* 1989;28(7):294–298.

189. Kaechele V, Wabitsch M, Thiere D, et al. Prevalence of gallbladder stone disease in obese children and adolescents: influence of the degree of obesity, sex, and pubertal development. *J Pediatr Gastroenterol Nutr* 2006;42(1): 66–70.

190. Kinugasa A, Tsunamoto K, Furukawa N, et al. Fatty liver and its fibrous changes found in simple obesity of children. *J Pediatr Gastroenterol Nutr* 1984;3(3):408–414.

191. Tominaga K, Kurata JH, Chen YK, et al. Prevalence of fatty liver in Japanese children and relationship to obesity. An epidemiological ultrasonographic survey. *Dig Dis Sci* 1995;40(9):2002–2009.

192. Tazawa Y, Noguchi H, Nishinomiya F, et al. Serum alanine aminotransferase activity in obese children. *Acta Paediatr* 1997;86(3):238–241.

193. Schwimmer JB, Deutsch R, Kahen T, et al. Prevalence of fatty liver in children and adolescents. *Pediatrics* 2006;118(4):1388.

194. Silvestri JM, Weese-Mayer DE, Bass MT, et al. Polysomnography in obese children with a history of sleep-associated breathing disorders. *Pediatr Pulmonol* 1993;16(2):124–129.

195. Marcus CL, Curtis S, Koerner CB, et al. Evaluation of pulmonary function and polysomnography in obese children and adolescents. *Pediatr Pulmonol* 1996;21(3):176–183.

196. Mallory GB Jr, Fiser DH, Jackson R. Sleep-associated breathing disorders in morbidly obese children and adolescents. *J Pediatr* 1989;115(6): 892–897.

197. Arens R, Muzumdar H. Childhood obesity and obstructive sleep apnea syndrome. *J Appl Physiol* 2010;108(2):436–444.

198. Tauman R, Gozal D. Obesity and obstructive sleep apnea in children. *Paediatr Respir Rev* 2006;7(4):247–259.

199. Kelsey JL. The incidence and distribution of slipped capital femoral epiphysis in Connecticut. *J Chronic Dis* 1971;23(8):567–578.

200. Kelsey JL, Acheson RM, Keggi KJ. The body build of patients with slipped capital femoral epiphysis. *Am J Dis Child* 1972;124(2):276–281.

201. Loder RT, Aronson DD, Greenfield ML. The epidemiology of bilateral slipped capital femoral epiphysis: a study of children in Michigan. *J Bone Joint Surg Am* 1993;75(8):1141–1147.

202. Wilcox PG, Weiner DS, Leighley B. Maturation factors in slipped capital femoral epiphysis. *J Pediatr Orthop* 1988;8(2):196–200.

203. Manoff EM, Banffy MB, Winell JJ. Relationship between body mass index and slipped capital femoral epiphysis. *J Pediatr Orthop* 2005;25(6):744–746.

204. Scott IU, Siatkowski RM, Eneyni M, et al. Idiopathic intracranial hypertension in children and adolescents. *Am J Ophthalmol* 1997;124(2):253–255.

205. Durcan FJ, Corbett JJ, Wall M. The incidence of pseudotumor cerebri: population studies in Iowa and Louisiana. *Arch Neurol* 1988;45(8):875–877.

206. Corbett JJ, Savino PJ, Thompson HS, et al. Visual loss in pseudotumor cerebri: follow-up of 57 patients from five to 41 years and a profile of 14 patients with permanent severe visual loss. *Arch Neurol* 1982;39(8):461–474.

207. Sugerman HJ, DeMaria EJ, Felton WL 3rd, et al. Increased intra-abdominal pressure and cardiac filling pressures in obesity-associated pseudotumor cerebri. *Neurology* 1997;49(2):507–511.

208. Balcer LJ, Liu GT, Forman S, et al. Idiopathic intracranial hypertension: relation of age and obesity in children. *Neurology* 1999;52(4):870–870.

209. Kesler A, Fattal-Valevski A. Idiopathic intracranial hypertension in the pediatric population. *J Child Neurol* 2002;17(10):745–748.

210. Willett WC, Manson JE, Stampfer MJ, et al. Weight, weight change, and coronary heart disease in women: risk within the "normal" weight range [see comments]. *JAMA* 1995;273(6):461–465.

211. Dietz WH. Childhood weight affects adult morbidity and mortality. *J Nutr* 1998;128(2 Suppl):411S–414S.

212. Srinivasan SR, Bao W, Wattigney WA, et al. Adolescent overweight is associated with adult overweight and related multiple cardiovascular risk factors: the Bogalusa Heart Study. *Metabolism* 1996;45(2):235–240.

213. Lauer RM, Clarke WR. Childhood risk factors for high adult blood pressure: the Muscatine Study. *Pediatrics* 1989;84(4):633–641.

214. Mossberg HO. 40-year follow-up of overweight children. *Lancet* 1989;2(8661):491–493.

215. Morrison JA, Glueck CJ, Horn PS, et al. Childhood predictors of adult type 2 diabetes at 9- and 26-year follow-ups. *Arch Pediatr Adolesc Med* 2010;164(1):53–60.

216. Must A, Jacques P, Dallal G, et al. Long-term morbidity and mortality of overweight adolescents. *New Engl J M* 1992;327(19):1350–1355.

217. Strauss R. Childhood obesity. *Curr Prob Pediatr* 1999;29(1):1–29.

218. Schonfeld-Warden N, Warden CH. Pediatric obesity: an overview of etiology and treatment. *Pediatr Clin N Am* 1997;44(2):339–361.

219. Lissner L, Odell P, D'Agostino R, et al. Variability of body weight and health outcomes in the Framingham population. *N Engl J Med* 1991;324(26):1839–1844.

220. Burt Solorzano CM, McCartney CR. Obesity and the pubertal transition in girls and boys. *Reproduction* 2010;140(3):399–410.

221. Brownell K. Effects of weight cycling on metabolism, health, and psychological factors. In: Brownell KD, Fairburn CG, eds. Eating *Disorders and Obesity: A Comprehensive Handbook*. New York, NY: Guilford; 1995:56–60.

222. Rzehak P, Meisinger C, Woelke G, et al. Weight change, weight cycling and mortality in the ERFORT male cohort study. *Eur J Epidemiol* 2007;22(10):665–673.

223. Taing KY, Ardern CI, Kuk JL. Effect of the timing of weight cycling during adulthood on mortality risk in overweight and obese postmenopausal women. *Obesity (Silver Spring)* 2012;20(2):407–4133.

224. Iribarren C, Sharp D, Burchfiel C, et al. Association of weight loss and weight fluctuation with mortality among Japanese American men. *N Engl J Med* 1995;333:686–692.

225. Stevens VL, Jacobs EJ, Sun J, et al. Weight cycling and mortality in a large prospective US study. *Am J Epidemiol* 2012;175(8):785–792.

226. Field AE, Malspeis S, Willett WC. Weight cycling and mortality among middle-aged or older women. *Arch Intern Med* 2009;169(9):881–886.

227. Wing R, Jeffery R, Hellerstedt W. A prospective study of effects of weight cycling on cardiovascular risk factors. *Arch Intern Med* 1995;155:1416–1422.

228. Graci S, Izzo G, Savino S, et al. Weight cycling and cardiovascular risk factors in obesity. Int *J Obes Relat Metab Disord* 2004;28(1):65–71.

229. National task force on the prevention and treatment of obesity. Weight Cycling. *JAMA* 1994;272(15):1196–202.

230. Jeffery RW. Does weight cycling present a health risk? *Am J Clin Nutr* 1996;63(3 Suppl):452S–455S.

231. Stunkard A, Sobal J. Psychosocial consequences of obesity. In: Brownell KD, Fairburn CG, eds. *Eating Disorders and Obesity: A Comprehensive Handbook.* New York, NY: Guilford; 1995;260–275.

232. Schwartz MB, Brownell KD. Obesity and body image. *Body Image* 2004;1(1):43–56.

233. Strauss RS. Childhood obesity and self-esteem. *Pediatrics* 2000;105(1):e15.

234. Petroni ML, Villanova N, Avagnina S, et al. Psychological distress in morbid obesity in relation to weight history. *Obes Surg* 2007;17(3):391–399.

235. Marchesini G, Cuzzolaro M, Mannucci E, et al. Weight cycling in treatment-seeking obese persons: data from the QUOVADIS study. *Int J Obes Relat Metab Disord* 2004;28(11):1456–1462.

236. Gortmaker SL, Must A, Perrin JM, et al. Social and economic consequences of overweight in adolescence and young adulthood. *N Engl J Med* 1993;329(14):1008–1012.

237. Puhl RM, Heuer CA. The stigma of obesity: a review and update. *Obesity* 2009;17(5): 941–964.

238. Hill J, Melanson E. Overview of the determinants of overweight and obesity: current evidence and research issues. *Med Sci Sports Exerc* 1999;31(11 Suppl):S515–S521.

239. McClure AC, Tanski SE, Kingsbury J, et al. Characteristics associated with low self-esteem among US adolescents. *Acad Pediatr* 2010;10(4):238–244.e2.

240. Griffiths LJ, Wolke D, Page AS, et al. Obesity and bullying: different effects for boys and girls. *Arch Dis Child* 2006;91(2):121–125.

241. Janssen I, Craig WM, Boyce WF, et al. Associations between overweight and obesity with bullying behaviors in school-aged children. *Pediatrics* 2004;113(5):1187–1194.

242. Thompson JW, Card-Higginson P. Arkansas' experience: statewide surveillance and parental information on the child obesity epidemic. *Pediatrics* 2009;124(Suppl 1):S73–S82.

243. Nihiser AJ, Lee SM, Wechsler H, et al. BMI measurement in schools. *Pediatrics* 2009;124(Suppl 1):S89–S97.

244. Maddi S, Khoshaba D, Persico M, et al. Psychosocial correlates of psychopathology in a national sample of the morbidly obese. *Obes Surg* 1997;7:397–404.

245. McGinnis J, Foege. Actual causes of death in the United States. *JAMA* 1993;270(18):2207–2212.

246. Allison DB, Fontaine KR, Manson JE, et al. Annual deaths attributable to obesity in the United States. *JAMA* 1999;282(16):1530–1538.

247. Calle EE, Thun MJ, Petrelli JM, et al. Body-mass index and mortality in a prospective cohort of U.S. adults. *N Engl J Med* 1999;341(15):1097–1105.

248. Manson J, Willett W, Stampfer M, et al. Body weight and mortality among women. *N Engl J Med* 1995;333(11):677–685.

249. Adams KF, Schatzkin A, Harris TB, et al. Overweight, obesity, and mortality in a large prospective cohort of persons 50 to 71 years old. *N Engl J Med* 2006;355(8):763–778.

250. Flegal KM, Kit BK, Orpana H, et al. Association of all-cause mortality with overweight and obesity using standard body mass index categories: a systematic review and meta-analysis. *JAMA* 2013;309(1):71–82.

251. Mckay B. Admitting errors, agency expected to revise findings; big health concerns remain. *Wall Street Journal*, 2004, A1.

252. Kolata G. Data on deaths from obesity is inflated, U.S. agency says. *New York Times*, Nov 24, 2004.

253. Mann CC. Public health. Provocative study says obesity may reduce U.S. life expectancy. *Science* 2005;307(5716):1716–1717.

254. Mokdad AH, Marks JS, Stroup DF, et al. Actual causes of death in the United States 2000 *JAMA* 2004;291(10):1238–1245.

255. Flegal KM, Graubard BI, Williamson DF, et al. Excess deaths associated with underweight, overweight, and obesity. *JAMA* 2005;293(15):1861–1867.

256. Ogden CL, Flegal KM, Carroll MD, et al. Prevalence and trends in overweight among US children and adolescents, 1999–2000. *JAMA* 2002;288(14):1728–1732.

257. Mckay B. Doctors debate how to gauge lifestyle's effect on mortality. *Wall Street Journal*, December 14, 2004, D6.

258. Yee D. *CDC Fixes Error in Figuring Obesity Risk.* Associated Press. 2005.

259. McKay B. CDC concedes it overstated obesity-linked deaths. *Wall Street Journal*, Jan 18, 2005.

260. Obesity death figures lowered. *Reuters Health*, January 18, 2005.

261. Obesity set "to cut US life expectancy." *Reuters*, February 2, 2005.

262. CDC again cuts estimate of obesity-linked deaths. *Associated Press*, April 19, 2005.

263. Mark DH. Deaths attributable to obesity. *JAMA* 2005;293(15):1918–1919.

264. Gregg W, Foote A, Erfurt JC, et al. Worksite follow-up and engagement strategies for initiating health risk behavior changes. *Health Educ Quart* 1990;17(4):455–478.

265. Mokdad AH, Marks JS, Stroup DF, et al. Correction: actual causes of death in the United States, 2000. *JAMA* 2005;293(3):293–294.

266. Gregg EW, Cheng YJ, Cadwell BL, et al. Secular trends in cardiovascular disease risk factors according to body mass index in US adults. *JAMA* 2005;293(15):1868–1874.

267. Flegal KM, Williamson DF, Pamuk ER, et al. Estimating deaths attributable to obesity in the United States. *Am J Public Health* 2004;94(9):1486–1489.

268. Flegal KM, Graubard BI, Williamson DF. Methods of calculating deaths attributable to obesity. *Am J Epidemiol* 2004;160(4):331–338.

269. Centers for Disease Control and Health: dangers of being overweight overstated. *Associated Press*, April 19, 2005.

270. Kolata G. Some extra heft may be helpful, new study says. *New York Times*, April 20, 2005.

271. So is obesity bad for you or not? *Reuters*, April 20, 2005.

272. Kolata G. Why thin is fine, but thinner can kill. *New York Times*, April 24, 2005.

273. Flegal KM. Estimating the impact of obesity. *Soz Praventivmed* 2005;50(2):73–74.
274. Neergaard L. Risks jump as obesity escalates. *Associated Press*, 2005. Washington.
275. Tanner L. Experts say obesity still a health risk. *Associated Press*, May 1, 2005.
276. Koplan JP. Attempts to downplay obesity ignore dangers. *Atlanta Journal-Constitution*, April 29, 2005.
277. Couzin JA. Heavyweight battle over CDC's obesity forecasts: how many people does obesity kill? *Science* 2005;5723:770–771.
278. Marchione M. CDC stresses obesity problem, faults study. *Associated Press*, June 2, 2005.
279. Hu FB, Willett WC, Stampfer MJ, et al. Calculating deaths attributable to obesity. *Am J Public Health* 2005;95(6):932; author reply, 932–933.
280. Flegal KM, Pamuk ER. Letter. Flegal et al. respond. *Am J Public Health* 2005;95(6):932–933.
281. Warner M. Striking back at the food police. *New York Times*, June 12, 2005.
282. JAMA News Releases. *Being Obese, Underweight, Associated with Increased Risk of Death*. April 19, 2005.
283. Masters RK, Reither EN, Powers DA, Yang YC, Burger AE, Link BG. The impact of obesity on US mortality levels: the importance of age and cohort factors in population estimates. *Am J Public Health* 2013;103(10):1895–1901.
284. Tsai AG, Williamson DF, Glick HA. Direct medical cost of overweight and obesity in the USA: a quantitative systematic review. *Obes Rev* 2011;12(1):50–61.
285. Thorpe KE, Howard DH. The rise in spending among Medicare beneficiaries: the role of chronic disease prevalence and changes in treatment intensity. *Health Aff (Millwood)* 2006;25(5):w378–w388.
286. Lightwood J, Bibbins-Domingo K, Coxson P, et al. Forecasting the future economic burden of current adolescent overweight: an estimate of the coronary heart disease policy model. *Am J Public Health* 2009;99(12):2230–2237.
287. Costello D. The price of obesity; beyond the health risks, the personal financial costs are steep, recent studies show. *Los Angeles Times*, August 1, 2005.
288. Zagorsky JL. Health and wealth: the late-20th century obesity epidemic in the U.S. *Econ Hum Biol* 2005;3(2):296–313.
289. Sturm R. The effects of obesity, smoking, and drinking on medical problems and costs. *Health Aff (Millwood)* 2002;21(2):245–253.
290. Thorpe KE, Florence CS, Howard DH, et al. The impact of obesity on rising medical spending. *Health Aff (Millwood)*. 2004;Suppl Web Exclusives:W4-480-6.
291. Thorpe KE. Factors accounting for the rise in health-care spending in the United States: the role of rising disease prevalence and treatment intensity. *Public Health* 2006;120(11):1002–1007.
292. Finkelstein E, Fiebelkorn C, Wang G. The costs of obesity among full-time employees. *Am J Health Promot* 2005;20(1):45–51.
293. Rosenwald MS. Why America has to be fat: a side effect of economic expansion shows up in front. *Washington Post*, Jan 22, 2006, F01.
294. Cheap food, societal norms and the economics of obesity. *Wall Street Journal* online. August 25, 2006. http://online.wsj.com/public/article/SB115634907472843442-_xrNV2M1Pwf8pAcQYUWEBITP1LQ_20060901.html.

295. Close RN, Schoeller DA. The financial reality of overeating. *J Am Coll Nutr* 2006;25(3):203–209.
296. Stevens J, Kumanyika SK, Keil JE. Attitudes toward body size and dieting: differences between elderly black and white women. *Am J Public Health* 1994;84:1322–1325.
297. Caldwell MB, Brownell KD, Wilfley DE. Relationship of weight, body dissatisfaction, and self-esteem in African American and white female dieters. *Int J Eat Disord* 1997;22(2):127–130.
298. Neff LJ, Sargent RG, McKeown RE. Black-white differences in body size perceptions and weight management practices among adolescent females. *J Adolesc Health* 1997;20:459–465.
299. Thompson SH, Sargent RG. Black and White women's weight-related attitudes and parental criticism of their childhood appearance. *Women Health* 2000;30:77–92.
300. Anderson LA, Eyler AA, Galuska DA, et al. Relationship of satisfaction with body size and trying to lose weight in a national survey of overweight and obese women aged 40 and older, United States. *Prev Med* 2002;35:390–396.
301. Perez M, Joiner TE Jr. Body image dissatisfaction and disordered eating in black and white women. *Int J Eat Disord* 2003;33:342–350.
302. Akan GE, Grilo CM. Sociocultural influences on eating attitudes and behaviors, body image, and psychological functioning: a comparison of African-American, Asian-American, and Caucasian college women. *Int J Eat Disord* 1995;18:181–187.
303. Ashworth M, Clement S, Wright M. Demand, appropriateness and prescribing of "lifestyle drugs": a consultation survey in general practice. *Fam Pract* 2002;19:236–241.
304. Lexchin J. Lifestyle drugs: issues for debate. *CMAJ* 2001;164:1449–1451.
305. Mitka M. Surgery for obesity: demand soars amid scientific, ethical questions. *JAMA* 2003;289:1761–1762.
306. Puhl R, Brownell KD. Ways of coping with obesity stigma: review and conceptual analysis. *Eat Behav* 2003;4:53–78.
307. Puhl RM, Brownell KD. Psychosocial origins of obesity stigma: toward changing a powerful and pervasive bias. *Obes Rev* 2003;4:213–227.
308. Latner JD, Stunkard AJ. Getting worse: the stigmatization of obese children. *Obes Res* 2003;11:452–456.
309. Kappagoda CT, Hyson DA, Amsterdam EA. Low-carbohydrate-high-protein diets: is there a place for them in clinical cardiology? *J Am Coll Cardiol* 2004;43:725–730.
310. Kong A, Beresford SA, Alfano CM, et al. Associations between snacking and weight loss and nutrient intake among postmenopausal overweight to obese women in a dietary weight-loss intervention. *J Am Diet Assoc* 2011;111:1898–1903.
311. Jenkins D, Wolever T, Vuksan V, et al. Nibbling versus gorging: metabolic advantages of increased meal fequency. *N Engl J Med* 1989;321:929–934.
312. Speechly D, Rogers G, Buffenstein R. Acute appetite reduction associated with an increased frequency of eating in obese males. *Int J Obes Relat Metab Disord* 1999;23:1151–1159.

313. Bellisle F, McDevitt R, Prentice A. Meal frequency and energy balance. *Br J Nutr* 1997;77(Suppl 1):s57–s70.

314. Drummond S, Crombie N, Kirk T. A critique of the effects of snacking on body weight status. *Eur J Clin Nutr* 1996;50:779–783.

315. Fox K. The influence of physical activity on mental well-being. *Public Health Nutr* 1999;2:411–418.

316. Miller W, Koceja D, Hamilton E. A meta-analysis of the past 25 years of weight loss research using diet, exercise or diet plus exercise intervention. *Int J Obes Relat Metab Disord* 1997;21(10):941–947.

317. US Preventive Services Task Force. *Behavioral Counseling in Primary Care to Promote a Healthy Diet. Recommendations and Rationale. Guide to Clinical Preventive Services.* 2nd ed. Washington, DC: Office of Disease Prevention and Health Promotion; 1996.

318. Moyer VA. Behavioral counseling interventions to promote a healthful diet and physical activity for cardiovascular disease prevention in adults: a US Preventive Services Task Force Recommendation Statement. *Ann Intern Med* 2012;157:367–372.

319. US Preventive Services Task Force. *Screening and Interventions to Prevent Obesity in Adults.* 2003. http://www.ahrq.gov/clinic/uspstf/uspsobes.htm. Accessed March 18, 2007.

320. Lin JS, O'Connor E, Whitlock EP, et al. Behavioral counseling to promote physical activity and a healthful diet to prevent cardiovascular disease in adults: a systematic review for the U.S. Preventive Services Task Force. *Ann Intern Med* 2010;153:736–750.

321. Ockene I, Hebert J, Ockene J, et al. Effect of physician-delivered nutrition counseling training and an office-support program on saturated fat intake, weight, and serum lipid measurements in a hyperlipidemic population: Worcester Area Trial for Counseling in Hyperlipidemia (WATCH). *Arch Intern Med* 1999;159:725–731.

322. Long BJ, Calfas KJ, Wooten W, et al. A multisite field test of the acceptability of physical activity counseling in primary care: project PACE. *Am J Prev Med* 1996;12(2):73–81.

323. Blackburn DG. Establishing an effective framework for physical activity counseling in primary care settings. *Nutr Clin Care* 2002;5(3):95–102.

324. Albright CL, Cohen S, Gibbons L, et al. Incorporating physical activity advice into primary care: physician-delivered advice within the activity counseling trial. *Am J Prev Med* 2000;18(3):225–234.

325. Kerse N, Elley CR, Robinson E, et al. Is physical activity counseling effective for older people? A cluster randomized, controlled trial in primary care. *J Am Geriatr Soc* 2005;53(11):1951–1956.

326. Petrella RJ, Koval JJ, Cunningham DA, et al. Can primary care doctors prescribe exercise to improve fitness? The Step Test Exercise Prescription (STEP) project. *Am J Prev Med* 2003;24(4):316–322.

327. Nawaz H, Adams M, Katz D. Weight loss counseling by health care providers. *Am J Public Health* 1999;89:764–767.

328. Tham M, Young D. The role of the general practitioner in weight management in primary care- a cross sectional study in general practice. *BMC Fam Pract* 2008;9:66.
329. Biener L, Heaton A. Women dieters of normal weight: their motives, goals, and risks. *Am J Public Health* 1995;85:714–717.
330. Nawaz H, Katz D, Adams M. Physician-patient interactions regarding diet, exercise and smoking. *Prev Med* 2000;31:652–657.
331. Wieland LS, Falzon L, Sciamanna CN, et al. Interactive computer-based interventions for weight loss or weight maintenance in overweight or obese people. *Cochrane Database Syst Rev* 2012;8:CD007675.
332. Spring B, Duncan JM, Janke EA, et al. Integrating technology into standard weight loss treatment: a randomized controlled trial. *JAMA Intern Med* 2013;173(2):105–111.
333. *Accelerating Progress in Obesity Prevention.* 2012. http://www.iom.edu/Reports/2012/Accelerating-Progress-in-Obesity-Prevention.aspx.
334. Wing RR, Jeffery RW. Food provision as a strategy to promote weight loss. *Obes Res* 2001;9:271S–275S.
335. Jeffery RW, Wing RR. Long-term effects of interventions for weight loss using food provision and monetary incentives. *J Consult Clin Psychol* 1995;63:793–796.
336. Rapoport L, Clark M, Wardle J. Evaluation of a modified cognitive-behavioural programme for weight management. *Int J Obes Relat Metab Disord* 2000;24(12):1726–1737.
337. Harvey-Berino J. The efficacy of dietary fat vs. total energy restriction for weight loss. *Obes Res* 1998;6:202–207.
338. Epstein LH. Family-based behavioural intervention for obese children. *Int J Obes Relat Metab Disord* 1996;20(Suppl 1):S14–S21.
339. Torgerson JS, Lissner L, Lindroos AK, et al. VLCD plus dietary and behavioural support versus support alone in the treatment of severe obesity: a randomised two-year clinical trial. *Int J Obes Relat Metab Disord* 1997;21(11):987–994.
340. Wadden T, Foster G, Letizia K. One-year behavioral treatment of obesity: comparison of moderate and severe caloric restriction and the effects of weight maintenance therapy. *J Consult Clin Psychol* 1994;62(1):165–171.
341. Buettner D. *The Blue Zones.* Washington, DC: National Geographic; 2008.
342. Welch HG, Schwartz L, Woloshin S. What's making us sick is an epidemic of diagnoses, *New York Times,* January 2, 2007.
343. The Affordable Care Act. Available from: https://www.healthcare.gov/.
344. Preventive Medicine Research Institute. *Ornish Programs Reimbursed by Medicare.* http://www.pmri.org/certified_programs.html. Accessed February 6, 2014.
345. Katz DL. Eat and run blog: school over scalpels. *US News & World Report.* 2013. http://health.usnews.com/health-news/blogs/eat-run/2013/01/11/school-over-scalpels.
346. Katz DL. Are our children "diseased"? *Childhood Obesity* 2014;10(1):1–3.

347. Galvez MP, Pearl M, Yen IH. Childhood obesity and the built environment. *Curr Opin Pediatr* 2010;22(2):202–207.

348. Friedman RR, Schwartz MB. Public policy to prevent childhood obesity, and the role of pediatric endocrinologists. *J Pediatr Endocrinol Metab* 2008;21(8):717–125.

349. Bleich SN, Segal J, Wu Y, Wilson R, Wang Y. Systematic review of community-based childhood obesity prevention studies. *Pediatrics* 2013;132(1):e201–e210.

350. *Online Weight Management Counseling for Healthcare Providers.* http://www.turnthetidefoundation.org/OWCH/index.htm.

351. *Weigh Forward.* http://www.rediclinic.com/weighforward/. Accessed February 7, 2014.

19

Sleep and Preventive Health—An Integrative Understanding and Approach

PARAM DEDHIA, MD

Introduction

Sleep is essential for health. As with nutrition and physical activity, sleep is among the cornerstones of optimal health and healing. It is the cornerstone of being well in our daily lives and of well-being as it relates to our mental and emotional health. As much as traditional medicine touted the vitality of sleep, contemporary medical education has increasingly embraced this concept. As sleep accounts for approximately one-third of our lives, the appreciation of its role in health and healing has been transparent to modern science only in recent decades. In these recent decades, we are driven to be a part of a nonstop lifestyle in which the quality and quantity of sleep may be casualties.

The role of sleep in the prevention of disease and illness has been extolled in folk remedies throughout the world. Beyond contemporary medicine's debate regarding the exact role of sleep, the weight of evidence has illuminated both the necessity and the benefits of sleep. The preventative medicine opportunity of sleep has been primarily supported by the observation that insufficient or disordered sleep is associated with serious disease, morbidity, and mortality. Moreover, poor sleep has demonstrated challenges to public health and safety. The perspective of sleep as preventive medicine is furthered by appreciating the two-way impact. By this, it is meant that poor sleep increases the risk of disease and illness, as well as the converse, that disease and illness disrupt sleep. This often creates a vicious cycle in which the accumulative effect is deepened morbidity and mortality. Modern medicine has developed treatments with a focus on pharmacology and interventions that have been helpful. Yet the burden and the growth of sleep challenges will require a frame shift into prevention by which integrative approaches will be the cornerstone.

In this chapter, the healthy obligation and significant opportunity for sleep will become transparent; optimal sleep as a key toward optimal prevention will become clear. To this end, the reader will appreciate the following:

- Epidemiology of sleep
- History of sleep and defining sleep in modern medicine
- Importance of sleep stages and cycles
- Need for quantity and quality of sleep
- Common sleep disorders
- Role of sleep in public safety and performance
- Association of disrupted or disordered sleep with disease and illness
- Interventions and treatments for disrupted and disordered sleep
  - Treatment of sleep-related breathing disorder
  - Treatment of Willis-Ekbom disease (formerly restless legs syndrome)
  - Treatment of insomnia
  - Integrative approaches and lifestyle habits for optimal sleep

Epidemiology of Sleep

The interest in sleep can be appreciated from four significant epidemiological perspectives.[1] First, sleep disorders negatively impact both short- and the long-term health. The more immediate effects reduce a sense of well-being and performance. Moreover, excessive daytime sleepiness is commonly experienced although not recognized and/or connected to poor sleep. Accumulated effects of disordered sleep include premature mortality, cardiovascular disease, hypertension, obesity, metabolic syndrome, diabetes and impaired glucose tolerance, immunosuppression, inflammation, cancer, cognitive impairment, and psychiatric disorders, such as anxiety and depression.[2] Second, there is a high prevalence of sleep problems. Insomnia is the most common specific sleep disorder, such that 30% of adults reports some form of insomnia in the past year[3] and 10% acknowledge chronic insomnia.[4,5,6] The prevalence of insomnia among women and older adults is even higher.[7,8] High prevalence of obstructive sleep apnea, characterized by a reoccurring air flow limitation during sleep, is observed in the general adult population between 5% and 25%, where it is twice as prevalent in women as compared to men.[9,10] Third, as the population has been aging and lifespans are longer, it is therefore noteworthy that older adults often take longer to fall asleep, wake more frequently during the night, experience lower sleep efficiency, and self-report poorer quality of sleep,[11-16] the incidence of sleep problems is increasing. The exponential growth of a 24/7 society providing and catering to day-and-night activities with increased access to mobile phones, media, and Internet has changed our ecosystems and thus has challenged opportunities toward achieving healthy sleep. Patient complaints of sleep have significantly increased over recent years, with increased prevalence of full-time workers experiencing short sleep (defined as less than 6 hours per night).[17,18] Shift work continues to expand to staff and service the around-the-clock societies leading to worsening circadian rhythm disorders, which often has a negative impact on health, healing, and performance. It is important to explain the myth that we need less sleep as we get older; it is found that sleep changes as we age such that slow-wave (or deep) sleep decreases and lighter sleep increases while night sleep disruptions and daytime sleepiness worsen, yet there may little insight into this, as it occurs insidiously. Moreover, the pandemic of health concerns such as obesity and the growing incidence of obstructive sleep apnea have had a bidirectional impact that worsens each of the illnesses in both poor and industrial countries.[19,20] Fourth, sleep problems are associated with accidents and human errors.[21] Thus, in turn, preventable causes of injury and death are unnecessarily promoted (see section "Public Safety and Performance").

History of Sleep and Defining Sleep in Modern Medicine

Medicine's interest in and understanding of sleep was minimal until the 1950s. Prior to the scientific innovations in measurements and metrics, it was difficult for many to appreciate sleep. Its importance was minimized as scientific inference was gleaned and based on casual observation. This still can be seen in the definition of "sleep" in the classic medical dictionary by Stedman:

> a natural periodic state of rest for the mind and body, in which the eyes usually close and consciousness is completely or partially lost, so that there is a decrease in bodily movement and responsiveness to external stimuli.[22]

Such a definition is only partially correct, as it omits the full understanding of sleep and health. To begin the appreciation of the vital importance of sleep, it is well to list its key features: (1) natural, (2) recurring, (3) unconsciousness, (4) inactivity of voluntary muscles, (5) reversible, and (6) essential. As observed by the cause and effect of neurotransmitters' innate response as a circadian rhythm over a 24-hour day, sleep is natural. The ebb and flow of the circadian rhythm's effect on neurochemistry orchestrates sleep as a recurring process. The total or partial unconsciousness sets the stage for significant internal processing and restoration that is enhanced by limiting the response to external stimuli. The nearly complete inactivity of voluntary muscles promotes physical growth and/or repair. Yet sleep is easily reversible and self-regulating, such that it allows us to engage with our environment as appropriate. In all, sleep is essential for survival. Sleep is no luxury, for it is vital and a key requirement for optimal health.

The key features of sleep are furthered by the emerging concepts and robust data on which Daniel Buysse proposed the "conceptual model of sleep health" (Figure 19.1).[23] With this, Buysse poses a helpful definition of sleep by highlighting its role in health and quality of life:

> Sleep health is a multidimensional pattern of sleep-wakefulness, adapted to individual, social, and environmental demands, that promotes physical and mental well-being. Good sleep health is characterized by subjective satisfaction, appropriate timing, adequate duration, high efficiency, and sustained alertness during waking hours.[23]

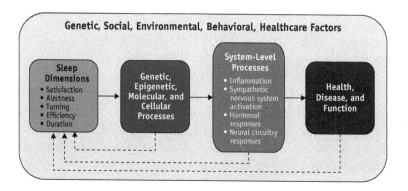

FIGURE 19.1 Conceptual model of sleep health. This model, similar to those proposed by many other authors, posits that various dimensions of sleep-wake function can affect distal outcomes of health and function. Intermediate processes may include epigenetic, molecular, and cellular processes that in turn affect systems-level processes. These processes, ranging from inflammation to altered function of neural circuits, are more proximally related to health outcomes. The model also recognizes that the relationships between sleep-wake function and molecular-, cellular-, systems-, and organism-level outcomes are reciprocal; just as sleep affects function and health, so too function and health influence sleep-wake function.

The casual view of sleep, as simply a dormant and passive unconsciousness with suspension of normal bodily activities, shifted as neurology laid the foundation of sleep using electroencephalograph (EEG). Initially, not knowing of all the connections to health and disease, this led many to minimize sleep complaints as only a psychological discussion when patients spoke of their sleep complaints. We know now that the brain is very active during sleep—vital restoration of the mind and body occurs with each night's rest. Sleep affects our daily functioning and is essential to our physical, mental, and emotional health. William Shakespeare insightfully and aptly described sleep as "nature's soft nurse."

THE IMPORTANCE OF SLEEP STAGES AND CYCLES

Healthy sleep demonstrates repeated oscillations between REM and non-REM stages of sleep through the night to constitute a sleep architecture that follows a repeating cycle approximately every 90 minutes. Healthy and restorative sleep typically consists of approximately five to six cycles of sleep. All stages do not need to be seen in every sleep cycle; however, optimal sleep needs all stages of sleep to occur through the entire sleep. Each sleep stage in any given sleep cycle accomplishes physiological functions to promote health of the body and mind. If sleep is disrupted, fragmented, or missing specific stages over the entire sleep night, then it is more likely for fatigue or daytime sleepiness to be experienced with disregard to whether sufficient amount of sleep was achieved or not.

NON-REM SLEEP

Non-REM sleep is composed of a continuum of three separate stages (stage1, stage 2, and stage 3) with each stage progressively "deeper" from a neurophysiological perspective. In non-REM, each "deeper" stage of sleep leads to further reductions in blood pressure and heart rate while rhythmic breathing patterns and heart rate are seen. Stages 1 and 2 are considered to be *light sleep*, from which we are more readily awakened or briefly aroused when compared to stage 3 sleep, which is referred to as *deep sleep*. In healthy sleep, stage 1 is the lightest stage and makes up only 5%–10% of the sleep night. Most often, it is the stage that we enter into when we fall asleep. It is often described as twilight sleep, in which we ebb and flow out of conscious awareness. Stage 2 of sleep is the typical sleep that we experience as well as the most common sleep stage, constituting 50% of a healthy sleep night. Stage 3 makes up between 15% and

25% of a healthy night of sleep and is *deep sleep*, from which it is difficult for us to be aroused or awakened as a result of the reduced receptiveness to external cues. Deep sleep is more likely to occur in the first half of the sleep night.

REM SLEEP

Dreams are famously associated with rapid eye movement. The truth is that dreamlike experiences of abstract sounds and images may occur in any stage of sleep. Those which we call *dreams* are those with a storyline; these are found in REM sleep. Approximately 20%–25% of the sleep night is REM sleep; REM typically starts 90 minutes from the time we fall asleep and then repeatedly occurs every 90 minutes, with each REM episode progressively getting longer. Thus, the relative amount of REM is more likely to be found in the second half of the night.

In REM there is relative atonia of the muscle throughout the body except for the eyes, heart, and diaphragm. A potential negative impact of this is observed in sleep-related breathing disorders, where obstructive sleep apnea may become worsened in REM. An airway obstruction is more challenged when the costal and accessory muscles of ventilation are essentially paralyzed, thereby creating a greater reliance on the diaphragm to drive airflow and ventilation. However, this atonia is of protective benefit to prevent the acting out of dreams that might otherwise harm us and/or our bed partners. The physical body is relatively slowed in REM, yet the brain-wave activity is similar to a brain that is awake, where heart rate is more rapid, blood pressure increases, breathing becomes less regular, and sexual arousal is more common.

RECOVERY SLEEP

All stages of sleep are important, yet there is an opportunity to cultivate stage 3 (deep sleep) and REM (dream) sleep through the adult years. These are the stages that are part of each night's recovery and they become amplified when sleep is deprived. Such recovery sleep occurs when deep sleep addresses physical repair and restoration. In stage 3 of sleep there is an increased blood supply to muscles as a result, while energy in the form of adenosine triphosphate (ATP) is restored and growth hormone is released to promote growth, development, and repair. There is a progressive reduction in stage 3 throughout adulthood. In REM, the limbic system, which processes emotions, is activated while the frontal cortex, which allows rational thinking, is subdued. This promotes the clearing of emotions.

Sleep patterns change as people age, and sleep disorders become more common. As many as 57% of older adults have reported complaints of poor sleep.[24-28] Changes in sleep architecture also occur with aging. In particular, sleep tends toward being less restorative, as older adults spend an increasing percentage of sleep in Stages 1 and 2 and a decreasing percentage of time in deep sleep (stage 3), and dream (REM) sleep.[29-31] Therefore, it is of great importance to seek opportunities to maintain healthy sleeping given that we have tendency toward less restorative sleep. As a result, awareness of sleep disorders and lifestyle factors that disrupt sleep is vital.

AMOUNT OF SLEEP NEEDED

Upon appreciating the importance of sleep stages, the typical follow-up inquiry seeks to know the amount of sleep that is needed. In general, the answer is the sleep time that permits us to be wide awake, alert, and energetic throughout the day. As this is true, it only begins the conversation when optimal sleep time is queried. The vast amount of the adult population requires about 8 hours of sleep, acknowledging that this does vary throughout our life and among people due to genetic predisposition. Without focusing on environmental cues such as light exposure and lifestyle habits, we see the underlying circadian rhythm is 24.2 hours long. This allows us to appreciate why most people are able to able to stay up later rather than seeking an earlier bedtime. This also influences travel across time zones, where we can more readily adjust to travel from West to East and acclimating to a later time. As a result of light exposure and cues from social interaction and environment, we become entrained into a 24-hour period.

As a starting point for the amount of sleep that is needed, the National Sleep Foundation Scientific Advisory Council has recommended sleep ranges for all age groups.[32]

- **Newborns (0–3 months)**: Sleep range narrowed to 14–17 hours each day
- **Infants (4–11 months):** Sleep range widened 2 hours to 12–15 hours
- **Toddlers (1–2 years):** Sleep range widened by 1 hour to 11–14 hours
- **Preschoolers (3–5):** Sleep range widened by 1 hour to 10–13 hours
- **School age children (6–13):** Sleep range widened by 1 hour to 9–11 hours
- **Teenagers (14–17):** Sleep range widened by 1 hour to 8–10 hours
- **Younger adults (18–25):** Sleep range is 7–9 hours

- **Adults (26–64):** Sleep range did not change and remains 7–9 hours
- **Older adults (65 +):** Sleep range is 7–8 hours

Optimal sleep for an individual varies from person to person and during their lifetime. Moreover, some adults do not fit into the guidelines for optimal sleep. Requiring more than 9 hours of sleep (being a "long sleeper") or needing less than 6 hours (being a "short sleeper") does not reflexively diagnose an individual with a sleep disorder. There are genetic predispositions that allow people to be outside of the recommended sleep parameters and have normal and healthy daytime functioning. Approximately 5%–10% of the adult populations are "long sleepers," and about 5% function well as "short sleepers."

Short sleep duration more commonly has been recognized for its connection with poor sleep and with poor health, yet both short and long sleep duration require further review, given that both may negatively impact health. Short sleep may be a result of insufficient opportunity to sleep or the result of disordered sleep that limits the ability to maintain sleep once the majority of sleep debt is remedied with some sleep. Long sleep duration may represent fragmented or inefficient sleep, thus requiring a person to establish a greater amount of bedtime to acquire actual sleep time.

An optimal night of quality of sleep necessitates spending enough time in the different stages of sleep—especially deep (stage 3) sleep and dream (REM) sleep. If society were aware of the optimal health and performance that can be promoted by optimal sleep quantity and quality, it would be a most important step toward promoting health via sleep. In clinical practice, it is found that some individuals seem to acclimate and *appear* well with their sleep despite achieving less than the recommended sleep. It may not be transparent if someone is a short or long sleeper even if they are without daytime complaints. External factors can promote and demand alertness as today's world is filled and propelled with artificial light and nonstop and increasing sets of imposed expectations and conveniences available 24 hours a day and 7 days a week. It is often surmised that the contemporary world has been actually getting less sleep over the past century. Many adults and teenagers are sleeping at least an hour less on average than 50 or 100 years ago;[33] and sleeping less than 6 hours or over 9 hours now accounts for about one-third of adults.[34]

Insufficient sleep is often termed "sleep deprivation" and leads to sleep debt (also called sleep deficit). This often results in varying expressions of mental, emotional, and physical fatigue. This is observed in difficulties in performing daily activities and those requiring high-level cognitive functions. Similar to the effects of ethanol, two of the effects of sleep deprivation are impaired judgement and reduced insight. Without awareness, or subconsciously denying, this may result in reduced alertness and functionality, which in turn creates serious implications. Although we are aware of our cognitive and physical deficits resulting from sleep debt in the short term, this awareness often fades over repeated nights of poor sleep leading to reduced alertness and functionality with continued sleep deprivation. Beyond reduced alertness and insight, symptoms of sleep deprivation include lapses in attention, poor short-term memory, errors by omission, reduced ability to multitask, irritable mood, aggressive behavior, or daytime sleepiness. Physical manifestations of sleep debt include impaired coordination, impaired reaction time, muscle fatigue, hand tremors, lowered body temperature, increased blood pressure, increased stress hormone levels, and increased heart rate variability. Sleep debt tends to accumulate. About 2 weeks of less than 6 hours sleep per night reduces alertness and performance to a level equivalent to a full 24 hours of sleep deprivation. A week or more of only 4 hours sleep each night creates errors on attention oriented tasks that is equivalent to 2–3 days without any sleep.[35]

Only sleep reverses the negative effects of sleep deprivation. Recovery from sleep loss depends on the accumulated amount of sleep loss. Following one night of inadequate sleep, the following night of sleep demonstrates the majority of recovery in the first night and essentially complete recovery by the third night of healthy sleep. Longer periods of sleep deprivation require longer periods of recovery. However, the amount of sleep time to recover is less than the total amount of sleep that was lost. This may occur over the period of 1 week if sleep time is given an unlimited opportunity. Recovery sleep is often referred to as *rebound sleep*, giving attention to the resultant variation in the staging of sleep. On the first night of sleep following a period of sleep deprivation, deep sleep (stage 3) is given priority to restore our physical functions by releasing more growth hormone and repairing the immune system. This is followed by an extension of REM sleep. When overall sleep and/or REM sleep is repeatedly disrupted, then earlier and longer REM is observed in rebound sleep. This is all given an opportunity to rebalance when sufficient quantity and quality of sleep are allowed to occur consistently.

Common Sleep Disorders

Sleep as one of our most essential needs requires both quality and quantity. Sleep disorders reduce the opportunity for optimal quality and quantity required for restful sleep and, as a result, can cause daytime sleepiness and dysfunction. Nearly all of us will experience some kind of sleep disorder during our lifetime. There are over 100 different types of sleep disorders ranging from difficulty sleeping at night to problems with excessive daytime sleepiness. For the purposes of this chapter, we focus on the most common sleep disorders.

"Sleep apnea" mostly commonly refers to obstructive sleep apnea (OSA), yet this may also refer to central sleep apnea (CSA). By far, OSA is the most common type of apnea and it is characterized by complete or partial collapse of the upper airway for 10 seconds or longer repeatedly throughout the night. Although all persons are submitted to relative relaxation of the soft tissues in the airway during sleep, in OSA, these tissues create an obstruction of the upper airway sufficient to limit airflow, and therefore, to disrupt sleep-related breathing. Moreover, when the airway is blocked, the drop in oxygen levels leads to an arousal that wakes us up long enough so we can take a normal breath. These awakenings are often brief, such there may be no awareness that they are occurring during sleep. This repeats during the night, and in severe sleep apnea this leads to 30 or more awakenings per hour over the entire sleep night. Even though the awakenings are usually very short, this fragmenting and interrupting of the sleep along with the reducing of oxygenation has a significant and negative impact on health.

Although snoring is often associated with obstructive sleep apnea, it simply may be a loud sound, as its relevance ranges from being a mild nuisance to a significant disruptor of sleep for a bed partner. It is the result of a partially occluded upper airway in which inhaled air is redirected from the lungs to the mouth. This creates a negative pressure that vibrates in the soft tissues of the palate. Not everybody who snores has OSA, and not everybody who has OSA snores. Snoring is a potential symptom but not a diagnosis of an underlying sleep disorder. In CSA, prolonged breathing pauses lead to both hypoventilation and hypoxemic syndromes. These are due to a dysregulation and lack of cuing from the central nervous system that would otherwise continue involuntary breathing. As a result, there is no drive to initiate and complete a breath for 10 seconds or longer. This fragments sleep quantity and quality similar to OSA, even though the mechanisms are different.

Periodic limb movement disorder (PLMD) is a sleep disorder characterized by rhythmic movements of the limbs that possibly fragments the quantity but more often disrupts the quality of sleep. A type of PLMD is Willis-Ekbom syndrome (previously referred to as restless legs syndrome). This sleep disorder is characterized as sensorimotor discord when resting or lying down to sleep. It is experienced as frequently repeating discomfort, aching, jerking, twitching, tingling, or creeping-crawling sensations, leading to an irresistible urge to move or shift the legs, arms, or torso.

Insomnia is the most common of all sleep complaints. It is a sleep disorder that is characterized by difficulty falling sleep, staying asleep, and/or experiencing restorative sleep for at least 1 month, which leads to daytime dysfunction or disturbance. Etiologies include poor sleep habits, stress, anxiety, depression, health condition(s), medication effect, late night eating, caffeine, nicotine, mental health condition, another medical diagnosis, and/or another sleep disorder.

Circadian rhythm disorders are disruptions to the internal body clock known as the circadian rhythm. This can present as delayed sleep phase disorder, in which the bedtime and wake up time are later, or advanced phase disorder, in which these times are earlier. This is a disorder when it disturbs quality of life as a result of sleep times not aligning with social opportunities or professional pursuits. Jet lag sleep problems are a form of a circadian disruption in which insomnia occurs as a result of change in time zones. Another circadian disruption has increasingly witnessed is shift work sleep disorder, in which sleep timing and opportunity are dysregulated due to working nights or rotating shifts.

Hypersomnia, or excessive sleepiness, is a condition when there is trouble staying awake during the day. A specific form of daytime sleepiness is narcolepsy, which is a neurological dysfunction controlling the sleep and wakefulness.

REM sleep behavior disorder (RBD) occurs when there is incomplete or absent paralysis that typically occurs during REM sleep. This may result in a person acting out a dream and thus is potentially harmful to the person sleeping or the bed partner.

Parasomnias are disruptive sleep disorders that can occur during arousals from REM sleep or partial arousals from non-REM sleep. Parasomnias include nightmares, night terrors, sleepwalking, and confusional arousals.

Public Safety and Performance

Sleep disorders impact individuals as well as the public at large. In recent decades, the burden of a nonstop 24-hours-a-day/7-days-a-week world has negatively impacted sleep as shift work continues to expand. Shift work often creates highly irregular sleep-wake schedules, and this has been found to contribute to poor health. Chronic exposure to shift work represents a serious challenge to health and healing by its connection with increased risk of obesity, metabolic syndrome, and type 2 diabetes[36-39]—shift workers and students also often show day-to-day variability in their sleep patterns. Young adults tend to have later bedtimes, but spend more time in bed for sleep on nonwork days compared to work days.[40] Similarly, following the transition to retirement, the older adult typically goes to bed later and sleeps longer than when they were working.[41] The impact of the difference in sleep timing between work days and free days is associated with increased body mass index, fat mass, and insulin resistance.[42-44] Hence, irregular sleep-wake timing may impact health, even in individuals who have never worked a night shift.[45]

Insomnia and poor sleep are major contributors to both unintentional fatal injuries in general as well as fatal motor vehicle injuries.[46] The lack of sleep is a factor in manmade errors and many accidents each year. The sleep debt is associated with an increased risk of accidents and injuries. In recent decades, the news headlines have reported industrial and transportation accidents that occurred at night or with limited amount of sleep. Culprit errors were found during the Chernobyl tragedy that occurred at 12:28 a.m., and the Three Mile Island accident was initiated at 4 a.m. The Exxon Valdez captain was not drunk but he had only slept 6 hours in the previous 48 hours. According to the National Transportation Safety Board, fatigue is a factor in 57% of deaths of truck drivers. The Libby Zion case brought national attention to the concerns with work hours of medical trainees and hospital-related errors.[47]

There is a higher risk of preventable injuries and accidents occurring on night shifts than on day shifts. This risk increases with the length of the work shift and the number of back-to-back night shifts worked. Traffic accidents are also more likely during nighttime hours. This surges around 2–3 a.m., when there is the greatest peak in sleep drive within circadian rhythm. The second surge in auto accidents coincides with the next-largest peak in sleep drive, which occurs in the midafternoon. An estimated 20% of all traffic accidents are, in part, due to drowsiness. A small shift, such as 1 hour less of sleep that is likely to occur with daylight-saving time each spring, has been associated with a 20% increase in motor vehicle accidents on the following Monday.

ASSOCIATION OF DISRUPTED OR DISORDERED SLEEP WITH DISEASE AND ILLNESS

Building on the appreciation of the underlying physiology of sleep and its inherent opportunities, the importance of sleep connects to not only the health of the public but also to vital opportunities of individuals for personal health and wellness. Sleep is associated with health and healing, whereas disrupted and disordered sleep is associated with disease and illness. The majority of medical literature has drawn the associations between premature all-cause mortality and both shorter (less than 7 hours) and longer sleep (more than 8 hours).[48,49,50] Research connects health and sleep by demonstrating the impact of sleep spanning the continuum of cellular health to organ systems. Moreover, sleep impacts health and healing at not only on the physical but also the mental and emotional level.

CARDIOVASCULAR HEALTH AND SLEEP

Atherosclerotic cardiovascular disease (ASCVD) is one of the most common diseases in industrial nations. Even with improved ability to diagnose and treat, ASCVD and its consequences are important contributors to morbidity and mortality. Therefore, it is necessary to go beyond the management of traditional ASCVD risk factors and seek other factors and comorbidities that might contribute to its development and progression. One such factor is sleep—and the focus on both poor quantity and quality of sleep.[51, 52] Once healthy sleep became a significant factor in heart health, the importance of sleep was firmly established in modern medicine. For this reason, we highlight the connections and correlations between sleep and ASCVD.

Decreased sleep time is associated with developing of cardiovascular diseases by way of endothelial dysfunction[53-58] leading to increased risk of inflammation, metabolic dysregulation of blood glucose, hypertension, stroke, coronary events, and sudden cardiac death.[59-61] And ASCVD, such as coronary heart disease, peripheral vascular disease, and stroke, is highly prevalent in obstructive sleep apnea.[62]

The underlying mechanisms that provoke ASCVD include hypoxemia, reoxygenation, hypercapnia, sympathetic activation, metabolic dysregulation, endothelial dysfunction, systemic inflammation, left atrial enlargement, acute cardiac stretch and diastolic dysfunction, left and right ventricular dilation, and hypercoagulability. As a result, sleep apnea—especially OSA, is associated with nocturnal nondipping of blood pressure, systemic hypertension, pulmonary hypertension, heart failure, arrhythmias, diabetes mellitus, renal disease, stroke, cardiac fibrosis through repeated remodeling, myocardial infarction, and sudden cardiac death.[63-68]

Inflammation significantly increases the risk of endothelial dysfunction and developing plaque in ASCVD.[69] Obstructive sleep apnea has been shown to increase inflammatory markers.[70] Moreover, OSA is a common condition in patients with ASCVD.[71-74] Obstructive sleep apnea with oxygen desaturation index ≥ 5 (number of oxygen desaturation events of 4% per hour) is independently associated with increased inflammatory activity in nonobese patients with coronary artery disease. The intermittent hypoxemia, as opposed to the number of apneas and hypopneas, is associated with enhanced inflammation.[75]

Patients with acute myocardial infarction and sleep-related breathing events have prolonged myocardial ischemia, less salvaged myocardium, and impaired left and right ventricular remodeling compared with those without sleep-related breathing events, all of which predispose to heart failure.[76] Several studies have identified that patients with acute myocardial infarctions have a high likelihood of OSA, with estimates ranging from 50% to 66%.[76-81]

Participants with untreated severe sleep-disordered breathing (defined as a apnea-hypopnea index > 30 breathing events per hour) were two-and-half times more likely to have an incident coronary heart disease or heart failure compared to those without sleep-disordered breathing.[82] Obstructive sleep apnea is highly prevalent in patients with cardiovascular disease, particularly heart failure. Approximately 35% to 60% of patients with heart failure have OSA,[83-87] and the presence of comorbid sleep apnea is associated with adverse outcomes including increased hospitalizations, morbidity, and mortality.[88-90]

There is a strong association between OSA and cardioembolic stroke. Cardioembolic strokes are more common in patients with OSA, even after adjusting for atrial fibrillation. There is a high incidence of paroxysmal atrial fibrillation in those with OSA.[91] Obstructive sleep apnea is 30% more common in people who have a stroke and is an independent risk factor for ischemic stroke.[92,93] Men with moderate to severe OSA are at a threefold higher risk of stroke.[94]

Furthermore, Willis-Ekbom disease (formerly restless legs syndrome) is independently associated with diastolic blood pressure.[95] Most epidemiologic studies,[96-98] though not all, have demonstrated that Willis-Ekbom disease is associated with cardiovascular disease, with higher risk among those who have frequent symptoms[98] and diagnosis for more than 3 years.[99, 100, 101]

SLEEP AND OBESITY

Today, we are witnessing two pandemics: increasing obesity[102] and increasing sleep disorders.[103] Obesity is reaching epidemic proportions throughout the developed world and is attributed largely to industrialization with reduced acute disease, increased food consumption,[104] and lowered levels of physical activity.[105] The role of sleep in obesity is becoming increasingly understood. Sleep deprivation and disorders have been hypothesized to contribute toward obesity by decreasing leptin, increasing ghrelin, and compromising insulin sensitivity.[106] There is a negative relationship between sleep duration and central adiposity. This has been recognized as a significant risk factor in the pathophysiology of OSA in adults. Furthermore, OSA is associated with increased body mass index.[107]

SLEEP AND METABOLIC SYNDROME

Obesity is a major risk factor not only for sleep apnea but also for cardiovascular and metabolic diseases. Metabolic syndrome is a cluster of risk factors that include central obesity, insulin resistance, hypertension, elevated triglyceride levels, and low high-density lipoprotein cholesterol levels,[108] and is associated with an increased risk for diabetes, cardiovascular events, and mortality in the general population.[108-110]

There is an independent association of OSA with the different components of metabolic syndrome, particularly insulin resistance, hypertension, and abnormal lipid metabolism.[111] The common association between OSA and obesity makes it difficult to separate the role each one plays in their metabolic consequences.[112,113] Nevertheless, OSA is associated with metabolic syndrome independently of central obesity with metabolic profile progressively worsened with increasing severity of OSA.[114] Sleep-disordered breathing and concurrent metabolic syndrome are synergistically associated with worse endothelial function. Individuals with both of these conditions appear to be at a significantly higher risk for cardiovascular disease complications.[115]

SLEEP AND DIABETES

In recent decades, type 2 diabetes has also reached epidemic proportions worldwide. The increasing prevalence of type 2 diabetes can be attributed to dramatic lifestyle changes in response to the industrialization of modern society that may not be limited to changes in our diet and physical activity.[116] As with cardiovascular disease, one such factor strongly associated with development and progression of type 2 diabetes is sleep. Although short sleep duration is more commonly observed than long sleep duration, both are noteworthy in regard to regulating blood glucose. Population studies have observed a U-shaped relationship between sleep duration and type 2 diabetes risk; those who self-report habitually sleeping less than 7 hours or more than 8 hours are at increased risk.[117] Decreased insulin sensitivity due to short sleep duration is observed among patients[118-121] and in laboratory studies.[122-127] Furthermore, when sleep time is extended in short sleepers, insulin sensitivity improves.[128] Strongly linked to the presence of obesity, the OSA syndrome is an independent risk factor for abnormalities of glucose metabolism ranging from simple impaired glucose tolerance to frank type 2 diabetes.[129]

SLEEP AND IMMUNOLOGY

Poor immune status or increased inflammation is related to poor quantity or quality of sleep. Inflammation may be observed when the immune system gets increasingly triggered. It is appropriate for the immune system to be turned on in the setting of infection or illness. It is increasingly appreciated that lifestyle practices, especially poor sleep, directly play a pivotal role in both inflammation and immunocompetence.[130-132]

Several studies have shown insufficient sleep may enhance the susceptibility to infection.[133-135] Shorter sleep duration prior to viral exposure was associated with increased susceptibility to the common cold.[136] Short sleep duration (less than 6 hours per night) and poor sleep continuity are associated with immunosuppression leading to chronic illnesses,[137-140] susceptibility to acute infectious illness,[141-143] and premature mortality.[144-147] Sleep deprivation results in diminished T cell proliferation,[148] shifts in T helper cell cytokine responses,[149,150] decreases in natural killer cell cytotoxicity,[151,152] and increased activation of proinflammatory pathways.[153-156] Furthermore, sleep deprivation and disorders have been found to induce increases in circulating levels of inflammatory markers, such as tumor necrosis factor-α (TNF-α),[153] C-reactive protein (CRP),[155] and interleukin-6 (IL-6),[157] with significant elevations occurring after only 1 night of sleep loss. Patients with both sleep apnea and nonapnea sleep disorders were associated with a higher risk for developing autoimmune diseases.[158] This results from chronic pattern of inflammation found in sleep disorders.[159,160] Brain health requires restorative function of sleep as focused on the glymphatic immune system, especially during REM sleep, as part of the restorative function of sleep is the removal of potentially neurotoxic waste that accumulates in the central nervous system during awake hours.[161]

As vaccinations have been a cornerstone of preventive medicine, it is therefore important to draw the connections between sleep and vaccinations. Sleep promotes antiviral immunity by supporting the adaptive immune response,[162] with evidence that experimental and naturalistic sleep loss is associated with poorer immunological memory after a vaccination.[163-165] One may not achieve the full benefit of the hepatitis B series or the hepatitis A and influenza vaccination followed by less than 6 hours of overnight sleep.

SLEEP AND CANCER

Emerging evidence links OSA with increased cancer incidence and worse cancer outcomes.[166-169] North American and European data sets suggest malignancy is more likely to occur in subjects with severe sleep-disordered breathing,[167,168] while animal models suggest that the mechanism is linked to intermittent hypoxia promoting tumor progression and metastasis.[170,171] The mechanisms underlying these adverse outcomes include chronic systemic inflammation, oxidative stress, and immune dysfunction.

Patients with OSA have significantly reduced levels of circulating invariant natural killer T (iNKT) cells, and hypoxia leads to impaired iNKT cell function. This may be helpful to explain the increased cancer risk reported in patients with OSA.[172] The iNKT cells are a select subset of innate T cells with a direct impact on cancer biology and autoimmune diseases.[173, 174] Moreover, iNKT cells have an anticancer response in the prevention of tumors and in the clearing of tumors,[175] by directly lysing cancer cells.[176] Furthermore, the number and function of circulating iNKT cells are reduced in cancer patients,[177,178] and therapeutic strategies aimed at restoring iNKT cell number and function have shown significant promise in the context of cancer immunotherapy.[179-183] Among these opportunities includes quantity and quality of sleep.

SLEEP AND MEMORY

Cognitive impairment and dementia together constitute a growing public health concern. Sleep disruption and excessive daytime sleepiness contribute to cognitive impairment as well as neurodegeneration[184-190]

The association between sleep and cognitive function in older adults has been established.[191-193] One key mechanism is nocturnal hypoxia, which in turn, decreases frontal lobe neuronal viability, and decreases hippocampal membrane turnover.[194] Another key mechanism includes sleep fragmentation, with more time in stage 1 sleep and less time in REM sleep. Both nocturnal hypoxia and sleep fragmentation in older adults are associated with incident Alzheimer's dementia and the rate of cognitive decline.[195,196] Specifically, sleep loss impairs cognitive functions ranging from attention and learning ability to verbal fluency and inhibitory control.[197-198]

Quantity of sleep is essential for memory, in part, by allowing for a healthy representation of all sleep stages—especially recovery sleep. Recovery sleep is also important for memory. In general, non-REM sleep, especially stage 3, is associated with improved episodic and declarative (factual) memory that was encoded during wakefulness,[199-205] while REM sleep is associated with gains in semantic and emotional memory.[206-208] As a result, non-REM sleep may function to consolidate specific memories, whereas REM sleep integrates these experiences into networks of generalized knowledge.[209,210]

SLEEP AND PAIN

Prevalence studies indicate high rates of comorbid chronic pain and insomnia in the aging population. Osteoarthritis, which affects approximately half of all persons age 65 years or older, is one of the most common comorbidities associated with poor sleep in the aging population.[211] In the general population, a majority of arthritis sufferers report pain during the night,[212] and pain secondary to arthritis is one of the most common factors predicting sleep disturbance.[213,214] Both insomnia and pain adversely affect physical function, mood, and cognition.[215,216] As poor sleep is associated with reduced pain thresholds and next-day pain reports,[217-220] interventions for both sleep and pain are necessary to improve both outcomes.[221]

MENTAL AND EMOTIONAL HEALTH

The World Health Organization has stated that mental illnesses are the leading causes of disability worldwide and account for over 30% of healthy years lost from noncommunicable diseases.[222] Depression alone is expected to be responsible for one-third of health years lost to disability from mental illness.[223] Impaired sleep occurring during psychiatric or medical disorders has a bidirectional and interactive relationship with and coexisting medical and psychiatric illnesses.[224,225]

Sleep disturbances—short sleep duration, long sleep duration, insomnia, poor sleep quality, alterations in sleep architecture and OSA—often precede, co-occur with, or result from the onset of depression.[226-233] More than 90% of patients with depression report some type of sleep disturbance[234,235] and those with OSA have nearly double the odds of depression compared to those without OSA.[236] There is a bidirectional relationship between Willis-Ekbom disease and a wide array of psychiatric conditions.[237] Sleep disturbances impair daytime functioning and quality of life, which in turn decreases adherence to treatments of the mental health conditions.[238] The importance of considering sleep disturbances in the context of mood disorders is highlighted by the fact that sleep disturbances are a risk factor for onset, exacerbation, and relapse of mood disorders.[239]

Interventions and Treatments for Disrupted and Disordered Sleep

Given the impact of disrupted and disorder sleep, the need for interventions and treatments is significant and important. Essentially the focus has been to address underlying etiologies and focus on improving outcomes. Modern medicine has made progress in treating some of the common sleep disorder: sleep-related breathing disorders, periodic limb movement disorders, and insomnia.

TREATMENT OF SLEEP-RELATED BREATHING DISORDERS

Given the significant challenges to morbidity and mortality as well as to quality of life, treatment of sleep apnea needs to be detailed and personalized. First and foremost, both a thorough clinical evaluation with an interdisciplinary team and sleep testing are required so a patient can be directed to appropriate and best treatment options. Proper patient selection increases the success of nonsurgical and surgical approaches.[240]

NONSURGICAL

Nonsurgical approaches for OSA begin with treating underlying medical conditions, positional therapy, and lifestyle modifications with focus on nutrition and exercise. Pharmacotherapy directed toward underlying allergic rhinitis or hypothyroidism may be helpful in combination with other therapies.[241,242] For CSA, narcotic medications may be a culprit cause, and thus it is necessary to review medications for alternative regimens. Depending on the results of the polysomnogram, positional therapy such as avoiding the supine sleep position can be efficacious.[243-247] Such an approach may improve snoring but also may either resolve or reduce the severity of sleep apnea. Typically, helpful lifestyle discussion prioritizes healthy body weight and judicious intake and timing of alcohol.

Nasal dilators and mandibular advancement devices demonstrate best results for mild and positional sleep apnea. Nasal dilators are for patients suffering from uncomplicated snoring and nasal obstruction. Mandibular advancing devices contract the genioglossus, and anteriorly forward both the mandible and hyoid bone to increase the oral airway during sleep.[248] Positive airway pressure (PAP) is the treatment of choice for moderate and severe sleep-disordered breathing including OSA, CSA, and sleep-related hypoventilation. The most common form—continuous positive airway pressure (CPAP)—maintains a continuous level of PAP in a spontaneously breathing patient. Other forms that provide noninvasive positive pressure ventilation include autoadjusting PAP (autoPAP), bilevel positive airway pressure (bilevel PAP), adaptive servoventilation (ASV), and volume-assured pressure support (VAPS).[249]

Continuous PAP uses a nearly continuous air pressure to promote an open airway during both inspiration and expiration. Autoadjusting PAP adjusts the pressure based on respiratory events while delivering the adjusted pressure throughout the respiratory cycle. An advantage of autoPAP is for those who require higher pressures in REM sleep or the supine position, but cannot tolerate the higher pressure through the entire night.[250] Bilevel PAP provides a higher pressure during inspiration and lower pressure during expiration, which may provide improved ventilation and ultimately greater tolerance and compliance, as high pressures may be difficult to tolerate. Some bilevel PAP devices provide a backup rate to address either weak or absent respiratory effort. Adaptive servoventilation is also a bilevel system during both inspiration and expiration, but it has the added sophistication of continuously changing the inspiratory pressure support on a breath-by-breath basis in order to achieve a target ventilation or flow for a more constant breathing pattern. This is especially important in the treatment of periodic breathing or Cheyne–Stokes respiration. An important contraindication of ASV therapy is regarding patients with symptomatic, chronic heart failure (New York Heart Association class 2-4) with reduced left ventricular ejection fraction $\leq 45\%$ and moderate to severe predominant CSA.[251] Finally, VAPS is a variable form of bilevel PAP that allows for more control of respiration by targeting volume or ventilation to be programmed. Indications for VAPS are those with combined periodic breathing and hypoventilation or patients with REM-related hypoventilation related to conditions like chronic obstructive pulmonary disease (COPD), neuromuscular disorders, or obesity, who may need different pressure support levels at different times.[252]

SURGICAL

The ultimate goal of surgical intervention for sleep-related breathing events is either to bypass upper airway obstruction or to increase the upper airway anatomical dimensions. Although not appropriate for all patients, surgical outcomes improve with site-specific surgery after detailed anatomical review.[253-261] Regardless of the chosen surgical approach to manage sleep apnea, constant reevaluation is necessary.

Surgery for moderate to severe OSA is an option for those who have failed CPAP. Surgical may not be definitive therapy but it may be a step toward reducing CPAP pressures to allow for compliance. To allow effective patient selection and site-specific surgery, drug-induced sedation endoscopy (DISE) is increasingly becoming the preferred and optimal evaluation.[262-264] Although a procedure at a single anatomical site can resolve symptoms, an increasing number of patients display multilevel obstruction and therefore require careful assessment and treatment.

Nasal surgery, including septoplasty, turbinate reduction, sinus surgery, and/or nasal valve surgery, can be efficacious for simple snorers and in facilitation of CPAP usage by reducing pressure requirements along with patient discomfort.[265-268]

Palatal surgery has been the most common surgery performed for sleep-related breathing disorders. This approach addresses the anatomy of the soft palate by removing excess tissue (e.g., uvula, soft palate, redundant pharyngeal mucosa, tonsils). Uvulopalatopharyngoplasty was developed by Fujita in the 1980s, but has significant associated morbidity and has fallen out of favor, as success rates for OSA are low.[269,270] In pediatric sleep apnea, adenotonsillectomy has been shown to improve apnea-hypopnea index and quality of life.[271-273]

Tracheostomy is rarely required, but remains the definitive treatment for OSA, as the upper airway is bypassed. Aside from tracheostomy, the highest success rates have been achieved by maxillo-mandibular advancement, which increases retropalatal and retroglossal dimensions.[274,275] Bariatric surgery may improve OSA, but typically does not resolve OSA or snoring.[276,277] A newer approach entails the surgical implantation of a hypoglossal nerve stimulator that is synchronized with inspiration when reduced upper airway muscle activity is the underlying etiology of OSA.[278,279]

TREATMENT OF PERIODIC LIMB MOVEMENTS (WILLIS-EKBOM DISEASE)

Therapeutic options for Willis-Ekbom disease, a neurosensorimotor disorder (better known by its previous name, restless legs syndrome) are contingent on the underlying etiology. The challenge lies within the varied causes that include both genetics and biochemical factors. Willis-Ekbom disease is a continuous spectrum with a major genetic contribution at one end and a major environmental or comorbid disease contribution at the other. It is suggested that the involved genes are significantly expressed in the primary form of the disease (idiopathic) but also are involved in the comorbidities that are the roots of the secondary forms of the disease.[280] In up to two-thirds of cases, genetic factors are considered to contribute to the etiology of Willis-Ekbom Disease.[281]

Whereas the most common secondary forms are linked to the biochemistry of iron deficiency, pregnancy, Parkinson's disease, and end-stage renal disease,[282] the list of associations include relative magnesium deficiency, B vitamin deficiencies, thyroid disorders, cardiovascular disease, arterial hypertension, diabetes, neuropathy, erectile dysfunction, arthritis, rheumatic illnesses, multiple sclerosis, migraine, fibromyalgia, depression, anxiety, mood disorder, attention-deficit hyperactivity disorder, liver disease, obesity, narcolepsy, and other sleep disorders.[283] Ultimately, most presentations of Willis-Ekbom disease are treated with pharmacology (dopamine agonists, gabapentin, or low-potency opioids).[284] Additional options seek to reduce the excessive periodic limb movement and their arousals by treating an accompanying sleep disorder, if present. A recently introduced approach enhances peripheral circulation with pneumatic compression or applies counterstimulation with vibration.[285]

TREATMENT OF INSOMNIA

Although more than half of primary care patients may experience insomnia, only about one-third report this problem to their physicians[286] and only 5% seek treatment.[287] The vast majority of persons with insomnia remain untreated.[288] Given the fast pace of primary care visits and the time needed to understand underlying etiology, it is not a surprise to know that two-thirds of patients with insomnia report a poor understanding of treatment options, and many turn to alcohol (28%) or untested over-the-counter remedies (23%).[289]

In this setting, the approaches may rely on use of prescribing pharmacology, resulting from the relatively short periods of time afforded to medical clinics to discuss underlying issues causing insomnia and patients living full lives with limited resources to delve deeper into root causes of insomnia. Nonbenzodiazapine receptor agonists such as eszopiclone and zolpidem, and the orexin antagonist suvorexant may improve short-term global and sleep outcomes for adults with insomnia disorder, but the comparative effectiveness and long-term efficacy of pharmacotherapies for insomnia are not known. Benzodiazepine hypnotics, melatonin agonists, and antidepressants in general populations and for most pharmacologic interventions in older adults may be helpful for select individuals but are without insufficient data to be widely helpful. In general, pharmacotherapy is intended for short-term use. Hypnotics may be associated with dementia, fractures, and major injury. The Food and Drug Administration warns about cognitive and behavioral changes, iatrogenic illness, or accidents including driving impairment, and other harms, and advises lower doses for females and older adults.[290,291]

Araújo and colleagues offer a framework to better address insomnia and its treatment. They categorize the issues as (1) experience of insomnia, (2) management of insomnia and (3) medicalization of insomnia. The main findings indicate that (1) insomnia is often experienced as a 24-hour problem and is perceived to affect several domains of life; (2) a sense of frustration and misunderstanding is very common among insomnia patients, which is possibly due to a mismatch between patients' and healthcare professionals' perspectives on insomnia and its treatment; (3) healthcare professionals pay more attention to sleep hygiene education and medication therapies and less to the patient's subjective experience of insomnia; and (4) healthcare professionals are often unaware of nonpharmacological interventions other than sleep hygiene education.[292]

The paradigm of therapy starts with etiology: comorbid insomnia due to another sleep disorder or a medical disorder that requires treatment of the underlying process; the more common psychophysiological insomnia requires cognitive and behavioral approaches. Herein is the opportunity to use cognitive-behavioral therapy for insomnia (CBT-I), which was been well-established as an evidence-based, efficacious treatment for insomnia.[293-296] Cognitive-behavioral therapy is commonly prescribed for depression, but clinical trials have shown it is also the most effective long-term solution for those with insomnia.

Positive effects of CBT-I on sleep quality are robust over time.[297,298] The treatment has been found to be efficacious in populations with a variety of comorbid medical conditions, including persons with comorbid insomnia,[299] comorbid psychiatric conditions,[300] and chronic pain.[301-305]

Also, CBT-I helps identify the negative attitudes and beliefs that hinder sleep, and replaces them with positive thoughts, effectively "unlearning" the negative beliefs.[306] The behavioral aspect of CBT focuses on helpful sleep habits and avoids unhelpful sleep behaviors. Behavioral techniques that may be recommended include stimulus control,[307] sleep restriction,[308] systemic desensitization,[309] sleep hygiene, sleep environment improvements, relaxation training,[310] parodoxical intention,[311] hypnosis,[312] and biofeeback.[313] Over a period of six to eight weekly sessions,[314-316] for most adults in either individualized or group-based administration, CBT-I has been shown to be effective[317-319] yet greatly underused in comparison to pharmacological approaches.

INTEGRATIVE AND PREVENTATIVE APPROACHES

First and foremost, the awareness and continued appreciation of the importance of sleep are essential for best health. Such awareness is the key to prevention. In our ever-expanding lives, we seek to expand the hours of day and as result, sleep is treated as a mere luxury. Sleep needs to be prioritized. Educating the public and our patients as to the fundamental need for quantity and quality of sleep cannot be overstated. As much as nutrition and exercise are appropriately highlighted for both health and healing, restorative sleep is prerequisite for optimal health and healing. In addition to positively impacting the physical body, sleep also promotes mental and emotional health. Furthermore, it is helpful to note that healthy sleep supports healthy eating and physical activity. Therefore, sleep both directly and indirectly benefits health. Conversely, disrupted and disordered sleep negatively impacts health and healing opportunities. In this chapter, we have presented sleep and its connection with both public health and personal wellness. Sleep is strongly correlated with cardiovascular disease, obesity, metabolic syndrome, diabetes, immune status, cancer, memory, pain control, mental health, and emotional health. It would be excessive to state that sleep is a single factor preventing these illnesses. Instead it is more helpful to urge the public and our patients to prioritize restorative sleep to reduce either the development or the progression of these diseases.

It is important to think of sleep beyond the time spent in bed. Thus, it is necessary to view the impact of the 24 hours of the day on sleep. By this, it is meant that our daytime lives impact our ability to get to sleep, stay asleep, and awake refreshed for the new day. The focus on lifestyle toward best health also can be applied toward best sleep. There are preventable causes of disrupted sleep when focusing on lifestyle: caffeine, alcohol, tobacco, eating patterns and food choices, light exposure, and exercise.

Caffeine is a common part of the lives of many, as witnessed by rituals of morning coffee or tea as well as the surge in energy drinks among younger adults. Unfortunately, caffeine has discernible impact on sleep that challenges opportunities for restorative sleep.[320] Caffeine blocks the adenosine receptor in the central nervous system, which is involved in sleep induction and the regulation of deep sleep. Caffeine has a half-life ranging from 3 to 7 hours depending on an individual's expression of the cytochrome p450 1A2 genotype. As much as coffee and tea are appropriately touted for their antioxidant benefits, the scheduling and quantity of caffeine is significant as it relates to timing and quality of sleep. According to the 2001 Sleep in America poll by the National Sleep Foundation, 43% of Americans are "very likely" to use caffeinated beverages to combat daytime sleepiness. This, in turn, creates a vicious cycle of poor sleep leading to daytime sleepiness, which leads to increased caffeine consumption. The opportunity is to focus on the timing and quantity of caffeine in our daily lives so that it can be helpful and not disrupt our best sleep.

Alcohol is commonly used around the world as a sleep aide.[321] Regrettably, this is neither helpful nor recommended based on its effects on sleep. Whereas in the short term, it helps induce sleep, this effect tapers in a series of days and weeks depending on the individual's hepatic clearance. The impact of ethanol on sleep staging demonstrates a reduction of quality of sleep in the second half of the sleep night. Alcohol has physiological effects on sleep such as airway relaxation and narrowing; hence, this negatively impacts sleep-related breathing such as OSA. There is a dose effect with ethanol on both its impact on sleep staging and the physiology of breathing during sleep. As with caffeine, the opportunity is to balance the timing and quantity of ethanol in our daily lives so that it does not interfere with healthy sleep.

Tobacco has multiple hazards toward optimal health. In particular, nicotine is usually discussed because of its addictive quality. However, it has significant effects that reduce the quantity and quality of sleep. Nicotine shifts the circadian rhythm by altering the expression of clock genes.[322] People who smoke tobacco are two and half times more like to have OSA. The limitation of airflow is in part due to the inflammatory effect on the nasal and oral airway.[323] Tobacco use leads to difficulty initiating sleep due to its stimulant and withdrawal effects.[324] Those who smoke tobacco are more likely to experience nonrestorative sleep due to more time spent in the light sleep stages as opposed to the deep and REM sleep stages.[325] It is appreciated that tobacco cessation is important for the health of the public as well as for individuals. Hence, the encouragement to be a former tobacco user can be furthered by appreciating its negative impact on sleep.

Eating patterns and food choices influence overall health as well as sleep health. Individuals consuming excessive numbers of calories report short sleep time and quality.[326] Concentrated carbohydrates such as sugars act as stimulants on the body and influence a wide range of neurotransmitter shifting that hinders the ability to fall asleep and stay asleep.[327] Individual variance in food tolerance, such as spicy foods and dairy, also impacts the ability to physically be soothed to be able to sleep. Large meals eaten close to bedtime typically disrupt sleep onset and/or sleep quality. As discussed earlier, poor sleep creates the hormonal and neurochemical basis for food cravings. Again, we see the vicious cycle of poor sleep leading to both overconsumption and poor food choices, which limits restorative sleep. The opportunity to support healthy nutrition also supports healthy sleep.

The world as we know it has expanded with artificial light and electronics. However, it has been at cost of sleep quantity and quality. Exposure to light, and especially blue light, acts on several non-image-forming (NIF) functions of the visual system. They impact sleep by directly acting on the sleep-wake cycle but also indirectly by influencing body temperature, hormonal balance, alertness, and cognitive processing—these, in turn, have a negative impact on sleep.[328] The NIF functions are maximally sensitive to blue wavelengths (460–480 nm), which in turn are involved in melatonin suppression, vigilance, and stimulating mental activity.[329,330] Blue light exposure 1–2 hours before bed reduces sleep onset, REM, and overall perception of sleep quality. Sources of blue light include artificial lighting and digital screens (televisions, computers, tablets, and phones). Herein lies the opportunity to honor the benefits that lighting and electronics have added to our lives, but there is a new opportunity to schedule the exposure to light so that healthy sleep can be promoted.

National Sleep Foundation's 2013 Sleep in America poll highlighted the association between exercise and better sleep. It is thought that a physically robust daytime uses our ATP resources such that the cleaving of the phosphate bonds results in a higher amount of adenosine by bedtime. Again, adenosine promotes sleep induction and deep sleep stages. Exercisers compared to non-exercisers are more likely to report restorative sleep. Poor sleep makes us less likely to exercise, which in turn leads to relative difficulty falling asleep, falling back asleep in the middle of the sleep night, and waking up too early.[331-333] Thus, there is a vicious cycle of reduced physical activity and reduced sleep. Although the timing of exercise has been widely debated, it is likely to be based on individual experience. Promoting daily physical activity also promotes nightly rest by way of healthy sleep.[334]

Integrative medical approaches ultimately bring together the best of modern medicine and traditional wisdom of lifestyle medicine. It is appreciated that the public is seeking quantity and quality of life—lifestyle medicine with appreciation of quantity and quality of sleep are essential toward this pursuit. The time-honored teaching of best medicine is rooted in taking a thorough and deep history and then aligning investigations and therapeutic offerings that are individualized to persons partnering with us. Whereas the histories are not always transparent toward the underlying challenge toward best sleep, investigations such as sleep studies are ripe with information but need to be applied to the context of a person's life. As some patients approach sleep via the modern medicinals and others via the proactive lifestyle route, the opportunity for integrative medicine is to educate and offer all persons as to the full spectrum of both opportunities toward best sleep. As medications are commonly prescribed or bought over-the-counter to promote sleep, they can be helpful for some in the short term. However, their benefits often wane over time. Moreover, pharmacology is only one approach and does not address the full spectrum of opportunities for best sleep. In addition to teaching or prescribing healthy lifestyle toward optimal sleep, integrative medicine is already positioned to translate this within the realms of modern medicine, which has adopted CBT with a focus on sleep hygiene as well as tests such as polysomnogram. Therefore this platform allows for understanding both underlying the lifestyle habits and medical conditions that influence an individual's sleep. On this platform, we can be build preventative approaches. Such preventative approaches can align toward maintaining optimal sleep as well as early detection of sleep disorders so that resulting medical ailments can be reduced or prevented. Again, sleep is no luxury for it is vital and a key factor for optimal health.

Conclusion

Healthy sleep is a cornerstone of healthy lifestyle and preventative medicine. Sleep that is healthy has both quantity of sleep and quality of sleep—this allows sleep to both physically reparative and emotionally restorative. To connect this sleep into both sick care and healthcare is to appreciate that there is a two-way impact: poor sleep increases the risk of disease and illness, and disease and illness disrupt and disorder sleep. This translates into a vicious cycle that creates both morbidity and mortality. Today's medicinal approaches to improve sleep primarily uses pharmacology and interventions. As much as these have been helpful, it is not comprehensive, and therefore it is not enough. If our patients and our communities were aware of the benefits of optimal sleep, it would be a most important step toward promoting health via sleep. Lifestyle and behavioral approaches for healthy sleep are a must, especially in our nonstop, expanding lives. With best sleep, we promote our best health.

References

1. Ferrie JE, Kumari M, Salo P, Singh-Manoux A, Kivimäki M. Sleep epidemiology: a rapidly growing field. *Int J Epidemiol* 2011;40(6):1431–1437.
2. Committee on Sleep Medicine and Research Board on Health Sciences Policy. *Sleep Disorders and Sleep Deprivation: An Unmet Public Health Problem*. Washington, DC: National Academies Press; 2006.
3. Ohayon MM. Epidemiology of insomnia: what we know and what we still need to learn. *Sleep Med Rev* 2002;6:97–111.
4. Ancoli-Israel S, Roth T. Characteristics of insomnia in the United States: results of the 1991 National Sleep Foundation Survey I. *Sleep* 1999;22(Suppl 2):S347–S353.
5. Mellinger GD, Balter MB, Uhlenhuth EH. Insomnia and its treatment: prevalence and correlates. *Arch Gen Psychiatry* 1985;42:225–232.
6. Brown WD. Insomnia: prevalence and daytime consequences. In: Lee-Chiong T, ed. *Sleep: A Comprehensive Handbook*. Hoboken, NJ: Wiley; 2006:93–98.
7. Lichstein KL, Durrence HH, Riedel BW, Taylor DJ, Bush AJ. *Epidemiology of Sleep: Age, Gender, and Ethnicity*. Mahwah, NJ: Erlbaum; 2002.
8. Brabbins CJ, Dewey ME, Copeland JR, Davidson IA. Insomnia in the elderly: prevalence, gender differences and relationships with morbidity and mortality. *Int J Geriatr Psychiatry* 1993;8:473–480.
9. Li C, Ford ES, Zhao G, Croft JB, Balluz LS, Mokdad AH. Prevalence of self-reported clinically diagnosed sleep apnea according to obesity status in men and women: National Health and Nutrition Examination Survey, 2005–2006. *Prev Med* 2010;51(1):18–23.
10. Young T, Palta M, Dempsey J, Skatrud J, Weber S, Badr S. The occurrence of sleep-disordered breathing among middle-aged adults. *N Engl J Med* 1993;328:1230–1235.
11. Buysse DJ, Reynolds CF, Monk TH, Hoch CC, Yeager AL, Kupfer DJ. Quantification of subjective sleep quality in healthy elderly men and women using the Pittsburgh Sleep Quality Index (PSQI). *Sleep* 1991;14:331–338.

12. Cochen V, Arbus C, Soto M, et al. Sleep disorders and their impacts on healthy, dependent, and frail older adults. *J Nutr Health Aging* 2009;13:322–329.

13. Unruh ML, Redline S, An M-W, et al. Subjective and objective sleep quality and aging in the Sleep Heart Health Study. *J Am Geriatr Soc* 2008;56:1218–1227.

14. Vitiello MV, Larsen LH, Moe KE. Age-related sleep change: gender and estrogen effects on the subjective-objective sleep quality relationships of healthy, noncomplaining older men and women. *J Psychosom Res* 2004;56:503–510.

15. Leger D, Roscoat E, Bayon V, Guignard R, Paquereau J, Beck F. Short sleep in young adults: insomnia or sleep debt? Prevalence and clinical description of short sleep in a representative sample of 1004 young adults from France. *Sleep Med* 2011;12(5):454–462.

16. Kronholm E, Partonen T, Laatikainen T, Peltonen M, Harma M, Hublin C, et al. Trends in self-reported sleep duration and insomnia-related symptoms in Finland from 1972 to 2005: a comparative review and re-analysis of Finnish population samples. *J Sleep Res* 2008;17:54–62.

17. Rowshan RA, Bengtsson C, Lissner L, Lapidus L, Bjorkelund C. Thirty-six-year secular trends in sleep duration and sleep satisfaction, and associations with mental stress and socioeconomic factors: results of the Population Study of Women in Gothenburg, Sweden. *J Sleep Res* 2010;19(3):496–503.

18. Knutson KL, Van CE, Rathouz PJ, DeLeire T, Lauderdale DS. Trends in the prevalence of short sleepers in the USA: 1975–2006. *Sleep* 2010;33(1):37–45.

19. Li C, Ford ES, Zhao G, Croft JB, Balluz LS, Mokdad AH. Prevalence of self-reported clinically diagnosed sleep apnea according to obesity status in men and women: National Health and Nutrition Examination Survey, 2005–2006. *Prev Med* 2010;51(1):18–23.

20. Sharma SK. Wake-up call for sleep disorders in developing nations. *Indian J Med Res* 2010;131:115–118.

21. Akerstedt T, Fredlund P, Gillberg M, Jansson B. A prospective study of fatal occupational accidents: relationship to sleeping difficulties and occupational factors. *J Sleep Res* 2002;11(1):69–71.

22. Stedman, TL. *Stedman's Medical Dictionary*. 28th ed. Philadelphia: Lippincott Williams & Wilkins; 2006.

23. Buysse DJ. Sleep health: can we define it? Does it matter? *Sleep* 2014;37(1):9–17.

24. Ancoli-Israel S, Kripke DF, Klauber MR, Mason WJ, Fell R, Kaplan O. Periodic limb movements in sleep in community-dwelling elderly. *Sleep* 1991;14:496–500.

25. Ferri R, Manconi M, Lanuzza B, et al. Age-related changes in periodic leg movements during sleep in patients with restless legs syndrome. *Sleep Med* 2008;9:790–798.

26. Claman DM, Redline S, Blackwell T, et al. Prevalence and correlates of periodic limb movements in older women. *J Clin Sleep Med* 2006;2:438–445.

27. Schubert CR, Cruickshanks KJ, Dalton DS, Klein BE, Klein R, Nondahl DM. Prevalence of sleep problems and quality of life in an older population. *Sleep* 2002;25:889–893.

28. Foley DJ, Monjan AA, Brown SL, Simonsick EM, Wallace RB, Blazer DG. Sleep complaints among elderly persons: an epidemiologic study of three communities. *Sleep* 1995;18:425–432.

29. Bliwise DL. Normal aging. In: Kryger MH, Roth T, Dement WC, eds. *Principles and Practice of Sleep Medicine*. 4th ed. Philadelphia, PA: Elsevier Saunders, 2005:24–38.

30. Feinsilver SH. Sleep in the elderly: what is normal? *Clin Geriatr Med* 2003;19:177–188.

31. Ohayon MM, Carskadon MA, Guilleminault C, Vitiello MV. Meta-analysis of quantitative sleep parameters from childhood to old age in healthy individuals: developing normative sleep values across the human lifespan. *Sleep* 2004;27:1255–1273.

32. Watson NF. Sleep duration: a consensus conference. *Sleep* 2015;38:5–6.

33. Roenneberg T. Chronobiology: the human sleep project. *Nature* 2013;498:427–428.

34. Schoenborn CA, Adams PE. Health behaviors of adults: United States, 2005–2007. *Vital Health Stat* 2010;10:1–132.

35. Van Dongen HP, Maislin G, Mullington JM, Dinges DF. The cumulative cost of additional wakefulness: dose-response effects on neurobehavioral functions and sleep physiology from chronic sleep restriction and total sleep deprivation. *Sleep* 2003;26(2):117–126.

36. Leproult R, Holmback U, Van Cauter E. Circadian misalignment augments markers of insulin resistance and inflammation, independently of sleep loss. *Diabetes* 2014;63:1860–1869.

37. Scheer FA, Hilton MF, Mantzoros CS, Shea SA. Adverse metabolic and cardiovascular consequences of circadian misalignment. *Proc Natl Acad Sci U S A* 2009;106:4453–4458.

38. De Bacquer D, Van Risseghem M, Clays E, Kittel F, De Backer G, Braeckman L. Rotating shift work and the metabolic syndrome: a prospective study. *Int J Epidemiol* 2009;38:848–854.

39. Pan A, Schernhammer ES, Sun Q, Hu FB. Rotating night shift work and risk of type 2 diabetes: two prospective cohort studies in women. *PLoS Med* 2011;8:e1001141.

40. Lo JC, Leong RL, Loh KK, Dijk DJ, Chee MW. Young adults' sleep duration on work days: differences between East and West. *Front Neurol* 2014;5:81.

41. Hagen EW, Barnet JH, Hale L, Peppard PE. Changes in sleep duration and sleep timing associated with retirement transitions. *Sleep* 2016 Mar 1;39(3):665–673.

42. Roenneberg T, Allebrandt KV, Merrow M, Vetter C. Social jetlag and obesity. *Curr Biol* 2012;22:939–943.

43. Parsons MJ, Moffitt TE, Gregory AM, et al. Social jetlag, obesity and metabolic disorder: investigation in a cohort study. *Int J Obes* 2015;39:842–848.

44. Wong PM, Hasler BP, Kamarck TW, Muldoon MF, Manuck SB. Social jetlag, chronotype, and cardiometabolic risk. *J Clin Endocrinol Metab* 2015;100:4612–4620.

45. Rajaratnam SM, Arendt J. Health in a 24-h society. *Lancet* 2001;358:999–1005.

46. Laugsand LE, Strand LB, Vatten LJ, Janszky I, Bjørngaard JH. Insomnia symptoms and risk for unintentional fatal injuries—the HUNT Study. *Sleep* 2014;37(11):1777–1786.

47. Kramer M. Sleep loss in resident physicians: the cause of medical errors? *Front Neurol* 2010;1:128.

48. Kapur VK, Redline S, Nieto FJ, Young TB, Newman AB, Henderson JA; Sleep Heart Health Research Group. The relationship between chronically disrupted sleep and healthcare use. *Sleep* 2002 May 1;25(3):289–96.

49. Gallicchio L, Kalesan B. Sleep duration and mortality: a systematic review and meta-analysis. *J Sleep Res* 2009;18:148–158.

50. Cappuccio FP, D'Elia L, Strazzullo P, Miller MA. Sleep duration and all-cause mortality: a systematic review and meta-analysis of prospective studies. *Sleep* 2010;33(5):585–592.

51. Cheung YY, Tai BC, Loo G, Khoo SM, Cheong KY, Barbe F, Lee CH. Screening for Obstructive Sleep Apnea in the Assessment of Coronary Risk. *Am J Cardiol* 2017 Apr 1;119(7):996–1002.

52. Arzt M, Hetzenecker A, Steiner S, Buchner S. Sleep-disordered breathing and coronary artery disease. *Can J Cardiol* 2015;31(7):909–917.

53. Sauvet F, Leftheriotis G, Gomez-Merino D, et al. Effect of acute sleep deprivation on vascular function in healthy subjects. *J Appl Physiol* 2010;108:68–75.

54. Dettoni JL, Consolim-Colombo FM, Drager LF, et al. Cardiovascular effects of partial sleep deprivation in healthy volunteers. *J Appl Physiol* 2012;113:232–236.

55. Takase B, Akima T, Uehata A, Ohsuzu F, Kurita A. Effect of chronic stress and sleep deprivation on both flow-mediated dilation in the brachial artery and the intracellular magnesium level in humans. *Clin Cardiol* 2004;27:223–227.

56. Sekine T, Daimon M, Hasegawa R, et al. The impact of sleep deprivation on the coronary circulation. *Int J Cardiol* 2010;144:266–267.

57. Kim W, Park HH, Park CS, Cho EK, Kang WY, Lee ES. Impaired endothelial function in medical personnel working sequential night shifts. *Int J Cardiol* 2011;151:377–378.

58. Khazaei M, Moien-Afshari F, Laher I. Vascular endothelial function in health and diseases. *Pathophysiology* 2008;15:49–67.

59. Gangwisch JE, Heymsfield SB, Boden-Albala B, et al. Short sleep duration as a risk factor for hypertension: analyses of the first National Health and Nutrition Examination Survey. *Hypertension* 2006;47:833–839.

60. Nagai M, Hoshide S, Kario K. Sleep duration as a risk factor for cardiovascular disease- a review of the recent literature. *Curr Cardiol Rev* 2010;6:54–61.

61. Hamazaki Y, Morikawa Y, Nakamura K, et al. The effects of sleep duration on the incidence of cardiovascular events among middle-aged male workers in Japan. *Scand J Work Environ Health* 2011;37:411–417.

62. Dong JY, Zhang YH, Qin LQ. Obstructive sleep apnea and cardiovascular risk: meta-analysis of prospective cohort studies. *Atherosclerosis* 2013;229:489–495.

63. Peppard PE, Young T, Palta M, Skatrud J. Prospective study of the association between sleep-disordered breathing and hypertension. *N Engl J Med* 2000;342:1378–1384.

64. Hla KM, Young T, Finn L, Peppard PE, Szklo-Coxe M, Stubbs M. Longitudinal association of sleep-disordered breathing and nondipping of nocturnal blood pressure in the Wisconsin Sleep Cohort Study. *Sleep* 2008;31:795–800.

65. Arzt M, Young T, Peppard PE, et al. Dissociation of obstructive sleep apnea from hypersomnolence and obesity in patients with stroke. *Stroke* 2010;41:e129–e134.

66. Iwasaki YK, Shi Y, Benito B, et al. Determinants of atrial fibrillation in an animal model of obesity and acute obstructive sleep apnea. *Heart Rhythm* 2012;9:1409–1416.

67. Orban M, Bruce CJ, Pressman GS, et al. Dynamic changes of left ventricular performance and left atrial volume induced by the Mueller maneuver in healthy young adults and implications for obstructive sleep apnea, atrial fibrillation, and heart failure. *Am J Cardiol* 2008;102:1557–1561.

68. Somers VK. AHA/ACCF Scientific Statement Sleep Apnea and Cardiovascular Disease. *Circulation* 2008;118:1080–1111.

69. Hansson GK. Inflammation, atherosclerosis, and coronary artery disease. *N Engl J Med* 2005;352:1685–1695.

70. Thunström E, Glantz H, Fu M, Yucel-Lindberg T, Petzold M, Lindberg K, Peker Y. Increased inflammatory activity in nonobese patients with coronary artery disease and obstructive sleep apnea. *Sleep* 2015;38(3):463–471.

71. Hla KM, Young T, Hagen EW, et al. Coronary heart disease incidence in sleep disordered breathing: the Wisconsin Sleep Cohort Study. *Sleep* 2015;38(5): 677–684.

72. Hansson GK. Inflammation, atherosclerosis, and coronary artery disease. *N Engl J Med* 2005;352:1685–1695.

73. Peppard PE, Young T, Palta M, Skatrud J. Prospective study of the association between sleep-disordered breathing and hypertension. *N Engl J Med* 2000;342:1378–1384.

74. Lui MM, Lam JC, Mak HK, et al. C-reactive protein is associated with obstructive sleep apnea independent of visceral obesity. *Chest* 2009;135:950–956.

75. Thunström E, Glantz H, Fu M, et al. Increased inflammatory activity in non-obese patients with coronary artery disease and obstructive sleep apnea. *Sleep* 2015;38(3):463–471.

76. Arzt M, Hetzenecker A, Steiner S, Buchner S. Sleep-disordered breathing and coronary artery disease. *Can J Cardiol* 2015;31(7):909–917.

77. Mehra R, Principe-Rodriguez K, Kirchner HL, Strohl KP. Sleep apnea in acute coronary syndrome: high prevalence but low impact on 6-month outcomes. *Sleep Med* 2006;7(6):521–528.

78. Lee CH, Khoo SM, Tai BC, et al. Obstructive sleep apnea in patients admitted for acute myocardial infarction: prevalence, predictors, and effect on microvascular perfusion. *Chest* 2009;135(6):1488–1495.

79. Skinner MA, Choudhury MS, Homan SD, Cowan JO, Wilkins GT, Tailor DR. Accuracy of monitoring for sleep-related breathing disorders in the coronary care unit. *Chest* 2005;127(1):66–71.

80. Bahammam A, Al-Mobeireek A, Al-Nozha M, Al-Tahan A, Binsaeed A. Behaviour and time-course of sleep disordered breathing in patients with acute coronary syndromes. *Int J Clin Pract* 2005;59(8):874–880.

81. Tsukamoto K, Ohara A. Temporal worsening of sleep-disordered breathing in the acute phase of myocardial infarction. *Circ J* 2006;70(12):1553–1556.

82. Hla KM, Young T, Hagen EW, et al. Coronary heart disease incidence in sleep disordered breathing: the Wisconsin Sleep Cohort Study. *Sleep* 2015;38(5):677–684.

83. Bitter T, Faber L, Hering D, et al. Sleep-disordered breathing in heart failure with normal left ventricular ejection fraction. *Eur J Heart Failure* 2009;11:602–608.

84. Ferreira S, Marinho A, Patacho M, et al. Prevalence and characteristics of sleep apnoea in patients with stable heart failure: results from a heart failure clinic. *BMC Pulm Med* 2010;10:9.

85. Herrscher TE, Akre H, Overland B, et al. High prevalence of sleep apnea in heart failure outpatients: even in patients with preserved systolic function. *J Cardiac Failure* 2011;17:420–425.

86. Oldenburg O, Lamp B, Faber L, et al. Sleep-disordered breathing in patients with symptomatic heart failure: a contemporary study of prevalence in and characteristics of 700 patients. *Eur J Heart Failure* 2007;9:251–257.

87. Zhao ZH, Sullivan C, Liu ZH, et al. Prevalence and clinical characteristics of sleep apnea in Chinese patients with heart failure. *Int J Cardiol* 2007;118:122–123.

88. Hammerstingl C, Schueler R, Wiesen M, et al. Impact of untreated obstructive sleep apnea on left and right ventricular myocardial function and effects of CPAP therapy. *PLoS One* 2013;8:e76352.

89. Kasai T, Narui K, Dohi T, et al. Prognosis of patients with heart failure and obstructive sleep apnea treated with continuous positive airway pressure. *Chest* 2008;133:690–696.

90. Pujante P, Abreu C, Moreno J, et al. Obstructive sleep apnea severity is associated with left ventricular mass independent of other cardiovascular risk factors in morbid obesity. *J Clin Sleep Med* 2013;9:1165–1171.

91. Lipford MC, Flemming KD, Calvin AD, et al. Associations between cardioembolic stroke and obstructive sleep apnea. *Sleep* 2015;38(11):1699–1705.

92. Yaggi HK, Concato J, Kernan WN, Lichtman JH, Brass LM, Mohsenin V. Obstructive sleep apnea as a risk factor for stroke and death. *N Engl J Med* 2005;353:2034–2041.

93. Munoz R, Duran-Cantolla J, Martinez-Vila E, et al. Severe sleep apnea and risk of ischemic stroke in the elderly. *Stroke* 2006;37:2317–2321.

94. Redline S, Yenokyan G, Gottlieb DJ, et al. Obstructive sleep apnea hypopnea and incident stroke: the Sleep Heart Health study. *Am J Respir Crit Care Med* 2010;182:269–277.

95. Dean DA, Wang R, Jacobs DR, et al. A Systematic assessment of the association of polysomnographic indices with blood pressure: the Multi-Ethnic Study of Atherosclerosis (MESA). *Sleep* 2015;38(4):587–596.

96. Lin CH, Sy HN, Chang HW, et al. Restless legs syndrome is associated with cardio/cerebrovascular events and mortality in end-stage renal disease. *Eur J Neurol* 2015;22:142–149.

97. Winter AC, Berger K, Glynn RJ, et al. Vascular risk factors, cardiovascular disease, and restless legs syndrome in men. *Am J Med* 2013;126:228–235.

98. Winkelman JW, Shahar E, Sharief I, Gottlieb DJ. Association of restless legs syndrome and cardiovascular disease in the Sleep Heart Health Study. *Neurology* 2008;70:35–42.

99. Winter AC, Schurks M, Glynn RJ, et al. Vascular risk factors, cardiovascular disease, and restless legs syndrome in women. *Am J Med* 2013;126:220–227.

100. Winter AC, Schurks M, Glynn RJ, et al. Restless legs syndrome and risk of incident cardiovascular disease in women and men: prospective cohort study. *BMJ Open* 2012;2:e000866.

101. Li Y, Walters AS, Chiuve SE, Rimm EB, Winkelman JW, Gao X. Prospective study of restless legs syndrome and coronary heart disease among women. *Circulation* 2012;126:1689–1694.

102. Stein CJ, Colditz GA. The epidemic of obesity. *J Clin Endocrinol Metabol* 2004;89:2522–2525.

103. Patel SR. Reduced sleep as an obesity risk factor. *Obes Rev* 2009 Nov;10 Suppl 2:61–8. doi: 10.1111/j.1467-789X.2009.00664.x. Review.

104. National Sleep Foundation. *2002 "Sleep in America" Poll.* Washington: National Sleep Foundation; 2001.

105. Eskin SB, Hermanson S. *Nutrition Labeling at Fast-Food and Other Chain Restaurants.* AARP Public Policy Institute. Issue Brief no. 71. http://assets.aarp.org/rgcenter/consume/ib71_nutrition.pdf. Accessed May 1, 2016.

106. Stein CJ, Colditz GA. The epidemic of obesity. *J Clin Endocrinol Metabol* 2004;89:2522–2525.

107. Gangwisch JE, Malaspina D, Boden-Albala B, et al. Inadequate sleep as a risk factor for obesity: analyses of the NHANES I. *Sleep* 2005;28(10):1289–1296.

108. Bonsignore MR, McNicholas WT, Montserrat JM, Eckel J. Adipose tissue in obesity and obstructive sleep apnoea. *Eur Respir J* 2012;39:746–767.

109. Alberti KG, Eckel RH, Grundy SM, et al. Harmonizing the metabolic syndrome: a joint interim statement of the International Diabetes Federation Task Force on Epidemiology and Prevention; National Heart, Lung, and Blood Institute; American Heart Association; World Heart Federation; International Atherosclerosis Society; and International Association for the Study of Obesity. *Circulation* 2009;120:1640–1645.

110. Ford ES, author. Risks for all-cause mortality, cardiovascular disease, and diabetes associated with the metabolic syndrome: a summary of the evidence. *Diabetes Care* 2005;28:1769–1778.

111. Ho JS, Cannaday JJ, Barlow CE, Mitchell TL, Cooper KH, FitzGerald SJ. Relation of the number of metabolic syndrome risk factors with all-cause and cardiovascular mortality. *Am J Cardiol* 2008;102:689–692.

112. Lam JC, Mak JC, Ip MS. Obesity, obstructive sleep apnoea and metabolic syndrome. *Respirology* 2012;17:223–236.

113. Lévy P, Bonsignore MR, Eckel J. Sleep, sleep-disordered breathing and metabolic consequences. *Eur Respir J* 2009;34:243–260.

114. Reichmuth KJ, Austin D, Skatrud JB, Young T. Association of sleep apnea and type II diabetes: a population-based study. *Am J Respir Crit Care Med* 2005;172:1590–1595.

115. Gasa M, Salord N, Fortuna AM, et al. Obstructive sleep apnoea and metabolic impairment in severe obesity. *Eur Respir J* 2011;38:1089–1097.

116. Korcarz CE, Stein JH, Peppard PE, Young TB, Barnet JH, Nieto FJ. Combined effects of sleep disordered breathing and metabolic syndrome on endothelial function: the Wisconsin Sleep Cohort study. *Sleep* 2014;37(10):1707–1713.

117. Qian J, Scheer FA. Circadian system and glucose metabolism: implications for physiology and disease. *Trends Endocrinol Metab* 2016;27(5):282–293.

118. Shan Z, Ma H, Xie M, et al. Sleep duration and risk of type 2 diabetes: a meta-analysis of prospective studies. *Diabetes Care* 2015;38:529–537.
119. Wong PM, Manuck SB, DiNardo MM, Korytkowski M, Muldoon MF. Shorter sleep duration is associated with decreased insulin sensitivity in healthy white men. *Sleep* 2015;38:223–231.
120. Matthews KA, Dahl RE, Owens JF, Lee L, Hall M. Sleep duration and insulin resistance in healthy black and white adolescents. *Sleep* 2012;35:1353–1358.
121. Darukhanavala A, Booth JN, Bromley L, et al. Changes in insulin secretion and action in adults with familial risk for type 2 diabetes who curtail their sleep. *Diabetes Care* 2011;34:2259–2264.
122. Robertson MD, Russell-Jones D, Umpleby AM, Dijk DJ. Effects of three weeks of mild sleep restriction implemented in the home environment on multiple metabolic and endocrine markers in healthy young men. *Metabolism* 2013;62:204–211.
123. Klingenberg L, Chaput JP, Holmbäck U, et al. Acute sleep restriction reduces insulin sensitivity in adolescent boys. *Sleep* 2013;36:1085–1090.
124. Donga E, van Dijk M, van Dijk JG, et al. Partial sleep restriction decreases insulin sensitivity in type 1 diabetes. *Diabetes Care* 2010;33:1573–1577.
125. Donga E, van Dijk M, van Dijk JG, et al. A single night of partial sleep deprivation induces insulin resistance in multiple metabolic pathways in healthy subjects. *J Clin Endocrinol Metab* 2010;95:2963–2968.
126. Buxton OM, Pavlova M, Reid EW, et al. Sleep restriction for 1 week reduces insulin sensitivity in healthy men. *Diabetes* 2010;59:2126–2133.
127. Schmid SM, Hallschmid M, Jauch-Chara K, et al. Disturbed glucoregulatory response to food intake after moderate sleep restriction. *Sleep* 2011;34:371–377.
128. Nedeltcheva AV, Kessler L, Imperial J, Penev PD. Exposure to recurrent sleep restriction in the setting of high caloric intake and physical inactivity results in increased insulin resistance and reduced glucose tolerance. *J Clin Endocrinol Metab* 2009;94:3242–3250.
129. Leproult R, Deliens G, Gilson M, Peigneux P. Beneficial impact of sleep extension on fasting insulin sensitivity in adults with habitual sleep restriction. *Sleep* 2015;38:707–715.
130. Frija-Orvoën E. Obstructive sleep apnea syndrome: metabolic complications. *Rev Mal Respir* 2016 Jun;33(6):474–483. pii: S0761-8425(16)00049-8.
131. Palma BD, Gabriel A Jr, Colugnati FA, Tufik S. Effects of sleep deprivation on the development of autoimmune disease in an experimental model of systemic lupus erythematosus. *Am J Physiol Regul Integr Comp Physiol* 2006;291:R1527–R1532.
132. Besedovsky L, Lange T, Born J. Sleep and immune function. *Pflugers Arch* 2012;463:121–137.
133. Dinges DF, Douglas SD, Hamarman S, Zaugg L, Kapoor S. Sleep deprivation and human immune function. *Adv Neuroimmunol* 1995;5:97–110.
134. Everson CA, Toth LA. Systemic bacterial invasion induced by sleep deprivation. *Am J Physiol Regul Integr Comp Physiol* 2000;278:R905–R916.
135. Cohen S, Doyle WJ, Alper CM, Janicki-Deverts D, Turner RB. Sleep habits and susceptibility to the common cold. *Arch Intern Med* 2009;169:62–67.

136. Kang JH, Lin HC. Obstructive sleep apnea and the risk of autoimmune diseases: a longitudinal population-based study. *Sleep Med* 2012;13:583–588.

137. Prather AA, Janicki-Deverts D, Hall MH, Cohen S. Behaviorally assessed sleep and susceptibility to the common cold. *Sleep* 2015;38(9):1353–1359.

138. Cappuccio FP, D'Elia L, Strazzullo P, Miller MA. Quantity and quality of sleep and incidence of type 2 diabetes: a systematic review and meta-analysis. *Diabetes Care* 2010;33:414–420.

139. Mallon L, Broman JE, Hetta J. Sleep complaints predict coronary artery disease mortality in males: a 12-year follow-up study of a middle-aged Swedish population. *J Intern Med* 2002;251:207–216.

140. Mallon L, Broman JE, Hetta J. High incidence of diabetes in men with sleep complaints or short sleep duration: a 12-year follow-up study of a middle-aged population. *Diabetes Care* 2005;28:2762–2767.

141. King CR, Knutson KL, Rathouz PJ, Sidney S, Liu K, Lauderdale DS. Short sleep duration and incident coronary artery calcification. *JAMA* 2008;300:2859–2866.

142. Patel SR, Malhotra A, Gao X, Hu FB, Neuman MI, Fawzi WW. A prospective study of sleep duration and pneumonia risk in women. *Sleep* 2012;35:97–101.

143. Cohen S, Doyle WJ, Alper CM, Janicki-Deverts D, Turner RB. Sleep habits and susceptibility to the common cold. *Arch Intern Med* 2009;169:62–67.

144. Cohen S, Doyle WJ, Skoner DP, Rabin BS, Gwaltney JM Jr. Social ties and susceptibility to the common cold. *JAMA* 1997;277:1940–1944.

145. Dew MA, Hoch CC, Buysse DJ, et al. Healthy older adults' sleep predicts all-cause mortality at 4 to 19 years of follow-up. *Psychosom Med* 2003;65:63–73.

146. Kripke DF, Garfinkel L, Wingard DL, Klauber MR, Marler MR. Mortality associated with sleep duration and insomnia. *Arch Gen Psychiatry* 2002;59:131–136.

147. Heslop P, Smith GD, Metcalfe C, Macleod J, Hart C. Sleep duration and mortality: the effect of short or long sleep duration on cardiovascular and all-cause mortality in working men and women. *Sleep Med* 2002;3:305–314.

148. Cappuccio FP, D'Elia L, Strazzullo P, Miller MA. Sleep duration and all-cause mortality: a systematic review and meta-analysis of prospective studies. *Sleep* 2010;33:585–592.

149. Bollinger T, Bollinger A, Skrum L, Dimitrov S, Lange T, Solbach W. Sleep-dependent activity of T cells and regulatory T cells. *Clin Exp Immunol* 2009;155:231–238.

150. Dimitrov S, Lange T, Tieken S, Fehm HL, Born J. Sleep associated regulation of T helper 1/T helper 2 cytokine balance in humans. *Brain Behav Immunity* 2004;18:341–348.

151. Sakami S, Ishikawa T, Kawakami N, et al. Coemergence of insomnia and a shift in the Th1/Th2 balance toward Th2 dominance. *Neuroimmunomodulation* 2002;10:337–343.

152. Irwin M, Mascovich A, Gillin JC, Willoughby R, Pike J, Smith TL. Partial sleep deprivation reduces natural killer cell activity in humans. *Psychosom Med* 1994;56:493–498.

153. Irwin M, McClintick J, Costlow C, Fortner M, White J, Gillin JC. Partial night sleep deprivation reduces natural killer and cellular immune responses in humans. *FASEB J* 1996;10:643–653.

154. Irwin M, Wang M, Campomayor CO, Collado-Hidalgo A, Cole S. Sleep deprivation and activation of morning levels of cellular and genomic markers of inflammation. *Arch Intern Med* 2006;166:1756–1762.

155. Irwin MR, Wang M, Ribeiro D, et al. Sleep loss activates cellular inflammatory signaling. *Biol Psychiatry* 2008;64:538–540.

156. Meier-Ewert HK, Ridker PM, Rifai N, et al. Effect of sleep loss on C-reactive protein, an inflammatory marker of cardiovascular risk. *J Am Coll Cardiol* 2004;43:678–683.

157. Moldofsky H, Lue FA, Davidson JR, Gorczynski R. Effects of sleep deprivation on human immune functions. *FASEB J* 1989;3:1972–1977.

158. Vgontzas AN, Zoumakis M, Bixler EO, Lin HM, Prolo P, Vela-Bueno A, Kales A, Chrousos GP. Impaired nighttime sleep in healthy old versus young adults is associated with elevated plasma interleukin-6 and cortisol levels: physiologic and therapeutic implications. *J Clin Endocrinol Metab* 2003 May;88(5):2087–2095.

159. Hsiao YH, Chen YT, Tseng CM, et al. Sleep disorders and increased risk of auto-immune diseases in individuals without sleep apnea. *Sleep* 2015;38(4):581–586.

160. Mullington JM, Simpson NS, Meier-Ewert HK, Haack M. Sleep loss and inflammation. *Best Pr Res Clin Endocrinol Metab* 2010;24:775–784.

161. Chung HY, Cesari M, Anton S, et al. Molecular inflammation: underpinnings of aging and age-related diseases. *Ageing Res Rev* 2009;8:18–30.

162. Xie L, Kang H, Xu Q, et al. Sleep drives metabolite clearance from the adult brain. *Science* 2013;342(6156):373–377.

163. Gangwisch JE, Heymsfield SB, Boden-Albala B, et al. Sleep duration associated with mortality in elderly, but not middle-aged, adults in a large US sample. *Sleep* 2008;31:1087–1096.

164. Lange T, Dimitrov S, Born J. Effects of sleep and circadian rhythm on the human immune system. *Ann N Y Acad Sci* 2010;1193:48–59.

165. Prather AA, Hall M, Fury JM, et al. Sleep and antibody response to hepatitis B vaccination. *Sleep* 2012;35:1063–1069.

166. Lange T, Perras B, Fehm HL, Born J. Sleep enhances the human antibody response to hepatitis A vaccination. *Psychosom Med* 2003;65:831–835.

167. Almendros I, Montserrat JM, Ramirez J, et al. Intermittent hypoxia enhances cancer progression in a mouse model of sleep apnoea. *Eur Respir J* 2012;39:215–217.

168. Nieto FJ, Peppard PE, Young T, Finn L, Hla KM, Farre R. Sleep-disordered breathing and cancer mortality: results from the Wisconsin Sleep Cohort Study. *Am J Respir Crit Care Med* 2012;186:190–194.

169. Campos-Rodriguez F, Martinez-Garcia MA, Martinez M, et al. Association between obstructive sleep apnea and cancer incidence in a large multicenter Spanish cohort. *Am J Respir Crit Care Med* 2013;187:99–105.

170. Almendros I, Wang Y, Becker L, et al. Intermittent hypoxia-induced changes in tumor-associated macrophages and tumor malignancy in a mouse model of sleep apnea. *Am J Respir Crit Care Med* 2014;189:593–601.

171. Almendros I, Montserrat JM, Torres M, et al. Obesity and intermittent hypoxia increase tumor growth in a mouse model of sleep apnea. *Sleep Med* 2012;13:1254–1260.

172. Almendros I, Montserrat JM, Torres M, et al. Intermittent hypoxia increases melanoma metastasis to the lung in a mouse model of sleep apnea. *Respir Physiol Neurobiol* 2013;186:303–307.

173. Gaoatswe G, Kent BD, Corrigan MA, et al. Invariant natural killer T cell deficiency and functional impairment in sleep apnea: links to cancer comorbidity. *Sleep* 2015;38(10):1629–1634.

174. Simoni Y, Diana J, Ghazarian L, Beaudoin L, Lehuen A. Therapeutic manipulation of natural killer (NK) T cells in autoimmunity: are we close to reality? *Clin Exp Immunol* 2013;171:8–19.

175. Bendelac A, Savage PB, Teyton L. The biology of NKT cells. *Annu Rev Immunol* 2007;25:297–336.

176. Kawano T, Cui J, Koezuka Y, et al. Natural killer-like nonspecific tumor cell lysis mediated by specific ligand-activated Valpha14 NKT cells. *Proc Natl Acad Sci U S A* 1998;95:5690–5693.

177. Kawano T, Nakayama T, Kamada N, et al. Antitumor cytotoxicity mediated by ligand-activated human V alpha24 NKT cells. *Cancer Res* 1999;59:5102–5105.

178. Tahir SM, Cheng O, Shaulov A, et al. Loss of IFN-gamma production by invariant NK T cells in advanced cancer. *J Immunol* 2001;167:4046–4050.

179. Lynch L, O'Shea D, Winter DC, Geoghegan J, Doherty DG, O'Farrelly C. Invariant NKT cells and CD1d(+) cells amass in human omentum and are depleted in patients with cancer and obesity. *Eur J Immunol* 2009;39:1893–1901.

180. Giaccone G, Punt CJ, Ando Y, et al. A phase I study of the natural killer T-cell ligand alpha-galactosylceramide (KRN7000) in patients with solid tumors. *Clin Cancer Res* 2002;8:3702–3709.

181. Nieda M, Okai M, Tazbirkova A, et al. Therapeutic activation of Valpha24 + Vbeta11 + NKT cells in human subjects results in highly coordinated secondary activation of acquired and innate immunity. *Blood* 2004;103:383–389.

182. Chang DH, Osman K, Connolly J, et al. Sustained expansion of NKT cells and antigen-specific T cells after injection of alpha-galactosylceramide loaded mature dendritic cells in cancer patients. *J Exp Med* 2005;201:1503–1517.

183. Schneiders FL, Scheper RJ, von Blomberg BM, et al. Clinical experience with alpha-galactosylceramide (KRN7000) in patients with advanced cancer and chronic hepatitis B/C infection. *Clin Immunol* 2011;140:130–141.

184. Hunn MK, Hermans IF. Exploiting invariant NKT cells to promote T-cell responses to cancer vaccines. *Oncoimmunology* 2013;2:4.

185. Pallier PN, Maywood ES, Zheng Z, et al. Pharmacological imposition of sleep slows cognitive decline and reverses dysregulation of circadian gene expression in a transgenic mouse model of Huntington's disease. *J Neurosci* 2007;27:7869–7878.

186. Kang JE, Lim MM, Bateman RJ, et al. Amyloid-beta dynamics are regulated by orexin and the sleep-wake cycle. *Science* 2009;326:1005–1007.

187. Bonnet MH. The effect of sleep fragmentation on sleep and performance in younger and older subjects. *Neurobiol Aging* 1989;10:21–25.

188. Tartar JL, Ward CP, McKenna JT, et al. Hippocampal synaptic plasticity and spatial learning are impaired in a rat model of sleep fragmentation. *Eur J Neurosci* 2006;23:2739–2748.

189. Tartar JL, McKenna JT, Ward CP, McCarley RW, Strecker RE, Brown RE. Sleep fragmentation reduces hippocampal CA1 pyramidal cell excitability and response to adenosine. *Neurosci Lett* 2010;469:1–5.

190. Bonnet MH. Performance and sleepiness as a function of frequency and placement of sleep disruption. *Psychophysiology* 1986;23:263–271.

191. Jaussent I, Bouyer J, Ancelin ML, et al. Excessive sleepiness is predictive of cognitive decline in the elderly. *Sleep* 2012;35(9):1201–1207.

192. Oosterman JM, van Someren EJ, Vogels RL, Van Harten B, Scherder EJ. Fragmentation of the rest-activity rhythm correlates with age-related cognitive deficits. *J Sleep Res* 2009;18:129–135.

193. Blackwell T, Yaffe K, Ancoli-Israel S, et al. Poor sleep is associated with impaired cognitive function in older women: the study of osteoporotic fractures. *J Gerontol A Biol Sci Med Sci* 2006;61:405–410.

194. Blackwell T, Yaffe K, Ancoli-Israel S, et al. Association of sleep characteristics and cognition in older community-dwelling men: the MrOS sleep study. *Sleep* 2011;34:1347–1356.

195. O'Donoghue FJ, Wellard RM, Rochford PD, et al. Magnetic resonance spectroscopy and neurocognitive dysfunction in obstructive sleep apnea before and after CPAP treatment. *Sleep* 2012;35(1):41–48.

196. Lim ASP, Kowgier M, Yu L, Buchman AS, Bennett DA. Sleep fragmentation and the risk of incident Alzheimer's disease and cognitive decline in older persons. *Sleep* 2013;36(7):1027–1032.

197. Blackwell T, Yaffe K, Ancoli-Israel S, Redline S, Stone KL; Osteoporotic Fractures in Men Study Group. Relationships between sleep stages and changes in cognitive function in older men: the MrOS Sleep Study. *Sleep* 2015;38(3):411–421.)

198. Killgore WD. Effects of sleep deprivation on cognition. *Prog Brain Res* 2010;185:105–129.

199. Goel N, Basner M, Rao H, Dinges DF. Circadian rhythms, sleep deprivation, and human performance. *Prog Mol Biol Transl Sci* 2013;119:155–190.

200. Diekelmann S, Born J. The memory function of sleep. *Nat Rev Neurosci* 2010;11:114–126.

201. Gais S, Plihal W, Wagner U, Born J. Early sleep triggers memory for early visual discrimination skills. *Nat Neurosci* 2000;3:1335–1339.

202. Wilhelm I, Rose M, Imhof KI, Rasch B, Büchel C, Born J. The sleeping child outplays the adult's capacity to convert implicit into explicit knowledge. *Nat Neurosci* 2013;16:391–393.

203. Marshall L, Helgadóttir H, Mölle M, Born J. Boosting slow oscillations during sleep potentiates memory. *Nature* 2006;444:610–613.

204. Ngo HV, Martinetz T, Born J, Mölle M. Auditory closed-loop stimulation of the sleep slow oscillation enhances memory. *Neuron* 2013;78:545–553.

205. Rasch B, Büchel C, Gais S, Born J. Odor cues during slow-wave sleep prompt declarative memory consolidation. *Science* 2007;315:1426–1429.

206. Diekelmann S, Büchel C, Born J, Rasch B. Labile or stable: opposing consequences for memory when reactivated during waking and sleep. *Nat Neurosci* 2011;14:381–386.

207. Rauchs G, Desgranges B, Foret J, Eustache F. The relationships between memory systems and sleep stages. *J Sleep Res* 2005;14:123–140.

208. Stickgold R. Sleep-dependent memory consolidation. *Nature* 2005;437:1272–1278.

209. Gujar N, McDonald SA, Nishida M, Walker MP. A role for REM sleep in recalibrating the sensitivity of the human brain to specific emotions. *Cereb Cortex* 2011;21:115–123.

210. Antrobus J. REM and NREM sleep reports: comparison of word frequencies by cognitive classes. *Psychophysiology* 1983;20:562–568.

211. Nielsen T. A review of mentation in REM and NREM sleep: "covert" REM sleep as a possible reconciliation of two opposing models. *Behav Brain Sci* 2000;23:851–866.

212. Sarzi-Puttini P, Cimmino MA, Scarpa R, et al. Osteoarthritis: An overview of the disease and its treatment strategies. *Semin Arthritis Rheum* 2005;35(Suppl 1):1–10.

213. Foley D, Ancoli-Israel S, Britz P, Walsh J. Sleep disturbances and chronic disease in older adults: Results of the 2003 National Sleep Foundation Sleep in America survey. *J Psychosom Res* 2004;56:497–502.

214. Blay SL, Andreoli SB, Gastal FL. Chronic painful physical conditions, disturbed sleep and psychiatric morbidity: results from an elderly survey. *Ann Clin Psychiatry* 2007;19:169–174.

215. Moffitt PF, Kalucy EC, Kalucy RS, Baum FE, Cooke RD. Sleep difficulties, pain and other correlates. *J Intern Med* 1991;230:245–249.

216. Kotlarz H, Gunnarsson CL, Fang H, Rizzo JA. Insurer and out-of-pocket costs of osteoarthritis in the US: evidence from national survey data. *Arthritis Rheum* 2009;60:3546–3553.

217. Ozminkowski RJ, Wang S, Walsh JK. The direct and indirect costs of untreated insomnia in adults in the United States. *Sleep* 2007;30:263–273.

218. Haack M, Lee E, Cohen DA, Mullington JM. Activation of the prostaglandin system in response to sleep loss in healthy humans: potential mediator of increased spontaneous pain. *Pain* 2009;145:136–141.

219. Lautenbacher S, Kundermann B, Krieg JC. Sleep deprivation and pain perception. *Sleep Med Rev* 2006;10:357–369.

220. Tiede W, Magerl W, Baumgärtner U, Durrer B, Ehlert U, Treede RD. Sleep restriction attenuates amplitudes and attentional modulation of pain-related evoked potentials, but augments pain ratings in healthy volunteers. *Pain* 2010;148:36–42.

221. Tang NK, Goodchild CE, Sanborn AN, Howard J, Salkovskis PM. Deciphering the temporal link between pain and sleep in a heterogeneous chronic pain patient sample: a multilevel daily process study. *Sleep* 2012;35:675–87A.

222. Smith MT, Haythornthwaite JA. How do sleep disturbance and chronic pain inter-relate? Insights from the longitudinal and cognitive-behavioral clinical trials literature. *Sleep Med Rev* 2004;8:119–132.

223. World Health Organization. *Global Status Report on Non-Communicable Diseases 2010*. Geneva: World Health Organization; 2011.

224. Bloom DE, Cafiero ET, Jane-Llopis E, et al. *The Global Economic Burden of Non-Communicable Diseases*. 2011. Geneva: World Economic Forum.

225. Gupta R, Zalai D, Spence DW, et al. When insomnia is not just insomnia: the deeper correlates of disturbed sleep with reference to DSM-5. *Asian J Psychiatr* 2014;12:23–30. Review.

226. Alvaro PK, Roberts RM, Harris JK. A systematic review assessing bidirectionality between sleep disturbances, anxiety, and depression. *Sleep* 2013;36(7):1059–1068.

227. BaHammam AS, Kendzerska T, Gupta R, et al. Comorbid depression in obstructive sleep apnea: an under-recognized association. *Sleep Breath* 2016;20(2):447–456.

228. Alcántara C, Biggs ML, Davidson KW, et al. Sleep disturbances and depression in the multi-ethnic study of atherosclerosis. *Sleep* 2016;39(4):915–925.

229. Tsuno N, Besset A, Ritchie K. Sleep and depression. *J Clin Psychiatry* 2005;66:1254–1269.

230. Baglioni C, Battagliese G, Feige B, et al. Insomnia as a predictor of depression: a meta-analytic evaluation of longitudinal epidemiological studies. *J Affect Disord* 2011;135:10–19.

231. Riemann D, Voderholzer U. Primary insomnia: a risk factor to develop depression? *J Affect Disord* 2003;76:255–259.

232. Cheng P, Casement MD, Chen CF, Hoffmann RF, Armitage R, Deldin PJ. Sleep-disordered breathing in major depressive disorder. *J Sleep Res* 2013;22:459–462.

233. Alvaro PK, Roberts RM, Harris JK. A systematic review assessing bidirectionality between sleep disturbances, anxiety, and depression. *Sleep* 2013;36:1059–1068.

234. Palagini L, Baglioni C, Ciapparelli A, Gemignani A, Riemann D. Rem sleep dysregulation in depression: state of the art. *Sleep Med Rev* 2013;17:377–390.

235. Fernandez-Mendoza J, Vgontzas AN, Kritikou I, Calhoun SL, Liao D, Bixler EO. Natural history of excessive daytime sleepiness: role of obesity, weight loss, depression, and sleep propensity. *Sleep* 2015;38:351–360.

236. Mendlewicz J, author. Sleep disturbances: core symptoms of major depressive disorder rather than associated or comorbid disorders. *World J Biol Psychiatry* 2009;10:269–275.

237. Sharafkhaneh A, Giray N, Richardson P, Young T, Hirshkowitz M. Association of psychiatric disorders and sleep apnea in a large cohort. *Sleep* 2005;28:1405–1411.

238. Mackie S, Winkelman JW. Restless legs syndrome and psychiatric disorders. *Sleep Med Clin* 2015;10(3):351–357, xv. doi: 10.1016/j.jsmc.2015.05.009. Epub 2015 Jun 27. Review.

239. Kamath J, Prpich G, Jillani S. Sleep disturbances in patients with medical conditions. *Psychiatr Clin North Am* 2015;38(4):825–841. doi: 10.1016/j.psc.2015.07.011. Epub 2015 Aug 21. Review.

240. Rumble ME, White KH, Benca RM. Sleep disturbances in mood disorders. *Psychiatr Clin North Am* 2015;38(4):743–759. doi: 10.1016/j.psc.2015.07.006. Review.

241. Virk JS, Kotecha B. Otorhinolaryngological aspects of sleep-related breathing disorders. *J Thorac Dis* 2016;8(2):213–223. doi: 10.3978/j.issn.2072-1439.2016.01.39.

242. Morin CM, Bootzin RR, Buysse DJ, Edinger JD, Espie CA, Lichstein KL. Psychological and behavioral treatment of insomnia: update of the recent evidence (1998-2004) *Sleep* 2006;29:1398–1414.

243. Stepanski EJ, Rybarczyk B. Emerging research on the treatment and etiology of secondary or comorbid insomnia. *Sleep Med Rev* 2006;10:7–18.

244. Joosten SA, Edwards BA, Wellman A, Turton A, Skuza EM, Berger PJ, Hamilton GS. The effect of body position on physiological factors that contribute to obstructive sleep apnea. *Sleep* 2015;38(9):1469–1478.

245. Lichstein KL. *Clinical Relaxation Strategies.* New York, NY: Wiley; 1988.

246. Spielman AJ, Caruso LS, Glovinsky PB. A behavioral perspective on insomnia treatment. *Psychiatr Clin North Am* 1987;10:541–553.

247. Morin CM, Azrin NH. Behavioral and cognitive treatments of geriatric insomnia. *J Consult Clin Psychol* 1988;56:748–753.

248. Morgenthaler T, Kramer M, Alessi C, et al. Practice parameters for the psychological and behavioral treatment of insomnia: an update; an American Academy of Sleep Medicine Report. *Sleep* 2006;29:1415–1419.

249. Pigeon WR, Crabtree VM, Scherer MR. The future of behavioral sleep medicine. *J Clin Sleep Med* 2007;3:73–79.

250. Hansford A. Thirty years of CPAP: a brief history of OSA. *ResMedica Clinical Newsletter.* 2011;14.

251. Rosen CL, Auckley D, Benca R, et al. A multisite randomized trial of portable sleep studies and positive airway pressure autotitration versus laboratory-based polysomnography for the diagnosis and treatment of obstructive sleep apnea: the HomePAP study. *Sleep* 2012;35(6):757–767.

252. *AASM Special Safety Notice: ASV Therapy for Central Sleep Apnea Patients with Heart Failure.* American Academy of Sleep Medicine. May 15, 2015.

253. Johnson KG, Johnson DC. Treatment of sleep-disordered breathing with positive airway pressure devices: technology update. *Med Devices (Auckl)* 2015;8:425–437.

254. Lin HC, Friedman M, Chang HW, et al. The efficacy of multilevel surgery of the upper airway in adults with obstructive sleep apnea/hypopnea syndrome. *Laryngoscope* 2008;118:902–908.

255. Elshaug AG, Moss JR, Hiller JE, et al. Upper airway surgery should not be first line treatment for obstructive sleep apnoea in adults. *BMJ* 2008;336:44–45.

256. Lim DJ, Kang SH, Kim BH, et al. Treatment of obstructive sleep apnea syndrome using radiofrequency-assisted uvulopalatoplasty with tonsillectomy. *Eur Arch Otorhinolaryngol* 2013;270:585–593.

257. Bowden MT, Kezirian EJ, Utley D, et al. Outcomes of hyoid suspension for the treatment of obstructive sleep apnea. *Arch Otolaryngol Head Neck Surg* 2005;131:440–445.
258. De Vito A, Frassineti S, Panatta ML, et al. Multilevel radiofrequency ablation for snoring and OSAHS patients therapy: long-term outcomes. *Eur Arch Otorhinolaryngol* 2012;269:321–330.
259. Iyngkaran T, Kanagalingam J, Rajeswaran R, et al. Long-term outcomes of laser-assisted uvulopalatoplasty in 168 patients with snoring. *J Laryngol Otol* 2006;120:932–938.
260. Randhawa PS, Cetto R, Chilvers G, et al. Long-term quality-of-life outcomes in children undergoing adenotonsillectomy for obstructive sleep apnoea: a longitudinal study. *Clin Otolaryngol* 2011;36:475–481.
261. Hultcrantz E, Harder L, Loord H, et al. Long-term effects of radiofrequency ablation of the soft palate on snoring. *Eur Arch Otorhinolaryngol* 2010;267:137–142.
262. Thatcher GW, Maisel RH. The long-term evaluation of tracheostomy in the management of severe obstructive sleep apnea. *Laryngoscope* 2003;113:201–204.
263. Croft CB, Pringle M. Sleep nasendoscopy: a technique of assessment in snoring and obstructive sleep apnoea. *Clin Otolaryngol Allied Sci* 1991;16:504–509.
264. Hewitt RJ, Dasgupta A, Singh A, et al. Is sleep nasendoscopy a valuable adjunct to clinical examination in the evaluation of upper airway obstruction? *Eur Arch Otorhinolaryngol* 2009;266:691–697.
265. De Vito A, Carrasco Llatas M, Vanni A, et al. European position paper on drug-induced sedation endoscopy (DISE). *Sleep Breath* 2014;18:453–465.
266. Kotecha B. The nose, snoring and obstructive sleep apnoea. *Rhinology* 2011;49:259–263.
267. Li HY, Lee LA, Wang PC, et al. Nasal surgery for snoring in patients with obstructive sleep apnea. *Laryngoscope* 2008;118:354–359.
268. Verse T, Maurer JT, Pirsig W. Effect of nasal surgery on sleep-related breathing disorders. *Laryngoscope* 2002;112:64–68.
269. Powell NB, Zonato AI, Weaver EM, et al. Radiofrequency treatment of turbinate hypertrophy in subjects using continuous positive airway pressure: a randomized, double-blind, placebo-controlled clinical pilot trial. *Laryngoscope* 2001;111:1783–1790.
270. Fujita S, Conway W, Zorick F, et al. Surgical correction of anatomic abnormalities in obstructive sleep apnea syndrome: uvulopalatopharyngoplasty. *Otolaryngol Head Neck Surg* 1981;89:923–934.
271. Sher AE, Schechtman KB, Piccirillo JF. The efficacy of surgical modifications of the upper airway in adults with obstructive sleep apnea syndrome. *Sleep* 1996;19:156–177.
272. Randhawa PS, Cetto R, Chilvers G, et al. Long-term quality-of-life outcomes in children undergoing adenotonsillectomy for obstructive sleep apnoea: a longitudinal study. *Clin Otolaryngol* 2011;36:475–481.
273. Swift AC. Upper airway obstruction, sleep disturbance and adenotonsillectomy in children. *J Laryngol Otol* 1988;102:419–422.

274. Marcus CL, Moore RH, Rosen CL, et al. A randomized trial of adenotonsillectomy for childhood sleep apnea. *N Engl J Med* 2013;368:2366–2376.

275. Faria AC, Xavier SP, Silva SN Jr, et al. Cephalometric analysis of modifications of the pharynx due to maxillo-mandibular advancement surgery in patients with obstructive sleep apnea. *Int J Oral Maxillofac Surg* 2013;42:579–584.

276. Hsieh YJ, Liao YF. Effects of maxillomandibular advancement on the upper airway and surrounding structures in patients with obstructive sleep apnoea: a systematic review. *Br J Oral Maxillofac Surg* 2013;51:834–840.

277. Faria AC, da Silva-Junior SN, Garcia LV, et al. Volumetric analysis of the pharynx in patients with obstructive sleep apnea (OSA) treated with maxillomandibular advancement (MMA). *Sleep Breath* 2013;17:395–401.

278. Haines KL, Nelson LG, Gonzalez R, et al. Objective evidence that bariatric surgery improves obesity-related obstructive sleep apnea. *Surgery* 2007;141:354–358.

279. Eastwood PR, Barnes M, Walsh JH, et al. Treating obstructive sleep apnea with hypoglossal nerve stimulation. *Sleep* 2011;34:1479–1486.

280. Kezirian EJ, Boudewyns A, Eisele DW, et al. Electrical stimulation of the hypoglossal nerve in the treatment of obstructive sleep apnea. *Sleep Med Rev* 2010;14:299–305.

281. Trenkwalder C, Allen R, Högl B, Paulus W, Winkelmann J. Restless legs syndrome associated with major diseases: a systematic review and new concept. *Neurology* 2016;86(14):1336–1343.

282. Nomura T, Nakashima K. Prevalence of restless legs syndrome. *Brain Nerve* 2009;61(5):515–521.

283. Ghorayeb I, Tison F. Epidemiology of restless legs syndrome. *Rev Neurol (Paris)* 2009;165(8-9):641–649.

284. Becker PM, Novak M. Diagnosis, comorbidities, and management of restless legs syndrome. *Curr Med Res Opin* 2014;30(8):1441–1460. doi: 10.1185/03007995.2014.918029. Epub 2014 May 9.

285. Nagandla K, De S. Restless legs syndrome: pathophysiology and modern management. *Postgrad Med J* 2013;89(1053):402–410.

286. Mitchell UH. Medical devices for restless legs syndrome: clinical utility of the Relaxis pad. *Ther Clin Risk Manag* 2015;11:1789–1794.

287. Shochat T, Umphress J, Israel AG, Ancoli-Israel S. Insomnia in primary care. *Sleep* 1999;22(Suppl 2):S359–S365.

288. Ancoli-Israel S, Roth T. Characteristics of insomnia in the United States: results of the 1991 National Sleep Foundation Survey. I. *Sleep* 1999;22(Suppl 2):S347–S353.

289. Mellinger GD, Balter MB, Uhlenhuth EH. Insomnia and its treatment: prevalence and correlates. *Arch Gen Psychiatry* 1985;42:225–232.

290. Ancoli-Israel S, Roth T. Characteristics of insomnia in the United States: results of the 1991 National Sleep Foundation Survey. I. *Sleep* 1999;22(Suppl 2):S347–S353.

291. Brasure M, MacDonald R, Fuchs E, et al. *Management of Insomnia Disorder.* Rockville, MD: Agency for Healthcare Research and Quality (US); 2015 Dec. Report No. 15(16)-EHC027-EF. AHRQ Comparative Effectiveness Reviews.

292. Wilt TJ, MacDonald R, Brasure M, et al. Pharmacologic treatment of insomnia disorder: an evidence report for a clinical practice guideline by the American College of Physicians. *Ann Intern Med* 2016:165(2):103–112.

293. Araújo T, Jarrin DC, Leanza Y, Vallières A, Morin CM. Qualitative studies of insomnia: current state of knowledge in the field. *Sleep Med Rev* 2017;31:58–69.

294. Espie CA. "Stepped care": a health technology solution for delivering cognitive behavioral therapy as a first line insomnia treatment. *Sleep* 2009;32:1549–1558.

295. McCurry SM, Logsdon RG, Teri L, Vitiello MV. Evidence-based psychological treatments for insomnia in older adults. *Psychol Aging* 2007;22:18–27.

296. Morin CM, Bootzin RR, Buysse DJ, Edinger JD, Espie CA, Lichstein K. Psychological and behavioral treatment of insomnia: update of the recent evidence (1998–2004). *Sleep* 2006;29:1398–1414.

297. Siebern AT, Manber R. New developments in cognitive behavioral therapy as the first-line treatment of insomnia. *Psychol Res Behav Manag* 2011;4:21–28.

298. Morin CM, Culbert JP, Schwartz SM. Nonpharmacological interventions for insomnia: a meta-analysis of treatment efficacy. *Am J Psychiatry* 1994;151:1172–1180.

299. National Institutes of Health State of the Science Conference Statement. Manifestations and management of chronic insomnia in adults. *Sleep* 2005;28:1049–1057.

300. Wu JQ, Appleman ER, Salazar RD, Ong JC. Cognitive behavioral therapy for insomnia comorbid with psychiatric and medical conditions: a meta-analysis. *JAMA Intern Med* 2015;175(9):1461–1472.

301. Sánchez-Ortuño MM, Edinger JD. Cognitive-behavioral therapy for the management of insomnia comorbid with mental disorders. *Curr Psychiatry Rep* 2012;14(5):519–528. doi: 10.1007/s11920-012-0312-9

302. Belleville G, Cousineau H, Levrier K, St-Pierre-Delorme M-E. Meta-analytic review of the impact of cognitive-behavior therapy for insomnia on concomitant anxiety. *Clin Psychol Rev* 2011;31:638–652.

303. Edinger JD, Olsen MK, Stechuchak KM, et al. Cognitive behavioral therapy for patients with primary insomnia or insomnia associated predominantly with mixed psychiatric disorders: a randomized clinical trial. *Sleep* 2009;32:499–510.

304. Morgan K, Gregory P, Tomeny M, David B, Gascoigne C. Self-help treatment for insomnia symptoms associated with chronic conditions in older adults: a randomized controlled trial. *J Am Geriatr Soc* 2012;60:1803–1810.

305. Rybarczyk B, Mack L, Harris JH, Stepanski E. Testing two types of self-help CBT-I for insomnia in older adults with arthritis or coronary artery disease. *Rehabil Psychol* 2011;56:257–266.

306. Smith MT, Huang MI, Manber R. Cognitive behavior therapy for chronic insomnia occurring within the context of medical and psychiatric disorders. *Clin Psychol Rev* 2005;25:559–592.

307. Davies D. A multiple treatment approach to the group treatment of insomnia. *Behav Psychotherapist* 1989;17:323–331.

308. Bootzin RR. A stimulus control treatment for insomnia. *Proceedings of the American Psychological Association* 1972;7:395–396.

309. Spielman AJ, Saskin P, Thorpy MJ. Treatment of chronic insomnia by restriction of time in bed. *Sleep* 1987;10:45–56.

310. Geer JH, Katkin ES. Treatment of insomnia using a variant of systematic desensitization: a case report. *J Abnorm Psychol* 1966;71:161–164.

311. Lick JR, Heffler D. Relaxation training and attention placebo in the treatment of severe insomnia. *J Consult Clin Psychol* 1977;45:153–161.

312. Frankl VE. *The Doctor and the Soul: From Psychotherapy to Logotherapy.* New York, NY: Knopf; 1955.

313. Anderson JA, Dalton ER, Basker MA. Insomnia and hypnotherapy. *J R Soc Med* 1979;72:734–739.

314. Hauri P. Treating psychophysiologic insomnia with biofeedback. *Arch Gen Psychiatry* 1981;38:752–758.

315. Lovato N, Lack L, Wright H, Kennaway DJ. Evaluation of a brief treatment program of cognitive behavior therapy for insomnia in older adults. *Sleep* 2014;37(1):117–126.

316. Morin C. *Insomnia: Psychological Assessment and Management.* New York, NY: Guilford Press; 1993.

317. Morin CM. Cognitive-behavioral approaches to the treatment of insomnia. *J Clin Psychiatry* 2004;65:33–40.

318. Germain A, Moul DE, Franzen PL, et al. Effects of a brief behavioral treatment for late-life insomnia: preliminary findings. *J Clin Sleep Med* 2006;2:403–406.

319. Irwin M, Cole J, Nicassio P. Comparative meta-analysis of behavioural interventions for insomnia and their efficacy in middle-aged adults and in older adults 55 + years of age. *Health Psychol* 2006;25:3–14.

320. Rybarczyk B, Lopez M, Benson R, Alsten C, Stepanski E. Efficacy of two behavioural treatment programs for comorbid geriatric insomnia. *Health Psychol* 2002;17:288–298.

321. Clark I, Landolt HP. Coffee, caffeine, and sleep: a systematic review of epidemiological studies and randomized controlled trials. *Sleep Med Rev* 2017 Feb;31:70–78.

322. Angarita GA, Emadi N, Hodges S, Morgan PT. Sleep abnormalities associated with alcohol, cannabis, cocaine, and opiate use: a comprehensive review. *Addict Sci Clin Pract* 2016;11(1):9.

323. Hwang JW, Sundar IK, Yao H, Sellix MT, Rahman I. Circadian clock function is disrupted by environmental tobacco/cigarette smoke, leading to lung inflammation and injury via a SIRT1-BMAL1 pathway. *FASEB J* 2014;28(1):176–194.

324. Kashyap R, Hock LM, Bowman TJ. Higher prevalence of smoking in patients diagnosed as having obstructive sleep apnea. *Sleep Breath* 2001;5(4):167–172.

325. McNamara JPH, Wang J, Holliday DB, et al. Sleep disturbances associated with cigarette smoking. *Psychol Health Med* 2014;19(4):410–419.

326. Zhang L, Samet J, Caffo B, et al. Power spectral analysis of EEG activity during sleep in cigarette smokers. *Chest* 2008;133:427–432.

327. Grandner MA, Jackson N, Gerstner JR, Knutson KL. Dietary nutrients associated with short and long sleep duration: data from a nationally representative sample. *Appetite* 2013;64:71–80.

328. Beebe DW, Simon S, Summer S, Hemmer S, Strotman D, Dolan LM. Dietary intake following experimentally restricted sleep in adolescents. *Sleep* 2013;36(6):827–834.

329. Cajochen C, Münch M, Kobialka S, et al. High sensitivity of human melatonin, alertness, thermoregulation, and heart rate to short wavelength light. *J Clin Endocrinol Metab* 2005;90(3):1311–1316.

330. Lockley SW, Evans EE, Scheer FA, Brainard GC, Czeisler CA, Aeschbach D. Short-wavelength sensitivity for the direct effects of light on alertness, vigilance, and the waking electroencephalogram in humans. *Sleep* 2006;29(2):161–168.

331. Daneault V, Hébert M, Albouy G, et al. Aging reduces the stimulating effect of blue light on cognitive brain functions. *Sleep* 2014;37(1):85–96.

332. Passos GS, Poyares DLR, Santana MG, Tufik S, de Mello MT. Is exercise an alternative treatment for chronic insomnia? *Clinics* 2012;67(6):653–659.

333. Guilleminault C, Clerk A, Black J, Labanowski M, Pelayo R, Claman D. Nondrug treatment trials in psychophysiologic insomnia. *Arch Intern Med* 1995;155(8):838–844.

334. Kline CE. The bidirectional relationship between exercise and sleep: implications for exercise adherence and sleep improvement. *Am J Lifestyle Medicine* 2014;8(6):375–379.

20

Midlife Transitions—The Integrative Preventive Medicine Approach to the Evaluation and Management of Menopause and Andropause

CYNTHIA GEYER, MD, AND STEVEN BREWER, MD

Menopause

Menopause refers to a narrow window of time, 12 months after the normal cessation of a woman's menses. The average age for menopause is 51, although the age of natural menopause can range from 40 to 55. The perimenopause, or menopause transition, can begin as early as a decade before a woman's last menstrual period; average onset is 6–8 years prior.[1] The early transition is characterized by wider fluctuations in estrogen production along with less consistent ovulation and progesterone production; eventually shifting to low levels of both hormones, usually with longer intervals between menses, until the final menstrual period. Symptoms can range from relatively few at one end of the spectrum to significant hot flashes, night sweats, disrupted sleep, heavy irregular periods, and decreased mood, which can negatively impact a woman's quality of life. Historically much of the conversation between women and their healthcare providers has centered on the discussion of whether they should take hormone replacement therapy (HRT), now commonly called hormone therapy (HT).

The following vignette illustrates common questions a woman in midlife may bring to her integrative and preventive medicine practitioner. A 49-year-old woman comes in for your opinion on HRT. Her periods have become more irregular, and she is noticing some hot flashes 4–5 times a day, which she describes as mild but noticeable. She is also waking up 2–3 times a night with night sweats, and is usually able to go back to sleep. However, she feels more fatigue and irritability in the daytime. She is concerned about HRT because her mother had breast cancer at 75. She read that bioidentical hormones are a more natural, safe approach, but she has received conflicting advice about whether she should take HT from her primary care physician and her gynecologist. She is seeking additional recommendations from you.

The pendulum of professional opinion has swung widely from recommending HT for most women, after the observational Nurses Health Initiative linked HT to lower risk of heart disease and osteoporosis, to strongly recommending against it after the randomized prospective Women's Health Initiative (WHI) found paradoxically higher cardiac events in addition to higher rates of breast cancer in women assigned to take HT.[2] Roughly two-thirds of the women in the WHI were 63 or older, representing a group likely to be physiologically different from most women entering menopause. This may have contributed to some of the negative findings related to cardiovascular risk: More recent subset analysis has found that outcomes differed by age. Key points that came from reanalysis:[3]

1. In women who started HT before the age of 70 or within 20 years of their last menstrual period, no increase in cardiovascular disease was seen.
2. In women who had no uterus and used conjugated equine estrogens only (ET), starting between the ages of 50 and 59, a trend toward fewer cardiovascular events was seen. Less coronary calcium was also seen.
3. Overall mortality was decreased in younger women on ET only.
4. Newer research adds more evidence that the form of HT used, the route of administration, and the timing of initiation in relation to a woman's last menstrual period all influence the potential benefit versus harm, particularly in regard to cardiovascular and thrombotic risk.[4-6] A recent observational study found that thrombotic risk from oral estradiol was much lower than from oral conjugated equine estrogens,[7] and no increased thrombotic risk was seen with either transdermal or intravaginal preparations.[8] Both the MESA and the ELITE trials add support for the timing hypothesis: earlier HT was associated with slower coronary calcium buildup and less carotid plaque buildup, respectively.[9,10]

As clinicians work with women in the menopause transition it is important to recognize the interplay among many different hormones beyond estrogen and progesterone with regard to symptoms. Insulin dysregulation,[11] subclinical thyroid disorders,[12] declining melatonin,[13,14] and production of catecholamines and cortisol in response to stress[15,16] all influence symptoms of the menopause transition and also play a role with the increased risk of diabetes, heart disease, and breast cancer in the post menopause. Disrupted sleep and increasing prevalence of sleep apnea may exacerbate weight gain, insulin resistance, and mood changes.[17] Emerging evidence implicates the gut microbiome[18,19] and exposure to endocrine-disrupting chemicals[20,21] as additional modulators of many aspects of the hormonal environment, particularly related to insulin and estrogen. Perhaps most significantly, the timing of menopause often coincides with many other life transitions for women. Children may be leaving home; women may be rethinking their long-term career or partner; they may grieve the loss of their parents or be dealing with their parents' health issues and functional decline; more peers and friends in their age group are facing cancer, heart disease, and other serious health concerns. A truly integrative approach takes all these factors into consideration in the partnership with each woman about the best individualized approach for her to reduce her symptoms, decide if hormones are right for her, and incorporate the lifestyle strategies that will not only reduce her risk of heart disease, osteoporosis, and breast cancer but also support her thriving in the post menopause.

These are key areas to explore with women in the conversation around the menopause transition (in addition to past medical and family history):

1. Symptoms such as hot flashes and night sweats: how often, how disruptive or not, any known triggers
2. Sleep: changes in ability to fall asleep/stay asleep; impact of night sweats on sleep; presence of snoring; daytime fatigue (see chapter 19)
3. Mood: irritability, weepiness, depression, feelings of helplessness, hopelessness; history of premenstrual or postpartum mood changes
4. Weight history and any recent changes
5. Libido: changes in sex drive, vaginal dryness, pain with vaginal penetration, decreased ability to attain orgasm; if still menstruating and sexually active with a male partner, use and type of contraception, satisfaction with method
6. If in a relationship: emotional and physical safety, shared interests, emotional connection, partner's physical and mental health
7. Community: who are her supports?
8. Concerns/fears/joys; thoughts and attitudes around aging
9. Thoughts/preferences/level of knowledge around HT

The preceding chapters have given excellent reviews on the integrative and preventive medicine approach to common clinical problems. What may be unique about women in the menopause transition is that for many, although their symptoms may get their attention, it may also be the first time they have started to think about aging and their risk of these common conditions. The menopause transition thus provides an opportune time to establish benchmarks in health and prioritize together the best lifestyle changes to help manage symptoms and lower risk of disease.

Helpful benchmarks:

1. Anthropometrics: height, weight, waist circumference, waist:hip ratio
2. Blood pressure
3. Fitness level—estimated or measured
4. Mammogram and breast tissue density
5. Bone density
6. Assessment of fat free mass, percent body fat and distribution (by caliper, bioimpedence analysis [BIA], DEXA scan), particularly for women with a lower BMI but elevated waist:hip ratio
7. Bone turnover/bone formation
8. Complete lipid profile with LDL and HDL size, remnant lipoproteins
9. hsCRP
10. Fasting glucose, insulin, (calculated HOMA-IR), Hgb A1c
11. TSH, free T4, free T3

It is also important for practitioners to understand their own opinions about HT and be open about any general biases they may have. In the wake of uncertainty, mixed study results and shifting professional guidelines about the long-term risks and benefits of HT, some healthcare practitioners have aligned on the side of generally recommending against HT while others have broadly recommended it for most of their patients. Being open about your opinions and also willing to explore the mindset of your patients fosters a relationship that allows a mutual exploration of the best approach for that particular person at a given point in time, consistent with her symptoms, concerns, goals, and attitudes. Establishing an open and respectful dialogue sets the stage for checking back in and modifying the approach over time as symptoms and goals change (and as new research about HT is published).

The potential pros and cons of HT have been extensively reviewed elsewhere. Hormone therapy remains the most effective treatment for the vasomotor symptoms of menopause, and also shows benefit for mood[22] and sleep. For women who do not have existing coronary artery disease, HT is likely to be safe (and may even lower risk) from a cardiovascular standpoint when initiated within a 6-year window from the last menstrual period. Because transdermal estrogens are less likely to have a negative impact on raising C-reactive protein (CRP), blood pressure, clotting factors and triglycerides, this is my preferred route of administration. Transdermal preparations are available as patches, creams, gels, and a mist.

"Bioidentical" is a term that has generated confusion for patients and practitioners. In its strictest definition, it refers to hormones that are identical on a molecular level to those endogenously produced (such as estradiol [E2], progesterone, and testosterone).[23] It is generally used in reference to compounded forms of sex hormones, which commonly use a combination of 70% estriol (E3) and 30% estradiol (E2). Standardized pharmaceutical preparations of bioidentical hormones (E2 and progesterone) are also available in a wide range of doses. Although the compounded versions are often marketed as "natural and safe," they are not regulated by the Food and Drug Administration and there has been a lack of studies looking at long-term outcomes. Estriol, the weakest of the three naturally occurring estrogens, has been touted as potentially providing benefits of estrogen without the risk of breast cancer. However, in human breast cancer cell lines, low levels of estriol were able to trigger a robust estrogenic response.[24] It is important for practitioners and their patients to recognize that even compounded HT is still HT: the same risk:benefit conversation is indicated.

In women with an intact uterus, unopposed estrogen is associated with an increased risk of hyperplasia of the uterine lining and with uterine cancer. Administering progestins mitigates that risk,[25] but progestins may also differentially affect cardiovascular risk factors, breast cancer risk,[26,27] and mood. Medroxyprogesterone, as opposed to progesterone, adversely affects endothelial function, lipids, and insulin sensitivity. In the WHI, higher rates of breast cancer were seen with combined conjugated equine estrogens (CEE) and medroxyprogesterone but not with unopposed CEE;[28] results from a prospective French cohort study named E3N did not find an elevation in breast cancer risk for women using estrogen and progesterone.[29] Both forms of progestins may negatively impact mood in susceptible women. Several regimens have been used to try and decrease total progesterone exposure while still protecting the lining of the uterus. Cycling progesterone, taking it the first 12 days of the month, is one option. Another is vaginal progesterone: In the recently reported ELITE trial, a 4% progesterone gel was administered vaginally on the first 12 days of each 30-day time frame. Although not FDA approved, dosing the 4% progesterone gel twice weekly on the day of changing an estradiol patch may also be acceptable. Until more long-term studies are done confirming the uterine protection of this latter regime, annual surveillance with a transvaginal ultrasound to look at the thickness of the endometrial lining would be reasonable. In my practice working with women who decide to try HT and for whom it is not contraindicated, I usually start with a low-dose FDA-approved standardized estradiol patch twice weekly and either nightly progesterone 100 mg (taking advantage of the potential soporific effects if there are sleep concerns)[30] or a 200-mg dose of progesterone orally on days 1–12 of 30 days. If a woman has a history of depression, premenstrual and/or postpartum depression, or does not tolerate the progesterone, vaginal administration of 200-mg progesterone or 4% progesterone gel can be done on days 1–12.

One of the biggest concerns with long-term HT is the potential for increased risk of breast cancer.[31] Understanding a woman's baseline risk of breast cancer is critical; one online risk calculator, based on the original Gail model and developed by the National Cancer Institute and the NSPI, is available at cancer.gov. Questions include age, ethnicity, onset of menarche, age of first live birth, prior history of breast cancer or chest radiation, known *BRCA* or other genetic risk, number of first-degree relatives with breast cancer, and history of breast biopsies/atypical hyperplasia. The Rosner-Colditz model[32] adds BMI, alcohol intake, and additional reproductive factors to the Gail model. Newer risk-prediction models are being developed that include common single nucleotide polymorphisms (SNPs) associated with elevated risk of breast cancer.[33] Other factors that increase risk of breast cancer include weight gain after menopause,[34] the presence of dense breast tissue,[35] high bone density,[36,37] insulin resistance,[38] and working night shifts (possibly due to lower melatonin).[39,40] Although less clear from the literature, certain dietary factors (low intake of fiber, omega-3's, fruits, and vegetables)[41,42] and exposure to persistent organic pollutants (POPs) or endocrine disrupting chemicals (EDCs)[43] may also influence risk. The higher the number of risk factors, the more a practitioner may elect to recommend against long-term HT (usually defined as >5 years).

If a woman chooses to try HT, addressing other potentially modifiable risk factors for breast cancer is crucial. The combination of HT and alcohol intake significantly increases risk.[44] Proposed mechanisms include alcohol's effect on decreasing estrogen metabolism, resulting in higher circulating estrogen in the bloodstream;[45] and increased needs for folic acid, a key cofactor for estrogen detoxification and DNA repair.[46,47] Incorporating regular physical activity; adopting a dietary pattern high in fiber, fruits and vegetables, and omega-3 fatty acids; and even reducing evening calorie intake and prolonging the overnight fasting interval may have beneficial effects on lowering insulin and insulin resistance, reducing inflammatory adipocytokines, supporting a more diverse gut microbiome, and increasing estrogen excretion.[48-52]

In addition to the association between weight gain and insulin resistance in the menopause transition with both higher rates of cardiovascular disease and breast cancer,[53] a deeper understanding of the relationship between insulin and menopausal symptoms is emerging.

1. Higher weight is associated with more vasomotor symptoms, and in turn a higher frequency of hot flashes is associated with higher glucose levels and insulin resistance, as estimated by the homeostasis model assessment of insulin resistance (HOMA-IR).[54,55]

2. In the WHI, weight loss significantly reduced hot flashes in women not on HT.[56] A more recent pilot study found that a behavioral approach to weight loss was effective in reducing hot flashes, and hot flash reduction was a major motivator to lose weight in 74% of the women studied.[57]

3. Weight gain adversely affects lipids, blood pressure, diabetes, and cardiovascular risk and can contribute to sleep apnea, which in turn exacerbates weight gain, insulin resistance, and dyslipidemia.

4. Arguably, addressing insulin resistance may be the most important hormonal modulation for women in an effort to improve symptoms and health outcomes in the transition and the postmenopausal years.

Women's desire for, and their ability to comfortably engage in, sexual activity may be impacted by the physical, emotional, and other changes of menopause. Many studies suggest that estrogen, not testosterone, has a larger impact on sexual desire.[58,59] Thinning of the vaginal epithelium and decreased lubrication may not occur until several years after the last menstrual period and can contribute to painful penetration. Those tissue changes along with alterations in vaginal flora and increase in vaginal pH may increase susceptibility to postcoital urinary tract or yeast infections. Attitudes about aging,[60] disrupted sleep and decreased energy, being uncomfortable with a changing body, and feeling emotionally distant from a partner[61] all impact a women's sexual desire. Vaginal estrogen is extremely effective in improving atrophy,[62] favorably impacting the vaginal microbiome,[63] and reducing urinary tract infections.[64] However, some women will absorb enough to elevate serum levels of estradiol, which may be a concern in women with a history of breast cancer.[65] A recent study found that daily intravaginal dehydroepiandrosterone (DHEA) 0.5% (6.5 mg) for 12 weeks resulted in an 86%–121% improvement in vaginal secretions along with improved integrity, color, and surface thickness of vaginal epithelium. Significant reduction in vaginal dryness and pain with sexual activity were also seen compared to placebo. Serum levels of DHEA and its metabolites, including testosterone, estradiol, and estrone, remained within normal postmenopausal limits. This appears to be an effective and safe option for treatment and management of vulvovaginal atrophy.[66] Vaginal DHEA received FDA approval for this indication in November 2016. In addition to addressing physiologic changes that can impact a woman's desire for and comfort with sexual activity, it is equally important to address relationship concerns and attitudes about aging. The American Academy of Sexuality Educators, Counselors and Therapists (www.aasect.org) is a resource for finding certified professionals for referral if indicated.

There are several nonhormonal modalities that may have benefit for relief of bothersome symptoms. Unfortunately, assessing efficacy of many commonly used therapies is hindered by lack of good-quality studies. It is important to recognize that "lack of evidence to support" a modality is not the same as "proof of ineffectiveness." That awareness needs to be balanced with the potential for harm. A comprehensive review of the comparative effectiveness and strength of evidence, along with potential risks, behind hormonal, nonhormonal pharmacologic, and supplemental and botanical therapies for menopausal symptoms was published by the Agency for Healthcare Research and Quality in March 2015, available at healthcare.ahrq.gov. In addition to HT, high-strength evidence shows the effectiveness of selective serotonin reuptake inhibitors (SSRIs) and serotonin-norepinephrine reuptake inhibitors (SNRIs) on vasomotor symptoms, anxiety and depression, and overall quality of life. The North American Menopause Society's (NAMS) position paper published the same year also cited level I evidence supporting the use of paroxetine salt,[67] currently the only FDA-approved nonhormonal treatment, for symptom relief.

The AHRQ's review found low-level evidence for the effectiveness of dietary or supplemental isoflavones. A more recent meta-analysis concluded that phytoestrogen supplementation, dietary and supplemental soy isoflavones (primarily genistein and daidzein), were moderately effective in reducing hot flashes and vaginal dryness, but not night sweats.[68] For a trial of soy isoflavone supplementation, a dose of 50 mg/d or higher should be used. A supplement containing s-equol (level II evidence according to NAMS) may be effective if women do not respond, since some women lack the gut bacteria that convert daidzein to s-equol. For red clover isoflavones, the usual dose is 80 mg/d.[69] Because of the phytoestrogenic effect of isoflavones, concerns have been raised about their safety in women with a history of breast cancer. A meta-analysis in 2013 concluded that isoflavone intakes in the doses typically used do not appear harmful and may even be associated with lower risk of breast cancer recurrence and mortality.[70]

Both reviews concluded that neither black cohosh nor dong quai, commonly used herbs, showed evidence for beneficial results. Limited evidence has shown improvements in symptoms using ERr731[71,72] (an extract from Rheum rhaponticum) and pycnogenol[73] (extract from pine bark). The dose for pycnogenol ranges from 30 to 100 mg/d. In higher doses (150 mg/d) pycnogenol has also shown beneficial effects in blood glucose, lipids, waist circumference, oxidative stress, and endothelial function.[74]

The NAMs position paper also cited level I evidence for cognitive-behavioral therapy and hypnotherapy as effective modalities for symptom relief. Mindfulness-based stress reduction was "recommended with caution," citing a need for additional studies; while acupuncture was not recommended. A more recent study found that telephone-based cognitive-behavioral therapy for insomnia was effective in improving sleep quality in women with vasomotor symptoms.[75] The Cochrane review found low-level evidence of benefit with acupuncture compared to placebo but not compared to sham acupuncture.[76] A more recent study of 190 women with breast cancer found significantly lower hot flash scores and improved quality of life in the group who received 10 acupuncture treatments plus an informational booklet on self-care compared to the women who only received the booklet. Differences remained significant 3 and 6 months after treatment.[77] Despite these conflicting recommendations, the low risk and possible effectiveness of acupuncture makes it a reasonable treatment for women to try, especially if HT is contraindicated.

Muscle mass begins to decrease in the 4th decade, and there is accelerated bone loss in the late menopause transition and the first years of the post menopause. Analysis of the Nationwide Inpatient Sample (NIS) between 2000 and 2011 found that for women age 55 and older, more were hospitalized for osteoporotic fractures than for myocardial infarction, stroke, and breast cancer, highlighting the significant impact bone loss has on healthcare costs and morbidity.[78] Hormone therapy can prevent the rapid phase of bone loss associated with the menopause transition, but the bone loss resumes upon discontinuation of HT. A preventive approach to minimize muscle and bone loss includes ensuring adequate dietary protein, calcium, magnesium, and vitamin D.[79-82] Although there is debate about the optimal level of vitamin D for bone health, maintaining levels in the 30–40 ng/mL range is a reasonable target, based on National Health and Nutrition Examination Survey (NHANES) data.[83] Higher adherence to a Mediterranean dietary pattern was associated with a 20% relative risk decrease in hip fractures and improved skeletal muscle mass and power.[84,85] Vitamin K2, produced by intestinal bacteria from vitamin K1 (present in dark leafy greens), may have a unique role in both reducing vascular calcification and improving bone mineral density by reducing undercarboxylated osteocalcin and promoting osteoblast differentiation.[86-90] Natto, a fermented soy product, provides the richest dietary source of vitamin K2, which is also found in aged and curd cheeses. Doses used in supplementation range from 45 to 100 μg daily. A combination of low-impact exercise and resistance training may both improve bone density and have other benefits related to reducing fracture risk: improved strength, maintenance of muscle mass, improved stability and balance, and reduction of falls.[91] A new bone balance index (BBI) using the ratio of bone turnover (measured by urinary N-telopeptide) to bone formation (serum osteocalcin) was found to predict women at risk for a faster decline in lumbosacral spine bone density and may prove to be a useful tool to identify women who need more intensive treatment and follow-up.[92] The strongest correlate of a more favorable BBI was a high BMI. On the other hand, since high bone density may predict higher than average risk of breast cancer, it becomes part of the risk:benefit equation in deciding about HT.

Regardless of whether a woman's initial decision is to try HT or to try alternative approaches to manage symptoms, encourage follow-up after a given period of time, such as 3–6 months, to review efficacy and side effects. If troublesome symptoms persist and HT is not desired or is contraindicated, a trial of an SSRI or SNRI may be offered. For women on HT whose symptoms have not responded, measuring an estradiol level may be helpful. If the level is extremely low, a higher dose of estradiol is reasonable. If the level is 40–100, efforts should be made to look for other contributors to symptoms if not already done. Reinforcement of exercise, stress reduction practices, quality and quantity of sleep, and a whole-foods diet can be done at each follow-up.

In summary, the menopause transition is a normal phase of a woman's life and there is tremendous variability in different women's experiences. Honoring the other life transitions that may coincide with changing hormones; "normalizing" the experience; framing it as an opportunity to reassess stress levels, dietary patterns, self-care, sleep habits, social support network, and quality of primary relationship; and individualizing recommendations with regular planned follow-up can ensure that women find what works best for them and reengage with the lifestyle strategies that contribute to lower risk of disease and improved quality of life through the menopause transition and beyond.

Andropause

Over the years much has been written about women's decreased production of hormones that result in multiple symptoms that we call menopause. Women have spent the last 50 plus years trying to treat these symptoms of menopause by using various hormonal and herbal therapies. The consequence of using these treatments has not always been good. There has been a potential of developing breast and uterine cancer.

Men have thought menopause is a "disease" that only women need to worry about. The reality is that men also have the potential of having lower levels of sex hormones. This has loosely been called andropause or late-onset hypogonadism. With scientific advances we have improved our understanding on how the male hormone system works. Men and women both go through changes as they age. One big difference seen with men compared to women is that men generally have a more gradual onset of hormonal changes. Men may notice difference in their libido or in their general mood over months and years where women will often notice changes emotionally in weeks and sometimes days.

So what really is andropause or the male version of female menopause? It is defined as a decrease in serum concentration of a man's testosterone level. The difference between female menopause and male andropause is that women generally have rather rapid loss of estrogen production from their ovaries. In men they generally have a more gradual decrease in their testosterone level or production of sperm as they age. The lower production of testosterone can cause many physical and emotional changes in the body.

Testosterone is responsible for the growth and development of the male reproductive system, but for these changes to take place, testosterone must first be converted to dihydrotestosterone. It is actually dihydrotestosterone that produces the male effects. During puberty with the higher production of testosterone and subsequently the higher level of dihydrotestosterone, the penis and testes increase in size. Testosterone also has an anabolic effect on the body. It increases muscle mass and promotes healthy bones by increasing bone density and mass. Other secondary sexual characteristics that are a result of increased testosterone production are facial, pubic, armpit, and chest hair.

There are basically two types of male andropause. The first is primary hypogonadism. This is where the problem is in the testes themselves. The levels of testosterone are decreased, and the production of sperm is often lower. It can be diagnosed by showing lower testosterone levels and a person's leutenizing hormone (LH) and/or follicle stimulating hormone (FSH) are above normal. The LH and FSH are the pituitary hormones whose job is to stimulate the testes to make testosterone and sperm. With secondary hypogonadism the testosterone and sperm count are low and the LH and/or FSH are normal or low. In this case the pituitary hormones, LH and FSH, are not producing enough to stimulate the testes effectively. This can be the result of a brain injury or a mass effect on the pituitary gland like a pituitary tumor.

There are several kinds of physical changes that can occur with andropause. One of the first physical changes that can occur is a decreased ability to obtain a spontaneous erection. Other physical findings are smaller testes and penis, hot flashes, decreased bone density, lower muscle mass, and lower sperm count. Also there can be an overall decrease in body hair. A secondary effect of andropause can be an increase in a man's percent body fat. With the loss of muscle mass that can occur with a decreased testosterone production, there is a decrease in caloric burn, which results in an increase in body fat.

There are psychological changes that can occur during andropause with lower testosterone levels. This first most obvious condition is a decrease in libido (sex drive). This can be such a gradual onset that men think that this is just a function of life and it is something to be expected. Other common psychological symptoms that men or their friends or significant others may notice is fatigue, depression, or a decreased ability to focus or concentrate.

There are various causes for decreased production of testosterone. Aging is the most common reason. As men age their testosterone production is lowered by 20% in their 60s, 30% in their 70s, and 50% in their 80s.[93] Other causes of decreased testosterone production can be seen with men who have a chronic illness. Some examples of that are diabetes, obesity, autoimmune diseases, cancers, HIV infections, and chronic kidney and liver disease. There are acquired causes of decreased testosterone production. This is seen with a direct injury to either the testicles or pituitary gland, if the individual has had the mumps virus, if the person drinks excessive alcohol (alcohol can have a direct toxic effect), or if the man has had systemic chemo or radiation therapy.

Having erectile dysfunction is the first thing that most people equate with a low testosterone level. This is an inability to maintain an erection more than 75% of the time during a sexual encounter. Certainly, low testosterone can be one of the causes of erectile dysfunction, however it is important to know that there are reasons other than low testosterone that can cause erectile dysfunction. These causes must be ruled out before any consideration for the use of testosterone is made. This can be seen with damage to the nerves that are involved in the ability to obtain an erection. To have an erection a man must have a psychological increased desire for sex. This information is sent down to the spinal cord from the brain to the thoracic spine 11 to lumbar spine 2. From that region of the spinal cord, a nerve fiber sends a signal to the iliac arteries (the major arteries that supply blood to the legs) to redirect a significant amount of blood flow to the penis to obtain an erection. Neurologic disease anywhere along this nerve path can cause erectile dysfunction. Some of these common neurologic diseases to the nerves include multiple sclerosis, spinal cord trauma, urological surgical procedures like prostate surgery, and nerve compression injuries that can occur with prolonged cycling. There are other metabolic causes of nerve damage that are seen in diseases such as diabetes. So any injury to these nerves can decrease the ability to have an erection.

Other causes of erectile dysfunction are disease states that can decrease the blood flow to the penis such as atherosclerosis (hardening of the arteries). The men most commonly seen with this condition are men who have the risk factors for cardiovascular disease. Those risk factors are a history of smoking, elevated cholesterol, increased blood sugars, lack of exercise, and elevated inflammatory rate (determined by a high C-reactive protein blood test). One of the most common causes of erectile dysfunction is medication. There are multiple medications that can do this. Many of the antidepressants are associated with erectile dysfunction. One antidepressant group in particular is the SSRIs (selective serotonin reuptake inhibitors). The first drug in this group was Prozac. These antidepressants increase the neurotransmitter serotonin, which is often low in depressed individuals. These drugs are excellent drugs in treating depression, however they may have the unfortunate side effect of lowering the ability to obtain an erection. Another common group of drugs associated with erectile dysfunction are many of the antihypertensive (blood pressure) medications. Two common types are the diuretics (the water pills) like the thiazide diuretics and beta-blockers. Other drugs known to cause erectile dysfunction are certain medications called 5-alpha reductase inhibitors. These drugs block the conversion of testosterone to dihydrotestosterone. These drugs are used to treat enlarged prostates and hair loss. Examples of these are Dutasteride and Finasteride.

Andropause usually begins for men in their 50s. This is a big transitional time in a man's life. This time is more than a decrease in testosterone, it has a lot of emotional transitions. Men at this age are often slowing down with their occupations and no longer are the young gunners trying to make a mark in their careers. It can be a difficult time emotionally because they are no longer the up-and-coming stars. Men have to emotionally deal with this slow-down phase, which can lead to a low level of depression. Because they cannot always accomplish what they have done in the past, men sometimes give up on many aspects in their lives, especially how they approach their fitness. In the past they may have focused on winning with their physical skills but now they may be having a hard time keeping up. For this reason they stop their physical fitness programs altogether. This causes weight gain and increases the risk of chronic ailments. Men need to acknowledge the physical limitations that occur with aging and andropause. They need to embrace and realize this is a fact of life then continue to exercise for the sake of maintaining health and not trying to keep up or compete with younger men. I have seen these phenomena over and over in my years of practicing medicine. Men constantly give up on their fitness program because they fall back in the pack and have slower and slower times with their exercise programs. They become so consumed about their inability to keep up that they completely give up on their health.

Another potential consequence of andropause is a loss of muscle mass. This is called sarcopenia. Testosterone is important in maintaining and the building up of muscles. With lower levels of testosterone there can be a 30% to 50% loss of muscle mass. This can lead to an inability to maintain balance, which can increase the risk of falls and subsequent injuries. These injuries can lead to more inactivity, which can lead to more loss of muscle mass and subsequently more falls and injuries. Men can acquiesce to this continual downward spiral with their health or they can fight it. One way to decrease muscle loss is to weight train. Resistance training (e.g., lifting weights) has been shown to not only slow down muscle loss but also actually increase muscle mass.[94] In addition, as we get older, over the age of 65, eating higher protein levels (25 to 30 grams per meal) has also been shown to help prevent muscle loss.[94]

If a man has significant sarcopenia (despite the fact that they are doing resistance training and have increased their protein intake) and/or has some of the consequences of low testosterone (less than 300 ng/dL) such as erectile dysfunction, decreased libido, or depression, and there are no correctable causes of decreases in testosterone production, then there can be consideration for the usage of prescriptive testosterone. Through the care and guidance of a physician who is familiar with the uses of testosterone and prescribes it only after nonpharmacologic treatments have been pursued, it may be prescribed for that man.

The decision whether or not to use testosterone is based on the potential benefits versus possible side effects of the medication. In making this decision, the first thing to note is at the time of the writing of this chapter, there has been no evidence that the use of therapeutic testosterone causes prostate cancer. It has however been shown to accelerate the growth of a prostate cancer if it already exists. For that reason it is important to obtain a prostate-specific antigen (PSA) and have a digital rectal exam prior to the use of testosterone. If the PSA is elevated, then the man needs to be worked up to rule out prostate cancer before testosterone can be started. If prostate cancer is found initially then testosterone cannot be started.

The use of testosterone can stimulate the growth of normal prostatic tissue, which can increase the size of the prostate. This can be a problem if the prostate is already enlarged. Prostatic enlargement has the potential of closing off the man's urinary flow. Symptoms associated with this are slow urinary stream, difficulty starting urination, urine retention, and getting up multiple times at night to urinate.

There are other potential physiologic problems associated with testosterone therapy. One is an increased production of red blood cells. This can lead to an increased risk for blood clots. Other problems are accelerated male pattern hair loss and the development of acne. Testosterone in addition can affect a person emotionally. It has been known to increase aggressive behavior. An important but controversial potential side effect of testosterone is cardiovascular disease. There have been conflicting reports on the risk of cardiovascular disease with the use of testosterone. Some studies have shown that if cardiovascular disease is already present, use of testosterone may cause progression of the disease.[95] This has been disputed by a later study that did not show an increase of cardiovascular disease.[96] The bottom line is that if a man has cardiovascular disease under the age of 65 or is over the age of 65 and is considering starting testosterone treatment, he should have a serious discussion with his doctor and possibly a consultation with a cardiologist prior to starting therapy.

Despite the potential side effects of testosterone, the benefits of testosterone may well be worth the risks. Summarizing, the possible benefits of testosterone include improved libido and possible reversal of erectile dysfunction. It may improve a man's depressed mood and chronic fatigue. Muscle mass can increase, which in turn may help lower body fat by increasing a man's metabolism and fitness capacity.

Andropause does not necessarily affect all men. It is not as inevitable as with women, who will all eventually have ovarian failure. If a man's testosterone level does not drop significantly, there may be little symptoms that are commonly seen with andropause.

In integrative medicine the question arises as to whether or not there are any alternatives to testosterone for the fatigue, decreased libido, and erectile dysfunction. There are many herbal and supplements advertised and sold for male enhancement. The regulation of such therapies is loosely regulated because they are considered supplements. Some of these therapies have had limited effectiveness. In this country dietary supplements have been touted as substitutes for prescription testosterone. These dietary supplements have contained androstenedione, dehydroepiandrosterone, and androstenediol. They are precursors to the endogenous production of testosterone. (With the Anabolic Steroid Control Act of 2004, androstenedione is now a schedule III controlled substance and therefore it is regulated by the FDA and requires a prescription.) The efficacy and safety of these prohormones are not well established, but they are promoted to have the same androgenic effects on building muscle mass and strength as anabolic-androgenic steroids. Studies have demonstrated repeatedly that acute and long-term administration of these oral testosterone precursors does not effectively increase serum testosterone levels and fails to produce any significant changes in lean body mass, muscle strength, or performance improvement compared with placebo.[97]

There are medications for the specific treatment of erectile dysfunction with or without testosterone. The most commonly used drugs are the phosphodiesterase-5 enzyme inhibitors. Two examples are sildenafil (Viagra) and tadalafil (Cialis). They work by increasing the blood flow to the penis. They have been helpful for a lot of men over the years, however they have potential side effects. The most common is a headache. These drugs work by dilating blood vessels to improve blood flow to the penis. The problem is that these medications are not selective for the blood flow to the penis. It can dilate other blood vessels, most notably the cerebral arteries. When this happens it has the potential of causing a vascular headache.

Phosphodiesterase-5 enzyme inhibitors do not have to be the only solution to erectile dysfunction. An integrative approach is to try other nonpharmacological approaches first. It has been shown that nonpharmacological, non-surgical therapies can reverse or improve erectile dysfunction in patients with organic, psychological, or mixed impairment. Among these therapies are life-style changes (losing weight, pelvic musculature strengthening, psychotherapy and/or psychoeducation, and improved sleep.[98]

If there is no obvious organic etiology for a man's erectile dysfunction, such as a neurologic or vascular compromise, this is called psychogenic erectile dysfunction. Studies have shown that this form of erectile dysfunction can be resolved in about a third of the time. These patients are generally older, more often living with their partner, and more frequently resigned with the diagnosis of psychogenic erectile dysfunction than the patients who did not resolve their psychogenic erectile dysfunction. A nonchalant or cooperative female partner's attitude to psychogenic erectile dysfunction improved the possibility of psychogenic erectile dysfunction resolution.[99] It is important to note that other studies have shown that psychogenic erectile dysfunction has been associated with disrupted childhood attachments. This group often has earlier onset of erectile dysfunction, a lower likelihood of being married, and higher rate of performance anxiety.[100]

Overall, andropause is different from female menopause. The onset of andropause is generally slower than menopause, and in some men it may not even occur. The symptoms of andropause compared to menopause are generally less dramatic and the length of onset of symptoms can be years, versus months, as seen with menopause. It is a physiologic change in the body that men should not fear but be educated on and understand as they get older. Being knowledgeable of andropause allows a man to take action against the potential negative effects of andropause. This can be done by increasing resistance training to compensate for the loss of muscle mass with lower testosterone production. They can also maintain a healthy lifestyle that may help compensate for loss of testosterone by exercising regularly (a minimum of 30 minutes a day more days than not), eating a diet low in animal fats and high in fruits and vegetables, learning to control stress and maintaining a healthy weight. Finally, if men do these healthy lifestyle changes and still have significant symptoms of andropause, they can discuss with their doctor the potential use of hormone replacement therapy.

References

1. Santoro N, Randolph JF. Reproductive hormones and the menopause transition. *Obstet Gynecol Clin North Am* 2011;38(3):455–466. doi:10.1016/j.ogc.2011.05.004.

2. Writing Group For The Women's Health Initiative Investigators. Risks and benefits of estrogen plus progestin in healthy postmenopausal women: principal results from the Women's Health Initiative randomized controlled trial. *JAMA* 2002;288(3):321–333. doi:10.1001/jama.288.3.321.

3. Gurney EP, Nachtigall MJ, Nachtigall LE, Naftolin F. The Women's Health Initiative trial and related studies: 10 years later: A clinician's view. *J Steroid Biochem* 2014;142:4–11. doi:10.1016/j.jsbmb.2013.10.009.

4. Reslan OM, Khalil RA. Vascular effects of estrogenic menopausal hormone therapy. *RRCT Rev Recent Clinical Trials* 2012;7(1):47–70. doi:10.2174/157488712799363253.

5. Monteiro R, Teixeira D, Calhau C. Estrogen signaling in metabolic inflammation. *Mediat Inflamm* 2014;2014:1–20. doi:10.1155/2014/615917.

6. Shufelt CL, Merz CNB, Prentice RL, et al. Hormone therapy dose, formulation, route of delivery, and risk of cardiovascular events in women. *Menopause* 2014;21(3):260–266. doi:10.1097/gme.0b013e31829a64f9.

7. Smith NL, Blondon M, Wiggins KL, et al. Lower risk of cardiovascular events in postmenopausal women taking oral estradiol compared with oral conjugated equine estrogens. *JAMA Intern Med* 2014;174(1):25. doi:10.1001/jamainternmed.2013.11074.

8. Bergendal A, Kieler H, Sundström A, Hirschberg AL, Kocoska-Maras L. Risk of venous thromboembolism associated with local and systemic use of hormone therapy in peri- and postmenopausal women and in relation to type and route of administration. *Menopause* 2016;23(6):593–599. doi:10.1097/gme.0000000000000611.

9. Hodis HN, Mack WJ, Henderson VW, et al. Vascular effects of early versus late postmenopausal treatment with estradiol. *N Engl J Med* 2016;374(13):1221–1231. doi:10.1056/nejmoa1505241.

10. Nezarat N. Poster Session, 2016 Annual Scientific Meeting Society for Cardiovascular Computed Tomography, as reported on *Medscape*, June 28, 2016.

11. Thurston RC, Khoudary SRE, Sutton-Tyrrell K, et al. Vasomotor symptoms and insulin resistance in the study of women's health across the nation. *J Clin Endocr Metab* 2012;97(10):3487–3494. doi:10.1210/jc.2012-1410.

12. Stuenkel CA. Subclinical thyroid disorders. *Menopause* 2015;22(2):231–233. doi:10.1097/gme.0000000000000407.

13. Toffol E, Kalleinen N, Haukka J, Vakkuri O, Partonen T, Polo-Kantola P. Melatonin in perimenopausal and postmenopausal women. *Menopause* 2014;21(5):493–500. doi:10.1097/gme.0b013e3182a6c8f3.

14. Walecka-Kapica E, Chojnacki J, Stępień A, Wachowska-Kelly P, Klupińska G, Chojnacki C. Melatonin and female hormone secretion in postmenopausal overweight women. *IJMS* 2015;16(1):1030–1042. doi:10.3390/ijms16011030.

15. Alexander JL, Dennerstein L, Woods NF, et al. Role of stressful life events and menopausal stage in wellbeing and health. *Expert Rev Neurother* 2007;7(Suppl 1):S93–113. Review. doi:10.1586/14737175.7.11s.s93.

16. Nosek M, Kennedy HP, Beyene Y, Taylor D, Gilliss C, Lee K. The effects of perceived stress and attitudes toward menopause and aging on symptoms of menopause. *J Midwifery Wom Heal* 2010;55(4):328–334. doi:10.1016/j.jmwh.2009.09.005.

17. Li Y, Gao X, Winkelman JW, et al. Association between sleeping difficulty and type 2 diabetes in women. *Diabetologia* 2016;59(4):719–727. doi:10.1007/s00125-015-3860-9.

18. Flores R, Shi J, Fuhrman B, et al. Fecal microbial determinants of fecal and systemic estrogens and estrogen metabolites: a cross-sectional study. *J Transl Med* 2012;10(1):253. doi:10.1186/1479-5876-10-253.

19. Paul B, Barnes S, Demark-Wahnefried W, et al. Influences of diet and the gut microbiome on epigenetic modulation in cancer and other diseases. *Clin Epigenet* 2015;7(1). doi:10.1186/s13148-015-0144-7.

20. Grindler NM, Allsworth JE, Macones GA, Kannan K, Roehl KA, Cooper AR. Persistent organic pollutants and early menopause in U.S. women. *PLoS One* 2015;10(1). doi:10.1371/journal.pone.0116057.

21. Vandenberg LN, Colborn T, Hayes TB, et al. Hormones and endocrine-disrupting chemicals: low-dose effects and nonmonotonic dose responses. *Endocr Rev* 2012;33(3):378–455. doi:10.1210/er.2011-1050.

22. Toffol E, Heikinheimo O, Partonen T. Hormone therapy and mood in perimenopausal and postmenopausal women. *Menopause* 2015;22(5):564–578. doi:10.1097/gme.0000000000000323.

23. Whelan AM, Jurgens TM, Trinacty M. Defining bioidentical hormones for menopause-related symptoms. *Pharmacy Practice (Internet)* 2011;9(1). doi:10.4321/s1886-36552011000100003.

24. Diller M, Schüler S, Buchholz S, Lattrich C, Treeck O, Ortmann O. Effects of estriol on growth, gene expression and estrogen response element activation in human breast cancer cell lines. *Maturitas* 2014;77(4):336–343. doi:10.1016/j.maturitas.2014.01.004.

25. Razavi P, Pike MC, Horn-Ross PL, Templeman C, Bernstein L, Ursin G. Long-term postmenopausal hormone therapy and endometrial cancer. *Cancer Epidem Biomar* 2010;19(2):475–483. doi:10.1158/1055-9965.epi-09-0712.

26. Asi N, Mohammed K, Haydour Q, et al. Progesterone vs. synthetic progestins and the risk of breast cancer: a systematic review and meta-analysis. *Syst Rev* 2016;5(1). doi:10.1186/s13643-016-0294-5.

27. Stanczyk FZ, Hapgood JP, Winer S, Mishell DR. Progestogens used in postmenopausal hormone therapy: differences in their pharmacological properties, intracellular actions, and clinical effects. *Endocr Rev* 2013;34(2):171–208. doi:10.1210/er.2012-1008.

28. Anderson GL, Limacher M, Assaf AR, Bassford T, Beresford SA, Black H, et al., Wassertheil-Smoller S; Women's Health Initiative Steering Committee. Effects of conjugated equine estrogen in postmenopausal women with hysterectomy. *JAMA* 2004;291(14):1701–1712. doi:10.1001/jama.291.14.1701.

29. Fournier A, Berrino F, Clavel-Chapelon F. Unequal risks for breast cancer associated with different hormone replacement therapies: results from the E3N cohort study. *Breast Cancer Res Treat* 2007;107(2):307–308. doi:10.1007/s10549-007-9604-x.

30. Caufriez A, Leproult R, L'hermite-Balériaux M, Kerkhofs M, Copinschi G. Progesterone prevents sleep disturbances and modulates GH, TSH, and melatonin

secretion in postmenopausal women. *Endocrinology* 2011;152(3):1193–1193. doi:10.1210/endo.152.3.zee1193a.

31. Colditz GA. Cumulative risk of breast cancer to age 70 years according to risk factor status: data from the Nurses' Health Study. *Am J Epidemiol* 2000;152(10):950–964. doi:10.1093/aje/152.10.950.

32. Rosner BA, Colditz GA, Hankinson SE, Sullivan-Halley J, Lacey JV, Bernstein L. Validation of Rosner–Colditz breast cancer incidence model using an independent data set, the California Teachers Study. *Breast Cancer Res Treat* 2013;142(1):187–202. doi:10.1007/s10549-013-2719-3.

33. Howell A, Anderson AS, Clarke RB, et al. Risk determination and prevention of breast cancer. *Breast Cancer Res* 2014;16(5). doi:10.1186/s13058-014-0446-2.

34. Munsell MF, Sprague BL, Berry DA, Chisholm G, Trentham-Dietz A. Body mass index and breast cancer risk according to postmenopausal estrogen-progestin use and hormone receptor status. *Epidemiol Rev* 2013;36(1):114–136. doi:10.1093/epirev/mxt010.

35. Huo CW, Chew GL, Britt KL, et al. Mammographic density—a review on the current understanding of its association with breast cancer. *Breast Cancer Res Treat* 2014;144(3):479–502. doi:10.1007/s10549-014-2901-2.

36. Chen Z, Arendell L, Aickin M, Cauley J, Lewis CE, Chlebowski R. Hip bone density predicts breast cancer risk independently of Gail score. *Cancer* 2008;113(5):907–915. doi:10.1002/cncr.23674.

37. Fraenkel M, Novack V, Liel Y, et al. Association between bone mineral density and incidence of breast cancer. *PLoS One* 2013;8(8). doi:10.1371/journal.pone.0070980.

38. Bermano G. A novel role for insulin resistance in the connection between obesity and postmenopausal breast cancer. *Int J Oncol* 2012. doi:10.3892/ijo.2012.1480.

39. Jia Y, Lu Y, Wu K, et al. Does night work increase the risk of breast cancer? A systematic review and meta-analysis of epidemiological studies. *Cancer Epidemiol* 2013;37(3):197–206. doi:10.1016/j.canep.2013.01.005.

40. Nooshinfar E, Safaroghli-Azar A, Bashash D, Akbari ME. Melatonin, an inhibitory agent in breast cancer. *Breast Cancer* 2016. doi:10.1007/s12282-016-0690-7.

41. Chlebowski RT. Nutrition and physical activity influence on breast cancer incidence and outcome. *Breast* 2013;22. doi:10.1016/j.breast.2013.07.006.

42. Goodwin PJ, Ambrosone CB, Hong C-C. Modifiable lifestyle factors and breast cancer outcomes: current controversies and research recommendations; improving outcomes for breast cancer survivors. *Adv Exp Med Biol* 2015:177–192. doi:10.1007/978-3-319-16366-6_12.

43. Reaves DK, Ginsburg E, Bang JJ, Fleming JM. Persistent organic pollutants and obesity: are they potential mechanisms for breast cancer promotion? *Endocr Related Cancer* 2015;22(2). doi:10.1530/erc-14-0411.

44. Hvidtfeldt UA, Tjønneland A, Keiding N, et al. Risk of breast cancer in relation to combined effects of hormone therapy, body mass index, and alcohol use, by hormone-receptor status. *Epidemiology* 2015;26(3):353–361. doi:10.1097/ede.0000000000000261.

45. Frydenberg H, Flote VG, Larsson IM, et al. Alcohol consumption, endogenous estrogen and mammographic density among premenopausal women. *Breast Cancer Res* 2015;17(1). doi:10.1186/s13058-015-0620-1.

46. Sellers TA, Kushi LH, Cerhan JR, et al. Dietary folate intake, alcohol, and risk of breast cancer in a prospective study of postmenopausal women. *Epidemiology* 2001;12(4):420–428. doi:10.1097/00001648-200107000-00012.

47. Baglietto L. Does dietary folate intake modify effect of alcohol consumption on breast cancer risk? Prospective cohort study. *BMJ* 2005;331(7520):807. doi:10.1136/bmj.38551.446470.06.

48. Friedenreich CM. Physical activity and breast cancer: review of the epidemiologic evidence and biologic mechanisms. *Clin Cancer Prevention Recent Results in Cancer Res* 2010:125–139. doi:10.1007/978-3-642-10858-7_11.

49. Goedert JJ, Jones G, Hua X, et al. Investigation of the association between the fecal microbiota and breast cancer in postmenopausal women: a population-based case-control pilot study. *JNCI* 2015;107(8). doi:10.1093/jnci/djv147.

50. Harris HR, Bergkvist L, Wolk A. Adherence to the World Cancer Research Fund/American Institute for Cancer Research recommendations and breast cancer risk. *Int J Cancer* 2016;138(11):2657–2664. doi:10.1002/ijc.30015.

51. Marinac CR, Sears DD, Natarajan L, Gallo LC, Breen CI, Patterson RE. Frequency and circadian timing of eating may influence biomarkers of inflammation and insulin resistance associated with breast cancer risk. *PLoS One* 2015;10(8). doi:10.1371/journal.pone.0136240.

52. Mckenzie F, Ferrari P, Freisling H, et al. Healthy lifestyle and risk of breast cancer among postmenopausal women in the European Prospective Investigation into Cancer and Nutrition cohort study. *Int J Cancer* 2014;136(11):2640–2648. doi:10.1002/ijc.29315.

53. Capasso I, Esposito E, Pentimalli F, et al. Homeostasis model assessment to detect insulin resistance and identify patients at high risk of breast cancer development: National Cancer Institute of Naples experience. *J Exp Clin Cancer Res* 2013;32(1):14. doi:10.1186/1756-9966-32-14.

54. Thurston RC, Sowers MR, Chang Y, et al. Adiposity and reporting of vasomotor symptoms among midlife women: the study of women's health across the nation. *Am J Epidemiol* 2007;167(1):78–85. doi:10.1093/aje/kwm244.

55. Thurston RC, Khoudary SRE, Sutton-Tyrrell K, et al. Vasomotor symptoms and insulin resistance in the study of women's health across the nation. *Obstet Gynecol Surv* 2013;68(2):113–114. doi:10.1097/01.ogx.0000427625.65263.23.

56. Kroenke CH, Caan BJ, Stefanick ML, et al. Effects of a dietary intervention and weight change on vasomotor symptoms in the Women's Health Initiative. *Menopause* 2012;19(9):980–988. doi:10.1097/gme.0b013e31824f606e.

57. Thurston RC, Ewing LJ, Low CA, Christie AJ, Levine MD. Behavioral weight loss for the management of menopausal hot flashes. *Menopause* 2015;22(1):59–65. doi:10.1097/gme.0000000000000274.

58. Cappelletti M, Wallen K. Increasing women's sexual desire: the comparative effectiveness of estrogens and androgens. *Horm Behav* 2016;78:178–193. doi:10.1016/j.yhbeh.2015.11.003.

59. Dennerstein L, Randolph J, Taffe J, Dudley E, Burger H. Hormones, mood, sexuality, and the menopausal transition. *Fertil Steril* 2002;77:42–48. doi:10.1016/s0015-0282(02)03001-7.

60. Kingsberg SA. The psychological impact of aging on sexuality and relationships. *J Women Health Gen-B* 2000;9(Suppl 1):33–38. doi:10.1089/152460900318849.

61. Dewitte M, Lankveld JV, Vandenberghe S, Loeys T. Sex in its daily relational context. *J Sex Med* 2015;12(12):2436–2450. doi:10.1111/jsm.13050.

62. Management of symptomatic vulvovaginal atrophy. *Menopause* 2013;20(9):886–887. doi:10.1097/gme.0b013e3182a15aa1.

63. Shen J, Song N, Williams CJ, et al. Effects of low dose estrogen therapy on the vaginal microbiomes of women with atrophic vaginitis. *Sci Rep* 2016;6:24380. doi:10.1038/srep24380.

64. Beerepoot M, Geerlings S. Non-antibiotic prophylaxis for urinary tract infections. *Pathogens* 2016;5(2):36. doi:10.3390/pathogens5020036.

65. Santen RJ. Vaginal administration of estradiol: effects of dose, preparation and timing on plasma estradiol levels. *Climacteric* 2014;18(2):121–134. doi:10.3109/13697137.2014.947254.

66. Labrie F, Archer DF, Koltun W, et al. Efficacy of intravaginal dehydroepiandrosterone (DHEA) on moderate to severe dyspareunia and vaginal dryness, symptoms of vulvovaginal atrophy, and of the genitourinary syndrome of menopause. *Menopause* 2016;23(3):243–256. doi:10.1097/gme.0000000000000571.

67. Nonhormonal management of menopause-associated vasomotor symptoms. *Menopause* 2015;22(11):1155–1174. doi:10.1097/gme.0000000000000546.

68. Franco OH, Chowdhury R, Troup J, et al. Use of plant-based therapies and menopausal symptoms. *JAMA* 2016;315(23):2554. doi:10.1001/jama.2016.8012.

69. Lipovac M, Chedraui P, Gruenhut C, et al. The effect of red clover isoflavone supplementation over vasomotor and menopausal symptoms in postmenopausal women. *Gynecol Endocrinol* 2011;28(3):203–207. doi:10.3109/09513590.2011.593671.

70. Fritz H, Seely D, Flower G, et al. Soy, red clover, and isoflavones and breast cancer: a systematic review. *PLoS One* 2013;8(11). doi:10.1371/journal.pone.0081968.

71. Hasper I, Ventskovskiy BM, Rettenberger R, Heger PW, Riley DS, Kaszkin-Bettag M. Long-term efficacy and safety of the special extract ERr 731 of Rheum rhaponticum in perimenopausal women with menopausal symptoms. *Menopause* 2009;16(1):117–131. doi:10.1097/gme.0b013e3181806446.

72. Heger M, Ventskovskiy BM, Borzenko I, et al. Efficacy and safety of a special extract of Rheum rhaponticum (ERr 731) in perimenopausal women with climacteric complaints. *Menopause* 2006;13(5):744–759. doi:10.1097/01.gme.0000240632.08182.e4.

73. Yang H-M, Liao M-F, Zhu S-Y, Liao M-N, Rohdewald P. A randomised, double-blind, placebo-controlled trial on the effect of Pycnogenol® on the climacteric syndrome in peri-menopausal women. *Acta Obstet Gynecol Scand* 2007;86(8):978–985. doi:10.1080/00016340701446108.

74. Belcaro G, Cornelli U, Luzzi R, et al. Pycnogenol® supplementation improves health risk factors in subjects with metabolic syndrome. *Phytother Res* 2013. doi:10.1002/ptr.4883.

75. Mccurry SM, Guthrie KA, Morin CM, et al. Telephone-based cognitive behavioral therapy for insomnia in perimenopausal and postmenopausal women with vasomotor symptoms. *JAMA Intern Med* 2016;176(7):913. doi:10.1001/jamainternmed.2016.1795.

76. Dodin S, Blanchet C, Marc I, et al. Acupuncture for menopausal hot flushes. *Cochrane DB Syst Rev* 2013. doi:10.1002/14651858.cd007410.pub2.

77. Lesi G, Razzini G, Musti MA, et al. Acupuncture as an integrative approach for the treatment of hot flashes in women with breast cancer: a prospective multicenter randomized controlled trial (AcCliMaT). *J Clin Oncol* 2016;34(15):1795–1802. doi:10.1200/jco.2015.63.2893.

78. Singer A, Exuzides A, Spangler L, et al. Burden of illness for osteoporotic fractures compared with other serious diseases among postmenopausal women in the United States. *Mayo Clin Proc* 2015;90(1):53–62. doi:10.1016/j.mayocp.2014.09.011.

79. Anagnostis P, Dimopoulou C, Karras S, Lambrinoudaki I, Goulis DG. Sarcopenia in post-menopausal women: is there any role for vitamin D? *Maturitas* 2015;82(1):56–64. doi:10.1016/j.maturitas.2015.03.014.

80. Castiglioni S, Cazzaniga A, Albisetti W, Maier J. Magnesium and osteoporosis: current state of knowledge and future research directions. *Nutrients* 2013;5(8):3022–3033. doi:10.3390/nu5083022.

81. Cosman F, Beur SJD, Leboff MS, et al. Clinician's guide to prevention and treatment of osteoporosis. *Osteoporos Int* 2014;25(10):2359–2381. doi:10.1007/s00198-014-2794-2.

82. Welch AA, Kelaiditi E, Jennings A, Steves CJ, Spector TD, Macgregor A. Dietary magnesium is positively associated with skeletal muscle power and indices of muscle mass and may attenuate the association between circulating c-reactive protein and muscle mass in women. *J Bone Miner Res* 2015;31(2):317–325. doi:10.1002/jbmr.2692.

83. Melamed ML, Michos ED, Post W, Astor B. 25-hydroxyvitamin D levels and the risk of mortality in the general population. *Arch Intern Med* 2008;168(15):1629–1637. doi:10.1001/archinte.168.15.1629.

84. Haring B, Crandall CJ, Wu C, et al. Dietary patterns and fractures in postmenopausal women. *JAMA Intern Med* 2016;176(5):645. doi:10.1001/jamainternmed.2016.0482.

85. Kelaiditi E, Jennings A, Steves CJ, et al. Measurements of skeletal muscle mass and power are positively related to a Mediterranean dietary pattern in women. *Osteoporos Int* 2016. doi:10.1007/s00198-016-3665-9.

86. Yamaguchi M, Weitzmann MN. Vitamin K2 stimulates osteoblastogenesis and suppresses osteoclastogenesis by suppressing NF-κB activation. *Int J Mol Med* 2011;27:3–14. doi:10.3892/ijmm.2010.562.

87. Kanellakis S, Moschonis G, Tenta R, et al. Changes in parameters of bone metabolism in postmenopausal women following a 12-month intervention period using dairy products enriched with calcium, vitamin D, and phylloquinone (vitamin K1) or menaquinone-7 (vitamin K2): the Postmenopausal Health Study II. *Calcif Tissue Int* 2012;90:251–262.

88. Iwamoto J. Vitamin K2 therapy for postmenopausal osteoporosis. *Nutrients* 2014;6:1971–1980.

89. Villa JK, Diaz MA, Pizziolo VR, Martino HS. Effect of vitamin K in bone metabolism and vascular calcification: a review of mechanisms of action and evidences. *Crit Rev Food Sci Nutr* [Epub July 20, 2016.] doi:10.1080/10408398.2016.1211616.

90. Cockayne S, Adamson J, Lanham-New S, Shearer MJ, Gilbody S, Torgerson DJ. Vitamin K and the prevention of fractures: systematic review and meta-analysis of randomized controlled trials. *Arch Intern Med* 2006;166:1256–1261.

91. Deutz NE, Bauer JM, Barazzoni R, et al. Protein intake and exercise for optimal muscle function with aging: recommendations from the ESPEN Expert Group. *Clin Nutr* 2014;33(6):929–936. doi:10.1016/j.clnu.2014.04.007.

92. Shieh A, Han W, Ishii S, Greendale GA, Crandall CJ, Karlamangla AS. Quantifying the balance between total bone formation and total bone resorption: an index of net bone formation. *J Clin Endocr Metab* 2016;101(7):2802–2809. doi:10.1210/jc.2015-4262.

93. Harman SM, Metter EJ, Tobin JD, Pearson J, Blackman MR. Longitudinal effects of aging on serum total and free testosterone levels in healthy men. Baltimore Longitudinal Study of Aging. *J Clin Endocr Metab* 2001;86(2):724.

94. De Spiegeleer A, Petrovic M, Boeckxstaens P, Van Den Noortgate N. Treating sarcopenia in clinical practice: where are we now? *Acta Clin Belg* 2016 Aug;71(4):197–205. doi: 10.1080/17843286.2016.1168064. Epub 2016 Apr 26.

95. Finkle WD, Greenland S, Ridgeway GK, et al. Increased Risk of Non-fatal Myocardial Infarction Following Testosterone Therapy Prescription in Men. *PLoS One* 2014;9:1: e85805. doi: 10.1371/journal.pone.0085805.

96. Basaria S, Harman SM, Travison TG, et al. Effects of testosterone administration for 3 years on subclinical atherosclerosis progression in older men with low or low-normal testosterone levels: a randomized clinical trial. *JAMA* 2015;314:6:570–581. doi: 10.1001/jama.2015.8881.

97. Smurawa, TM, Congeni, JA. Testosterone precursors: use and abuse in pediatric athletes. *Pediatr Clin North Am* 2007;54(4):787–796, xii.

98. Simopoulos, T. Male erectile dysfunction: integrating psychopharmacology and psychotherapy. *Gen Hosp Psychiatry* 2013;35(1):33–38. doi: 10.1016/j.genhosppsych.2012.08.008. [Epub 2012 Oct 6.]

99. Cavallini G. Resolution of erectile dysfunction after an andrological visit in a selected population of patients affected by psychogenic erectile dysfunction. *Asian J Androl* 2017;19(2):219–222.

100. Rajkumar RP. The impact of disrupted childhood attachment on the presentation of psychogenic erectile dysfunction: an exploratory study. *J Sex Med* 2015;12(3):798–803. doi: 10.1111/jsm.12815. Epub 2015 Jan 8.

21

Transforming Pain Management Through the Integration of Complementary and Conventional Care

HEATHER TICK, MA, MD, AND ERIC B. SCHOOMAKER, MD, PHD

In Taoism there's a famous saying that goes, "The Tao that can be spoken is not the ultimate Tao." Another way you could say that, although I've never seen it translated this way, is, "As soon as you begin to believe in something, then you can no longer see anything else." The truth you believe in and cling to makes you unavailable to hear anything new. (Pema Chodron,

Awakening Loving-Kindness[1]

Definition

As its hallmark, complementary integrative pain management (CIPM) offers patient-centered care that is inclusive of and collaborative with all appropriate disciplines and strategies—conventional and complementary—for the benefit of the patient. It then follows that it is multidisciplinary and team based. Patient self-actualization and self-care is essential. Its goal is health creation, and it is driven by patient priorities.

HISTORICAL PERSPECTIVE

Healthcare professionals enter medicine to help people; we do not enroll in medical, dental, nursing, or other schools with the intention of harming patients. Nevertheless, there is abundant evidence that many of us cause a lot of harm. Some of this harm is due to outright blunders, but most of it is just the side effects of products and procedures we routinely prescribe or practice. The 1999 Institute of Medicine (IOM)[1] report, *To Err Is Human*,[2] and the works of Starfield,[3] James,[4] and most recently Mackery,[5] present the alarming statistics of morbidity and mortality caused by conventional medicine. Even the most favorable analysis of these statistics is grim, and ranks medical care as the third-leading cause of death in the United States. This is deeply disturbing and should be totally unacceptable.

The prevailing management strategy in the field of pain treatment has contributed heavily to these statistics. Deaths from nonsteroidal anti-inflammatory drugs (NSAIDs) alone exceed those from HIV/AIDS.[6] Unfortunately, while these data on NSAIDS have been available for nearly a decade, the treating community has failed to adjust their prescribing practices.[7] The FDA has recently intensified warnings about the adverse cardiac effects of NSAIDs and amended recommendations to warn about their wholesale use, but we are aware that even when good evidence-based or recommended practices are available, there are serious deficits in their application.[8]

The overprescription of opioids for chronic noncancer pain has caused an even more worrisome epidemic. The use of these drugs causes tolerance, leading to escalating doses, which too often has dire consequences.[9-13] There are now more deaths in the United States from accidental prescription opioid overdose than from highway accidents in the majority of states. Prescription opioids are responsible for more deaths than cocaine and heroin combined. This is especially alarming when we consider the recent resurgence of heroin addiction through the gateway of oxycodone and other prescription narcotics.[14] Moreover, these opioids seem to have contributed very little toward actually helping our nation's chronic pain problem. Doctors in the United States prescribe 50 times more opioids than the rest of the entire world combined, yet the prevalence of pain in the United States is *increasing* and there is likely to be increasing disability associated with chronic pain.[15]

So how did well-intentioned doctors get pain treatment so wrong? To answer this, we have to look back at the origins of modern pain medicine. In the 1950s, a prominent anesthesiologist, John Bonica, recognized that pain is a biopsychosocial disease, and together with Bill Fordyce, a psychologist, began developing theories for pain treatment. In 1961, Bonica founded the first multidisciplinary pain program at the University of Washington. He had a novel idea: Pain management required its own set of skills and its own field of study and patients were best treated by a team of professionals. Until this time, pain was treated by the specialty that claimed authority over the area that hurt—orthopedic pain was treated by orthopedists, pelvic pain by urologists and gynecologists, and so on. Bonica's model still survives as the best way to manage complex pain.[16]

Dr. Bonica was an anesthesiologist, a scholarly pursuit that positioned him well to understand how drugs and procedural interventions could be used but gave the future field of pain management a bias toward anesthetic principles and practices. For this reason, most academic pain clinics are based in anesthesiology departments. This match, however, is only a partial fit. On the one hand, anesthesiologists have created enormous advancements in the safety and effectiveness of general anesthesia and analgesia during surgery. Regional anesthesia has further improved surgical outcomes and safety while providing effective pain relief as a result of major trauma or during procedures. These techniques translate well into interventional pain treatments. On the other hand, anesthesiology practice is based on a consultation model in which patients are referred by clinicians who have already done most of the diagnostics and patient assessment. Unlike the clinical and business models of other disciplines—such as internists and primary care practitioners—who come into the patient relationship with a disciplined agnosticism about what the problem is and from whence symptoms emanate, the models of anesthesiology are based on managing a problem—such as sedating a patient for surgery whose principal condition has already been sorted out by others. The very fact that the majority of pain clinic patients are referred from other entry care sites introduces a selection bias into the patients these pain management specialists are treating. They rarely see the newer pain patients, but rather are consulted for the more resistant, complex cases. This selection bias and the frequency with which pain patients are referred for consultation to specialty pain clinics and then often return to their referring clinic or primary clinical manager translates into several errors in comprehensive management of the problem or problems. There may be an inaccurate assessment of the meaning of pain within the context of the patients' lives; the best approach to managing the pain (medications and anesthesia-based interventions); and the duration of the response to any treatment initiated in terms of subjective pain relief, its impact on patient function and comorbidity, such as sleep disturbances, mood issues (anxiety, depression, etc.), activity, and the like.

In addition, most anesthesiology-based pain programs, for practical reasons (e.g., time management, therapeutic target, financial practice models, etc.) do not focus on detailed physical examination and diagnostic reasoning, which should be considered fundamental to pain management. This skill is well established in the training programs of many other practitioners, including osteopaths, chiropractors, physical therapists, sports medicine physicians, and physical medicine and rehabilitation doctors. This may put the pain-managing anesthesiologist at a relative disadvantage. This is not a reflection on their motivations, desire to help or formidable grasp of complex science-based anesthetic modalities, but a reflection of the realities of healthcare delivery in a busy anesthesiology and pain practice. While the anesthesiology skill sets translate very well for acute pain and trauma, chronic pain demands a broader skill set and ultimately a different business model.

Bonica understood the importance of integrating nonanesthesiologist physical or manual therapy skills and disciplines into the field of pain management, and his original *comprehensive functional restoration program* did just that. Sadly, this integration lasted only until the workload- and business-driven culture of medicine led to reduced insurance coverage of these treatments. Most pain clinic business models remain financially viable by performing large numbers of procedures. Now, few of the comprehensive multidisciplinary programs remain, and Bonica's novel and effective idea, his independent field of pain management, has lost much of its depth and diversity in most current practice environments.

TWO CONVENTIONAL APPROACHES TO PAIN

All of this has led conventional medicine to two main approaches to pain. Both groups embrace the influence of central sensitization, and promote analgesics and pain-modifying drugs such as antidepressants and anticonvulsants. One approach addresses the physical causes of pain with interventions including injections, nerve blocks, epidurals, tissue ablations, spinal cord stimulators and pain pumps. In situations of acute tissue injury and damage these procedures can save life and limb and reduce suffering. Evidence from combat-related acute pain management suggests that wounding-associated long-term secondary emotional and mental health problems such as post-traumatic stress disorder (PTSD) are also reduced by timely application of these techniques as close to the point of injury as possible.[17] Once there is "chronification" of pain, interventions through blocks and other injections can also be very helpful in carefully selected patients who meet evidence-based criteria such as those put forward by the Spine Intervention Society (SIS, formerly ISIS—International Spine Intervention Society).[18] All indications are, however, that the pain community as a whole does not apply careful patient selection criteria and overuses these potentially risky and costly strategies.

The second approach focuses on behavioral strategies. Chronic pain is not so much about tissue injury and nociception but is now better understood as a very patient-specific brain disorder.[19] As a consequence, those who employ this second approach see psychology as the main determinant of chronic pain. Pain centers that employ this strategy deal more with the psychological, spiritual, social, and symbolic aspects of pain, and often develop strong partnerships with psychology and psychiatry departments as well as social work in those few centers that have funding. Neuroscience research, specifically in the areas of neuroplasticity and the central nervous system sensitized by past trauma, depression, anxiety, anger, and frustration, has deepened these collaborations. While these partnerships have led to useful advances in behavioral treatments for pain, they also often oversimplify the issue by failing to fully explore the contributions of predisposing, precipitating, and perpetuating physical factors.

At the end of the day, neither of these two treatment paradigms has stellar outcomes in returning people with chronic pain to functional lives. As mentioned earlier, this is because most of the tools used by our most prevalent pain models were developed for the care of acute conditions. These tools allow for a focused assessment, a rapid diagnosis, and an algorithm for treatment that is designed to act like a "silver bullet" striking at the core of the problem. If a patient is in an emergency room suffering from a heart attack, this approach can be very successful during the short window of exposure we have. It allows the patient to survive the acute episode, but the optimal strategy for long-term care of chronic heart disease must be considerably different. This is also true of acute and chronic pain conditions, between which the difference is not just timeline; it is also the lack of a clear target to hit with an isolated, less-than-comprehensive therapy. The treatment goal of rapid alleviation of signs and symptoms in the acute situation, whether it is for pain or heart disease, will be detrimental to long-term function and even survival if the root causes of the chronic condition are not ultimately addressed. In fact, even when dealing with only acute pain conditions, our limited tools can lead us astray by directing us to choose a diagnosis and commit to a long-term therapeutic approach, which sometimes reduces our list of possible pain generators. This leads us to seek panaceas—the proverbial "silver bullets" fired at the wrong targets. It launches a vicious cycle.

In some cases, our good intentions to quickly relieve suffering may get in the way of what is best for the long run by leading us to focus on the wrong things. For example, in an effort to highlight the importance of pain, our conventional medical community has dubbed pain the "fifth vital sign." The Joint Commission added to this by requiring repeated evaluations of patients' pain intensity using the conventional Visual Analogue Scale (VAS). This caused a single metric—a number on an 11-point scale—to become the focus of the pain visit. But as the *NEJM* perspective article "Pain Intensity Scores: Are We Chasing the Wrong Metric?"[20] outlines, this strategy is not helping. We now treat pain scores as if they were thermometer readings, where each numerical benchmark demands specific actions. This completely ignores the lack of meaningful correlations between pain scores and the multifaceted function of patients. Chronic pain practitioners have long realized that these scores can vary in inexplicable ways, and are not useful benchmarks for treatment. Some people with 8/10 pain can function in their daily lives and some people with 3/10 pain cannot.

Perhaps the goal of chasing lower pain scores originally derived from the anesthesiology perspective that optimal pain relief is its complete ablation (i.e., the anesthetized patient), but we know now that it is unrealistic to think we can eliminate the perception of pain entirely and it may be both unnecessary and potentially injurious. Although the initial intention of this numeric assessment of pain intensity may have been good, this strategy has continually focused the chronic pain conversations on the complete elimination of perceived pain, and has led increasingly to reliance on opioid use. This has shifted us away from more useful parameters of the patient's progress toward functional restoration. The pharmaceutical industry has been relentless in its marketing to practitioners and patients—who have both been very receptive to the message—with claims that chronic opioid use is effective, that there are advantages to long-acting opioids, that escalating doses is safe, and that pain patients cannot become addicted to opioids. None of these claims is supported by evidence.[21] Ironically, the medical community's major reliance on the use of chronic opioids has led to a second round of drug interventions for the *complications* of opioids, from reversing opioid-induced constipation; to treating opioid-related hormonal imbalance, mood, and sleep disturbance; to managing overdoses.

It appeals to all doctors' good intentions to think we can help any patient quickly and definitively. We live in an impatient, quick-fix society; our patients often demand it; and we are no less susceptible to that mentality—especially when faced with the distress and disability associated with pain. As practitioners, we take pride in our ability to administer *precision medicine* that is tailored for a specific patient and clinical problem, and we idealize the model of a highly selective therapeutic agent. These are perhaps best represented by a well-selected antibiotic that cures a highly sensitive bacterial infection without side effects, complications, or the emergence of pathogen resistance. Newer generations of more selective immunologic-based therapies for autoimmune disorders and cancers also exhibit these idealized features. Drugs, procedures, and surgery have all seen a rise in popularity because they give us "something to do," and they are sold with the allure of rapid and definitive results. The outcomes, however, increasingly do not match our expectations.

The conventional medical community hoped that intervention would be its savior, but now, with evidence abounding, we should know better. A review of the definition of "precision medicine" will also remind us that it is "an innovative approach to disease prevention and treatment that takes into account individual differences in people's genes, environments, and lifestyles."[22]

But the practice and general public's focus on precision medicine appears to have only focused on the chemistry of our genes and the agents that interact with genes and gene products and not the highly variable environmental and lifestyle differences among all of us.

Drugs and procedures alone, though they are used increasingly, do not improve chronic pain, and interventions and patient functionality have all too often had an inverse relationship.[23-25] Often, proponents of drugs and intervention, including the leading pain specialists, the pharmaceutical industry, and patients themselves, invoke a trump card—our moral imperative to relieve pain. But, the truth is, outcomes of our best efforts for treatment cannot be guaranteed, whether treating pain or treating cancer and diabetes. Our moral imperative should actually be to relieve suffering (not pain), to optimize human potential and growth on all levels, to provide our best level of care, while adhering to the premier imperative: "First, do no harm." Our goal should be to "Do good while doing no harm."

Regardless of how our model of care ended up missing the mark for so many chronic pain patients and leading to so much collateral harm, it is clear we need a different approach. Over the past few decades, there has been a growing consensus of authorities and organizations calling for a culture change in the practice of both general and pain medicine. In 2013, the IOM published a report titled *US Healthcare in International Perspective: Shorter Lives and Poorer Health*, which affirms that America is doing healthcare wrong, and declares that there is no need to wait for more studies before making significant changes.[26] One key topic of culture change is an emphasis on *health*, which the World Health Organization defines as, "a state of complete physical, social and mental well-being and not merely the absence of disease or infirmity."[27] Douglas Wood, director of strategy and policy at the Mayo Center for Innovation, described this when he wrote, "We will realize fairly quickly that we need to change the focus of the health care industry to creating health, not just producing health care."[28] To that effect, the Accountable Care Act has recognized the need to expand the contributions of nonstandard strategies, and introduced a nondiscrimination clause that directs insurers to cover a wide variety of complementary and alternative healthcare practitioners who previously had little or no insurance funding.

With specific regard to pain medicine, the IOM's *Relieving Pain in America*[29] and the report from the Army Surgeon General's Task Force[30] agree that we need more than minor adjustments to our current practices. This consensus is also reflected in the recommendations of the recent *National Pain Strategy*,[31] as well as the new guidelines for opioid use from the Centers for Disease Control and Prevention (CDC). The message across the board is clear: Not only have we not reduced pain and suffering, we have added to it, and that status quo is no longer acceptable.[32] The time has come for culture change.

A Fundamental Change in the Approach to Chronic Pain Management

COMPLEMENTARY AND INTEGRATIVE HEALTH AND MEDICINE

So what does culture change look like? As with all major shifts in the framework for our thinking and our understanding of practice, even when founded on solid scientific evidence, there will be naysayers, some of whom will be authority figures. Many doctors and other leaders of the current practices have built their careers on familiar, widely and long-held premises, and it is very difficult for them to accept new science paradigms that shift those premises and therefore their lives' work. (An important limitation to acceptance of a new approach is that our present tools for evaluating favorable outcomes of our treatment of chronic pain, the VAS scale and workload-based models of care as described earlier, are woefully deficient.) At a recent meeting, pioneering authorities on the role of central sensitization in chronic pain stated that they thought the focus on inflammation and the microbiome was misguided. These doctors had very impressive curriculum vitaes but, then again, so too did the famous mathematician and physicist Lord Kelvin, who made the 1895 assertion, "heavier-than-air-flying machines are impossible."

Only a few years ago, other authorities could not imagine a place in medicine for neuroplasticity. Now, neuroplasticity is taught in medical schools, but has still barely touched standard clinical practice. Perhaps the lesson here is that old habits die hard, but they do die. After all, what would our travel plans look like if they had all listened to Lord Kelvin?

Thomas Kuhn in *The Structure of Scientific Revolutions*[33] describes the process of scientific progress, where a system of thought progresses with accumulation of scientific explanations and anomalies until a new paradigm that asks different questions causes changes to the rules of the game. This is precisely the process that faces conventional medicine at this juncture: Asking more of the same questions will not solve the present crisis in healthcare or paincare. A truly innovative paradigm is needed. As Don Berwick discussed in his keynote address to the 2015 annual meeting of the Institute of Healthcare Improvement, we need to move beyond "fixing the flat tire . . . and making the car more reliable." We need innovation, which "abandons the car and creates an airplane."[34]

Integrative medicine (IM) asks different questions. It can teach us at least two new strategies that will be essential for bringing lasting, meaningful change to our failed pain care system. The first has to do with the cornerstone of conventional medical practice—diagnosis. It is helpful to think of our current system as a game of connect the dots, where each dot is a data point. When these dots, such as imaging, blood tests, electrodiagnostics, and limited details of a physical exam or patient history, describe a shape, we give that shape a name, which is our diagnosis. Although rapid diagnosis is fully justified in acute care and life-saving situations, this process has become so ingrained in our thinking and the business model of medical practices that it is very easy to forget that a diagnosis is merely an agreed on construct that permits us to provide a coherent framework for understanding some important concerns. These concerns are the dizzying array of states of health and more often, pathology; to outline an expected clinical course, and/or to categorize our treatment options. While these categories are useful for organization, they eliminate individual characteristics by ignoring many of the dots, which are essential individual characteristics that give clues to the complex etiologies of chronic pain conditions. The diagnosis also leads to an expectation of clinical outcome, which, though it may be our best guess at the time, is often assumed to have absolute (or authoritative) predictive value. Generic diagnoses also neglect positive outliers assuming that they are irrelevant in the majority of patients, thus missing potential therapeutic options. Integrative medicine sees diagnosis as the starting point of the puzzle, not the end point, and seeks positive outliers as exemplars to be studied.

CONNECTING THE DOTS

A more significant problem with our game of collecting dots is that it focuses our attention on the dots, and away from what current science tells us is more important, the connections among the dots and the connectors. If the dots are data points, the connectors are context. And while the dots are static, the connectors are dynamic; they are constantly moving, filling in the endless blanks between dots that often appear completely unrelated today, but may be correlated tomorrow. The connections are the critical intersections among the genome, environment, and lifestyle used to describe precision medicine. Some connections are intellectual constructs—relationships among variables. Others identify more physical, biochemical, and other material linkages. It was by focusing on these connectors that medical science revealed that multiple sclerosis (MS) is primarily an immune disorder and not a neurological one;

that part of the microbiome, *Helicobacter pylori*, causes recurrences of duodenal ulcers; and that both physical or psychological stressors can affect the same biochemical, proinflammatory cascade in the body. By weaving between and among and through the dots, these connectors demonstrate far more complex and unique situations than our traditional diagnoses can express, and therefore a more complete, albeit more complicated, picture of a patient's health. We can probably all think of a patient whose data points told us a different story from their context. Examples include the patient whose spinal magnetic resonance imaging (MRI) images looked terrible but who had very good function, or the patient with a hemipelvis who was taught to walk even though they were missing key parts. Integrative medicine does exactly what its name suggests; it focuses on the integration of parts. In other words, IM is all about the connectors.

It should not be surprising that many of the body's most notable connectors have been misunderstood or overlooked in the past; their roles are more difficult to define than those of most individual body parts. In a study of medical error, Graber et al[35] found that failure to adequately synthesize data was the most significant cognitive contributor to adverse outcomes. It is easier to focus on the dots. The microbiome, as mentioned earlier, is a mass of microorganisms located mainly in the gut that affects digestion, the immune system, and mood. Although it was 100 years ago that the Nobel laureate Élie Metchnikoff drew much attention to the microbiome by declaring it a major determinant of health, over 90% of all papers about the microbiome were written in just the past decade. It is likely that the medical community largely ignored this connector for so long because of the amorphousness of "a mass of microorganisms." This was coupled with a bias that microorganisms are largely pathogens, not symbiotic agents of health and well-being. Nevertheless, we now know just how important the microbiome is to a patient's health, and how easily it can be affected by both endogenous and environmental factors, including drugs, chemicals, and the foods and foodlike substances of the modern diet.[36-41]

Another notable connector, fascia, has long been misconstrued as an inert structure with no dynamic function. It was thought to simply define and delineate boundaries, but studies now suggest it is more about connection than delineation, and acts as a crucial means of force transmission.[42-44] Fascial fibers surround each myocyte and create a fine, three-dimensional network of crisscrossing strands that connect many structures in the body and are constantly being remodeled. Fascial pathways connect the right and left sides of the body, upper and lower limbs, and all internal organs, including the brain, which helps to explain many previously unexplained symptoms.

The process of inflammation also serves as a connector that has generally been considered a troublemaker and the root cause of most chronic disease. It is a bodywide reaction that affects every tissue type, and its chemical mediators circulate throughout the body, linking immune responses to blood clotting; to renal, pulmonary, and cardiac function; and to a range of other organ functions and dysfunctions. It explains why certain patterns of disease are often found in clusters in individual patients. But there is also a lesser-addressed, positive side to inflammation; it is the first step in healing. The tissue response to inflammation draws in platelets, white blood cells, and fibroblasts, all of which fight infection and heal damaged tissues. Unfortunately, our pharmaceutical anti-inflammatory drugs reduce both the negative and positive effects of inflammation and are therefore often more harmful than helpful.[45-47]

Neuroplasticity, the process by which experiences change the nervous system, was not recognized as a connector for a long time. Experiences that cause neuroplastic changes include injuries, activities, thoughts, and attitude changes, all of which can alter the connections within the nervous system, affecting the cellular function of many sites and even change their structure. The process of *central sensitization*, which is the most commonly discussed part of neuroplasticity in chronic pain settings, was initially regarded as a one-way black hole of altered nervous system function that exacerbated an individual's sensitivity to normal stimuli, caused pain, and reduced function. The latest science, however, demonstrates the possibility of ongoing changes that can reverse this process. There is a tremendous capacity for the positive influences of neuroplasticity to enhance function of the psychosomatic system.[48-53] Influences as disparate as exercise and consuming turmeric can enhance the formation of new brain cells throughout life, and learning any type of new skill increases new synapse formation in the brain giving our cognitive functions more resiliency.

Epigenetics is a connector between the effects of the environment, lifestyle choices, and current experience and the more static genome. Epigenetics is the process of methylation, acetylation, and other processes, that influences DNA transcription and translation, thereby altering gene expression rather than DNA sequencing. Epigenetics has transformed our thinking about determinants of health. Altered gene expression is proving to have great impact on health outcomes.[54,55]

SALUTOGENESIS

Integrative medicine can also inform and guide our management of chronic pain with a second revision to our fundamental notions of human health. Integrative medicine has a *focus on health*, as opposed to a disease focus. From medical and professional school education onward, we are oriented to states of disordered physiologic and behavioral function; we are generally taught to spend most of our efforts reacting to pathological findings. In other words, we focus on the factors that cause disease far more than we do those that create and maintain health. This despite the obvious fact that the body spends almost continuous activity healing and sustaining health. Research studies on healthy lifestyles tell us that the opposite approach yields far better results.[56-58] Aaron Antonovsky coined the term "salutogenesis" to describe this inherent capacity to heal, sending us searching for ways to create positive conditions in which healing can take place, also known as optimal healing environments (OHE). These OHEs can be summed up as environments "in which the social, psychological, spiritual, physical, and behavioral components of health care are oriented toward support and stimulation of healing and the achievement of wholeness.[59,60] "In looking at human health and illness in this way, the practice of medicine becomes both more daunting and more invigorating, as all of a patient's interconnected health and illness factors become possible points of intervention in the process of salutogenesis.

As was already discussed, IM is all about the connections and connectors, which include more than just the anatomical and physiological ones listed above. An OHE is a wider-angle lens through which we can consider not just the microconnectors, like the microbiome, but also the equally important macroconnectors, such as the relationship of the patient to the practitioner, to the system of medicine, and even to the community and the environment as a whole. While conventional medicine pays little attention to these macroconnectors, emerging science tells us that they are crucial, and that it is not by accident that ancient healers and folk healers and shamans in many cultures today enlist the help of their entire village in their medical practice.

Foundational Elements to Improving Patient Outcomes

We now know that lifestyle choices have a more profound impact on population health outcomes than genetics and all our medical management interventions combined. While genetics accounts for 20%–30% of our health outcomes, epigenetics—our environment and what we eat, drink, think, feel, and do—accounts for 70%–80%. Lifestyle choices affect which of our genes are turned on or off,[60] which influences overall health outcomes by changing host susceptibility to disease and the ability to heal. The European Prospective Investigation into Cancer and Nutrition–Potsdam Study (EPIC) evaluated the effects of four lifestyle factors on health—never smoking, a BMI under 30, physical activity for at least 3.5 hours a week, and eating a healthy diet that includes vegetables, fruit, whole grain bread, and low meat consumption. The study followed 23,000 people for 7.8 years and demonstrated that those with all four factors at baseline had a 78% lower overall risk of developing a chronic disease. More specifically, these individuals reduced their risk of diabetes by 93%, myocardial infarction by 81%, strokes by 50%, and cancer by 36%. All of these diseases and, in fact, all of the chronic diseases that were tracked in EPIC can impact pain. These findings are particularly significant when compared to the results of interventions; there are no drugs or procedures that come anywhere close to producing these benefits. Recognizing the impact of lifestyle choices on health is the key to culture change within our healthcare system, and is an effective platform for changing the conversation around chronic pain.

NUTRITION

Most chronic disease is fostered by an acidic[61,62] and proinflammatory environment in the body. Nutrition plays a crucial role in this; with every meal eaten, food choices either increase or decrease inflammation in the body. All too often, healthy choices are difficult for people to make, either because healthy foods are not available (or affordable), or because education about optimal nutrition is lacking. In the United States, politics and business have worked together to make processed foods cheaper than fresh, whole, unprocessed foods. Subsidies to huge corporations support the growing of grains, which are used to create relatively cheap, mass-produced meat (consuming much of these grains) and processed foods, while vegetables remain expensive and even inaccessible in some parts of the country. The US Department of Agriculture (USDA), which issues food recommendations for the nation, has a stated mission that focuses more on economic innovation than health.[63] In fact, the USDA has issued food recommendations that support the use of heavily processed foods containing high levels of sugar and refined carbohydrates devoid of nutritional value, against the advice of its own nutritional advisers.[64,65] This strategy has led us to an epidemic of chronic illness and obesity. It is estimated that one in three Americans will become diabetic in their lifetime—a figure that increases to one in two for Hispanics, African Americans, and Native Americans. Record numbers of preteens are obese, diabetic, or showing signs of coronary artery disease. In an outrageously profitable business model, cheaply priced fast foods create ample customers for hospitals, insurance companies, and pharmaceutical companies. And pharmaceutical companies win in two ways; drugs are used without prescription in animal food production as well as with prescription to treat the human health consequences of the Standard American Diet (SAD). This diet is dominated by processed foods—almost 80% of which contain added sugar[66]—and is high in calories, unhealthy fats, refined carbohydrates and sugar, salt, and chemicals such as pesticides, stabilizers, antibiotics, and preservatives. Fiber, vitamins, minerals, and antioxidants are missing from the SAD (sad, indeed), which serves up nutritional deficiencies despite excess calories.[67] It is no coincidence that many chronic pain patients eat very unhealthy diets; with the increasing prevalence of obesity, cardiovascular disease, and diabetes come the complications of other chronic diseases and pain syndromes.

Studies evaluating the influence of diet on inflammatory markers show that diets high in fiber, healthy oils, vegetables, and fruit but low in sugars, starchy carbohydrates, and unhealthy oils can reduce inflammation and disease.[68-71] Thus, by increasing or decreasing inflammation, food choices influence the brain and body function much as the contents of a fuel tank influence how well a car runs, or the quality of soil influences how well a plant grows.[72-74]

Paradoxically, many doctors who hesitate to prescribe supplements and restricted diets for fear of harming patients do not hesitate to prescribe drugs for pain or inflammation, or other drugs to lower cholesterol, blood pressure, or blood sugar. The CDC statistics are very clear on the relative risks of food and supplements versus drugs—the greater potential for harm is with drugs.[75-78] But while these prescribing trends are paradoxical, they are also perfectly understandable; we are all more comfortable with what we know. The 4-year curriculum at most conventional medical schools allocates thousands of hours to learning about pharmacologic agents, and only a few hours (if any) to nutrition. Often, graduates not only are ill-prepared to advise patients on the subject of nutrition but also do not even know how to eat well themselves. We know that doctors who smoke are less likely to stress smoking cessation to their patients,[79] and we can assume that this same relationship applies to doctors who have other unhealthy habits or who lack healthy ones, such as eating a healthy diet. After all, it is not a logical stretch to assume that those healthy living elements we feel are important in our own lives, such as diet, exercise, and sleep, are also considered important in the lives of our patients.

What distinguishes an unhealthy diet from a healthy one? All diets consist of *macronutrients*—protein, fat, simple carbohydrates, and complex carbohydrates—which provide the calories in our food, and *micronutrients*—vitamins, minerals, enzymes, and antioxidants. An unhealthy diet is an unbalanced one, and, in America, that tends to mean an overconsumption of macronutrients and an insufficient intake of micronutrients. On average, an American consumes 150 pounds of sugar and 150 pounds of refined flour every year, and over one-third of their calories comes from junk food.[80] Americans tend to eat too much animal protein,[81] but neglect vegetable protein and have a high intake of processed grains,[82] resulting in the overconsumption of unhealthy fats, but a very low intake of unprocessed fruits, vegetables, beans, legumes, nuts, seeds, whole grains, herbs, and spices, which is why we lack fiber and micronutrients.

Walter Willett—professor of epidemiology and nutrition and chairman of the Department of Nutrition at Harvard T. H. Chan School of Public Health, and one of the most frequently cited medical authors who publishes extensively on diet and its effects on well-being and longevity—has outlined the evidence for the health-promoting effects of a proper diet, and provides an alternative food pyramid to *My Plate*—the latest recommendation from the USDA. The base of Willett's pyramid is composed of whole grains and plant oils, followed at the next tier by unlimited vegetables and 2–3 fruits per day. Nuts and legumes are next, followed by fish, poultry, and eggs, and then dairy or calcium supplementation. At the very top of the pyramid are red meats, butter, sweets, and "white foods," meaning white bread, pasta, potatoes, and rice.[83] These should be used sparingly.

Moderate use of coffee, tea, wine, and dark chocolate has been shown to be beneficial because of their antioxidant content. When consuming these products, however, it is important to be aware of their source and quality, as all of them tend to be produced with heavy usage of pesticides, and are sometimes chemically altered. The Environmental Working Group[84] is a nonprofit organization that compiles lists of sources and contaminants and makes them available to the public.

Processed grains and sweetened foods are called high–glycemic index (GI) foods because they cause a rapid rise in blood sugar (BS) followed by an insulin spike. Low-GI foods, on the other hand, produce only small fluctuations in BS and insulin. Large fluctuations in BS and insulin begin the path to insulin resistance and diabetes, accompanied by an increase in inflammation, which, as already mentioned, is a factor in the development of most known chronic degenerative diseases.[85-87] These include medical and psychiatric disorders such as, metabolic syndrome, diabetes, cardiovascular disease, cancer, autoimmune disorders, schizophrenia, and depression, all of which have adverse effects on health and life expectancy and can complicate the experience of pain. High-GI foods are also addictive, which leads to overeating.[88] Furthermore, processed foods, grains, and animal products promote low tissue pH, which reduces the activity of essential physiological enzyme reactions and mitochondrial energy production in the body and itself is a cause of pain.[89,90] Green vegetables, lentils, and most fruits raise tissue pH to more optimal levels.

In addition, processed and high-GI foods adversely affect the microbiome.[91] Artificial sweeteners, such as aspartame and sucralose, and many common occurring chemicals, pesticides, and food additives also harm this *crucial connector* discussed earlier. While the microbiome only weighs about 6 lbs, its cells outnumber our human cells 10 to 1 and it has incredibly diversity—it contains 100 times more DNA than our human DNA.[92] The balance of this genetic diversity greatly impacts human health and disease; it affects the absorption of nutrients, causes or prevents excessive gut permeability, affects the function of the immune system, may be responsible for some forms of abdominal pain, and can stimulate unhealthy fermentation within the gut. For example, we have known since the 1990s that gut bacterial imbalances can cause abnormal colonic fermentation, which can present itself as irritable bowel syndrome.[93] Martin Blaser in *Missing Microbes*, outlines the health consequences of the loss of diversity in the microbiome due to modern diet, drugs, and chemicals.

Besides an unhealthy diet, other factors that can disrupt the microbiome include many non-life-saving drugs such as NSAIDs, proton pump inhibitors (PPIs), antibiotics, steroids, and hormones. These drugs can also cause significant morbidity, mortality, and micronutrient depletion,[94-99] and these changes can impact pain.

While it is important to eat a healthy diet, we are also not just what we eat; we are what we ingest, digest, and absorb. In the nutritional process, the digestive system is supposed to play the role of gatekeeper; as digestion takes place, the gut wall is supposed to act as a pathway for needed nutritional molecules to be absorbed into the body, and as a barrier to toxic ones and pathogens. Recent research shows, however, that inflamed intestinal mucosa can lead to increased gut permeability, which allows the entry of bacteria, toxics, and partially digested nutrients. Eighty percent of the immune system lies adjacent to the gut, which enables rapid reactions to immunogenic substances crossing the mucosal barrier. In the case of *increased permeability*, absorption of pathogens and immunogenic molecules leads to increased bodywide inflammation, and may enable the development of autoimmune disorders in susceptible individuals.[100,101] Increased permeability was once called *leaky gut* by nontraditional practitioners, before it was finally validated and accepted by mainstream science and medicine. Of course, increased permeability is just one of many factors that affect proper digestion. Another essential component is sufficient stomach acid, which triggers gastric emptying, stimulates the secretion of digestive enzymes, and enables absorption of many minerals, vitamin B12, and protein.[102]

Most Americans tend not to absorb enough nutrients, because of both a patent lack of nutrition and digestive problems. And while a whole-foods diet, properly digested, will always be the best basis for nutritional sufficiency, supplements such as multivitamins can be regarded as an insurance policy to provide a baseline level of nutrients. This can guard against fluctuations in health and food intake that may increase need or decrease the supply of nutrients.[103]

As with food, the health risks associated with nutritional supplements are minimal. Although the safety profiles of nutritional supplements must continue to be monitored and evaluated, the National Poison Data System, which tracks deaths from drugs and supplements, reported no deaths due to vitamins A, B, C, D, E, or any other vitamin, and no deaths attributable to amino acid or other dietary supplements in their 2010 report.[104] There have, however, been recent reports of adverse effects from supplements tainted with pharmaceuticals. The National Center for Complementary and Integrative Health (NCCIH) provides a website that lists drug-tainted supplements.[105,106] These supplements are mostly those used for body building, weight loss, and sexual performance,[107] and are not embraced by IM practitioners. This issue of contamination, while important for public safety, is one of quality control and reflects the adverse effects of the contaminating drugs, not the underlying supplements.[108,109] This problem of quality control is also apparent in situations where the ingredients of supplement bottles are found to differ from their labels.[110]

Although nutritional supplements should generally be considered safe, as with all things, there are specific micronutrients or supplements that can adversely interact with certain states of health and disease.

There are many vitamins, minerals, antioxidants and botanicals that can benefit pain patients. Those reviewed here are some of the most studied and readily available, and have demonstrated effectiveness in improving inflammation, pain, and healing.[111-113] Micronutrients also have an impact on the comorbidity of depression and anxiety, which have been shown to exacerbate pain. A series of clinical trials repeated in many countries has linked micronutrient and fish oil supplements to reduced levels of violence in prisoners and of delinquency in children. These trials that link nutritional status to psychological status are of particular interest when we consider that psychological states have already been linked to adverse outcomes in pain.[114,115]

Vitamin D

The population of the northern hemisphere is generally vitamin D deficient,[116,117] and those deficits are even more profound in chronic pain populations on both sides of the equator.[118-120] Vitamin D supplements have been shown to improve pain as well as improve muscle strength in men and women.[121,122] Vitamin D functions more as a hormone than as a vitamin and is necessary for every system and cell type that has been studied so far. Deficiencies are associated with inflammation and susceptibility to illness, and sufficient levels are necessary for a healthy immune system. Deficiencies are more common in the elderly, the obese, and those who have more skin pigmentation. Testing of serum 25OH vitamin D is the best way to gauge the optimal amount needed, because gastrointestinal absorption, states of inflammation, and other factors cause some patients to require high levels of supplementation to achieve optimal serum levels. It is generally regarded as safe for people to take 2,000 IU per day orally, and the No Adverse Effect Level (NOAL), an international standard, has been set at 4,000 IU daily.[123]

Omega-3 Oils

The omega-3 oils (n-3) and omega-6 (n-6) polyunsaturated fatty acids (PUFAs) are essential nutrients that we must get from our diet. North Americans generally ingest too much n-6 and insufficient n-3. *Linoleic acid* is the predominant n-6 that promotes inflammation, and the main source is from vegetable oils. The n-3s are *docosahexaenoic acid* (DHA) and *eicosapentaenoic acid* (EPA), found in fish, organic free-range eggs, and even grass-fed beef, and *alpha-linolenic acid* (ALA), from plants such as flax. The n-3s promote anti-inflammatory physiology and are being studied for treatment of a wide variety of conditions (headache, rheumatoid arthritis, discogenic pain, and others) with positive outcomes ranging from reduced pain, reduced needs for analgesic medications, and improved quality of life indicators.[124-128] The doses used are in the range of 3,000–4,000 mg of combined EPA and DHA, which can usually be found in 6,000–8,000 mg of fish oil.

B Vitamins

The B vitamins are coenzymes for reactions essential for fundamental cellular function—particularly in adenosine triphosphate (ATP) production and detoxification. Increasingly, research is looking at the connection between inefficient mitochondrial function and damage to mitochondrial DNA as underlying defects in chronic pain states, including myalgias, neuropathic pain, fibromyalgia, and chronic fatigue.[129-134] Many of the B vitamins act as methyl donors in the processes of mitochondrial protein and nucleic acid synthesis and methionine and glutathione metabolism. Deficiencies of the Bs negatively affect many systems: neurologic, hematologic, cardiovascular, bone metabolism, and many aspects of muscle function.

B12

Deficiency of this B vitamin has been most studied in connection with homo-cysteine damage to the endothelium in the development of hyperalgesia. The mitochondrial electron transport chain is ATP dependent and is being studied in relation to neuropathic pain—specifically the effect of reactive oxygen species (ROS) on chronic regional pain syndrome (CRPS). There may be common mechanisms in mitochondrial myopathies and fibromyalgia where mitochondria are adversely affected by substrate and cofactor deficiencies as well as inhibition by drugs and industrial chemicals.[135,136]

B12 deficiencies have long been known to cause neurological dysfunction and chronic pain. Absorption from food sources depends on adequate stomach acid and intrinsic factor and declines with age. B12 tissue levels are likely more significant than serum levels and may be better correlated with methyl-malonic acid (MMA) and homocysteine levels. In both active treatment arms of a double blind, placebo-controlled, crossover trial, Mauro[137] found that daily B12 injections in pain patients with normal B12 levels resulted in reduced pain scores and analgesic use. A British study[138] found that preservation of brain value correlated positively with B12 levels within the normal range in 61- to 87-year-olds without cognitive impairment. The normal values for B12 in Japan have a much higher range than in the United States, and there are controversies regarding the best way to assess B12 sufficiency.[139,140] There is growing recognition that fatigue, depression, and nonspecific lack of wellness may accompany insufficient levels of B12.

A month-long trial of 1,000 mcg sublingually, taken daily, may produce improved symptoms of pain, insomnia, and fatigue. This route of administration avoids injections while still bypassing any impairment in gastrointestinal absorption. If not effective, a trial of self-administered daily injections may be tried.

Vitamin C

A powerful antioxidant and cofactor, vitamin C is essential for tissue repair and adaptation to stress. It is needed for the production of hormones, neurotransmitters, bone, and collagen, which are all important to physical and psychological well-being and healing.[141] Vitamin C increases iron absorption, and higher serum vitamin C levels are associated with lower blood lead levels. Unlike most animals, we humans cannot produce vitamin C, which makes it an essential nutrient that must be consumed. Vitamin C needs vary from day to day based on stress levels, physical activity, injury, and sickness. A 70-kg goat makes 13 g of vitamin C per day and more when stressed.[142] A moderate dose is 2,000 mg per day. Current research is reevaluating our vitamin C needs for optimal health.

Magnesium

Magnesium is one of the most common nutritional deficiencies in the American diet.[143] It is an intracellular mineral, like calcium, and levels are likewise tightly regulated. Our bones and muscles act as reservoirs of magnesium, and these reservoirs can be depleted without changing serum test levels, which may appear to be normal. Magnesium plays a role in over 300 essential metabolic reactions.[144,145,] It is needed for synthesis of protein, DNA, RNA, glutathione, carbohydrates, and lipids. It also plays a role in cell signaling, optimal bone density, collagen production, and regulation of serum glucose.[146] It controls the rate of nerve firing and is an excellent muscle relaxant. People with fibromyalgia, nocturnal leg cramps, high blood pressure, and cardiac arrhythmias are often magnesium deficient. Magnesium should be the first line choice for bodywide inflammation,[147] muscle cramps, spasms, myofascial tightness, and trigger points. Magnesium can reduce migraine frequency[148] and the cramping and pain of irritable bowel syndrome,[149] can improve sleep,[150] and is now being studied for its role in neuropathic pain.[151]

Some forms of magnesium are better absorbed by the body, and are therefore better distributed to tissues, than others. These forms include chloride, glycinate, citrate, and ascorbate. Other forms, such as oxide, hydroxide, or sulfate, are not well absorbed by the gut and are more likely to cause diarrhea. Patients should take as much of a good-quality magnesium as can be tolerated with the goal of producing 1–2 easy-to-pass bowel movements per day. The daily dose may vary from a few hundred milligrams to much higher doses for those with severe deficiencies. The result of overdose is diarrhea, which stops when the dose is lowered.

Glutathione Precursors

There is growing literature on the role of mitochondrial dysfunction in the development of chronic neuropathic and inflammatory pain. A review paper by Sui highlights "five major mitochondrial functions" that impact chronic pain (the mitochondrial energy generating system, ROS generation, mitochondrial permeability transition pore, apoptotic pathways, and intracellular calcium mobilization).[152,153] Most of us rolled our eyes when we had to memorize the

Krebs cycle, but its relevance to daily practice is becoming ever more apparent. It turns out, mitochondria are another crucial connector, which maybe should not come as a surprise; cellular energy production and detoxification are obviously cornerstones of any healthy body.

In our society, sensational problems often receive far more notice than common ones. For example, while severe mitochondrial disorders capture our attention because they are life threatening, we do not pay much mind to lesser forms of mitochondrial dysfunction caused by damage to mitochondrial DNA because they are far more common. Similarly, extreme lead poisoning in Flint, Michigan, makes the headlines, but reports on ASTDR.gov about the association between lead levels *within the normal range* and delayed development, learning disorders, and behavioral disorders goes unheeded. Likewise, it is well-recognized that nutritional supplementation helps the severe neurological and psychiatric disorders caused by untreated vitamin B12 deficiency, while the studies that show reduced levels of violence in prisoners given nutritional supplementation are not being acted on.

These three examples are not random. Problems of mitochondrial dysfunction, exposures to even low levels of toxics, and nutritional deficiencies all affect the efficiency of the Krebs cycle and the inability of mitochondrial DNA to recover from oxidative damage. This damage is caused by high-energy particles called *free radicals* that interact with the components of cells at many of sites, including DNA, lipids, cell membranes, and proteins like intracellular enzymes. Free radicals act by stealing electrons. Free radicals are caused by external agents such as smoking, exposure to toxics, and radiation including cosmic rays or internal processes of normal metabolism. And while each of our cells suffers millions of "hits" every day by free radicals, mitochondria are particularly susceptible to oxidative damage because they generate free radicals during normal function and also suffer from exogenous free radical attack. When this damage accumulates, it becomes *oxidative stress*, causes inflammation, and plays a role in degenerative disease. For this reason, mitochondria create an enormous need for *antioxidants*, which are electron donors that repair the damage caused by free radicals. Antioxidants will help to prevent mitochondrial dysfunction, which is suspected of playing a role in neuropathic pain as well as fatigue in multisystem disorders.[154] Unfortunately, some of the very agents we look to for solutions—drugs—also interfere with mitochondrial function through the disruption of glutathione pathways. The most effective solution is therefore a nutritional one.

Glutathione is a key survival antioxidant that recycles other antioxidants and is essential for mitochondrial and liver enzyme detoxification function.[155] Methylation is a metabolic process that is necessary for mitochondrial energy production, detoxification, and free radical damage repair. These nutritionally dependent processes are important players in some pain syndromes. High levels of homocysteine from deficient methylation and deficiencies of glutathione can create macrovascular damage, and thus cause coronary heart disease[156] Microvascular damage is now being recognized from the same causes and may be a mechanism causing neuropathy and hyperalgesia.[157-160] Single nucleotide polymorphisms of the MTHFR gene that can cause reduced levels of methylation are being studied in conditions that will impact pain medicine. There are animal studies demonstrating the benefits of antioxidants such as vitamins C and E and coenzyme Q10 (CoQ10 or ubiquinone) on chronic pain. Milk thistle is an antioxidant and free radical scavenger that raises the intracellular glutathione levels studied in many different disease models, including thallassemia,[161] diabetes,[162] drug-induced liver injury,[163] and more. N-acetylcysteine (NAC) stimulates phase II liver enzymes, disarms free radicals, and repairs damaged DNA. It also helps the liver produce glutathione.[164] In addition, NAC protects the body against a wide variety of toxics, including heavy metals, which it binds into complexes so they can be excreted from the body.

Oxidative phosphorylation (OXPHOS) reactions are critical reactions on the inner mitochondrial membrane: OXPHOS defects reduce mitochondrial ATP production, and "can theoretically give rise to any symptom, in any organ or tissue, at any age, with any mode of inheritance."[165] Medication-induced mitochondrial damage and disease has been associated with many common medications including NSAIDS, Aspirin, acetaminophen, antidepressants, local anesthetics, anxiolytics, antipsychotics, statins, oral hypoglycemic agents, and anticonvulsants.[166,167] There is a growing body of research looking at subtle and acquired OXPHOS disorders secondary to environmental toxics and many drug exposures. These last two facts might explain why clinical medicine is lagging behind the science. Though we may be used to complex patient scenarios, it is a leap to get our heads around the idea that "any symptom, any system" can be caused or affected by mitochondrial dysfunction. If we then take away most of the drugs we commonly use to help people because they may be contributing to the problem, common practice protocols become impossible. While this would be a wearisome treatment model to embrace, it is at least worth our awareness and consideration in the area of difficult-to-understand pain syndromes. At the bare minimum, we should explore exposures to heavy metals and common toxics and avoid non-life-saving polypharmacy. Supporting mitochondrial function with antioxidants has been shown to be effective in improving ATP production. Positive effects have been shown with CoQ10, ascorbic acid, vitamin E, riboflavin, thiamine, niacin, vitamin K (phylloquinone and menadione), and carnitine.[168] CoQ10 should be considered essential for anyone on a statin drug, since HMGcoA reductase enzyme reduces CoQ10 production. CoQ10 is essential for mitochondrial function, and deficiency may result in muscle (including heart muscle) and nerve dysfunction.

Turmeric and Ginger

Turmeric and ginger come from the botanically related plants curcuma longa, and Zingiber[169-171] respectively. They have anti-inflammatory properties, which are at least in part due to the disruption the cyclooxygenase-2 (COX2) pathway at many points leading to a more nuanced influence on inflammation. Ginger and the main active ingredient of turmeric (curcumin)[172,173] have similar effects as pharmaceutical NSAIDs but without the harmful side effects. Other actions, besides COX2 inhibition, are being studied. It has been found that turmeric root plays a role in the preservation of cognitive function, which may be partly due to neurogenesis[174] through the promotion of stem cell differentiation. This seems to be a property of the whole root—either fresh or dried as a spice—and not the extracts of curcuminoids. Turmeric also inhibits phase I liver enzymes and activates phase II.

Systematic reviews of both turmeric (root and extracts) and ginger have significant beneficial effects on pain and function in osteoarthritis.[175] Clinical trials have shown curcumin reduces perioperative pain[176,177] and reduces the need for other analgesics. A 2009 review of hundreds of studies on turmeric and its use for a variety of complaints concluded, "turmeric appears to outperform many pharmaceuticals in its effects against several chronic debilitating diseases, and does so with virtually no serious adverse side effects."[178]

Cinnamon

This spice is being shown to inhibit inflammatory cytokines and has been studied in rheumatoid arthritis and dysmenorrhea. It also reduces blood sugar levels and insulin resistance through its "insulin-like" mechanism that allows glucose to bypass the insulin receptor on myocytes. Chromium and magnesium also optimize blood sugar levels and can impact pain states by reducing inflammation and general health complications that accompany insulin resistance.[178]

Quercetin

Quercetin is a plant-derived flavonoid that has antioxidant and analgesic effects.[179] Glucosamine and chondroitin have been shown to be beneficial for cartilage healing and preservation in osteoarthritis.[180]

Given the importance of the microbiome for overall heath as well as the multiple challenges that modern living presents for the microbiome, it is prudent to recommend fermented foods to replenish the microflora, and probiotics (beneficial bacteria) and prebiotics (nutrients that nourish the microbiota) when there are known exposures to adverse circumstances.

There are many different types of elimination diets that can be useful for patients to try. A systematic use of an elimination diet can help sort out reactions people have to foods, food additives, or even pesticides and contaminants. Gluten intolerance has been called an underrecognized trigger for headaches and a cause for uncontrollable blood sugars in some diabetics. One percent of the population has Celiac disease, and 10% have genetically determined gluten intolerance. (REF) There seems to be increasing levels of gluten intolerance continent-wide, and the reasons for this are unclear. In North America, there is very heavy use of pesticides on most nonorganic grains, and many pain patients feel better with a trial of restriction of gluten or all grains.

Nightshades are a family of plants that have long been recognized as a source of joint pain and stiffness in some animals and people. A 6-week trial off nightshades—tomatoes, potatoes, all peppers except white and black peppercorns, and eggplant—may improve some patients' pain.

Nutrition research seldom looks like drug research. Drugs have dramatic therapeutic effects as well as the potential for dramatic side effects. Nutrients work more subtly, slowly, and physiologically than drugs because they are naturally occurring substances that our bodies are programmed to recognize, utilize, and excrete appropriately. Of course, there are rare metabolic disorders, allergies, and intolerances to foods that can cause adverse reactions in a small group of people.

Nutrients work synergistically with each other, and while drug-style randomized-controlled trials of isolated nutrients over a short period of time have provided some information, the major impact diet has on health occurs when overall nutritional status improves.

People rarely get drug deficiencies but they regularly get nutritional deficiencies. The 2004 *JAMA* article concludes, "Poor diet and physical inactivity account for four hundred thousand deaths, or 16.6 percent of total deaths, per year in the United States."[181] Our heavily processed, high-GI diet causes diabetes, depression, cardiovascular disease, and obesity, all of which are risk factors for adverse outcomes in the cases of painful conditions and the procedures used to treat them.

EMERGING AREAS OF NUTRITIONAL LINKS TO PAIN SYNDROMES

New research is pointing to immune dysfunction, beyond the obvious autoimmune disorders, as a player in clinical pain syndromes. This way of thinking connects distinct tissue types, distant anatomical sites, and varied physiological functions, all potentially affected by immune activation, and accounts for some of the complex and confusing syndromes we see. For example, there is a relationship of mast cell activation with interstitial cystitis and chronic pancreatitis. Experimental pain models have demonstrated that activated macrophages can cause the release of inflammatory mediators tumor necrosis factor alpha (TNF alpha), interleukin 1-beta (IL-1beta), nerve growth factor (NGF), nitric oxide (NO), and prostanoids, all of which can cause clinically relevant pain pathology.[182] There is mounting evidence that industrial food additives are adversely affecting intestinal tight junctions, leading to increased gut permeability. This is a suspected mechanism that can lead to the observed increase prevalence of autoimmune disorders,[183] many of which are pain associated. Recently discovered lymphatic connections to the brain are revealing a more extensive role for the immune system in both the function and dysfunction of the brain.[184] The blood-brain barrier is increasingly seen as less of a protective barrier.

Xenobiotics are foreign chemical substances, many of which are neurotoxic or endocrine disruptors. Many of them find their way into our food and water supplies. Neutrophils may be playing a role in nerve injury leading to hyperalgesia,[185] secondary to both injury and xenobiotic attack. These circulating leukocytes respond to injury by migrating to the site of inflammation and moving into the nervous system.[186] This raises interesting possibilities for understanding the development of sensitized pain states and the possibility that xenobiotic substances are possible initiators of these reactions. This may help explain why we seem to have an epidemic of ill health and intractable pain states. There have been over 75,000 new chemicals introduced into the environment between 1960 and 2000, and most of them have not been subjected to safety studies. Heavy metals, especially mercury, lead, cadmium, and arsenic, are frequently found in modern humans, and can interfere with many metabolic processes.[187] Some groups have very high risk of exposure to multiple chemicals. These groups include farm workers, residents living close to chemical plants, chemical industry workers, and the military. The aging water infrastructure in most large cities contains lead, which is a known neurotoxin.

Unfortunately, we have not been systematically looking for xenobiotic exposure in our chronic pain patients, and so we give them diagnoses that may be very incomplete, and therefore miss effective solutions. This makes Malcolm Gladwell's observation especially salient: "We have, as human beings, a storytelling problem. We're a bit too quick to come up with explanations for things we don't really have an explanation for."[188]

The Connection Between Mind and Body

Both popular Western notions of health and disease and the conventional medical system that attempts to prevent, diagnose, and manage disease suffers from a nearly 300-year-old "mind-body dualism" that has been attributed to Rene Descartes. The brain and all body systems use a single instantaneous communication network mediated by the same molecules.[189] There is a multidirectional communication system between the cerebral cortex, limbic system, and hypothalamic-pituitary-adrenal axis that is both influenced by and sends output to the periphery, which includes all organs, endocrine glands, the immune system, and the central and peripheral nervous systems (somatic, sympathetic, and parasympathetic). There are modulations from mind to brain to body and back again. Recent scientific advances are disrupting the mind and body schism of Descartes, and indicate that connections between these two spheres are unavoidable in the effective management of chronic conditions, especially chronic pain syndromes. This field of medicine has been called mind-body medicine (MBM) or psychoneuroendocrine immunology. This is closely related to the field of biofield science, which is "an emerging field of study that aims to provide a scientific foundation for understanding the complex homeodynamic regulation of living systems."[190] Biofields are "endogenously generated fields, which may play a significant role in information transfer processes that contribute to an individual's state of mental, emotional, physical, and spiritual wellbeing." Biofield treatment of pain could be "bottom-up" processes, such as reductions in cellular inflammation or nociceptive signaling and/or "top-down" processes such as cortical nociceptive control mechanisms.

The concept of biofields places us in the context of the world of physics.[191] Physicists tell us that we, like all observable matter, consist of more empty space than solid matter, with numerous electromagnetic connections among the "dots" that make up the subatomic and atomic particles. Biofields may lie within these connections or at a larger more macroscopic dimension. Looking at chronic pain through the lens of a united mind-body/biofield makes it obvious that there can be unintended and very poorly understood repercussions to any intervention we make when we chase isolated features of a pain syndrome, such as nociception, mood, or sleep disturbances. For example when we raise serotonin or norepinephrine, what are the repercussions for the dopaminergic reward system? A comprehensive, integrative approach could set its goal on endpoints that enhance health rather than merely ameliorate symptoms.

Mind-body medicine practices can interrupt the cycle of stress and thereby improve a patient's sense of well-being and resilience to all manner of stressors.[192] Stress is proinflammatory. The stress response (fight or flight) shuts down many nonessential bodily functions such as digestion, immune response, and reproductive functions; it shrinks the hypothalamus and has a net proinflammatory effect on many tissues.[193] This explains many of the symptoms accompanying pain syndromes and indicates possible treatment strategies. Mind-body medicine techniques, through their effects on mind-brain-body physiology, are cost-effective interventions to mitigate the effects of chronic stress (Box 21.1). Kabat-Zinn and others showed that a mindfulness-based meditation practice by a treatment group decreased pain-related drug use, improved activity levels, and increased self-esteem relative to the control group. At the 15-month follow-up in Kabat-Zinn's study, the improvements continued and there was a high level of compliance with ongoing meditation practice.[194-200] Other studies, including a trial at the Ford Motor Plant for back pain have found mind-body interventions useful as adjunctive therapy to ameliorate pain, to enhance treatment response, and to reduce drug use and costly, risky interventions.[201]

The 2009 Nobel Prize in Medicine recognized the research on "caps" on strands of chromosome or telomeres and the enzyme that maintains them, telomerase. Shortened telomeres are associated with reduced longevity, and chronic stress was shown to cause accelerated telomere shortening and therefore premature aging.[202] Research has also shown that meditation and a healthy lifestyle can preserve the length of telomeres.[203]

Many mind-body therapies are disdainfully referred to as placebo effects. This comes from the long history of placebos being used as representatives of no active treatment, to which drug activity was being compared. But the issue is far more complex than this. When Kaptchuk used a placebo intervention as

Box 21.1

Mind-body strategies include meditation, guided imagery, biofeedback, yoga, tai chi, qi gong, and other mindfully done movement and any practice that creates a relaxation response or affects the autonomic nervous system.

the active arm of an irritable bowel syndrome (IBS) study—in which patients were told they were receiving an inactive pill that sometimes improves symptoms—he found that the placebo caused a statistically significant improvement.[204] Placebo and the placebo effects are an emerging area of study that represents the ill-understood effects of the treatment and the context of treatment. Being in pain is stressful, and interacting with the pain care system has been called one big *nocebo* experience due to the stressful aspects of interacting with the healthcare system. An essential element of the OHE is the reduction of stress that has the potential for improving the suffering associated with chronic pain.

CENTRAL SENSITIZATION AND MOVEMENT

Non-neuronal cells in the central nervous system (CNS), such as microglia, have been shown to both contribute to and resolve damage in the CNS. Microglia have a surveillance function in their resting state,[205] but when activated they can cause damage to peripheral nerves or the CNS, leading to persisting pain states and heightened responses to stimuli. This state is called *sensitization* and has been demonstrated both peripherally and in the CNS. Hyperalgesia (the experience of severe pain in response to an uncomfortable stimulus) and allodynia (severe pain response to a nonpainful stimulus)[206] have long been recognized as sensitization states associated with sympathetic nervous system dysfunction. Microglial activation has been shown to be a factor in their development. In addition there are now many experimental models and studies showing that there is a connection between peripheral and central sensitization; psychological stress can both lead to a centrally mediated pain sensitization and enhance the peripheral effects centrally. Somatic pain and sensitized peripheral nerves and nociceptors can cause central sensitization, which further heightens the experience of pain. It is a two-way street. Clinically, it is unclear how to distinguish peripheral from central sensitization in all instances, and they can be co-occurrent.[207,208] The work of Cannon[209] and Rosenblueth *The Supersensitivity of Denervated Structures: A Law of Denervation*[210] dates back to the 1940s, but has been overlooked in the current conversations about sensitization. This work adds another dimension to this complex process.

Once the centralized process is established, there can be output from the CNS to diverse areas of the body, which helps to explain the symptom complexes of multiple seemingly disconnected systems affected by pain including muscle pain, bladder irritability, and intestinal cramps. The dysfunctions may be interconnected through central sensitization. Pharmacologic solutions for these symptom complexes have only been partially effective.

To further expand on the bidirectional nature of central pain sensitization, current clinical focus on central sensitization looks mostly at how the brain affects the body by sensitizing it to pain. But there is the other half of the equation—the influence of the body on the function of the brain. A succession of small physical injuries can accumulate and reach a tipping point resulting in pain, impairment, or disability. In these cases the onset of symptoms seems sudden and out of proportion to the stimulus. This is because once a threshold is met, the reactions are no longer linear: this can be explained by the reorganized, sensitized peripheral and central nervous system. By the time the person is symptomatic their myofascial system and nervous system have made significant accommodations and the body in pain causes changes in C-fiber excitability (called wind-up), alters function of the dorsal horn neurons, and augments nociceptive reflexes.[211] The somatosensory cortex also becomes reorganized, resulting in altered sensory perception and movement initiation and effectively creating a movement disorder.[212-214] Other reactions include cocontractions of opposing muscle groups and the loss of fine motor coordination. Movement can then become awkward, inefficient, and increasingly painful. This disorder of movement can explain muscle fatigue and exercise intolerance in chronic pain patients. How this process evolves in any one individual patient is difficult to explore because usually the injuries are in the distant past or are too subtle to be detected by usual examination and imaging techniques. There are therapists who address movement and can be very valuable as part of pain clinic treatment teams. Physical therapists Shirley Sahrmann in the United States and O'Sullivan in Australia have a robust interest in movement-based contributors to pain and using movement retraining as a treatment strategy.[215,216]

Many people in chronic pain develop fear of movement. This kinesiophobia is exacerbated by nonindividualized, formulaic practices in physical therapy that often allow for visits that are too few and too short to address the issues of maladaptive movement patterns of chronic pain patients. The difficulty of arriving at clear explanations for many pain syndromes leaves patients and practitioners uncertain and confused about whether a painful activity is harmful (pain that indicates ongoing tissue damage) or merely hurtful (painful movement that is not causing increased damage). Movement and exercise have many well-known benefits by stimulating positive changes in mood, anxiety, cardiovascular health, breathing patterns, tissue oxygenation and detoxification through sweat, improved parasympathetic and sympathetic tone, the release of endorphins and other communication molecules, increased strength, and better sleep. Exercising any part of the body affects the entire body, and movement improves patients' resilience and promotes increased neuron production and synapse formation in the brain.[217-219] The American

Physical Therapy Association recently recognized movement as a system within the body. "The human movement system comprises the anatomic structures and physiologic functions that interact to move the body or its component parts." [220]

Without proper guidance, patients who are chronically injured often accomplish movements by using unsustainable movement patterns for the task. Understanding optimal muscle recruitment patterns and the compensatory patterns that develop secondary to pain and injury may explain exercise intolerance. Therapists trained in the details of optimal muscle recruitment patterns and compensatory adaptations can teach patients to recruit and train patterns that can be sustainable over the long term, but much of standard physical therapy education does not cover this material. Ancient exercises such as yoga, tai chi, and qi gong can be useful at retraining movement patterns. The movement therapies such as Alexander, Feldenkreis, and Bartinieff techniques are also helpful. Chiropractors, osteopaths, and kinesiologists also bring experts to this area of functional restoration.

In summary, because pain augmentation and abnormal patterns of movement develop due to contributions from the central nervous system and the peripheral nervous system, and are influenced by physical and psychological factors, potential treatments can come from any of these areas, thus reinforcing the interconnectedness of the system of systems that we are. This leads us back to the Bonica model of team-based care, which draws strength from the diversity of its interprofessional team.

Everybody in Healthcare Is a Pain Practitioner—Or Should Be

Most medical visits are initiated because of a pain complaint. The most common reason that people seek out complementary and integrative medicine (CIM) and integrative practitioners also involves a pain complaint. [221] Yet pain education in medical schools has for decades been acknowledged to be inadequate. [222-225] This has led to a gap in services that in turn has led patients to seek out other types of practitioners. Another gap filled by CIM is the attention paid to whole patient [226]—body, mind, and spirit rather than just the narrow biological diagnosis, and the opportunity to address factors such as nutritional status, poorly managed stress, social supports, coping skills, ergonomics, and exercise.

We are faced with growing numbers of disabled people with pain, and the situation is financially unsustainable. The situation is perpetuated by a workforce of professionals of different disciplines that is not organized into collaborative, cooperative, interprofessional teams whose efforts are based on whatever is best for the patient. The adversarial insurance system exacerbates this problem by tying compensation for health claims and disability to particular structural abnormalities and diagnoses while denying coverage for many disciplines. Many of these disciplines are expert at coaching patients in self-care strategies, thus empowereing them to take control of their health. An internal locus of control or self-efficacy is a positive prognostic indicator for improvement.[227-228] These barriers discourage diversity in the treatment options available for complex pain problems. Shifting to team-based, interprofessional care can improve our ability to provide more diverse responses to address the complexity.

Symptom control in CIM is a positive byproduct of improving health and lifestyle changes. Self-care by the patient becomes the cornerstone, and primary care and specialty/subspecialty care practitioners all play critical roles. The complementary integrative healthcare (CIH)/CIM approaches should be "front-loaded" as soon as possible in the acute and early chronic pain phases to promote self-care and self-actualization and to avoid potential injurious medications and procedures. Patients are often pleasantly surprised to shift their focus and see themselves as a person pursuing health rather than fleeing symptoms. This shift makes primary care practices the ideal setting in which to address most pain care. The use of nonconventional CIH/CIM practices are common worldwide and even in the United States and Canada there is an increasing demand for IM care despite very poor or even no insurance reimbursement. The World Health Organization estimates that 80% of the population of the southern hemisphere receives at least part of their primary care from nonallopathic practitioners. In some first world countries the use of this type of care already exceeds 75%.[229]

Perhaps we should regard our body as we do our dental care or our cars: we need to be assessed regularly for degenerative changes and to have preventative maintenance. This shift in focus would make it easier to think of health-promoting, movement-based solutions to physical pain rather than palliative drugs and procedures. This would encourage the use of surgical repair only when there is imminent irreversible loss of function because it is only rarely effective to alleviate pain.

Case Study in CIH/CIM Approach to Chronic Pain

What do these two IM habits look like in practice? Let us look at the case of Jennifer, a 46-year-old woman with a fibromyalgia (FM) diagnosis. Six years ago, she was injured in Afghanistan while in the military. Her right arm was broken and required a plate with pins, screws, and skin grafting to treat the initial injury. After the accident, she went to physical therapy, which helped her regain her arm function, but her pain eventually got worse, despite continued sessions. She subsequently developed extreme fatigue and muscle pain in her neck, shoulders, and back. The physical therapy then seemed to be making her worse. Finally, she stopped therapy and was given her FM diagnosis, but she does not know how that diagnosis helps her. Before the accident, she had been an active runner, but now, with each passing year, she has less capacity for exercise. These days, she gets headaches and muscle cramps, does not sleep well, is tired all the time, craves sugar and starchy foods, and gets particularly sleepy after eating. She sometimes gets dizzy and sometimes has diarrhea. She also has patches of dry skin with red bumps.

She works as an accountant, but is struggling to keep her job, as her manager is no longer happy with her performance. She used to work in a toxic environment exposed to persistent organic pollutants. She also has a past history of abuse. She has stopped seeing her friends because they do not understand how ill she feels, and she hates feeling like a complainer. This has led her to feel lonely and isolated.

Her x-rays show that she has reduced lordosis in the cervical and lumbar spine. Her blood work is normal, and her gastrointestinal assessment reveals normal stool cultures and no parasites. Her physical exam reveals a normal neurological exam with no weakness, and normal reflexes. The rash has been called a "nonspecific dermatitis," and the muscle cramps come and go but are worse at night and are being called "restless leg syndrome." One of her doctors recommended a cholecystectomy even though the work-up for gall bladder disorders only showed a mildly shrunken gall bladder. She has had epidural steroid injections, facet blocks, and it has been noted that her symptoms are too widespread to respond to a spinal cord simulator. She was tried on a dozen different drugs, including several antidepressants of different classes, gabapentinoids, proton pump inhibitors (PPIs), muscle relaxants, and opioids, which made her feel drugged. She eventually stopped all of them because they did not help, and she did not like feeling sedated.

Jennifer feels frustrated with her situation and with her diagnosis, and perhaps rightfully so. The label of FM gives us very little information on how a person got to such a state, or how to help them. It does not give the clarity that some other diagnoses do, such as pneumococcal pneumonia, which provides a clear target for treatment, some insight into prognosis, and an expected trajectory for recovery. With a clear target, we can act like sharpshooters and, most of the time, the drug or procedure we pick will work. But FM is not a clear target, and adding a series of other vague diagnoses, such as central sensitization, postural orthostatic tachycardia syndrome (POTS), irritable bowel, eczema or

506 INTEGRATIVE PREVENTIVE MEDICINE

rosacea, does not make it any more of one. A drug, or two, or 10 may improve some of the symptoms listed above, but are unlikely to move this patient any closer toward health and functional restoration.

Using the two principle approaches discussed above, an IM physician would start by broadening the discussion with Jennifer past her diagnosis, and then by applying the least harmful interventions and the ones most closely aligned to Jennifer's own physiology, which will support the capacity of her body to heal itself. Box 21.2 shows Jennifer's immediate to-do list, which would be tailored in 1–2 months to fit her updated status.

Notably, most of these interventions require Jennifer's active engagement. There is no magic bullet here that will "fix" the problem. Patients have been trained to seek out medical advice looking for answers, and we in medicine have been trained to feel inadequate when we do not have those answers. In most sciences, such as engineering and physics, the scientist defines the problem before they are expected to come up with solutions. But sometimes the best we as *medical practitioners* can do is to explain to our patients that healing is a path and that, while we cannot walk it for them, we will coach, guide, encourage, and accompany them on their journey.

The management of Jennifer's FM diagnosis after her severe physical injury is only one example of an approach that works for many other types of chronic pain associated with other conditions, including post-spinal-surgery pain, headaches, chronic musculoskeletal pain from accidents, degenerative arthritis, pelvic pain, inflammatory bowel disorders, and the recent epidemic of pancreatitis, to name just a few. Even when invasive interventions and surgeries *are* necessary, approaching the patient to improve health and healing is advisable and will lead to better outcomes. Just as when building a house we need proper materials, when helping someone heal we need an understanding of the patient's physiology, resilience, and context for healing —nutritional status, physical conditioning, psychological and social stressors, the effectiveness of their circulation, and their ability to effectively excrete waste materials and environmental toxics including drugs. This is especially true with invasive procedures that are a major challenge to the body which is a homeostatic, dynamic system of systems. Efforts to improve health habits before and after procedures may improve outcomes.

This IM approach and the focus on salutogenesis require time and effort, and, in an ideal setting, integrative pain medicine is practiced with interprofessional teams that use all appropriate healthcare strategies and disciplines. In the case of chronic pain, there are many individual patient characteristics that help clarify the predisposing, precipitating, and perpetuating factors that contribute to their condition, and a broad treatment team will make it easier to address as many of those characteristics as possible. Of course, perspectives

Box 21.2

- Sleep at least 8 hours every night, which impacts mood, healing, memory, and the hypothalamic-pituitary axis.
- Begin gentle yoga stretching or tai chi and a gradual increase of exercise such as walking. Exercise improves metabolic function as well as mood and balance of the sympathetic and parasympathetic system.
- Eat an anti-inflammatory diet. Reduce caffeine, sugar, and refined foods, and move toward a whole foods, plant-based diet that includes healthy oils. Also, avoid foods that bother her.
- Stress management strategies.
- Remove chemicals from her environment, such as cleaning fluids, parabens, phthalates, pesticides, and food additives. These irritants and contaminants may interfere with the function of many systems, including the microbiome, mito-chondrial energy production, and hormone balance.
- Take Epsom salt baths, which contain magnesium that can be absorbed through the skin. Afterward, apply almond oil or coconut oil to the skin. Almond oil is anti-inflammatory.
- Take magnesium supplements according to her bowel tolerance (until she has 1–2 easy to pass bowel movements per day). Magnesium affects muscle relaxation, neurotransmitter production, and blood sugar control, and daily bowel evacua-tion releases the toxics in the bowel, both endogenously produced and from the environment.
- Drink 1–2 teaspoon(s) of apple cider vinegar before meals to improve gastric emp-tying and pancreatic enzyme secretion.
- Take vitamin D to maintain serum levels in the top third of the normal range. Vitamin D deficiency is very common in pain patients.
- Take omega-3 fish oils and turmeric, which decrease inflammation and therefore pain.
- Stop all PPIs, NSAIDs and topical steroids, as well as any other unnecessary non-life-saving drugs that only offer symptomatic relief.
- Conduct additional assessments to determine optimal use of exercise and movement-based therapies. Sleep apnea, depression, anxiety, and PTSD screen-ings are also needed.
- In the short term, some medications may be considered for relief of symptoms, especially insomnia, depression, anxiety, and PTSD. Some of these drugs only work for a short time, and there should be specific goals for starting them and a plan in place to assess their effectiveness and eventually discontinue them. Pain-modifying drugs may be considered, but it is important to remember that all drugs have metabolites and side effects. Adding a cocktail of drugs is only occasionally indicated.

- She needs to be assessed for any continuing effects of PTSD. Her history of abuse, whether family violence, verbal abuse, or sexual abuse, can have a profound influence on her overall pain experience and suffering. Her entire healthcare team will need to be aware of which factors can be triggers for her.
- Her healthcare team would have improved transparency and visibility of all that is done by and for Jennifer through a shared medical record.
- The pain team that is recommending alterations in medications that affect pain such as the NSAIDs and PPIs need to communicate with the prescribing providers.

will inevitably vary among team members; the diversity of observations and inputs, in the end, is for the patient's benefit. In addition, as integrative strategies such as nutrition- and movement-based therapies often require the patient's active engagement, the patient should be considered a member of the care team—the centerpiece of the team's focus and strategy.

Pain has been and always will be a major challenge to humanity. It has been with us since the beginning of the human experience. But its persistence and our inability to interrupt its impact on ongoing suffering and disability is because our most prevalent models of care are using limited tools. We have narrowed the aperture of our approach to pain management—especially chronic pain management—to a very narrow avenue. The current system of pain management prioritizes treatments in a therapeutic order[230]—high-impact, high-risk interventions with high rates of associated morbidity and mortality—that is counterproductive. Correcting this requires that we prioritize salutogenesis and health creation. By reserving risky drugs and interventions as last resorts, we can deliver more personalized care, achieve more sustainable results, and reduce the harm caused by the medical system.

Additionally, patients need to be active partners in a new system that takes their priorities and values into account. This system will change the implied contract with our patients, and will not allow business models to dictate the pathways of care. A resetting of priorities is in order: "If not now, when? If not you, who?"[231]

System Transformation

For acute and chronic pain to be effectively managed in a fashion that "Does Good While Not Doing Harm" there is a need for a fundamental transformation in how we conceptualize pain, how we organize our approaches to the patients' needs, the role of the patient and principal supports, the range of provider skills needed, and our business model for sustaining a new system of prevention, mitigation, and management. These changes require systemwide cultural revisions, not simply transactional modifications at the point of care delivered. This transformation to integrative pain care that brings evidence-based complementary and conventional modalities together requires a quantum leap. We must undergo a reversal of the current conceptual, clinical, and business models where nontraditional services are tried almost as an afterthought when all else has failed. Using complementary practices as a "last-ditch effort" in well-established chronic pain has seriously biased the perceived utility of these approaches.

The current system reinforces illness behavior, since every transaction is predicated on a diagnosis of some dysfunction (i.e., the ticket into the appointment is a complaint). The brief appointment times do not allow for a full exploration of the state of the person who is reduced to being a patient, who is attended by the medical expert—"the sage on the stage"—at the convenience of the system. The system is good at creating and maintaining people as "customers" in a commercial transaction, overlooking our fiduciary responsibility to serve the patient's needs without attention to material reward or betterment of the practitioner or care system. The result is that everyone suffers—the patient, the provider, the family, the community—large and small. The standard for the industry right now prioritizes administrative needs and neglects both the patients and the healthcare providers. In addition to the earlier mentioned health hazards generated by the system of medical care, nearly 50% of doctors are experiencing burnout and they kill themselves three times more often than other professionals.[232] Transformation requires that we shift away from many of the assumptions, paradigms, and systems of practice that have led us into our current problems.

EARLY SYSTEM ADOPTERS: THE VETERANS HEALTH ADMINISTRATION AND MILITARY HEALTH SYSTEM

There have been isolated examples of early adopters of integrative pain care delivered by interprofessional teams since the 1990s. But military medicine and veterans' healthcare in the United States—centering increasingly on interagency coordination through the work of groups such as the Defense and Veterans Center for Integrative Pain Management (DVCIPM)—are changing their culture with the large-scale adoption of these strategies. The recommendations of the Military Health System (MHS) Review and Veterans Health Administration (VHA) Pain Management Directive are in line with other federal pain management initiatives including the National Pain Strategy, the

IOM Report "Pain in America," and the CDC guidelines that recommend the inclusion of nontraditional health services with interprofessional teams. As in civilian medicine, chronic pain and its management have been recognized as problematic by the Department of Defense and Veterans Affairs health services. The military and VHA have been more proactive than civilian medicine in addressing the problems arising from use of opioids—lack of effectiveness with chronic use, the morbidity and mortality with high doses, and the risk of dependence, addiction, and diversion—responding with a mandate for cultural transformation within their system of care. The use in the MHS and VHA of such therapies as chiropractic, yoga, massage, acupuncture, and lifestyle coaching are recognized as vital in these communities for the treatment of pain due to the evidence basis for their effectiveness, their robust patient acceptance, and broad safety margin.

The military has adopted a tiered pain management strategy pioneered early in the VHA ("Stepped Care Model"), where initial pain management implementation strategies are coordinated within the primary care setting or Patient Centered Medical Home (PCMH).[233,234] For more complex cases there is the opportunity for comanagement in conjunction with a regional Interdisciplinary Pain Management Center (IPMC) using consultation, collaboration, and educational opportunities. While emphasis is placed on pain care being managed in the primary care setting, the system fully allows for referrals to the regional IPMC and functional restoration programs. Such a model is very dependent on adequate education of primary care providers, enhanced through the use of the Extension for Community Healthcare Outcomes (ECHO) program developed by the University of New Mexico.[235,236] Finally, there is the inclusion of nonconventional disciplines providing evidence-based approaches such as yoga, massage, music therapy, tai-chi, chiropractic, and acupuncture, in the compensation equations. These nonconventional providers who have long been told they are "bad for business" in the setting of fee for service, drug- and procedure-based medicine, are "good for business" in an accountable care setting.[237]

COLLABORATIVE PILOT PROGRAMS IN INTEGRATIVE COMPREHENSIVE PAIN MANAGEMENT

Recent attempts to explore the lessons gleaned from leading civilian integrative care programs as well as from the military and veterans care systems have employed all of the foundational elements described in the previous sections: a reconceptualization of what causes and perpetuates pain; the essential role of the patient in self-care and self-actualization; a team-based, multidisciplinary approach integrating the best of CIH/CIM with conventional pain care to tailor to the patients' unique needs; and a sustainable business model for providing care. One such effort, under the auspices of the Samueli Institute, used an Institute for Healthcare Improvement "breakthrough collaborative" approach.[238] The process began with the establishment of clear goals and patient-focused outcomes, benchmarked the initial state of achieving these goals, and then iteratively applied a learning model to launch initiatives and measure improvements—or stalled efforts—to improve desired outcomes. These and other transformational experiences reinforce the individual, site-specific nature of a successful comprehensive pain management approach and the need for organization-wide buy-in for the plan to succeed.

Conclusion

Our collective maturation and more granular understanding of the complex nature of acute and chronic pain are providing great promise for a transformational breakthrough in how pain can be prevented, mitigated, and ultimately managed. Ironically, the advent of more advanced neuroimaging, including studies that combine structure with function; of genomic and proteomic biomarker studies; and of systems analysis of the many connections that maintain the health of an individual and restore that health in the event of injury or illness has reinforced the need for a full integration of emerging technologies with proven conventional modalities and millennia-old complementary practices. But what is needed is a major overhaul in our cognitive and organizational approaches to pain care. As Albert Einstein famously observed, "We cannot solve our problems with the same thinking we used when we created them."[239]

What is apparent is that there are essential elements of this transformational effort. Beginning with the aforementioned reformulation of our notions of pain generation and the transition from acute to chronic pain, we have outlined these foundational aspects of the least elements of what must occur. Engagement of the patient as the best advocate for self-healing and preservation of health is fundamental and essential. Embracing sound healthy habits, including exercise, a nutritional diet, sleep, and assisted self-inquiry and/or observation of the individuated links between pain and its associated suffering and disability are needed. Everyone within the support system of each patient and everyone involved in providing care to the patient becomes a pain practitioner on a patient-centered, multidisciplinary team of complementary and conventional providers. All must be cognizant of the close connection between mind and body and how their effort to intervene—or disciplined withholding of intervention—contributes to relieving the suffering and comorbidity associated with pain.

The experience in military and veterans' healthcare is influencing the movement toward transformation within civilian care as well. Integral to this process is a shift in how to think of the determinants of pain in the context of overall health, how to assess or measure the effectiveness of treatments, evaluate cost-benefit ratios, and openly incorporate team-based interventions including nonconventional ones as an integral part of care rather than as an afterthought. This allows for the synergistic effects of multiple approaches and individualized care. The importance of coordinated messaging, which focuses on function and enables patient empowerment, is key to the transformation of care. Health creation is the new goal, and it cannot be achieved if we only focus on diagnoses.

We stand at a unique place in the history of the understanding, management, and relief of suffering and disability associated with one of the cardinal experiences in human life—pain. It is as important as the first synthesis of morphine, the discovery of the anesthetic properties of ether, the mapping of the somatosensory cortex and John Bonica's and Bill Fordyce's introduction of comprehensive team-based pain care. In concert with these significant milestones, the intellectual and practical requirements will necessitate a transformation in how we think, work, reward, and measure our progress. "The proper management of pain remains, after all, the most important obligation, the main objective, and the crowning achievement of every physician". . . in fact, of us all.[240]

References

1. Chödrön, Pema. *Awakening Loving-Kindness*. Shambala. 1996
2. Institute of Medicine. *To Err Is Human*. Washington, DC: National Academy of Sciences Press; 2000.
3. Starfield B. Is US health really the best in the world? *JAMA* 2000;284(4):483. doi:10.1001/jama.284.4.483.
4. James JT. A new, evidence-based estimate of patient harms associated with hospital care. *J Patient Saf* 2013;9(3):122–128.
5. Makary MA, Daniel M. Medical error—the third leading cause of death in the US. *BMJ* 2016:i2139. doi:10.1136/bmj.i2139.
6. Singh G. Gastrointestinal complications of prescription and over-the-counter non-steroidal anti-inflammatory drugs. *Am J of Ther* 2000;7(2):115–122. doi:10.1097/00045391-200007020-00008.
7. Lanas A, Garcia-Tell G, Armada B, Oteo-Alvaro A. Prescription patterns and appropriateness of NSAID therapy according to gastrointestinal risk and

cardiovascular history in patients with diagnoses of osteoarthritis. *BMC Medicine* 2011;9(1). doi:10.1186/1741-7015-9-38.

8. McGlynn EA, Asch SM, Adams J, et al. The quality of health care delivered to adults in the United States. *New Engl J Med* 2003;348(26):2635–2645. doi:10.1056/nejmsa022615.

9. Schoomaker E, Buckenmaier C. Call to action: "If not now, when? If not you, who?" *Pain Med* 2014;15(S1):S4–S6. doi:10.1111/pme.12385.

10. Hay JL, White JM, Bochner F, Somogyi AA, Semple TJ, Rounsefell B. Hyperalgesia in opioid-managed chronic pain and opioid-dependent patients. *J Pain* 2009;10(3):316–322. doi:10.1016/j.jpain.2008.10.003.

11. Volkow ND, Frieden TR, Hyde PS, Cha SS. Medication-assisted therapies— tackling the opioid-overdose epidemic. *New Engl J Med* 2014;370(22):2063–2066. doi:10.1056/nejmp1402780.

12. Manchikanti L, Helm S 2nd, Fellows B, et al. Opioid epidemic in the United States. *Pain Physician* 2012;15:ES9–ES38.

13. Alexander GC, Kruszewski SP, Webster DW. Rethinking opioid prescribing to protect patient safety and public health. *JAMA* 2012;308:1865–1866.

14. Quinones S. *Dreamland the story of America's new* opiate *epidemic:* the *true tale of America's Opiate epidemic.* United States: Bloomsbury Academic USA; 2015.

15. Deyo RA, Mirza SK, Turner JA, Martin BI. Overtreating chronic back pain: Time to back off? *J Am Board Fam Med* 2009;22(1):62–68. *Spine Journal.* 2010;10(6):568. doi:10.1016/j.spinee.2010.04.022.

16. Institute of Medicine Committee on Advancing Pain Research, Care, and Education. *Relieving Pain in America: Blueprint for Transforming Prevention, Care, Education, and Research.* Washington, DC: National Academies Press; 2011.

17. Kearns MC, Ressler KJ, Zatzick D, Rothbaum BO. Early interventions for PTSD: a review. *Depress Anxiety* 2012;29(10):833–842. doi:10.1002/da.21997.

18. https://www.spineintervention.org/?page=S5_EBM

19. Interagency Pain Research Coordinating Committee. *National Pain Strategy: A Comprehensive Population Health-Level Strategy for Pain.* Washington, DC: Department of Health and Human Services; 2015. https://iprcc.nih.gov/docs/HHSNational_Pain_Strategy.pdf; p. 16, Box 2

20. Ballantyne JC, Sullivan MD. Intensity of chronic pain: the wrong metric? *New Engl J Med* 2015;373(22):2098–2099. doi:10.1056/nejmp1507136.

21. Chou R, Turner JA, Devine EB, et al. The effectiveness and risks of long-term opioid therapy for chronic pain: a systematic review for a national institutes of health pathways to prevention workshop. *Ann Inter Med* 2015;162(4):276. doi:10.7326/m14-2559.

22. *White House Press Release on the President's Precision Medicine Initiative Release.* January 30, 2015. https://www.whitehouse.gov/the-press-office/2015/01/30/fact-sheet-president-obama-s-precision-medicine-initiative.

23. Manchikanti L, Pampati V, Falco FJ, Hirsch JA. An updated assessment of utilization of interventional pain management techniques in the Medicare population: 2000–2013. *Pain Physician* 2015 Mar–Apr;18(2):E115–27.

24. Manchikanti L, Parr A, Singh V, Fellows B. Ambulatory surgery centers and interventional techniques: a look at long-term survival. *Pain Physician* 2011;14:E177–E215.

25. Manchikanti L, Pampati V, Falco FJE, Hirsch JA. Growth of spinal interventional pain management techniques. *Spine* 2013;38(2):157–168. doi:10.1097/brs.0b013e318267f463.

26. Institute of Medicine. *Shorter Lives Poorer Health: Panel on Understanding Cross-National Health Differences Among High-Income Countries.* Washington, DC: National Academy of Sciences Press; 2013.

27. http://www.who.int/trade/glossary/story046/en/. Accessed April 26, 2016.

28. Stempniak, Marty. *The Patient Experience.* American Hospital Association's Hospitals and Health Networks. April 2013. http://www.hhnmag.com/articles/6407-the-patient-experience.

29. Institute of Medicine. *Relieving Pain in America: A Blueprint for Transforming Prevention, Care, Education, and Research.* Washington, DC: The National Academy of Sciences Press; 2011.

30. Office of the Army Surgeon General, Pain Management Task Force. *Final Report: Providing a Standardized DoD and VHA Vision and Approach to Pain Management to Optimize the Care for Warriors and Their Families.* Washington, DC: US Army; May 2010. http://www.regenesisbio.com/pdfs/journal/Pain_Management_Task_Force_Report.pdf.

31. Interagency Pain Research Coordinating Committee. *National Pain Strategy: A Comprehensive Population Health-Level Strategy for Pain.* Washington, DC: Department of Health and Human Services. 2015.https://iprcc.nih.gov/docs/HHSNational_Pain_Strategy.pdf

32. Rudd RA, Aleshire N, Zibbell JE, Gladden RM. Increases in Drug and Opioid Overdose Deaths—United States, 2000–2014. *MMWR Morb Mortal Wkly Rep* 2016 Jan 1;64(50–51):1378–1382.

33. Kuhn TS, Hacking I. *The Structure of Scientific Revolutions.* 4th ed. Chicago: University of Chicago Press; May 11, 2012.

34. https://createvalue.org/wp-content/uploads/2013/12/Berwick-Keynote-IHI-National-Forum-7Dec20111.pdf

35. Graber ML, Franklin N, Gordon R. Diagnostic error in internal medicine. *Arch Intern Med* 2005;165(13):1493. doi:10.1001/archinte.165.13.1493.

36. Mazmanian SK, Round JL, Kasper DL. A microbial symbiosis factor prevents intestinal inflammatory disease. *Nature* 2008;453(7195):620–625. doi:10.1038/nature07008.

37. Gilbert JA, Quinn RA, Debelius J, et al. Microbiome-wide association studies link dynamic microbial consortia to disease. *Nature* 2016;535(7610):94–103. doi:10.1038/nature18850.

38. Turnbaugh PJ, Ley RE, Hamady M, Fraser-Liggett CM, Knight R, Gordon JI. The human microbiome project. *Nature* 2007;449(7164):804–810. doi:10.1038/nature06244.

39. Christian LM, Galley JD, Hade EM, Schoppe-Sullivan S, Kamp Dush C, Bailey MT. Gut microbiome composition is associated with temperament during early childhood. *Brain Behav Immun* 2015;45:118–127. doi:10.1016/j.bbi.2014.10.018.

40. Blaser MJ. *Missing* Microbes: *How the Overuse of Antibiotics Is Fueling Our Modern Plagues.* New York, NY: Henry Holt; 2014.

41. National Institutes of Health. *Human Microbiome Project.* n.d. http://common-fund.nih.gov/hmp/overview. Accessed August 8, 2016.

42. Langevin HM. Connective tissue: A body-wide signaling network? *Med Hypotheses* 2006;66(6):1074–1077. doi:10.1016/j.mehy.2005.12.032.

43. Langevin HM, Churchill DL, Wu J, Badger GJ, Yandow JA, Fox JR, Krag MH. Evidence of connective tissue involvement in acupuncture. *FASEB J* 2002 Jun;16(8):872–874.

44. Krause F, Wilke J, Vogt L, Banzer W. Intermuscular force transmission along myofascial chains: a systematic review. *J Anat* 2016;228(6):910–918. doi:10.1111/joa.12464.

45. Huang KC, Huang TW, Yang TY, Lee MS. Chronic NSAIDs Use Increases the Risk of a Second Hip Fracture in Patients After Hip Fracture Surgery: Evidence From a STROBE-Compliant Population-Based Study. *Medicine (Baltimore)* 2015 Sep;94(38):e1566.

46. Sandberg O, Aspenberg P. Different effects of indomethacin on healing of shaft and metaphyseal fractures. *Acta Orthop* 2015;86(2):243–247. doi:10.3109/17453674.2014.973328.

47. Jeffcoach DR, Sams VG, Lawson CM, et al. Nonsteroidal anti-inflammatory drugs' impact on nonunion and infection rates in long-bone fractures. *J Trauma Acute Care* 2014;76(3):779–783. doi:10.1097/ta.0b013e3182aafeod.

48. Thayer JF, Sternberg E. Beyond heart rate variability: Vagal regulation of allostatic systems. *Ann NY Acad Sci* 2006;1088(1):361–372. doi:10.1196/annals.1366.014.

49. Remen RN. Practicing a medicine of the whole person: an opportunity for healing. *Hematol Oncol Clin N* 2008;22(4):767–773. doi:10.1016/j.hoc.2008.04.001.

50. Ornish D, Lin J, Daubenmier J, et al. Increased telomerase activity and comprehensive lifestyle changes: a pilot study. *Lancet Oncol* 2008;9(11):1048–1057. doi:10.1016/s1470-2045(08)70234-1.

51. Epel ES, Blackburn EH, Lin J, et al. Accelerated telomere shortening in response to life stress. *P Natl A Sci* 2004;101(49):17312–17315. doi:10.1073/pnas.0407162101.

52. Jacobs TL, Epel ES, Lin J, et al. Intensive meditation training, immune cell telomerase activity, and psychological mediators. *Psychoneuroendocrino* 2011;36(5):664–681. doi:10.1016/j.psyneuen.2010.09.010.

53. Weihs KL, Enright TM, Simmens SJ. Close relationships and emotional processing predict decreased mortality in women with breast cancer: preliminary evidence. *Psychosom Med* 2008;70(1):117–124. doi:10.1097/psy.0b013e31815c25cf.

54. Weinhold B. Epigenetics: the science of change. *Environ Health Persp* 2006;114(3):A160–A167. doi:10.1289/ehp.114-a160.

55. Simmons D. *Epigenetic Influence and Disease.* 2008.http://www.nature.com/scitable/topicpage/epigenetic-influences-and-disease-895. Accessed August 12, 2016.

56. Healthy living is the best revenge. *Arch Intern Med* 2009;169(15):1355. doi:10.1001/archinternmed.2009.237.

57. Koertge J, Weidner G, Elliott-Eller M, et al. Improvement in medical risk factors and quality of life in women and men with coronary artery disease in the multicenter lifestyle demonstration project. *Am J Cardiol* 2003;91(11):1316–1322. doi:10.1016/s0002-9149(03)00320-5.

58. Dod HS, Bhardwaj R, Sajja V, et al. Effect of intensive lifestyle changes on endothelial function and on inflammatory markers of atherosclerosis. *Am J Cardiol* 2010;105(3):362–367. doi:10.1016/j.amjcard.2009.09.038.

59. Jonas WB, Chez RA. Toward optimal healing environments in health care. *J Altern Complem Med* 2004;10(1):1–6. doi:10.1089/1075553042245818.

60. Ornish D, Magbanua MJM, Weidner G, et al. Changes in prostate gene expression in men undergoing an intensive nutrition and lifestyle intervention. *P Natl A Sci* 2008;105(24):8369–8374. doi:10.1073/pnas.0803080105.

61. Schwalfenberg GK. The alkaline diet: IS there evidence that an alkaline pH diet benefits health? *J Environ Public Health* 2012;2012:1–7. doi:10.1155/2012/727630.

62. Drake VJ. *Inflammation*. Oregon State University, Linus Pauling Institute; 2010. http://lpi.oregonstate.edu/mic/health-disease/inflammation

63. https://www.usda.gov/our-agency/about-usda

64. Light L. *What to Eat: The Ten Things You Really Need to Know to Eat Well and Be Healthy*. New York: McGraw Hill; 2006.

65. Nestle M, Michael P. *Food Politics: How the Food Industry Influences Nutrition and Health*. 1st ed., University of California Press, 2013.

66. Ng SW, Slining MM, Popkin BM. Use of caloric and noncaloric sweeteners in US consumer packaged foods, 2005–2009. *J Acad Nutr Diet* 2012;112(11):1828–1834.e6. doi:10.1016/j.jand.2012.07.009.

67. Mokdad AH. Actual causes of death in the United States, 2000. *JAMA* 2004;291(10):1238. doi:10.1001/jama.291.10.1238.

68. Estruch R, Ros E, Salas-Salvadó J, et al. Primary prevention of cardiovascular disease with a Mediterranean diet. *New Engl J Med* 2013;368(14):1279–1290. doi:10.1056/nejmoa1200303.

69. Liu H-Q, Qiu Y, Mu Y, et al. A high ratio of dietary n-3/n-6 polyunsaturated fatty acids improves obesity-linked inflammation and insulin resistance through suppressing activation of TLR4 in SD rats. *Nutr Res* 2013;33(10):849–858. doi:10.1016/j.nutres.2013.07.004.

70. Kiecolt-Glaser JK. Stress, food, and inflammation: psychoneuroimmunology and nutrition at the cutting edge. *Psychosom Med* 2010;72(4):365–369. doi:10.1097/psy.0b013e3181dbf489.

71. Ford ES, Bergmann MM, Kröger J, Schienkiewitz A, Weikert C, Boeing H. Healthy living is the best revenge: findings from the European Prospective Investigation into Cancer and Nutrition-Potsdam study. *Arch Intern Med* 2009 Aug 10;169(15):1355–1362.

72. Barnard ND, Cohen J, Jenkins DJ, et al. A low-fat vegan diet and a conventional diabetes diet in the treatment of type 2 diabetes: a randomized, controlled, 74-wk clinical trial. *Am J Clin Nutr* 2009;89(5):1588S–1596S. doi:10.3945/ajcn.2009.26736h.

73. Eves A, Gesch B. Food provision and the nutritional implications of food choices made by young adult males, in a young offenders' institution. *J Hum Nutr Diet* 2003;16(3):167–179. doi:10.1046/j.1365-277x.2003.00438.x.

74. Berkow SE, Barnard ND, Saxe GA, Ankerberg-Nobis T. Diet and survival after prostate cancer diagnosis. *Nutr Rev* 2008;65(9):391–403. doi:10.1111/j.1753-4887.2007. tb00317.x.

75. Angell M. *The Truth About Drug Companies*. Penguin Random House; 2004. New York.

76. Bronstein AC, Spyker DA, Cantilena LR Jr, Rumack BH, Dart RC. 2011 Annual report of the American Association of Poison Control Centers' National Poison Data System (NPDS): 29th Annual Report. *Clin Toxicol (Phila)* 2012 Dec;50(10):911–1164.

77. Light DW, Lexchin J, Darrow JJ. Institutional corruption of pharmaceuticals and the myth of safe and effective drugs. *J Law Med Ethics* 2013;41(3):590–600. doi:10.1111/jlme.12068.

78. https://nccih.nih.gov/health/supplements/wiseuse.htm, accessed 8/8/2016.

79. Hallett R. Intervention against smoking and its relationship to general practitioners' smoking habits. *J R Coll Gen Pract* 1983;33:565–567.

80. *How Much Sugar Do You Eat? You May Be Surprised*. New Hampshire Department of Health and Human Services. https://www.google.com/search?q=how+much+sugar+do+you+eat&ie=utf-8&oe=utf-8Accessed 8/13/2016.

81. Campbell TC. *The Mystique of Protein and Its Implications*. Ithaca, NY: T. Colin Campbell Center for Nutrition Studies; 2014. http://nutritionstudies.org/mystique-of-protein-implications/ Accessed August 12, 2016.

82. de Punder K, Pruimboom L. The dietary intake of wheat and other cereal grains and their role in inflammation. *Nutrients* 2013;5(3):771–787. doi:10.3390/nu5030771.

83. Willett W. *Eat, Drink and Be Healthy: The Harvard Medical School Guide to Healthy Eating*. New York: Simon & Schuster; 2001.

84. Environmental Working Group. www.ewg.org.

85. Egger G. In search of a germ theory equivalent for chronic disease. *Prev Chronic Dis* 2012;9:E95. Epub 2012 May 10.

86. Minihane AM, Vinoy S, Russell WR, et al. Low-grade inflammation, diet composition and health: current research evidence and its translation. *Brit J Nutr* 2015;114(7):999–1012. doi:10.1017/S0007114515002093.

87. Barclay A, Petocz P, McMillan-Price J, et al. CD1-1 glycemic index, glycemic load and diabetes risk: a meta-analysis. *Diabetes Res Clin Pr* 2008;79:S30–S31. doi:10.1016/s0168-8227(08)70722-8.

88. Moss M. *Salt Sugar Fat: How the Food Giants Hooked Us*. New York: Random House; 2014; Paperback edition.

89. Schwalfenberg GK. The alkaline diet: is there evidence that an alkaline pH diet benefits health? *J Environ Public Health* 2012;2012:1–7. doi:10.1155/2012/727630.

90. Marcus NJ, Mense S. Muscle pain: pathophysiology, evaluation and treatment. In: Bajwa ZH, Wooten J, Warfield CA, eds. *Principles and Practice of Pain Medicine*. (3rd ed.). 2017; McGraw Hill Education, ISBN 978-0-07-176683-8.

91. National Institutes of Health. *Human Microbiome Project*. Bethesda, MD: Author; 2013. http://commonfund.nih.gov/hmp/overview. Accessed July 27, 2016.

92. Wenner M. Humans carry more bacterial cells than human ones. New York: *Nature Publishing Group*; 2007. http://www.scientificamerican.com/article/strange-but-true-humans-carry-more-bacterial-cells-than-human-ones/.

93. King T, Elia M, Hunter J. Abnormal colonic fermentation in irritable bowel syndrome. *Lancet* 1998;352(9135):1187–1189. doi:10.1016/s0140-6736(98)02146-1.

94. Yang YX, Metz DC. Safety of proton pump inhibitor exposure. *Gastroenterology* 2010;139(4):1115–1127. doi:10.1053/j.gastro.2010.08.023.

95. Russell RM, Golner BB, Krasinski SD. Effect of antacid and H2 receptor antagonists on the intestinal absorption of folic acid. *J Lab Clin Med* 1988;112:458–463.

96. Sturniolo GC, Montino MC, Rossetto L, et al. Inhibition of gastric acid secretion reduces zinc absorption in man. *J Am Coll Nutr* 1991;10(4):372–375. doi:10.1080/07315724.1991.10718165.

97. Karadima V, Kraniotou C, Bellos G, Tsangaris GT. Drug-micronutrient interactions: food for thought and thought for action. *EPMA J* 2016;7(1). doi:10.1186/s13167-016-0059-1.

98. Schatz RA, Zhang Q, Lodhia N, Shuster J, Toskes PP, Moshiree B. Predisposing factors for positive D-xylose breath test for evaluation of small intestinal bacterial overgrowth: a retrospective study of 932 patients. *World J Gastroenterol* 2015;21(15):4574–4582. doi: 10.3748/wjg.v21.i15.4574.

99. Folkers K, Langsjoen P, Willis R, et al. Lovastatin decreases coenzyme Q levels in humans. *P Natl A Sci* 1990;87(22):8931–8934. doi:10.1073/pnas.87.22.8931.

100. Rogers GB. Germs and joints: the contribution of the human microbiome to rheumatoid arthritis. *Nat Med* 2015;21(8):839–841. doi:10.1038/nm.3916.

101. Tejesvi MV, Arvonen M, Kangas SM, et al. Faecal microbiome in new-onset juvenile idiopathic arthritis. *Eur J Clin Microbiol* 2015;35(3):363–370. doi:10.1007/s10096-015-2548-x.

102. Yang YX, Metz DC. Safety of proton pump inhibitor exposure. *Gastroenterology* 2010;139(4):1115–1127. doi:10.1053/j.gastro.2010.08.023.

103. Fairfield KM, Fletcher RH. Vitamins for chronic disease prevention in adults. *JAMA* 2002;287(23):3116. doi:10.1001/jama.287.23.3116.

104. Bronstein AC, Spyker DA, Cantilena LR, Green JL, Rumack BH, Dart RC. 2010 annual report of the American association of poison control centers' national poison data system (NPDS): 28th annual report. *Clin Toxicol* 2011;49(10):910–941. doi:10.3109/15563650.2011.635149.

105. USUHS Consortium for Health And Military Performance (CHAMP)'s Human Performance Resource Center (HPRC) and Operation Supplement Safety (OPSS).

106. http://hprc-online.org/dietary-supplements/opss/operation-supplement-safety-OPSS/high-risk-supplement-list. Accessed August 10, 2016.

107. https://nccih.nih.gov/news/alerts. Accessed July 31, 2016.

108. http://www.vox.com/a/supplements/the-hidden-drugs-in-your-favorite-supplements. Accessed July 31, 2016.

109. Alerts and Advisories. https://nccih.nih.gov/news/alerts, Accessed July 27, 2016.

110. http://www.usp.org/dietary-supplements/overview. Accessed July 27, 2016.

111. National Center for Complementary and Alternative Medicine. *Dietary and Herbal Supplements.* Bethesda MD: National Center for Complementary and Alternative Medicine (NCCAM); 2013. http://nccam.nih.gov/health/supplements. Accessed July 31, 2016.

112. Johnson RL, Foster S, Lowdog T, Kiefer D. *National Geographic Guide to Medicinal Herbs: The World's Most Effective Healing Plants.* Washington, DC: National Geographic Society; 2012.

113. Tick H. *Holistic Pain Relief.* Novato, CA: New World Library; 2013.

114. Sullivan MD, Howe CQ. Opioid therapy for chronic pain in the United States: promises and perils. *Pain* 2013;154:S94–S100. doi:10.1016/j.pain.2013.09.009.

115. Chou R, Turner JA, Devine EB, et al. The effectiveness and risks of long-term opioid therapy for chronic pain: a systematic review for a national institutes of health pathways to prevention workshop. *Ann Intern Med* 2015;162(4):276. doi:10.7326/m14-2559.

116. Holick MF. Vitamin D deficiency. *New Engl J Med* 2007;357(3):266–281. doi:10.1056/nejmra070553.

117. Melamed ML, Michos ED, Post W, Astor B. 25-Hydroxyvitamin D levels and the risk of mortality in the general population. *Arch Intern Med* 2008;168(15):1629–1637. doi:10.1001/archinte.168.15.1629.

118. Plotnikoff GA, Quigley JM. Prevalence of severe hypovitaminosis D in patients with persistent, nonspecific musculoskeletal pain. *Mayo Clin Proc* 2003;78(12):1463–1470. doi:10.4065/78.12.1463.

119. Macfarlane GJ. An excess of widespread pain among south Asians: are low levels of vitamin D implicated? *Ann Rheum Dis* 2005;64(8):1217–1219. doi:10.1136/ard.2004.032656.

120. Al Faraj S, Al Mutairi K. Vitamin D deficiency and chronic low back pain in Saudi Arabia. *Spine* 2003;28(2):177–179. doi:10.1097/00007632-200301150-00015.

121. de Torrente de la Jara G. Musculoskeletal pain in female asylum seekers and hypovitaminosis D3. *BMJ* 2004;329(7458):156–157. doi:10.1136/bmj.329.7458.156.

122. Grimaldi AS, Parker BA, Capizzi JA, et al. 25(OH) vitamin D is associated with greater muscle strength in healthy men and women. *Med Sci Sport Exer* 2013;45(1):157–162. doi:10.1249/mss.0b013e31826c9a78.

123. Holick MF. Vitamin D deficiency. *New Engl J Med* 2007;357(3):266–281. doi:10.1056/nejmra070553.

124. Ramsden CE, Mann JD, Faurot KR, et al. Low omega-6 vs. Low omega-6 plus high omega-3 dietary intervention for chronic daily headache: protocol for a randomized clinical trial. *Trials* 2011;12(1). doi:10.1186/1745-6215-12-97.

125. Ramsden CE, Faurot KR, Zamora D, et al. Targeted alteration of dietary n-3 and n-6 fatty acids for the treatment of chronic headaches: a randomized trial. *Pain* 2013;154(11):2441–2451. doi:10.1016/j.pain.2013.07.028.

126. Lee YH, Bae SC, Song GG. Omega-3 polyunsaturated fatty acids and the treatment of rheumatoid arthritis: a meta-analysis. *Arch Med Res* 2012;43(5):356–362.

127. Goldberg RJ, Katz J. A meta-analysis of the analgesic effects of omega-3 polyunsaturated fatty acid supplementation for inflammatory joint pain. *Pain* 2007;129(1–2):210–223.

128. Maroon JC, Bost JW. Omega-3 fatty acids (fish oil) as an anti-inflammatory: an alternative to nonsteroidal anti-inflammatory drugs for discogenic pain. *Surg Neurol* 2006;65(4):326–331.

129. Ferrari LF, Levine JD. Alcohol consumption enhances antiretroviral painful peripheral neuropathy by mitochondrial mechanisms. *Eur J Neurosci* 2010;32(5):811–818. doi:10.1111/j.1460-9568.2010.07355.x.

130. Joseph EK, Levine JD. Mitochondrial electron transport in models of neuropathic and inflammatory pain. *Pain* 2006;121(1):105–114. doi:10.1016/j.pain.2005.12.010.

131. Kim HK, Park SK, Zhou J-L, et al. Reactive oxygen species (ROS) play an important role in a rat model of neuropathic pain. *Pain* 2004;111(1):116–124. doi:10.1016/j.pain.2004.06.008.

132. Joseph EK, Levine JD. Caspase signalling in neuropathic and inflammatory pain in the rat. *Eur J Neurosci* 2004;20(11):2896–2902. doi:10.1111/j.1460-9568.2004.03750.x.

133. Shin CY, Shin J, Kim B-M, et al. Essential role of mitochondrial permeability transition in vanilloid receptor 1-dependent cell death of sensory neurons. *Mol Cell Neurosci* 2003;24(1):57–68. doi:10.1016/s1044-7431(03)00121-0.

134. Morris G, Berk M, Galecki P, Walder K, Maes M. The neuro-immune pathophysiology of central and peripheral fatigue in systemic immune-inflammatory and neuro-immune diseases. *Mol Neurobiol* 2015;53(2):1195–1219. doi:10.1007/s12035-015-9090-9.

135. Neustadt J, Pieczenik SR. Medication-induced mitochondrial damage and disease. *Mol Nutr Food Res* 2008;52(7):780–788. doi:10.1002/mnfr.200700075.

136. Myhill S, Booth N, McLaren-Howard J. Targeting mitochondrial dysfunction in the treatment of Myalgic Encephalomyelitis/Chronic Fatigue Syndrome (ME/CFS)—a clinical audit. *Int J Clin Exp Med* 2013;6(1):1–15. http://www.ijcem.com/ISSN:1940-5901/IJCEM1207003. Accessed November 28, 2016.

137. Mauro GL, Martorana U, Cataldo P, et al. Vitamin B12 in low back pain: a randomised, double-blind, placebo-controlled study. *Eur Rev Med Pharmacol Sci* 2000;4(3):53–58.

138. Vogiatzoglou A, Refsum H, Johnston C, et al. Vitamin B12 status and rate of brain volume loss in community-dwelling elderly. *Neurology* 2008;71(11):826–832. doi:10.1212/01.wnl.0000325581.26991.f2.

139. Carmel R. Biomarkers of cobalamin (vitamin B-12) status in the epidemiologic setting: a critical overview of context, applications, and performance characteristics of cobalamin, methylmalonic acid, and holotranscobalamin II. *Am J Clin Nutr* 2011;94(1):348S–358S. doi:10.3945/ajcn.111.013441.

140. Goodman M, Chen XH. Are U.S. lower normal B12 limits too low? *J Am Geriatr Soc* 1996;44(10):1274–1275. doi:10.1111/j.1532-5415.1996.tb01389.x.

141. *Vitamin C.* Corvalis: Oregon State University, Linus Pauling Institute; 2013. http://lpi.oregonstate.edu/mic/vitamins/vitamin-C. Accessed July 13, 2016.

142. Stone I. Homo sapiens ascorbicus: a biologically corrected robust human mutant. *Med Hypotheses* 1979;5:711–722.

143. Whang R. Magnesium deficiency: pathogenesis, prevalence, and clinical implications. *Am J Med*1987;82(3):24–29. doi:10.1016/0002-9343(87)90129-x.

144. *Magnesium.* Linus Pauling Institute; 2016. http://lpi.oregonstate.edu/infocenter/minerals/magnesium/. Accessed August 10, 2016.

145. Seelig M. Cardiovascular consequences of magnesium deficiency and loss: pathogenesis, prevalence and manifestations: magnesium and chloride loss in refractory potassium repletion. *Am J Cardiol* 1989;63(14):G4–G21. doi:10.1016/0002-9149(89)90213-0.

146. Rondón LJ, Privat AM, Daulhac L, et al. Magnesium attenuates chronic hypersensitivity and spinal cord NMDA receptor phosphorylation in a rat model of diabetic neuropathic pain. *J Physiol* 2010;588(21):4205–4215. doi:10.1113/jphysiol.2010.197004.

147. Kim DJ, Xun P, Liu K, et al. Magnesium intake in relation to systemic inflammation, insulin resistance, and the incidence of diabetes. *Diabetes Care* 2010;33(12):2604–2610. doi:10.2337/dc10-0994.

148. Demirkaya S, Vural O, Dora B, Topcuoglu MA. Efficacy of intravenous magnesium sulfate in the treatment of acute migraine attacks. *Headache: J Head and Face Pain* 2001;41(2):171–177. doi:10.1046/j.1526-4610.2001.111006171.x.

149. Murakami K, Sasaki S, Okubo H, Takahashi Y, Hosoi Y, Itabashi M. Association between dietary fiber, water and magnesium intake and functional constipation among young Japanese women. *Eur J Clin Nutr* 2007;61(5):616–622.

150. Nielsen FH, et al. Magnesium supplementation improves indicators of low magnesium status and inflammatory stress in adults older than 51 years with poor quality sleep. *Magnes Res* 2010;23(4):158–168.

151. Brill S, Sedgwick PM, Hamann W, di Vadi PP. Efficacy of intravenous magnesium in neuropathic pain. *Brit J Anaesth* 2002;89(5):711–714. doi:10.1093/bja/89.5.711.

152. Sui B, Xu T, Liu J, et al. Understanding the role of mitochondria in the pathogenesis of chronic pain. *Postgrad Med J* 2013;89(1058):709–714. doi:10.1136/postgradmedj-2012-131068.

153. Ames BN, Shigenaga MK, Hagen TM. Oxidants, antioxidants, and the degenerative diseases of aging. *P Natl A Sci* 1993;90(17):7915–7922. doi:10.1073/pnas.90.17.7915.

154. Morris G, Berk M, Walder K, Maes M. Central pathways causing fatigue in neuroinflammatory and autoimmune illnesses. *BMC Med* 2015;13(1):28. doi:10.1186/s12916-014-0259-2.

155. Marí M, Morales A, Colell A, García-Ruiz C, Fernández-Checa JC. Mitochondrial glutathione, a key survival antioxidant. *Antioxid Redox Sign* 2009;11(11):2685–2700. doi:10.1089/ars.2009.2695.

156. Rimm EB. Folate and vitamin B6 from diet and supplements in relation to risk of coronary heart disease among women. *JAMA* 1998;279(5):359. doi:10.1001/jama.279.5.359.

157. Zheng LQ, Zhang HL, Guan ZH, Hu MY, Zhang T, Ge SJ. Elevated serum homocysteine level in the development of diabetic peripheral neuropathy. *Genet Mol Res* 2015;14(4):15365–15375. doi:10.4238/2015.november.30.14.

158. Övey İS, Nazıroğlu M. Homocysteine and cytosolic GSH depletion induce apoptosis and oxidative toxicity through cytosolic calcium overload in the

hippocampus of aged mice: Involvement of TRPM2 and TRPV1 channels. *Neuroscience* 2015;284:225–233. doi:10.1016/j.neuroscience.2014.09.078.

159. Merchant AT, Hu FB, Spiegelman D, Willett WC, Rimm EB, Ascherio A. The use of B vitamin supplements and peripheral arterial disease risk in men are inversely related. *J Nutr* 2003;133(9):2863–2867.

160. Areti A, Yerra V, Komirishetty P, Kumar A. Potential therapeutic benefits of main-taining mitochondrial health in peripheral neuropathies. *Curr Neuropharmacol* 2016;14(6):593–609. doi:10.2174/1570159x14666151126215358.

161. Alidoost F, Gharagozloo M, Bagherpour B, et al. Effects of silymarin on the proliferation and glutathione levels of peripheral blood mononuclear cells from β-thalassemia major patients. *Int Immunopharmacol* 2006;6(8):1305–1310. doi:10.1016/j.intimp.2006.04.004.

162. Soto C, Recoba R, Barrón H, Alvarez C, Favari L. Silymarin increases antioxi-dant enzymes in alloxan-induced diabetes in rat pancreas. *Comp Biochem Phys C* 2003;136(3):205–212. doi:10.1016/s1532-0456(03)00214-x.

163. Luangchosiri C, Thakkinstian A, Chitphuk S, Stitchantrakul W, Petraksa S, Sobhonslidsuk A. A double-blinded randomized controlled trial of silymarin for the prevention of antituberculosis drug-induced liver injury. *BMC Complem Altern M* 2015;15(1):334. doi:10.1186/s12906-015-0861-7.

164. Lauterburg BH, Corcoran GB, Mitchell JR. Mechanism of action of N-acetylcysteine in the protection against the hepatotoxicity of acetaminophen in rats in vivo. *J Clin Invest* 1983;71(4):980–991. doi:10.1172/jci110853.

165. Munnich A, Rustin P. Clinical spectrum and diagnosis of mitochondrial disor-ders. *Am J Med Genet* 2001;106(1):4–17. doi:10.1002/ajmg.1391.

166. Neustadt J, Pieczenik SR. Medication-induced mitochondrial damage and dis-ease. *Mol Nutr Food Res* 2008;52(7):780–788. doi:10.1002/mnfr.200700075.

167. Amacher D. Drug-associated mitochondrial toxicity and its detection. *Curr Med Chem* 2005;12(16):1829–1839. doi:10.2174/0929867054546663.

168. Marriage BJ, Clandinin MT, Macdonald IM, Glerum DM. Cofactor treatment improves ATP synthetic capacity in patients with oxidative phosphorylation disorders. *Mol Genet Metab* 2004;81(4):263–272. doi:10.1016/j.ymgme.2003.12.008.

169. Bartels EM, Folmer VN, Bliddal H, et al. Efficacy and safety of ginger in osteo-arthritis patients: a meta-analysis of randomized placebo-controlled trials. *Osteoarthr Cartilage* 2015;23(1):13–21. doi:10.1016/j.joca.2014.09.024.

170. Terry R, Posadzki P, Watson LK, Ernst E. The use of ginger (Zingiber officinale) for the treatment of pain: a systematic review of clinical trials. *Pain Med* 2011;12(12):1808–1818. doi:10.1111/j.1526-4637.2011.01261.x.

171. Lantz RC, Chen GJ, Sarihan M, Sólyom AM, Jolad SD, Timmermann BN. The effect of extracts from ginger rhizome on inflammatory mediator production. *Phytomedicine* 2007;14(2-3):123–128. doi:10.1016/j.phymed.2006.03.003.

172. Kuptniratsaikul V, Thanakhumtorn S, Chinswangwatanakul P, Wattanamongkonsil L, Thamlikitkul V. Efficacy and safety of Curcuma domestica extracts in patients with knee osteoarthritis. *J Altern Complem Med* 2009;15(8):891–897. doi:10.1089/acm.2008.0186.

173. Jurenka JS. Anti-inflammatory properties of curcumin, a major constituent of Curcuma longa: a review of preclinical and clinical research. *Altern Med Rev* 2009;14(2):141–153.

174. Hucklenbroich J, Klein R, Neumaier B, et al. Aromatic-turmerone induces neural stem cell proliferation in vitro and in vivo. *Stem Cell Res Ther* 2014;5(4):100. doi: 10.1186/scrt500.

175. Altman RD, Marcussen KC. Effects of a ginger extract on knee pain in patients with osteoarthritis. *Arthritis Rheum* 2001;44(11):2531–2538. doi:10.1002/1529-0131(200111)44:11<2531::aid-art433>3.0.co;2-j.

176. Agarwal KA, Tripathi CD, Agarwal BB, Saluja S. Efficacy of turmeric (curcumin) in pain and postoperative fatigue after laparoscopic cholecystectomy: a double-blind, randomized placebo-controlled study. *Surg Endosc* 2011;25(12):3805–3810. doi:10.1007/s00464-011-1793-z.

177. Kuptniratsaikul V, Thanakhumtorn S, Chinswangwatanakul P, Wattanamongkonsil L, Thamlikitkul V. Efficacy and safety of Curcuma domestica extracts in patients with knee osteoarthritis. *J Altern Complem Med* 2009;15(8):891–897. doi:10.1089/acm.2008.0186.

178. Duke JA. The garden pharmacy: turmeric, the queen of COX-2-inhibitors. *Alternative Complem Ther* 2007;13(5):229–234. doi:10.1089/act.2007.13503.

179. Valério DA, Georgetti SR, Magro DA, et al. Quercetin reduces inflammatory pain: inhibition of oxidative stress and cytokine production. *J Nat Prod* 2009;72(11):1975–1979. doi:10.1021/np900259y.

180. Towheed T, Maxwell L, Anastassiades TP, et al. Glucosamine therapy for treating osteoarthritis. *Cochrane DB Syst Rev* 2005;2: CD002946. doi: 10.1002/14651858. CD002946.pub2.

181. Mokdad AH. Actual causes of death in the United States, 2000. *JAMA* 2004;291(10):1238. doi:10.1001/jama.291.10.1238.

182. Marchand F, Perretti M, McMahon SB. Role of the immune system in chronic pain. *Nat Rev Neurosci* 2005;6(7):521–532. doi:10.1038/nrn1700.

183. Lerner A, Matthias T. Changes in intestinal tight junction permeability associated with industrial food additives explain the rising incidence of autoimmune disease. *Autoimmun Rev* 2015;14(6):479–489. doi:10.1016/j.autrev.2015.01.009.

184. Louveau A, Harris TH, Kipnis J. Revisiting the mechanisms of CNS immune privilege. *Trends Immunol* 2015;36(10):569–577. doi:10.1016/j.it.2015.08.006.

185. Perkins NM, Tracey DJ. Hyperalgesia due to nerve injury: role of neutrophils. *Neuroscience* 2000;101(3):745–757. doi:10.1016/s0306-4522(00)00396-1.

186. Marchand F, Perretti M, McMahon SB. Role of the immune system in chronic pain. *Nat Rev Neurosci* 2005;6(7):521–532. doi:10.1038/nrn1700.

187. Bridges CC, Zalups RK. Molecular and ionic mimicry and the transport of toxic metals. *Toxicol Appl Pharm* 2005;204(3):274–308. doi:10.1016/j.taap.2004.09.007.

188. Gladwell M. *Blink: The Power of Thinking Without Thinking*. New York and Boston: Back Bay Books, Little Brown; 2007:69.

189. *Pert C. Candace, PhD*. Website. http://candacepert.com. Accessed August 5, 2016.

190. Rubik B, Muehsam D, Hammerschlag R, Jain S. Biofield science and healing: history, terminology, and concepts. *Global Adv Health and Med* 2015;4(Suppl):8–14. doi:10.7453/gahmj.2015.038.suppl.

191. Jain S, Hammerschlag R, Mills P, et al. Clinical studies of biofield therapies: summary, methodological challenges, and recommendations. *Global Adv Health and Med* 2015;4(Suppl):58–66. doi:10.7453/gahmj.2015.034.suppl.

192. Thayer JF, Sternberg E. Beyond heart rate variability: vagal regulation of allostatic systems. *Ann NY Acad Sci* 2006;1088(1):361–372. doi:10.1196/annals.1366.014.

193. Sapolsky R. *Why Zebras Don't Get Ulcers: A Guide to Stress, Stress-Related Diseases, and Coping.* New York, NY: Henry Holt; 2004.

194. Kabat-Zinn J, Lipworth L, Burney R. The clinical use of mindfulness meditation for the self-regulation of chronic pain. *J Behav Med* 1985;8(2):163–190. doi:10.1007/bf00845519.

195. Cherkin DC, Sherman KJ, Balderson BH, et al. Effect of mindfulness-based stress reduction vs cognitive behavioral therapy or usual care on back pain and functional limitations in adults with chronic low back pain. *JAMA* 2016;315(12):1240. doi:10.1001/jama.2016.2323.

196. Cash E et al. Mindfulness meditation alleviates fibromyalgia symptoms in women: results of a randomized clinical trial. *Ann Behav Med* 2015;49(3):319–330. doi: 10.1007/s12160-014-9665-0.

197. Chiesa A, Serretti A. Mindfulness-based stress reduction for stress management in healthy people: a review and meta-analysis. *J Altern Complem Med* 2009;15(5):593–600. doi:10.1089/acm.2008.0495.

198. Morone NE, Greco CM, Weiner DK. Mindfulness meditation for the treatment of chronic low back pain in older adults: a randomized controlled pilot study. *Pain* 2008;134(3):310–319. doi:10.1016/j.pain.2007.04.038.

199. Schmidt S, Grossman P, Schwarzer B, Jena S, Naumann J, Walach H. Treating fibromyalgia with mindfulness-based stress reduction: Results from a 3-armed randomized controlled tria. *Pain* 2011;152(2):361–369. doi:10.1016/j.pain.2010.10.043.

200. McCubbin T. Mindfulness-based stress reduction in an integrated care delivery system: one-year impacts on patient-centered outcomes and health care utilization. *Permanente Journal* November 2014:4–9. doi:10.7812/tpp/14-014.

201. Kimbrough E, Lao L, Berman B, Pelletier KR, Talamonti WJ. An integrative medicine intervention in a Ford motor company assembly plant. *J Occup Environ Med* 2010;52(3):256–257. doi:10.1097/jom.0b013e3181d09884.

202. Epel ES, Blackburn EH, Lin J, et al. Accelerated telomere shortening in response to life stress. *P Natl A Sci* 2004;101(49):17312–17315. doi:10.1073/pnas.0407162101.

203. Jacobs TL, Epel ES, Lin J, Blackburn EH, Wolkowitz OM, Bridwell DA, et al. Intensive meditation training, immune cell telomerase activity, and psychological mediators. *Psychoneuroendocrinol* 2011;36:664–681.

204. Kaptchuk TJ, Friedlander E, Kelley JM, et al. Placebos without deception: a randomized controlled trial in irritable bowel syndrome. *PLoS One* 2010;5(12):e15591. doi:10.1371/journal.pone.0015591.

205. Paolicelli RC, Gross CT. Microglia in development: linking brain wiring to brain environment. *Neuron Glia Biol* 2011;7(01):77–83. doi:10.1017/s1740925x12000105.
206. Marchand F, Perretti M, McMahon SB. Role of the immune system in chronic pain. *Nat Rev Neurosci* 2005;6(7):521–532. doi:10.1038/nrn1700.
207. Sigfried Mense, personal communication.
208. Chen X, Green PG, Levine JD. Stress enhances muscle nociceptor activity in the rat. *Neuroscience* 2011;185:166–173. doi:10.1016/j.neuroscience.2011.04.020.
209. Walter Bradford Cannon, Chair of the Department of Physiology at Harvard Medicial School. http://hms.harvard.edu/departments/medical-education/student-services/academic-societies-hms/walter-bradford-cannon-society/walter-bradford-cannon. Accessed July 31, 2016.
210. Cannon WB, Rosenbluth A. *The Supersensitivity of Denervated Structures.* New York, NY: MacMillan; 1949.
211. Gold MS, Gebhart GF. Nociceptor sensitization in pain pathogenesis. *Nat Med* 2010;16(11):1248–1257. doi:10.1038/nm.2235.
212. Coq J-O, Barr AE, Strata F, et al. Peripheral and central changes combine to induce motor behavioral deficits in a moderate repetition task. *Exp Neurol* 2009;220(2):234–245. doi:10.1016/j.expneurol.2009.08.008.
213. Napadow V, Liu J, Li M, et al. Somatosensory cortical plasticity in carpal tunnel syndrome treated by acupuncture. *Hum Brain Mapp* 2006;28(3):159–171. doi:10.1002/hbm.20261.
214. Dhond RP, Ruzich E, Witzel T, et al. Spatio-temporal mapping cortical neuroplasticity in carpal tunnel syndrome. *Brain* 2012;135(10):3062–3073. doi:10.1093/brain/aws233.
215. Sahrmann S. *Diagnosis and Treatment of Movement Impairment Syndromes.* Philadelphia, PA: Mosby; 2013.
216. O'Sullivan P. It's time for change with the management of non-specific chronic low back pain. *Brit J Sport Med* 2011;46(4):224–227. doi:10.1136/bjsm.2010.081638.
217. Voss MW, Vivar C, Kramer AF, van Praag H. Bridging animal and human models of exercise-induced brain plasticity. *Trends Cogn Sci* 2013;17(10):525–544. doi:10.1016/j.tics.2013.08.001.
218. Kramer AF, Hahn S, Cohen NJ, et al. Ageing, fitness and neurocognitive function. *Nature* 1999;400(6743):418–419. doi:10.1038/22682.
219. Gill SJ, Friedenreich CM, Sajobi TT, et al. Association between lifetime physical activity and cognitive functioning in middle-aged and older community dwelling adults: Results from the brain in motion study. *J Int Neuropsych Soc* 2015;21(10):816–830. doi:10.1017/s1355617715000880.
220. http://www.apta.org/MovementSystem/. Accessed July 17, 2016.
221. Nahin RL, Barnes PM, Stussman BJ, Bloom B. Costs of complementary and alternative medicine (CAM) and frequency of visits to CAM practitioners: United States, 2007. *Natl Health Stat Report* 2009 Jul 30;(18):1–14.
222. Mezei L, Murinson BB. Pain education in north American medical schools. *J Pain* 2011;12(12):1199–1208. doi:10.1016/j.jpain.2011.06.006.

223. Watt-Watson J, McGillion M, Hunter J, et al. A survey of prelicensure pain curricula in health science faculties in Canadian universities. *Pain Res Manag* 2009;14(6):439–444. doi:10.1155/2009/307932.

224. Loeser JD. Five crises in pain management. *Pain Clin Updates* 2012;20:1–4.

225. Tauben DJ, Loeser JD. Pain education at the university of Washington school of medicine. *J Pain* 2013;14(5):431–437. doi:10.1016/j.jpain.2013.01.005.

226. Rakel D, Weil A. Philosophy of integrative medicine. In: Rakel D, ed. *Integrative Medicine*. 3rd ed. Philadelphia: Elsevier; 2011:2–11.

227. Turner JA, Anderson ML, Balderson BH, Cook AJ, Sherman KJ, Cherkin DC. Mindfulness-based stress reduction and cognitive behavioral therapy for chronic low back pain: similar effects on mindfulness, catastrophizing, self-efficacy, and acceptance in a randomized controlled trial. *Pain* 2016 Nov;157(11):2434–2444.

228. Cherkin DC, Sherman KJ, Balderson BH, et al. Effect of mindfulness-based stress reduction vs cognitive behavioral therapy or usual care on back pain and functional limitations in adults with chronic low back pain. *JAMA* 2016;315(12):1240. doi:10.1001/jama.2016.2323.

229. World Health Organization. *WHO Launches the First Global Strategy on Traditional and Alternative Medicine*. Geneva: World Health Organization; 2002. www.who.int/mediacentre/news/releases/release38/en/. Accessed July 30, 2016.

230. Zeff JL, Snider P, Myers S, DeGrandpre Z. A hierarchy of healing: the therapeutic order: a unifying theory of naturopathic medicine. In: Pizzorno JE, Murray M, eds. *Textbook of Natural Medicine*. Livingston, MO: Churchill; 2013:18–33.

231. Schoomaker E, Buckenmaier C. Call to action: "If not now, when? If not you, who?" *Pain Med* 2014;15(S1):S4–S6. doi:10.1111/pme.12385.

232. Shanafelt TD, Hasan O, Dyrbye LN, Sinsky C, Satele D, Sloan J, West CP. Changes in Burnout and Satisfaction With Work-Life Balance in Physicians and the General US Working Population Between 2011 and 2014. *Mayo Clin Proc* 2015 Dec;90(12):1600–1613.

233. Dobscha SK, Corson K, Perrin NA, et al. Collaborative care for chronic pain in primary care. *JAMA* 2009;301(12):1242. doi:10.1001/jama.2009.377.

234. Von Korff M. Stepped care for back pain: activating approaches for primary care. *Ann Intern Med* 2001;134(9 Part 2):911. doi:10.7326/0003-4819-134-9_part_2-200105011-00016.

235. Arora S, Thornton K, Murata G, et al. Outcomes of treatment for hepatitis C virus infection by primary care providers. *New Engl J Med* 2011;364(23):2199–2207. doi:10.1056/nejmoa1009370.

236. Katzman JG, Comerci G, Boyle JF, et al. Innovative telementoring for pain management: project ECHO pain. *J Contin Educ Health* 2014;34(1):68–75. doi:10.1002/chp.21210.

237. Herman PM, Poindexter BL, Witt CM, Eisenberg, DM. Are complementary therapies and integrative care cost-effective? A systematic review of economic evaluations. *BMJ Open* 2012:2(5). Piie001046. PMID 22945962.

238. http://samueliinstituteblog.org/collaborative-focus-pain-management/#more-974. Accessed August 4, 2016.
239. http://www.brainyquote.com/quotes/quotes/a/alberteins121993.html
240. Bonica J. *The Management of Pain*. 1st ed. 1954. https://www.amazon.com/Management-Pain-Analgesic-Diagnosis-Prognosis/dp/B0000CIPHO/ref=sr_1_1?ie=UTF8&qid=1498758858&sr=8-1&keywords=Bonica+J.+The+Management+of+Pain

22

Integrative Medicine and Public Policy

JOSEPHINE P. BRIGGS, MD

Introduction

Integrative medicine represents both a challenge to conventional medical care and an opportunity for change. The challenge arises from the familiar concerns about shortcomings in our conventional ways of caring for patients. The last few decades have seen enormous strides in our ability to change the course of many chronic diseases. Cardiovascular disease, kidney disease, many cancers—the care we can offer today for many of these conditions is measurably and often dramatically better than it was 20 or 30 years ago. But the demands and pace of modern medicine are omnipresent, and the subjective experience of patients is not improving. The criticisms of conventional care are familiar: Care is disease-centric rather than patient-centric; poor coordination results in costly redundancies like duplicate tests; and our conventional methods of care fail to effectively engage patients in more effective self-care. It is clear there will be no simple answers to these challenges. Integrative medicine offers a philosophy of care that is patient-centric, and a strategy to address some of these widely acknowledged shortcomings of the standard modes for delivery of care. The centerpiece of integrative medicine is a strategy to more effectively engage patients in their own care.

Other chapters in this book discuss the specific modalities that are being integrated into care by integrative medicine providers, as well as the integrative medicine approach to prevention and treatment of specific diseases and symptoms. In this chapter we summarize the public resources supporting the development of integrative medicine and some of the policy and regulatory implications of the model of integrative care that starts with the personal perspective of the patient.

Encouraging Patient Self-Education

A major change in healthcare delivery is the changing dialogue between the patient and healthcare providers. The practice of integrative medicine incorporates an acknowledgment that an important starting point for all discussion is the identification of the elements of health most important to the patient.

Patient self-education is playing an increasing role in the dialogue with healthcare providers. The availability of extensive Internet resources providing information about health and disease—both reliable and unreliable—has had dramatic impact on the conversations between doctors and patients. The impact of these sources of information is felt in almost all patient encounters. Physicians often feel concerned about these resources and stretched to provide reliable information in the time constraints of short clinical visits. Patients need information about what resources to trust and guidance in distinguishing reliable information from marketing. Listed in Table 22.1 are the major federal public health websites that provide general information about health and disease. Table 22.2 provides a list of websites from both the private and public sectors that focus on complementary health practices. Healthcare providers need to be able to provide guidance to the availability of helpful resources and help patients distinguish reliable Web information from questionable sources.

An interest in complementary health practices is often recognized by integrative medicine providers as a useful step in self-care, not a barrier to good care. It has been well documented that patients do not consistently inform physicians about an interest in complementary health practices or in the use of dietary supplements.[1,2] Failure to open this conversation creates a barrier to identification of possible adverse effects of combining some dietary supplements, particularly herbal agents, with certain conventional pharmaceutical agents. Drug-drug interactions are probably an even greater concern, since Americans, particularly older Americans, take many pharmaceutical agents concomitantly, including conventional drugs, over-the-counter medicines, and dietary supplements.

Research on Complementary Practices and the Development of an Evidence-Base for the Practice of Integrative Medicine

As discussed in earlier chapters in this textbook, most integrative practitioners incorporate a variety of complementary approaches into the care they offer patients. The evidence for the effectiveness of these interventions is

Table 22.1 Federal Public Health Resources for General Information About Health and Disease

Centers for Disease Control and Prevention (CDC)	The Centers for Disease Control and Prevention's website provides information for consumers about specific diseases and conditions, as well as safe and healthy living. http://www.cdc.gov/DiseasesConditions/ http://www.cdc.gov/HealthyLiving/
National Institutes of Health (NIH)	The National Institutes of Health website provides evidence-based information on a wide array of health topics, as well as links to science-based health and wellness resources for communities, information on clinical research trials, and tips for talking with your doctor. http://www.nih.gov/health-information http://www.nih.gov/health-information/science-based-health-wellness-resources-your-community http://www.nih.gov/health-information/nih-clinical-research-trials-you http://www.nih.gov/institutes-nih/nih-office-director/office-communications-public-liaison/clear-communication/talking-your-doctor
National Library of Medicine, MedlinePlus	The National Library of Medicine's MedlinePlus website offers reliable, evidence-based information on health, wellness, disorders, and conditions as well as on drugs and supplements. The site also provides health videos on topics such as anatomy, body systems, and surgical procedures. https://www.nlm.nih.gov/medlineplus/healthtopics.html https://www.nlm.nih.gov/medlineplus/druginformation.html https://www.nlm.nih.gov/medlineplus/videosandcooltools.html
US Department of Agriculture (USDA)	The US Department of Agriculture's Center for Nutrition Policy and Promotion provides information on healthful eating, including dietary guidelines and tools to help consumers reduce their risk of chronic disease and maintain a healthy weight. http://www.cnpp.usda.gov/dietary-guidelines http://www.cnpp.usda.gov/supertracker http://www.whatscooking.fns.usda.gov/
Substance Abuse and Mental Health Services Administration (SAMHSA)	SAMHSA's website provides information on prevention and early intervention strategies to reduce the impact of mental illness and substance use disorders in America's communities. http://www.samhsa.gov/prevention http://www.samhsa.gov/topics

Table 22.2 Private and Public Sector Resources on Complementary Health Approaches

Cochrane Collaboration Complementary Medicine Reviews	This website offers rigorous systematic reviews of mainstream and complementary health interventions using standardized methods. It includes more than 300 reviews of complementary health approaches. Complete reviews require institutional or individual subscription, but summaries are available to the public. http://www.cochrane.org
Mayo Clinic	Providing reliable, evidence-based information for consumers, these Web resources on complementary, alternative, and integrative health offer an overview of the evidence on specific approaches and information on herbs and supplements. http://www.mayoclinic.org/healthy-lifestyle/consumer-health/in-depth/alternative-medicine/art-20045267 http://www.mayoclinic.org/healthy-lifestyle/consumer-health/in-depth/health-tip/art-20049034 http://www.mayoclinic.org/drugs-supplements
National Library of Medicine, MedlinePlus MedlinePlus All Herbs and Supplements MedlinePlus Complementary and Integrative Medicine	These National Library of Medicine (NLM) Web pages provide an A–Z database of evidence-based information on herbal and dietary supplements and basic facts about complementary and integrative approaches https://www.nlm.nih.gov/medlineplus/druginformation.html https://www.nlm.nih.gov/medlineplus/complementaryandintegrativemedicine.html
NIH National Center for Complementary and Integrative Health (NCCIH)	The National Institutes of Health NCCIH website contains consumer information on many aspects of complementary and integrative health approaches. Downloadable information sheets include brief summaries of complementary approaches and uses and risks of herbal and dietary supplements. http://www.nccih.nih.gov
NIH Office of Dietary Supplements (ODS)	The National Institutes of Health ODS website offers resources to strengthen the public's knowledge of dietary supplements. Its resources include publications on specific supplements, consumer safety, and decision-making. https://ods.od.nih.gov/
US Food and Drug Administration (FDA) Consumer Information on Dietary Supplements	The FDA website offers safety information and consumer tips on dietary supplements and links to alerts, as well as information on the Dietary Supplement Health and Education Act (DSHEA) of 1994, the regulatory role the FDA plays, and manufacturers' responsibilities. http://www.fda.gov/ForConsumers/default.htm http://www.fda.gov/ForConsumers/ProtectYourself/default.htm

incomplete but is expanding rapidly. Excellent resources to assess the state of the current evidence are the systematic reviews performed by the Cochrane Collaboration, which includes reviews on approximately 300 complementary and integrative medicine topics (http://www.cochrane.org). While these resources are valuable, the methods place heavy reliance on randomized trials, which generally compare two similar modalities, or the intervention with a control. With rare exceptions the available evidence often does not provide answers to the practical questions faced by clinicians, such as comparisons between the risks and benefits of conventional pharmaceuticals and integrative approaches. This shortcoming in the evidence base is not confined to complementary health approaches or integrative medicine. Recent reviewers have commented that many of the practices used in conventional care, perhaps as many as half, also lack a solid evidence base.[3,4] Similarly, there is a shortage of trials that compare exercise with drugs.[5]

Nonetheless, the evidence base is growing. Pain management provides an informative example of the way complementary approaches are becoming part of an evidence-based integrative approach to care. Evidence-based algorithms for care of patients with chronic pain increasingly acknowledge and incorporate nonpharmacologic practices that until recently have not been part of standard conventional care.[6] A useful example is the management of back pain, as shown in Figure 22.1. In addition, several guidelines that may be useful in the diagnosis and management of pain are listed in Box 22.1.

Ultimately, making the best choices about policies for healthcare requires access to high-quality evidence to guide those choices. Health policy makers increasingly acknowledge the need for standardized and critical analysis of the level of evidence to guide the development of policy and inform personal choices. The assessment of evidence for guidelines on clinical treatments will almost certainly continue to rely heavily on randomized clinical trials. Prevention poses different challenges, however. The approach to the development of standards for preventive modalities is largely led by the US Prevention Task Force (USPTF), and under the Affordable Care Act, their guidelines influence reimbursement decisions. With rare exceptions, approaches to prevention, such as screening tests, have not been tested by large randomized trials, in large part because the sample size requirements make such trials overly expensive and impractical. The USPTF relies on the development of a chain of evidence, relying on a mix of data from randomized trials and observational data to establish quantitative estimates of risks and benefits. This approach is potentially applicable to the systematic study of prevention approaches in integrative medicine. Methods to study complex interventions while retaining the rigor created by randomization include cluster-randomized trials or trials

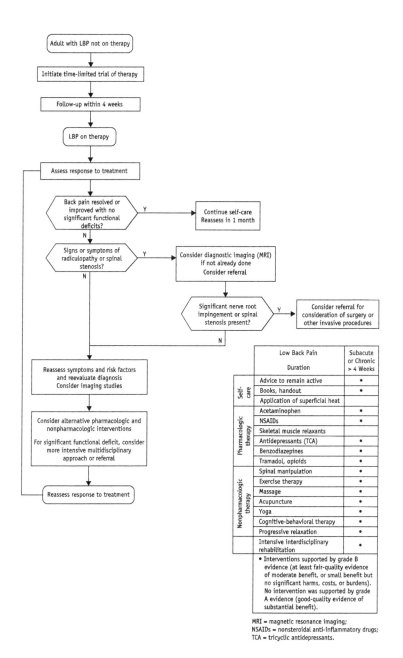

FIGURE 22.1 Management of Nonspecific Chronic Low-Back Pain
Source: Adapted from reference 6.

Box 22.1 Pain Management Guidelines

- CDC Guideline for Prescribing Opioids for Chronic Pain (CDC)
- Chiropractic Management of Fibromyalgia Syndrome: Summary of Clinical Practice *(Council on Chiropractic Guidelines and Practice Parameters)*
- Diagnosis and Treatment of Low-Back Pain *(Annals of Internal Medicine)*
- Low Back Pain: Clinical Practice Guidelines Linked to the International Classification of Functioning, Disability, and Health *(Journal of Orthopaedic and Sports Physical Therapy)*
- Management of the Acute Migraine Headache *(American Family Physician)*
- NSAIDs and Other Complementary Treatments for Episodic Migraine Prevention in Adults *(Neurology)*
- Osteopathic Manipulative Treatment for Low-Back Pain *(Journal of the American Osteopathic Association)*
- Pain Management Task Force Final Report *(Office of the Army Surgeon General)*
- Practice Parameter: Evidence-Based Guidelines for Migraine Headache *(Neurology)*
- Treatment of Osteoarthritis of the Knee *(AAOS)*

---

that incorporate a randomized approach to staged implementation.[7] The NIH Health Care Systems Research Collaboratory (http://www.nihcollaboratory. org) is pioneering the development of these approaches.

Professional Standards for Integrative Medicine and for Complementary Healthcare Providers

A patchwork of regulations and standards governs the practice of integrative medicine and care provided by associated healthcare providers. In the United States, medical licensure is the responsibility of state government. The development of standards for medical subspecialties is the responsibility of professional accrediting organizations or commissions recognized by the US Department of Education (ED).[8] Standards for professional education and curriculum standards are largely established by commissions also overseen by the ED.

Integrative medicine is a subspecialty in transition. Some practitioners have viewed the goal of integrative medicine as a change in the process of care applicable to all specialties, and have argued that subspecialization would not serve the broader goals of promotion of change across all medical practices. However, in the last 3 to 5 years, some leaders in integrative medicine have concluded that a formal subspecialty designation is desirable and have established the American Board of Integrative Medicine (ABOIM) under the aegis to the American Board of Physician Specialties. They have established the following definition:[9]

> The ABOIM defines integrative medicine as the practice of medicine that reaffirms the importance of the relationship between practitioner and patient, focuses on the whole person, is informed by evidence, and makes use of all appropriate therapeutic approaches, healthcare professionals and disciplines to achieve optimal health and healing.

The ABOIM has established criteria for accreditation of fellowship programs and credentialing integrative physician providers including specification of the training requirements and development of examinations. Currently, 23 fellowship programs are accredited in the United States.[9]

Not surprisingly, there is even greater state-to-state variation in the approaches to licensure of complementary practitioners. Furthermore, healthcare providers vary in how they approach the credentialing of practitioners of complementary modalities. The complexities and uncertainties around credentialing complementary practices remain a barrier to their effective integration with conventional medicine.

At present five forms of complementary practice—chiropractic, therapeutic massage, naturopathy, homeopathy, and acupuncture and traditional Chinese medicine—are subject to some form of licensure requirements or educational requirements. Mind and body practices including meditation, biofeedback, and other relaxation techniques and meditative exercise forms such as yoga, tai chi, or qi gong are not subject to licensure requirements in any state. Practitioners of integrative health generally place emphasis on a team-based model of care, integrating a variety of clinical disciplines, including nutritionists, exercise therapists, and behavioral coaches and psychologists. Many nurses and physical therapists integrate these complementary approaches in their practices, either by obtaining expertise themselves or by referral. Nurses, in particular, have been early proponents of integrative medicine policy. For example, the Gillette Nursing Summit in 2002 was convened to "identify common concerns and a set of core recommendations that would enable nurses to provide leadership in this emerging field" of integrative health. Recommendations on integrative medicine that stemmed from this meeting covered areas of research, education, clinical care, and policy.[10]

CHIROPRACTIC

Chiropractic care is currently licensed in all 50 states and the District of Columbia and is reimbursed by Medicare.[11,12] Licensure standards are largely determined by the main chiropractic professional organizations: the American Chiropractic Association, the Federation of Chiropractic Licensing Boards, and the Council on Chiropractic Education.[11] Two years of undergraduate training and 4 years of professional training at an accredited institution are required for licensure, and most states require the successful completion of the standardized board examination; the discipline does not have a postgraduate training requirement. Many states require chiropractors to earn annual continuing education credits to maintain their licenses. There is some state-to-state variability in scope of practice; chiropractors are, in general, not authorized to prescribe drugs or perform surgery, but in most states, they may dispense or sell dietary supplements.[11,13,14]

THERAPEUTIC MASSAGE

Massage therapists are the most numerous of the regulated complementary health practitioner groups and the most rapidly growing.[15] Insurance coverage of massage therapy has been mandated in the state of Washington since 1995,[16] and massage therapists are increasingly incorporated into conventional health practices.[17] Forty-two states impose some regulation of massage therapy, and although there is no consistency, typical requirements include 500 hours of training in an accredited postsecondary institution.[15] The American Massage Therapy Association is generally recognized as the leading professional organization; it established an ED-recognized Commission on Massage Therapy Accreditation (COMTA), which has accredited approximately 100 schools.[18] Most massage schools are not accredited, however, and many states have no licensure requirements.[11]

NATUROPATHY

Naturopathy or naturopathic medicine is currently licensed in 15 states and the District of Columbia, although the profession is actively seeking licensure in a number of other states.[19] There are five accredited educational institutions in the United States. Licensure requires completion of a 4-year postbaccalaureate program with a curriculum that includes medical science and traditional naturopathic training. Although not required, many graduates complete a year or more of postgraduate training.[16] All states that license naturopaths consider them to be doctors or physicians with the title of doctor of naturopathic medicine (ND) or naturopathic physician (NP).[20]

HOMEOPATHY

Homeopathy has been practiced in the United States since the 19th century, but licensure as a homeopathic practitioner is available only in three states (Arizona, Connecticut, and Nevada) and then only to licensed physicians.[11] Some states include homeopathy within the scope of practice of other fields, including chiropractic, naturopathy, and physical therapy,[11] and some lay and professional providers self-identify as homeopathic practitioners,[12] making estimates of the number of practitioners uncertain.

ACUPUNCTURE AND TRADITIONAL CHINESE MEDICINE

Acupuncture was first licensed in Nevada, Oregon, and Maryland in 1973, and it is currently licensed in 42 states and the District of Columbia, with licensure standards varying widely but generally including 3 years of accredited training and successful completion of a standardized examination.[11] The ED-recognized Accreditation Commission for Acupuncture and Oriental Medicine is the main accreditation body.[21] In 31 states, acupuncture is expressly included in MD and DO licensure; 11 states require additional training for physicians performing acupuncture.[11]

Costs of Complementary and Alternative Medical Care and Reimbursement Practices

The most recent data suggest that most complementary health practices are paid for out of pocket.[22] (See Figure 22.2.) Total out-of-pocket spending for complementary approaches in 2012 was $30.2 billion—$28.3 billion for adults and $1.9 billion for children—representing 9.2% of all out-of-pocket spending by Americans on healthcare and 1.1% of total healthcare spending.[22]

There is wide variation between insurance plans in the coverage of complementary interventions. Section 2706 of the Affordable Care Act contains the following provision: "A group health plan and a health insurance issuer offering group or individual health insurance coverage shall not discriminate

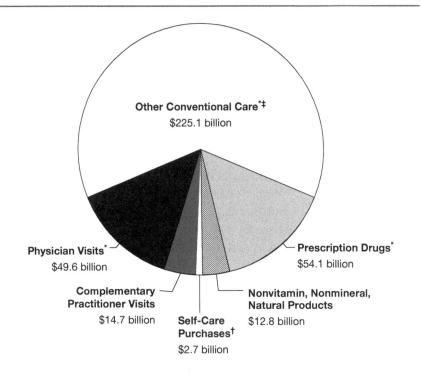

FIGURE 22.2 Out-of-Pocket Spending, 2012

*National Health Expenditure Data for 2012. US Department of Health and Human Services, Centers for Medicare and Medicaid Services Website. https://www.cms.gov/Research-Statistics-Data-and-systems/Statistics-Trends-and-reports/NationalHealthExpendData/ index.html. Accessed March 31, 2016.

†Self-Care Purchases includes, for example, homeopathic medicines and self-help materials, such as books or CDs related to complementary health topics.

‡Other conventional care includes dental care, nursing homes, home healthcare, non-drug medical products, hospital care, and other professional services.

Source: Nahin RL, Barnes PM, Stussman BJ. *Expenditures on Complementary Health Approaches: United States, 2012.* National Health Statistics Reports. Hyattsville, MD: National Center for Health Statistics. 2016.

with respect to participation under the plan or coverage against any health care provider who is acting within the scope of that provider's license of certification under the applicable State law."[23]

This provision for coverage of care is limited to licensed providers and does not impact on payment for interventions such as yoga classes or training in meditation that are not provided by licensed providers.

Several studies have brought the methods of cost-effective analysis to study the impact of complementary and integrative medicine on overall healthcare costs.[24] By and large, these analyses suggest that coverage of complementary and integrative health, when available, is not necessarily associated with an increase in health costs.[25]

Conclusion

Integrative medicine offers opportunities to more effectively engage patients in their own healthcare by encouraging self-education and guiding patients to credible sources of information. In addition to patients, healthcare providers and health policy makers require access to rigorous evidence and a critical analysis of evidence to make the best decisions—those that will impact patients and policy. The regulations and standards that govern the practice of integrative medicine vary widely, as do the licensing and credentialing of complementary health practitioners—a barrier to their effective integration with conventional medicine. Another barrier that impacts full integration is the variation in insurance coverage of specific complementary approaches, and as a consequence, patients must pay for most complementary health interventions out-of-pocket.

References

1. Chao MT, Wade C, Kronenberg F. Disclosure of complementary and alternative medicine to conventional medical providers: variation by race/ethnicity and type of CAM. *J Natl Med Assoc* 2008;100(11):1341–1349.
2. Mehta DH, Gardiner PM, Phillips RS, McCarthy EP. Herbal and dietary supplement disclosure to health care providers by individuals with chronic conditions. *J Altern Complement Med* 2008;14(10):1263–1269.
3. Tricoci P, Allen JM, Kramer JM, Califf RM, Smith SC Jr. Scientific evidence underlying the ACC/AHA clinical practice guidelines. *JAMA* 2009;301:831–834.
4. Institute of Medicine. Chapter 2—The need for better medical evidence. In: McLellan MB, McGinnis JM, Nabel EG, Olsen LM, eds. *Evidence-Based Medicine and the Changing Nature of Healthcare: 2007 IOM Annual Meeting Summary.* Washington, DC: National Academies Press; 2008. http://ncbi.nlm.nih.gov/books/NBK52829. Accessed February 16, 2016.
5. Naci H, Ioannidis JPA. Comparative effectiveness of exercise and drug interventions on mortality outcomes: metaepidemiological study. *BMJ* 2013;347:f5577.
6. Chou R, Qaseem A, Snow V, et al. Clinical practice guideline from the American College of Physicians and the American Pain Society. *Ann Intern Med* 2007;147(7):478–491.
7. Dreischulte T, Donnan P, Grant A, Hapca A, McCowan C, Guthrie B. Safer prescribing—a trial of education, informatics, and financial incentives. *N Engl J Med* 2016;374:1053–1064.

8. US Department of Education. *FAQs About Accreditation.* http://ope.ed.gov/accreditation/FAQAccr.aspx. Accessed February 22, 2010.

9. American Board of Integrative Medicine Website. http://www.abpsus.org/integrative-medicine. Accessed March 30, 2016.

10. Leading the Way: The Gillette Nursing Summit on Integrated Health and Healing. May 30–31, 2002. St. Paul, Minnesota, USA. *Altern Ther Health Med* 2003;9(Suppl 1):3A–10A.

11. Eisenberg DM, Cohen MH, Hrbek A, et al. Credentialing complementary and alternative medical providers. *Ann Intern Med* 2002;137:965–973.

12. Federation of Chiropractic Licensing Boards. *Questions and Answers About Professional Regulation and the Chiropractic Profession.* 2007. http://www.fclb.org/Resources/ConsumerInformation/tabid/485/Default.aspx. Accessed February 23, 2010.

13. Cooper RA, Laud P, Dietrich CL. Current and projected workforce of nonphysician clinicians. *JAMA* 1998;280:788–794.

14. Cooper RA, McKee HJ. Chiropractic in the United States: trends and issues. *Milbank Q* 2003;81:107–138.

15. US Department of Labor, Bureau of Labor Statistics. *Occupational Outlook Handbook, 2010–2011 Edition.* http://www.bls.gov/oco/. Accessed February 22, 2010.

16. Cherkin DC, Deyo RA, Sherman KJ, et al. Characteristics of licensed acupuncturists, chiropractors, massage therapists, and naturopathic physicians. *J Am Board Fam Pract* 2002;15:378–390.

17. Nedrow A. Status of credentialing alternative providers within a subset of U.S. academic health centers. *J Altern Complement Med* 2006;12:329–335.

18. Commission on Massage Therapy Accreditation. http://www.comta.org/about.php. Accessed February 22, 2010.

19. Association of Accredited Naturopathic Medical Colleges. *Naturopathic Doctor Licensure.* http://www.aanmc.org/careers/naturopathic-doctor-licensure.php. Accessed February 22, 2010.

20. Cooper RA. Health care workforce for the twenty-first century: the impact of nonphysician clinicians. *Annu Rev Med* 2001;52:51–61.

21. Accreditation Commission for Acupuncture and Oriental Medicine. http://www.acaom.org. Accessed February 22, 2010.

22. Nahin RL, Barnes PM, Stussman BJ. Expenditures on complementary health approaches: United States, 2012. National Health Statistics Reports. Hyattsville, MD: National Center for Health Statistics. 2016

23. The Center for Consumer Information and Insurance Oversight, the Centers for Medicare and Medicaid Services. https://www.cms.gov/CCIIO/Resources/FAct-Sheets-and-FAQs/aca_implementation_faqs15.html. Accessed March 30, 2016.

24. Herman PM, Poindexter BL, Witt CM, Eisenberg DM. Are complementary therapies and integrative care cost-effective? A systematic review of economic evaluations. *BMJ Open* 2012;2(5).

25. Martin BI, Gerkovich MM, Deyo RA, et al. The association of complementary and alternative medicine use and health care expenditures for back and neck problems. *Med Care* 2012;50(12):1029–1036.

INDEX

Page numbers followed by b, *f,* or *t* indicate a box, figure or table on the associated page.